Clinical Diagnosis and Management of COPD

Clinical Diagnosis and Management of COPD

Editor: Denver Cox

AMERICAN
MEDICAL PUBLISHERS
www.americanmedicalpublishers.com

AMERICAN
MEDICAL PUBLISHERS
www.americanmedicalpublishers.com

Cataloging-in-Publication Data

Clinical diagnosis and management of COPD / edited by Denver Cox.
p. cm.
Includes bibliographical references and index.
ISBN 979-8-88740-588-9
1. Lungs--Diseases, Obstructive. 2. Lungs--Diseases, Obstructive--Diagnosis.
3. Lungs--Diseases, Obstructive--Treatment. 4. Lungs--Diseases.
5. Respiratory organs--Obstructions. I. Cox, Denver.
RC776.O3 C55 2023
616.24--dc23

American Medical Publishers,
41 Flatbush Avenue,
1st Floor, New York,
NY 11217, USA

ISBN 979-8-88740-588-9 (Hardback)

Contents

Preface

Over the recent decade, advancements and applications have progressed exponentially. This has led to the increased interest in this field and projects are being conducted to enhance knowledge. The main objective of this book is to present some of the critical challenges and provide insights into possible solutions. This book will answer the varied questions that arise in the field and also provide an increased scope for furthering studies.

Chronic obstructive pulmonary disease (COPD) refers to a type of chronic inflammatory lung disease in which airflow of the lungs is blocked. The two common conditions that cause COPD are chronic bronchitis and emphysema. There are several signs and symptoms of COPD, such as wheezing, coughing, mucus production and difficulty in breathing, while doing daily activities and mild exercise. Lung cancer, heart disease, metabolic syndrome, depression and a number of other diseases are more likely to occur in COPD patients. Spirometry is a widely used and reliable approach for diagnosing this medical condition. The treatments of COPD include pulmonary rehabilitation, corticosteroids, smoking cessation, inhaled bronchodilators and vaccinations. Lung transplantation, long-term oxygen therapy and lung volume reduction may be advantageous in some cases. The aim of this book is to present researches that have transformed the diagnosis and management of COPD. It is appropriate for students seeking detailed information in this area as well as for experts.

I hope that this book, with its visionary approach, will be a valuable addition and will promote interest among readers. Each of the authors has provided their extraordinary competence in their specific fields by providing different perspectives as they come from diverse nations and regions. I thank them for their contributions.

Editor

1

Oral Health-Related Quality of Life in Patients with Chronic Respiratory Diseases

Simin Li[1†]*, Wanchen Ning*[1†]*, Wei Wang*[1†]*, Dirk Ziebolz*[2]*, Aneesha Acharya*[3]*, Gerhard Schmalz*[2‡]*, Jianjiang Zhao*[4*‡]*, Shaohong Huang*[1*‡] *and Hui Xiao*[1*‡]

[1] Stomatological Hospital, Southern Medical University, Guangzhou, China, [2] Department of Cariology, Endodontology and Periodontology, University Leipzig, Leipzig, Germany, [3] Dr. D. Y. Patil Dental College and Hospital, Dr. D. Y. Patil Vidyapeeth, Pune, India, [4] Shenzhen Stomatological Hospital, Southern Medical University, Shenzhen, China

***Correspondence:**
Shaohong Huang
hsh.china@tom.comz
Jianjiang Zhao
zjj2521@sina.com
Hui Xiao
zzmmxh@126.com

† These authors share first authorship
‡ These authors share senior authorship

Background: This systematic review evaluates the oral health-related quality of life (OHRQoL) of patients with chronic respiratory diseases.

Methods: A systematic literature search was performed based on the PubMed, Medline, Web of Science, and Scopus, using the search terms: "oral health-related quality of life" and "respiratory disease" or "lung" and "oral health-related quality of life." Full-text articles published until June 30, 2021 and reporting any OHRQoL measurement in children or adults with a chronic respiratory disease or condition were included and analyzed qualitatively.

Results: A total of seven out of 44 studies were included, of which four studies examined adults and three studies investigated children. The respective diseases were chronic obstructive pulmonary disease (COPD) ($n = 2$), sleep apnea ($n = 2$), severe asthma ($n = 1$), cystic fibrosis ($n = 1$), and lung transplantation ($n = 1$). Four studies confirmed a worse OHRQoL in the respiratory diseased group compared to healthy controls. The overall OHRQoL was reduced in the included studies. Oral health, health-related quality of life, and disease-related parameters were rarely examined with regard to OHRQoL.

Conclusion: Patients with chronic respiratory diseases show a reduced OHRQoL. Oral health should be fostered in these individuals to support their OHRQoL.

Keywords: oral health, oral health-related quality of life, respiratory disease, lung, COPD

BACKGROUND

Chronic diseases affecting the respiratory system cover a broad variety of different conditions; thereby, lifestyle or risk factor-associated, high prevalent diseases, such as chronic obstructive pulmonary disease (COPD), exist (1) alongside with very rare genetic diseases, such as cystic fibrosis (2). Other examples of respiratory diseases are asthma, which is a highly prevalent condition with primarily an autoimmune cause (3) or sleep apnea or sleep-disordered breathing as a complex and multifactorial condition (4). Especially, if breathlessness occurs, chronic respiratory diseases can be related to a high morbidity and a negative impact on the quality of life of affected patients (5). Additionally, chronic respiratory diseases, such as COPD, can lead to different comorbidities and physical deconditioning, decreasing the health-related quality of life (HRQoL) of patients suffering from these diseases (6).

Oral health is often reported to be affected by respiratory diseases in respective patients; a recent meta-analysis showed that patients with asthma as well as COPD showed an association to the presence of periodontal diseases (7). Besides a direct association, medications, e.g., asthma medication including bronchodilators, corticosteroids, or anticholinergic drugs inhaled by the patients can increase the risk of dry mouth, dental caries, dental erosion, periodontal diseases, and oral candidiasis (8, 9). Especially for severely diseased patients, such as patients with cystic fibrosis or COPD, oral bacteria related to dental and periodontal diseases can also colonize the lungs, increasing the risk for complications (10, 11). Additionally, patients with obstructive sleep apnea, which is completely different from the other respiratory diseases described here, show affected oral health conditions as well as the relationship between oral diseases and the underlying disorder; this is heterogeneous, but obvious for both the children and adults (12). In the complex relationship between oral and respiratory health, the multifactorial character of oral diseases, as well as the anatomic proximity of the oropharyngeal and respiratory tract could be relevant.

A particular issue of interest in this context is the oral HRQoL (OHRQoL). As a part of the general HRQoL, the OHRQoL reflects the perceived affection of HRQoL by conditions related to the oral cavity including teeth, mouth, or dentures (13, 14). In other groups of systemically diseased patients, the OHRQoL showed interesting and clinically relevant results. For example, patients with rheumatic diseases show an impaired OHRQoL, whereby rheumatic disease-related parameters might be major influential factors (15). On the other hand, patients after solid organ transplantation were supposed to undergo a "response shift" of the perception of OHRQoL, i.e., reduced awareness of their insufficient oral health status (16). Considering the impaired oral health, reduced general HRQoL alongside the anatomic proximity between the oral cavity and the respiratory system, the OHRQoL of patients with different respiratory diseases appears a topic of clinical interest. Therefore, this study evaluates the OHRQoL of patients with chronic respiratory diseases. It was hypothesized that these patients would show a reduced OHRQoL.

METHODS

This study was performed in full accordance with the Preferred Reporting Items for Systematic Reviews and Meta-Analyses (PRISMA) (17).

Patients, Intervention, Comparison, and Outcome (PICO) Question

The PICO question was as follows: "Do patients with severe respiratory diseases show a reduced OHRQoL?". Thereby, "patients" were individuals with chronic respiratory diseases. The aspect "intervention" was not defined because it was expected to primarily include cross-sectional studies. "Comparison" was a healthy control group, if applicable. Otherwise, values should be compared to reference values or other groups of patients with systemic diseases. Finally, "outcome" was any applied OHRQoL measurement. The hypothesis was formed that the OHRQoL of patients with chronic respiratory diseases would be worse than in healthy individuals.

Eligibility Criteria

For inclusion in this study, several inclusion criteria were formulated:

- Publication until 30th of June, 2021.
- Examination of children or adults with a chronic respiratory disease or condition.
- Reporting of any OHRQoL measurement.
- Full text in English language.

Search Strategy

In July 2021, a systematic literature search was performed by two different and independent reviewers. As databases for literature search, the PubMed, Medline, Web of Science, and Scopus were chosen, using the search terms: "oral health-related quality of life" and respiratory disease or lung and "oral health-related quality of life." A manual search based on the references of findings complemented the systematic literature search. All the findings were checked and screened for their eligibility.

Data Extraction

After all the articles were screened and checked, qualitative data extraction was applied. Thereby, different issues were extracted from the respective articles.

- Form of respiratory disease, year of publication, number of participants, study type, age, gender, and smoking.
- Presence and characteristics of a healthy control group.
- Oral health findings, if applicable.
- Oral HRQoL assessment including the form of measurement and results.
- Potential relationship between OHRQoL and general parameters, disease-related parameters, or oral health findings, if applicable.
- Subscales of the OHRQoL measurements, if applicable.

Two independent reviewers executed the whole process of systematic search and study selection as well as qualitative analysis. Only studies explicitly reporting OHRQoL of patients with chronic respiratory diseases were considered within this study.

Quality Assessment

The 11-item checklist from the Agency for Healthcare Research and Quality (AHRQ) for cross-sectional studies was applied for quality assessment of the included studies (18). The answers "no" or "unclear" were rated as 0 and the answer "yes" was rated as 1 point for each question to

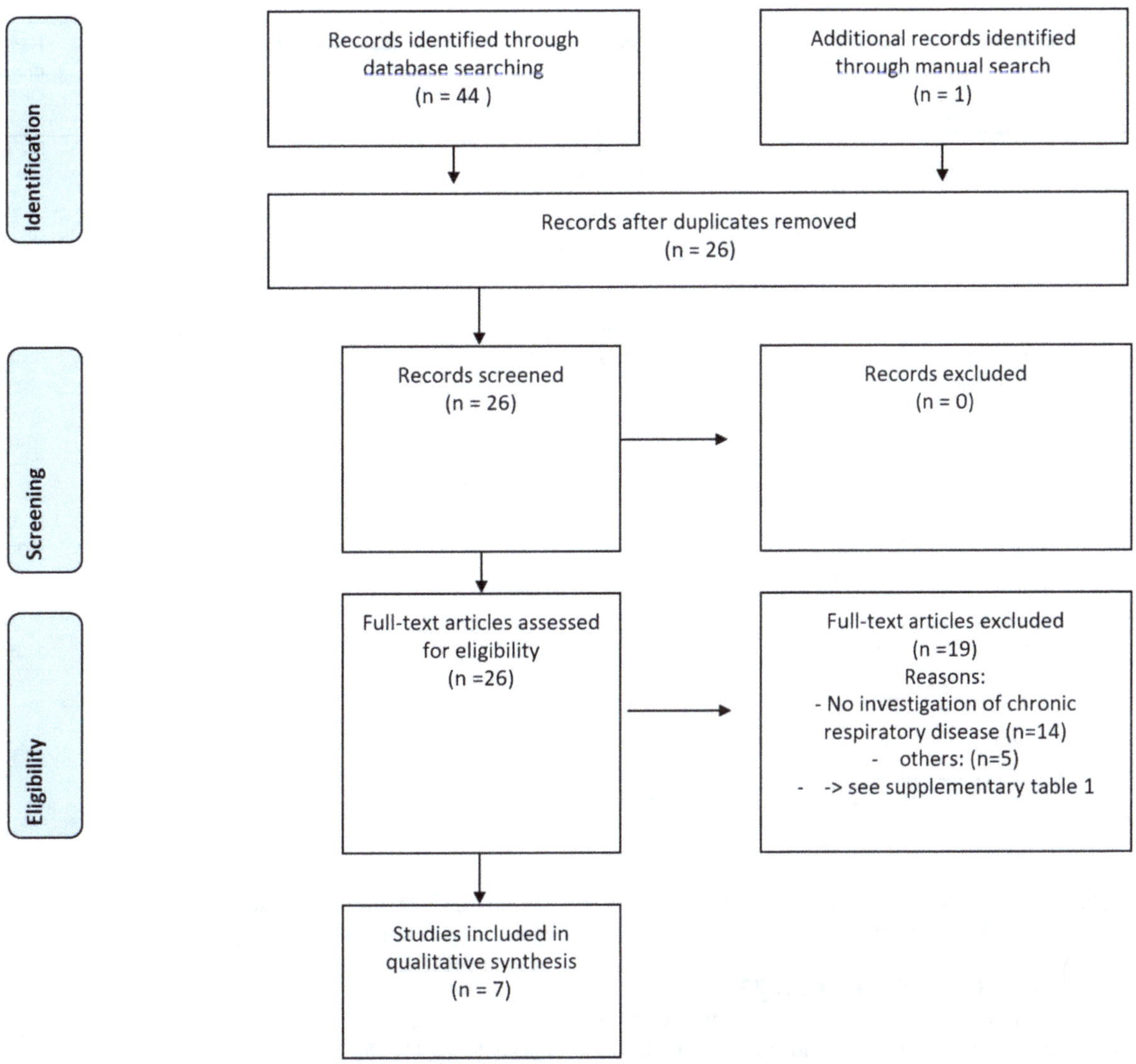

FIGURE 1 | The Preferred Reporting Items for Systematic Reviews and Meta-Analyses (PRISMA) diagram for the systematic review process in this study (17).

estimate a score for the respective quality of the studies. A sum score of all the questions of 0–3 indicated low quality, 4–7 indicated moderate quality, and a score of 8–11 indicated high quality of this study. The quality appraisal was conducted by two independent reviewers, whereby any disagreements were discussed and resolved in the whole author group.

RESULTS

Search Findings

The PRISMA diagram, reflecting the findings of the systematic search, is given in **Figure 1**. Out of 44 database search findings, 26 full-text articles were assessed for their eligibility. During this, 19 articles were excluded (**Supplementary Table 1**). Finally, seven studies were included in the qualitative analysis.

Characteristics of the Included Studies

Out of the seven studies, two studies were on patients with COPD (19, 20), while each one study was on cystic fibrosis (21), lung transplantation (22), sleep-disordered breathing (23), obstructive sleep apnea (24), and severe asthma (25). Three studies were performed in children (21, 23, 24), while four studies were conducted in adult patients (19, 20, 22, 25). All the included studies had either a cross-sectional or an observational design. The healthy control group was examined in five of the included studies (20, 22–25). A full overview of the study characteristics is shown in **Table 1**.

Quality Assessment

Quality appraisal revealed that three studies were of high quality (19, 20, 23), while four studies were elevated with moderate

TABLE 1 | Overview of the included studies.

Author, year	Disease	Country	No. of patients	Study type	Subjects mean age in years	Smoking	Male (%)	Healthy control group for OHRQoL
Saltness et al. (19)	COPD	Norway	100	Monocentric cross-sectional study	65.9 ± 10.1	39%	56%	No
Patrick et al. (21)	Cystic fibrosis	USA	39	Multicentric cross-sectional	43.6% 8–12 years, 56.4% 13–17 years	n/a	53%	No
Schmalz et al. (22)	Lung transplantation	Germany	60	Monocentric cross-sectional study	54.03 ± 9.97	0%	50%	Yes: $n = 70$, age: 55.44 ± 8.54 years, 37% male
Gaeckle et al. (20)	COPD	USA	20	Monocentric prospective observational study (follow-up: 60 days)	60 (56–68)	50%	60%	Yes: $n = 10$, age: 54.5 (50-60) years, 60% male
Grillo et al. (23)	Sleep-disordered breathing	Italy	61	Monocentric cross-sectional study	12.4 ± 3.1	16.4%	54.1%	Yes: $n = 61$, age: 11.9 ± 2.8 years, 50.8% male
Tamsas et al. (24)	Obstructive sleep apnoea	USA	31	Monocentric cross-sectional study	12.8 ± 3.1	14%	52%	Yes: $n = 36$, age: 11.8 ± 2.2 years, 55% male
Brasil-Oliveira et al. (25)	Severe asthma	Brazil	40	Monocentric cross-sectional study	51.8 ± 10.8	0%	15%	Yes: $n = 50$, age: 48.2 ± 12.4 years, 42% male

Values are presented as the mean values ± SD, mean values (range), or percentages.
OHRQoL, oral health-related quality of life; n/a, not applicable; COPD, chronic obstructive pulmonary disease.

quality (21, 22, 24, 25) according to the AHRQ criteria for cross-sectional studies (18) (**Table 2**).

Oral Health Records and Findings

Reporting of oral health data was not very comprehensive in the majority of included studies. One study did not report on any oral health conditions of the participants (21). The four studies including adults reported on remaining teeth (19, 20, 22, 25). Moreover, four studies reported on dental as well as periodontal conditions, whereby the assessment method was quite different (22–25). The detailed oral health findings, if applicable, are shown in **Table 3**.

Oral Health-Related Quality of Life Measurements and Results

The four adult studies applied the Oral Health Impact Profile-14 (OHIP-14) for OHRQoL assessment, showing mean values between 1.7 and 12 points in sum scale (**Figure 2**) (19, 20, 22, 25). The three other studies applied the Child OHIP (COHIP), reporting average sum scores between 23.2 and 67.5 points (**Figure 3**) (21, 23, 24). Four studies (each two in children and adults) reported a worse OHRQoL in the respiratory disease compared to the healthy control group (20, 23–25), while only one study an adult lung transplant recipients did not show a difference against a healthy control (22). Associations between OHRQoL and HRQoL, disease-related parameters, or oral health conditions were rarely examined and reported, respectively (**Table 4**). Only one study examining adults (25) and two studies examining children (21, 24) reported on subscales of the OHIP-14 or the COHIP, respectively (**Table 5**).

DISCUSSION

This study hypothesized that patients with chronic respiratory diseases would show a reduced OHRQoL. Based on the findings of the literature search, this hypothesis can be confirmed, but several disease-specific and methodological issues need further discussion. Thereby, the following will provide: (I) an interpretation of the reduced OHRQoL in patients with chronic respiratory diseases in general and with respect to the different diseases, (II) a discussion of the applied methods alongside with (III) recommendations for further study in this field to strengthen the body of evidence and strive some clinical implications.

(I) Altogether, the OHRQoL of patients suffering from systemic diseases can be discussed controversially because several heterogeneous phenomena, depending on the form of the disease and/or therapy, exist. It is known that oral health can affect general HRQoL (26) and that reduced HRQoL can negatively affect OHRQoL (13, 27). Patients with severe chronic diseases or conditions, e.g., rheumatic diseases or hemodialysis show a reduced OHRQoL caused by their general disease burden including pain and impact on their daily life (15, 28). Thereby,

TABLE 2 | Quality assessment of the included studies according to the Agency for Healthcare Research and Quality (ARHQ) (18).

Item	Saltnes et al. (19)	Patrick et al. (21)	Schmalz et al. (22)	Gaeckle et al. (20)	Grillo et al. (23)	Tamasas et al. (24)	Brasil-Oliveira et al. (25)
(1) Define the source of information (survey, record review)	Yes	Yes	Yes	Yes	Yes	Yes	Yes
(2) List inclusion and exclusion criteria for exposed and unexposed subjects (cases and controls) or refer to previous publications	Yes	No	Yes	Yes	Yes	Yes	Yes
(3) Indicate time period used for identifying patients	Yes	No	Yes	Yes	Yes	No	Yes
(4) Indicate whether or not subjects were consecutive if not population-based	Yes	Yes	Yes	Yes	Yes	Yes	Yes
(5) Indicate if evaluators of subjective components of study were masked to other aspects of the status of the participants	No	No	No	No	No	No	No
(6) Describe any assessments undertaken for quality assurance purposes (e.g., test/retest of primary outcome measurements)	Yes	NA	Yes	Yes	Yes	NA	Yes
(7) Explain any patient exclusions from analysis	Yes	NA	NA	Yes	Yes	NA	NA
(8) Describe how confounding was assessed and/or controlled.	Yes	Yes	U	Yes	Yes	Yes	Yes
(9) If applicable, explain how missing data were handled in the analysis	NA	Yes	NA	NA	NA	NA	NA
(10) Summarize patient response rates and completeness of data collection	Yes	Yes	Yes	Yes	Yes	Yes	Yes
(11) Clarify what follow-up, if any, was expected and the percentage of patients for which incomplete data or follow-up was obtained	NA	NA	NA	Yes	NA	NA	NA
Total score	8	5	6	9	8	5	7

the OHIP-14 values for patients with respiratory diseases in this study were similar as for rheumatic diseased patients or individuals undergoing renal replacement therapy (15, 28). Thus, the HRQoL impairment due to the general disease could be one reason for the reduced OHRQoL in this study; especially, severely diseased individuals with proceeded COPD, cystic fibrosis, and severe asthma are impaired in their everyday life and show affected HRQoL (29–31). Thereby, both severe symptoms, such as breathlessness, as well as mental health issues, such as anxiety or depression, can affect HRQoL outcomes (6, 31), potentially

TABLE 3 | Oral health parameters and respective main results if they presented as the mean values ± SD, means (range), or percentages in the included studies.

References	Tooth loss, remaining teeth, dentures	Dental diseases, caries, dental treatment need	Oral hygiene indices	Periodontal parameters, periodontal treatment need	Further oral health parameters
Saltness et al. (19)	44% <20 teeth	n/a	n/a	n/a	9% hyposalivation, 39% oral health problems
Patrick et al. (21)	n/a	n/a	n/a	n/a	n/a
Schmalz et al. (22)	M-T: 8.17 ± 5.82*	DMF-T: 20.53 ± 5.09, D-T: 0.82 ± 1.85, F-T 11.55 ± 4.57	n/a	98% moderate to severe periodontitis	n/a
Gaeckle et al. (20)	Number of teeth: 16.5 (8.5–23.5)	n/a	PI: 2.2 (1.5–2.8)	n/a	n/a
Grillo et al. (23)	n/a	DMFS: 13.6 ± 4.7, dmfs: 8.5 ± 2.3	n/a	PPD: 2.4 ± 0.5, BOP: 0.9 ± 0.2	n/a
Tamsas et al. (24)	n/a	dmfs: 5.1 ± 8.5, DMFS: 15.2 ± 11.8	n/a	BOP: 87%, PPD mean 2.7 ± 1.3	Comprehensive information on oropharyngeal morphology reported
Brasil-Oliveira et al. (25)	M-T: 7.9 ± 7.2,	D-T: 1.4 ± 2.0, F-T: 4.2 ± 3.7, DMF-T: 13.5 ± 6.5	n/a	Periodontitis: 92.5%	Reduced salivary flow: 80%

*M-T, missing teeth; D-T, decayed teeth; F-T, filled teeth; DMF-T, decayed-, missing-, and filled teeth index; PI, plaque index; GI, gingival index; PPD, periodontal probing depth; n/a, not applicable; *inclusion criterion: at least 6 remaining teeth.*

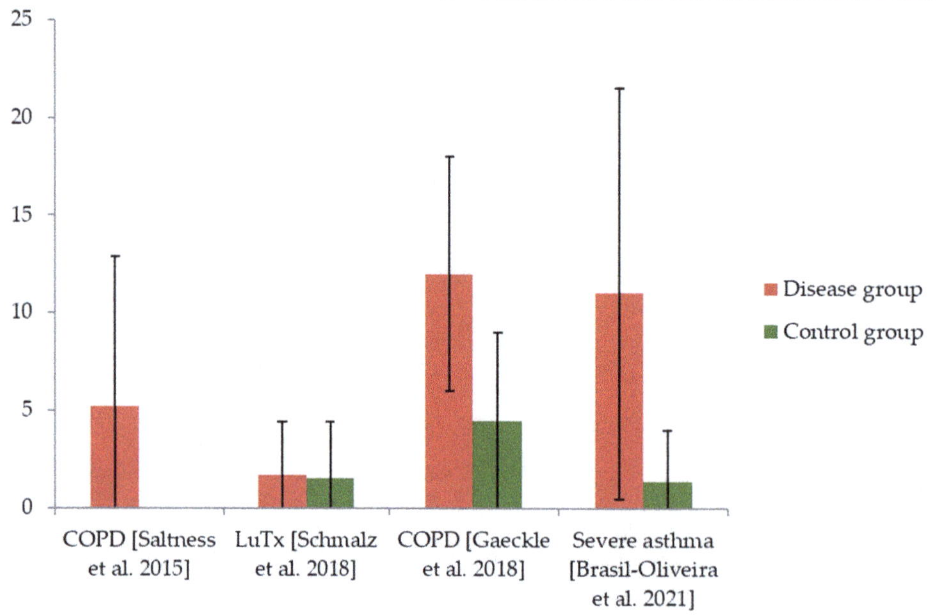

FIGURE 2 | The Oral Health Impact Profile (OHIP) values of included studies on adults and values for healthy controls, if applicable.

affecting OHRQoL of patients. A special position within this study is obstructive sleep apnea or sleep-disordered breathing, respectively. Although this is not an exclusive respiratory disease, it has been included in this study because it is a chronic condition affecting the respiratory system and is of high relevance for the dentist because oral health issues are common in these individuals (12). These sleep disorders lead to complex suffering of the patients, with an impairment of quality of life in both children and adults (12, 32). Furthermore, oral appliances for therapy or wearing an oxygen mask overnight could affect

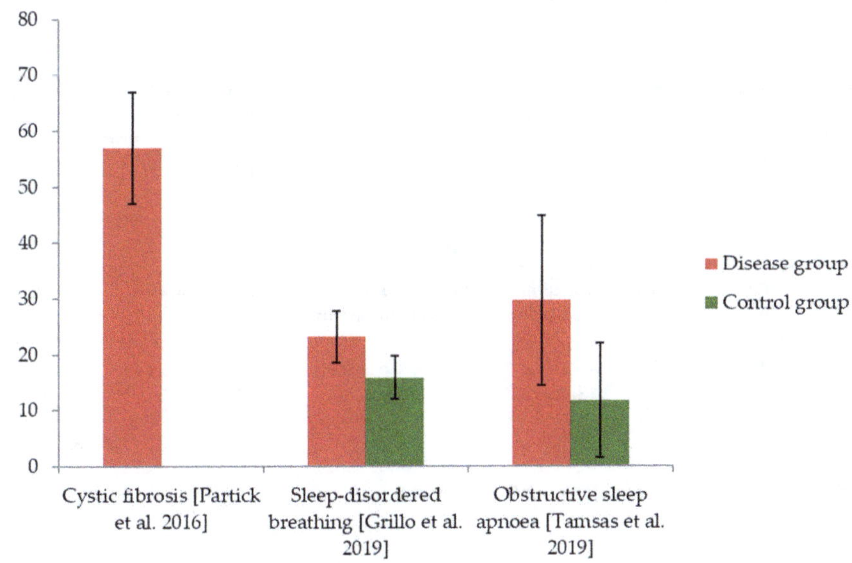

FIGURE 3 | The Child OHIP (COHIP) values for children in included studies and of healthy controls, if applicable.

TABLE 4 | Applied assessments for OHRQoL and relevant results for the included studies.

References	Assessment of OHRQoL	OHRQoL worse than healthy control (HC)	Association/correlation between OHRQoL and general HRQoL	Association/correlation between OHRQoL and oral health	Association and/or correlation between OHRQoL and disease-related parameters
Saltness et al. (19)	OHIP 14: 5.2 ± 7.7	n/a	Higher OHIP 14 related to worse MCS SF-36	Oral health problems related to poorer OHRQoL	n/a
Patrick et al. (21)	COHIP: A: 57.0 ± 10.0, B: 67.5 ± 14.2	n/a	n/a	n/a	Number of medications correlated with better COHIP
Schmalz et al. (22)	OHIP 14: 1.70 ± 2.70	No, OHIP 14: 1.54 ± 2.86	n/a	No associations detected	No
Gaeckle et al. (20)	OHIP 14: 12 (6–18.5)	Yes, OHIP 14: 4.5 (0–8)	n/a	n/a	No
Grillo et al. (23)	COHIP: 23.2 ± 4.6	Yes, COHIP: 15.9 ± 3.8	n/a	Malocclusion	Mallampati class and Obesity correlated with worse COHIP
Tamsas et al. (24)	COHIP: 29.7 ± 15.2	Yes, COHIP: 11.8 ± 10.2	n/a	n/a	n/a
Brasil-Oliveira et al. (25)	OHIP 14: 11.0 ± 10.5 (mild-to-moderate asthma: 6.2 ± 7.4)	Yes, OHIP 14: 1.4 ± 2.6	Higher OHIP 14 correlation with better PCS and MCS of SF-36	n/a	n/a

OHRQoL, oral health-related quality of life; n/a, not applicable; OHIP, Oral Health Impact Profile; COHIP, Child OHIP; PCS, physical compound summary; MCS, mental compound summary; SF-36, Short Form 36 Health Survey Questionnaire.

OHRQoL of respective individuals. Only one patient group, i.e., patients after lung transplantation, what rather represents a therapy than a respiratory disease, showed unaffected OHRQoL (22). It is known that patients after organ transplantation show a response shift, whereby oral health issues are pushed into the background because of the general disease burden (16, 33).

TABLE 5 | Subscales of OHRQoL in the included studies, if applicable.

	OHIP 14						
References, disease	**Functional limitation**	**Physical pain**	**Psycho-social discomfort**	**Physical disability**	**Psycho-logical disability**	**Social disability**	**Handicap**
Brasil-Oliveira et al. (25)	1.2 ± 2.0*	3.0 ± 2.4*	1.8 ± 2.5*	2.1 ± 2.3*	2.6 ± 2.3*	1.1 ± 0.8	0.6 ± 1.6
	OHIP 14						
References, disease	**Oral hgealth well-being**	**Functional well being**	**Social-emotional well-being**	**School environment**	**Self-image**	**Global health**	
Patrick et al. (21)**	A: 19.3 ± 4.3, B: 21.9 ± 6.4	A: 7.7 ± 1.4, B: 8.2 ± 3.2	A: 10.1 ± 3.1, B: 13.4 ± 5.2*	A: 4.5 ± 0.9, B: 4.9 ± 2.2	A: 12.3 ± 3.9, B: 14.8 ± 2.8*	A: 3.8 ± 1.6, B: 4.6 ± 1.4	
Tamasas et al. (24)	14.1 ± 5.5*	3.7 ± 3.0*	3.5 ± 5.6*	1.0 ± 1.7	7.3 ± 5.5*	n/a	

*The results are given as the mean values ± SD or otherwise as percentages. OHIP, Oral Health Impact Profile. *significant different from control. **Group A: 8–12 years (n = 17); group B: 13–17 years (n = 22).*

While this is the reason for the unaffected OHRQoL of patients after lung transplantation, the other groups did not show this response shift phenomenon. A reasonable explanation for that appears the anatomic proximity between the airways and the oral cavity. Moreover, the association between oral diseases and the included respiratory conditions and/or the respective medication (7–12) could explain the affected OHRQoL. Altogether, the reduced OHRQoL of patients with chronic respiratory diseases appears expedient, but complex. However, the reporting of oral health conditions and HRQoL in the included studies was inconsistent. However, the association between COPD (19) and severe asthma (25) with HRQoL supports the upper mentioned interpretation. The affected OHRQoL of patients with chronic respiratory diseases appears of clinical significance because appropriate management of oral conditions of these systemically ill patients will be needed to positively affect their quality of life. Therefore, sufficient multidisciplinary dental care concepts might be needed, as already demanded for other groups of at-risk patients (15, 16, 28). Until now, there is no specific approach available for a respective dental care concept. It is known that a simple allocation to the dentist does not significantly decrease the dental treatment need of patients with severe general diseases (34). Moreover, respective patients need to receive psychosocial support and sensibilization within a multidisciplinary care concept (16). Therefore, it appears of high importance to apply an individualized, prevention-oriented, and patient-centered dental care concept, focusing on the risk and needs of respective patients (35).

(II) The included studies applied two different methods for OHRQoL assessment, according to the age of included participants. For adult patients, the short form of the OHIP-14 was chosen, which is a validated questionnaire-based tool (36, 37). This questionnaire allows assessing the OHRQoL by 14 different questions, which can be answered on a five-point scale between 0 and 4, where higher values indicate worse OHRQoL. As a patient-reported outcome, the OHRQoL is part of the evidence-based dentistry, and applying the OHIP-14 allows conclusions on the impairment of the domains, such as oral function, psychosocial impact, oral pain, and orofacial appearance (14, 38). Although the OHIP-14 is a validated and commonly used instrument, it is not specific for generally diseased individuals, what potentially limits this method in that case (15, 16, 28). The other measurement, which was applied for children, was the COHIP. This instrument is also validated and was found to present reliable results by the assessment of 34 items and five conceptually distinct subscales: oral health, functional well-being, social/emotional well-being, school environment, and self-image (39). Similar as for the OHIP-14, higher values represent a worse OHRQoL. Thereby, the assessment of the OHRQoL of children is difficult because children often have difficulties to express their concerns in clinical environments and they are largely influenced by socioenvironmental factors of their family and caregivers (40, 41). Although the COHIP findings perceived by the caregivers are sometimes reported, this was not considered in this study because it was aimed to exclusively display the perspective of patient. Within the included studies, the COHIP values between children and parents did not differ in a clinically relevant manner, so it seems reasonable to omit this issue in this study (23, 24). Accordingly, the applied OHRQoL measurement appears reasonable in the included studies, but the major flaw appears the rarely applied investigation on the relationship between OHRQoL and HRQoL, disease-related parameters, and, particularly, oral health.

(III) Some recommendations can be provided for future study in the field. The comprehensive assessment of oral health parameters and their consideration as an influential factor in patients with respiratory diseases would be helpful to evaluate this issue. Additionally, assessment of HRQoL alongside with disease-specific parameters as well as mental problems or conditions would help to gain a deeper understanding. Thereby, the different dimensions/subcategories of OHRQoL measurement should be addressed. Multicenter, prospective study designs, especially considering any dental or medical intervention, would also bring benefit to the understanding of

OHRQoL and possibilities to its improvement in patients with respiratory diseases. Reference values and minimal important differences to interpret the clinical relevance of the data would also be of research interest in this study. Altogether, the body of evidence with respect to OHRQoL of patients with chronic respiratory diseases is quite weak, making more study in the field recommendable.

STRENGTHS AND LIMITATIONS

This is the first systematic study in this field. The methodology was sound, according to the PRISMA guidelines, and included a quality appraisal of the included studies. This quality appraisal revealed that the included studies were of moderate-to-high quality. The main points of criticism were missing blinding of examination and no consideration of any follow-up in most studies. Altogether, the included studies can be seen as of appropriate quality because the most relevant issues of quality appraisal were addressed by those investigations. The inclusion of such a heterogeneous combination of diseases and of children and adults together limits the comparability of findings. On one hand, the different diseases can cause different intra- and extraoral effects, potentially affecting OHRQoL of patients. For example, COPD and asthma are associated with periodontitis (7), while other included respiratory diseases are not associated with periodontitis. Periodontitis leads to reduced OHRQoL (42), what might be of relevance in the respective diseases, which are related to periodontal conditions. As this is just one potential example for the heterogeneity of the included diseases, the comparability of respective studies in this study is very limited. However, this study aimed to gain insight into the OHRQoL of patients with chronic respiratory diseases and not directly to compare the different diseases to each other. Similarly, the rationale for including children and adults together can be seen critically. Thereby, a direct comparison between the disease groups was not possible; but, due to the low number of studies on OHRQoL of the respective patient groups, it was decided to include studies on children, too. Of course, it is not possible to compare adults and children suffering from different respiratory diseases. To allow a comprehensive view on the OHRQoL of patients with chronic respiratory diseases, the inclusion appears reasonable, irrespective of the heterogeneity. Only seven studies were considered within this study, limiting the ability to draw meaningful conclusion. Moreover, the analysis was just qualitative. The low number of included studies is an important limitation, but is also an important result. The search terms were quite broad and a very comprehensive manual literature search was applied, checking the reference lists of all the included studies. Thereby, no additional findings could be detected. Therefore, this field of study appears understudied, yet, requiring an increased audience in the future. For this, this study provided several recommendations for future study in the field. More study will be necessary to gain insight into the OHRQoL of patients with respiratory diseases; this study can provide a basis for future study in the field.

CONCLUSION

Patients with chronic respiratory diseases show a reduced OHRQoL. This could be caused by a higher prevalence of oral diseases and underlying disease burden that need further clarification in future studies. An interdisciplinary dental care to support oral health and OHRQoL could be recommendable in individuals with chronic respiratory diseases.

AUTHOR CONTRIBUTIONS

SL, WN, and WW conceptualized the research, conducted a systematic review, analyzed and interpreted the results, and wrote the manuscript. DZ and AA participated in data analysis and interpretation and revised the manuscript. GS, JZ, SH, and HX administrated and supervised the whole research project. All the authors have read and approved the final version of the manuscript.

REFERENCES

1. Mannino DM, Buist AS. Global burden of COPD: risk factors, prevalence, and future trends. *Lancet.* (2007) 370:765–73. doi: 10.1016/S0140-6736(07)61380-4
2. Ratjen F, Bell SC, Rowe SM, Goss CH, Quittner AL, Bush A. Cystic fibrosis. *Nat Rev Dis Primers.* (2015) 1:15010. doi: 10.1038/nrdp.2015.10
3. Stern J, Pier J, Litonjua AA. Asthma epidemiology and risk factors. *Semin Immunopathol.* (2020) 42:5–15. doi: 10.1007/s00281-020-00785-1
4. Lin J, Suurna M. Sleep Apnea and Sleep-Disordered Breathing. *Otolaryngol Clin North Am.* (2018) 51:827–33. doi: 10.1016/j.otc.2018.03.009
5. Booth S, Johnson MJ. Improving the quality of life of people with advanced respiratory disease and severe breathlessness. *Breathe.* (2019) 15:198–215. doi: 10.1183/20734735.0200-2019
6. Fiorentino G, Esquinas AM, Annunziata A. Exercise and chronic obstructive pulmonary disease (COPD). *Adv Exp Med Biol.* (2020) 1228:355–68. doi: 10.1007/978-981-15-1792-1_24
7. Gomes-Filho IS, Cruz SSD, Trindade SC, Passos-Soares JS, Carvalho-Filho PC, Figueiredo ACMG, et al. Periodontitis and respiratory diseases: A systematic review with meta-analysis. *Oral Dis.* (2020) 26:439–46. doi: 10.1111/odi.13228
8. Thomas MS, Parolia A, Kundabala M, Vikram M. Asthma and oral health: a review. *Aust Dent J.* (2010) 55:128–33. doi: 10.1111/j.1834-7819.2010.01226.x
9. Gani F, Caminati M, Bellavia F, Baroso A, Faccioni P, Pancera P, et al. Oral health in asthmatic patients: a review: asthma and its therapy may impact on oral health. *Clin Mol Allergy.* (2020) 18:22. doi: 10.1186/s12948-020-00137-2
10. Coffey N. O' Leary F, Burke F, Roberts A, Hayes M. Periodontal and oral health status of people with Cystic Fibrosis: a systematic review. *J Dent.* (2020) 103:103509. doi: 10.1016/j.jdent.2020.103509
11. Bansal M, Khatri M, Taneja V. Potential role of periodontal infection in respiratory diseases—a review. *J Med Life.* (2013) 6:244–8
12. Huynh NT, Emami E, Helman JI, Chervin RD. Interactions between sleep disorders and oral diseases. *Oral Dis.* (2014) 20:236–45. doi: 10.1111/odi.12152
13. Reissmann DR, John MT, Schierz O, Kriston L, Hinz A. Association between perceived oral and general health. *J Dent.* (2013) 41:581–9. doi: 10.1016/j.jdent.2013.05.007
14. Reissmann DR. Methodological considerations when measuring oral health-related quality of life. *J Oral Rehabil.* (2021) 48:233–45. doi: 10.1111/joor.12983

15. Schmalz G, Patschan S, Patschan D, Ziebolz D. Oral-health-related quality of life in adult patients with rheumatic diseases—a systematic review. *J Clin Med.* (2020) 9:1172. doi: 10.3390/jcm9041172
16. Schmalz G, Garbade J, Kollmar O, Ziebolz D. Does oral health-related quality of life of patients after solid organ transplantation indicate a response shift? Results of a systematic review. *BMC Oral Health.* (2020) 20:356. doi: 10.1186/s12903-020-01350-w
17. Moher D, Liberati A, Tetzlaff J, Altman DG, The PRISMA Group. Preferred reporting items for systematic reviews and meta-analyses: the PRISMA statement. *PLoS Med.* (2009) 6:e1000097. doi: 10.1136/bmj.b2535
18. Rostom A, Dubé C, Cranney A, Saloojee N, Sy R, Garritty C, et al. *Celiac disease. Evidence Reports/Technology Assessments, No. 104. Agency for Healthcare Research and Quality (US) (2004).* Available online at: https://www.ncbi.nlm.nih.gov/books/NBK35156/ (accessed September 2004).
19. Saltnes SS, Storhaug K, Borge CR, Enmarker I, Willumsen T. Oral health-related quality-of-life and mental health in individuals with chronic obstructive pulmonary disease (COPD). *Acta Odontol Scand.* (2015) 73:14–20. doi: 10.3109/00016357.2014.935952
20. Gaeckle NT, Heyman B, Criner AJ, Criner GJ. Markers of dental health correlate with daily respiratory symptoms in COPD. *Chronic Obstr Pulm Dis.* (2018) 5:97–105. doi: 10.15326/jcopdf.5.2.2017.0159
21. Patrick JR, da Fonseca MA, Kaste LM, Fadavi S, Shah N, Sroussi H. Oral Health-related quality of life in pediatric patients with cystic fibrosis. *Spec Care Dentist.* (2016) 36:187–93. doi: 10.1111/scd.12162
22. Schmalz G, Wendorff H, Marcinkowski A, Weinreich G, Teschler H, Haak R, et al. Oral health related quality of life depending on oral health and specific factors in patients after lung transplantation. *Clin Respir J.* (2018) 12:731–7. doi: 10.1111/crj.12625
23. Grillo C, La Mantia I, Zappala G, Cocuzza S, Ciprandi G, Andaloro C. Oral health in children with sleep-disordered breathing: a cross-sectional study. *Acta Biomed.* (2019) 90(7-S):52–9. doi: 10.23750/abm.v90i7-S.8661
24. Tamasas B, Nelson T, Chen M. Oral health and oral health-related quality of life in children with obstructive sleep apnea. *J Clin Sleep Med.* (2019) 15:445–52. doi: 10.5664/jcsm.7672
25. Brasil-Oliveira R, Cruz ÁA, Souza-Machado A, Pinheiro GP, Inácio DDS, Sarmento VA, et al. Oral health-related quality of life in individuals with severe asthma. *J Bras Pneumol.* (2020) 47:e20200117. doi: 10.36416/1806-3756/e20200117
26. Haag DG, Peres KG, Balasubramanian M, Brennan DS. Oral conditions and health-related quality of life: a systematic review. *J Dent Res.* (2017) 96:864–74. doi: 10.1177/0022034517709737
27. Sischo L, Broder HL. Oral health-related quality of life: what, why, how, and future implications. *J Dent Res.* (2011) 90:1264–70. doi: 10.1177/0022034511399918
28. Schmalz G, Patschan S, Patschan D, Ziebolz D. Oral health-related quality of life in adult patients with end-stage kidney diseases undergoing renal replacement therapy—a systematic review. *BMC Nephrol.* (2020) 21:154. doi: 10.1186/s12882-020-01824-7
29. Hodkinson A, Bower P, Grigoroglou C, Zghebi SS, Pinnock H, Kontopantelis E, et al. Self-management interventions to reduce healthcare use and improve quality of life among patients with asthma: systematic review and network meta-analysis. *BMJ.* (2020) 370:m2521. doi: 10.1136/bmj.m2521
30. Akinci B, Aslan GK, Kiyan E. Sleep quality and quality of life in patients with moderate to very severe chronic obstructive pulmonary disease. *Clin Respir J.* (2018) 12:1739–46. doi: 10.1111/crj.12738
31. Cronly JA, Duff AJ, Riekert KA, Fitzgerald AP, Perry IJ, Lehane EA, et al. Health-related quality of life in adolescents and adults with cystic fibrosis: physical and mental health predictors. *Respir Care.* (2019) 64:406–15. doi: 10.4187/respcare.06356
32. Pauletto P, Réus JC, Bolan M, Massignan C, Flores-Mir C, Maia I, et al. Association between obstructive sleep apnea and health-related quality of life in untreated adults: a systematic review. *Sleep Breath.* (2021) 11:1–7. doi: 10.1007/s11325-021-02323-1
33. Schmalz G, Garbade J, Sommerwerck U, Kollmar O, Ziebolz D. Oral health-related quality of life of patients after solid organ transplantation is not affected by oral conditions: results of a multicentre cross-sectional study. *Med Oral Patol Oral Cir Bucal.* (2021) 26:e437–44. doi: 10.4317/medoral.24277
34. Ziebolz D, Friedrich S, Binner C, Rast J, Eisner M, Wagner J, et al. Lack in Periodontal Care of Patients Suffering from Severe Heart Diseases-Results after 12 Months Follow-Up. *J Clin Med.* (2020) 9:352. doi: 10.3390/jcm9020352
35. Schmalz G, Ziebolz D. Changing the Focus to the Whole Patient instead of One Oral Disease: The Concept of Individualized Prevention. *Adv Prev Med.* (2020) 2020:6752342. doi: 10.1155/2020/6752342
36. Slade GD, Spencer AJ. Development and evaluation of the oral health impact profile. *Community Dent Health.* (1994) 11:3–11.
37. Slade GD. Derivation and validation of a short-form oral health impact profile. *Community Dent Oral Epidemiol.* (1997) 25:284–90. doi: 10.1111/j.1600-0528.1997.tb00941.x
38. John MT, Rener-Sitar K, Baba K, Celebić A, Larsson P, Szabo G, et al. Patterns of impaired oral health-related quality of life dimensions. *J Oral Rehabil.* (2016) 43:519–27. doi: 10.1111/joor.12396
39. Broder HL, McGrath C, Cisneros GJ. Questionnaire development: face validity and item impact testing of the Child Oral Health Impact Profile. *Community Dent Oral Epidemiol.* (2007) 35 Suppl 1:8–19. doi: 10.1111/j.1600-0528.2007.00401.x
40. de Paula JS, Ambrosano GM, Mialhe FL. Oral Disorders, Socioenvironmental Factors and Subjective Perception Impact on Children's School Performance. *Oral Health Prev Dent.* (2015) 13:219–26. doi: 10.3290/j.ohpd.a32672
41. Scott JM, Gadbury-Amyot CC, Hoffman AM, Simmer-Beck ML. Associations of self-reported oral health quality of life with actual oral health status in children. *J Dent Hyg.* (2021) 95:57–66.
42. Fuller J, Donos N, Suvan J, Tsakos G, Nibali L. Association of oral health-related quality of life measures with aggressive and chronic periodontitis. *J Periodontal Res.* (2020) 55:574–80. doi: 10.1111/jre.12745

2

Compare the Effect of Inhaled Corticosteroids and Systemic Corticosteroids on Sputum Microbiome of AECOPD

*Nan Ma, Yujing Qi, Xiaona Liang, Jing Bai, Jingmin Deng, Meihua Li and Zhiyi He**

Department of Pulmonary and Critical Care Medicine, First Affiliated Hospital of Guangxi Medical University, Nanning, China

***Correspondence:**
Zhiyi He
zhiyi-river@163.com

Background: To observe the effects of inhaled corticosteroids (ICS) and systemic corticosteroids (SCS) on the sputum microbiology of patients with AECOPD.

Methods: The 16S rRNA sequencing results for sputum samples from 36 admitted AECOPD patients were analyzed using ICS or SCS on the basis of standard treatment; sputum samples were collected before and after treatment for 1 day, 7, and 14 days.

Results: After 7 days of SCS treatment, the bacterial abundance of *Sorangium, Acidibacter,* and *Fretibacterium* decreased at the genus level. After 14 days of SCS treatment, the bacterial abundance of *Prevotella_2, Bergeyella, Corynebacterium_1*, and *Ruminococcaceae_UCG-014* was decreased at the genus level, and an increase in the bacterial abundance of the Clostridiales_vadinBB60_group was observed at the family level. The linear discriminant analysis effect size (LEfSe) algorithm showed that after treatment for 14 days, *Sphingobacterium* increased in the SCS group, and Corynebacterium_1 (genus level), Bacillales (order level), and Lactobacillales (order level) decreased in the ICS group. However, the abundance of the above bacteria in each group of samples was <1%, suggesting that the two treatments may have similar effects on bacterial abundance. Alpha diversity analysis results showed that there was no significant difference in the ACE index, Chao1 index, Shannon index, or Simpson index between the ICS group and the SCS group. Beta diversity analysis showed that there was little difference in bacterial diversity among each group. BugBase predicted that although bacteria containing mobile elements in the SCS group decreased significantly compared with those in patients using ICS after treatment for 14 days, these two treatments had similar effects on other phenotype categories assigned to the bacterial contents.

Conclusions: Our results show that ICS and SCS have remarkably similar effects on the sputum microbiome of AECOPD patients.

Keywords: chronic obstructive pulmonary disease, acute exacerbation, inhaled corticosteroids, systemic corticosteroids, sputum microbiome

INTRODUCTION

Chronic obstructive pulmonary disease (COPD) is a common respiratory disease that is characterized by persistent symptoms and impaired lung function due to small airway obliteration and alveolar destruction and is related to a chronic inflammatory response in the lungs (1, 2). The exacerbation of airway inflammation and disease progression during acute exacerbation of COPD have been demonstrated to be related to changes in the lung microbiology (3). The effects of acute exacerbation of COPD on airway microbiology mainly consist of the imbalance of airway microbiology and changes in microecological diversity (1, 3, 4).

Glucocorticoids are widely used to treat a variety of pulmonary inflammatory diseases and have become first-line therapies for COPD (5). An enhanced systemic inflammatory response is a pathological characteristic of AECOPD, and glucocorticoids show anti-inflammatory effects in patients with AECOPD. Systemic glucocorticoids (SCS) are recommended by guidelines for the treatment of AECOPD (5, 6), and SCS improve oxygenation, the risk of early relapse, treatment failure, and the length of hospitalization (5, 7, 8). The Global Initiative for Chronic Obstructive Lung Disease notes that therapy with inhaled corticosteroids (ICS) is equally as effective as SCS during the acute exacerbation of COPD (9). The current study demonstrated that 6–8 mg of corticosteroids administered by nebulized inhalation provides benefits and short-term clinical outcomes similar to those of systemic corticosteroids (10). In the treatment of AECOPD, the advantage of ICS lies in the lower incidence of adverse events than SCS (11), such as impairment of systemic immunity, infection, steroid diabetes, and osteoporosis (10).

Corticosteroid treatment of AECOPD has significant effects on microbiome composition, and treatment with SCS alone and without antibiotics can increase Proteobacteria, Bacteroides, and Firmicute abundance (12). One-year treatment with ICS increases the total bacterial load in the sputum of COPD patients and changes the microbiome composition (13). Local inflammation in AECOPD is related to changes in the microbiota, characterized by reduced microbial diversity (14, 15). Treatment with SCS alone decreased microbial alpha diversity in AECOPD (1). Long-term use of ICS in COPD patients is positively correlated with beta diversity of the upper airway microbiota (16). However, whether there are different effects of ICS and SCS on the sputum microbiome during the treatment of AECOPD remains poorly understood. This study investigated the bacterial load and microbial diversity and aimed to compare the effects of ICS and SCS on the sputum microbiome in patients with AECOPD.

MATERIALS AND METHODS

Ethical Approval

This study was approved by the Ethics Committee of the First Affiliated Hospital of Guangxi Medical University in 2017 (number: 2017KY-E-024). All subjects provided written informed consent before enrollment, and all subjects could withdraw from the study at any time.

Patients

Thirty-six patients with AECOPD meeting the diagnostic criteria of GOLD (17) were enrolled in the present study. There are no antibiotic treatment before patients admitted to hospital. The inclusion criteria of patients were as follows: (1) patients were more than 50 years old and had a history of smoking or smoking exposure; (2) patients were diagnosed with acute exacerbation of COPD that requires additional treatment; (3) patients had no history of asthma, tuberculosis, cystic fibrosis, obliterative bronchiolitis, pulmonary embolism, diffuse panbronchiolitis (DPB), and no complications with acute respiratory failure, acidosis, cancer, or serious heart, liver, or kidney disease; and (4) patients were able to undergo pulmonary function tests or venipuncture.

Study Design

Patients with AECOPD were randomly assigned to the ICS group and SCS group, patients in the ICS group received inhaled budesonide (2 mg Tid for 5 days), and patients in the SCS group were treated with systemic methylprednisolone (methylprednisolone acetate injectable suspension 40 mg Qd for 5 days). Therapy with corticosteroids was based on standard treatments, including long-acting muscarinic antagonists (LAMAs), long-acting beta-adrenergic receptor agonists (LABA), broad-spectrum antibiotics, and low-flow oxygen, according to local treatment guidelines for AECOPD (17).

Sputum Sampling and Microbiome Analysis

As per the inclusion criteria, sputum samples were collected for all patients on the 1st, 7th, and 14th mornings before

TABLE 1 | Major clinical characteristics of patients in the cohort upon admission.

	ICS group (n = 18)	SCS group (n = 18)	p-value
Age (year)	67.72±6.95	66.47±7.4	0.609
Smoke (pack-years)	90.44±85.02	62.29±21.67	0.195
BMI (kg/m^2)	22.17±2.36	21.70±2.70	0.589
FEV1%pred	39.17±17.48	37.70±16.29	0.799
FEV1/FVC	44.29±16.44	43.14±13.92	0.824
CAT	20.17±4.32	18.47±3.78	0.226
WBC	8.87±1.72	8.96±1.93	0.875
NEU	6.58±1.26	6.78±1.07	0.619
Gender			0.471
Male	14	11	
Female	4	7	
GOLD			
D	9	9	
C	5	5	
B	4	3	
mMRC			
3	2	4	
2	8	8	
1	8	5	

glucocorticoid use and ICS/SCS treatment. To collect induced sputum, 3% sterile NaCl solution was inhaled by nebulizer for 15 min, and taked the induced sputum, it was the same as those introduced in our previous paper (18). And bacterial 16S rRNA gene detection were also the same as our previous paper (18).

Bioinformatic and Statistical Analysis

Usearch software (v.10.0.240) was used to identify unique tags and to discard excess tags, and tags with more than 97% similarity were clustered into operational taxonomic units (OTUs) by Usearch (19–21). Krona taxonomy visualization and petals diagrams were used to analyze the relative proportions of different OTUs for different classification levels (22). Metastats software was used to analyze bacteria with different abundances at the family and genus levels (23). Linear discriminant analysis effect size (LEfSe) was used to determine which OTUs had differences between the groups under different biological conditions. LEfSe is suitable for the discovery and interpretation of multilevel biological identification and characteristics, such as species taxonomy pedigrees (24). The Shannon sparse curve was drawn using the Shannon index, which is used to evaluate whether the amount of sequencing data is sufficient to cover all bacterial species and reflect the species richness in the sample (25, 26). Alpha diversity was calculated on the basis of the gene profile for each sample based on the Shannon, Chao1, Simpson, and ACE indices. Alpha diversity estimates

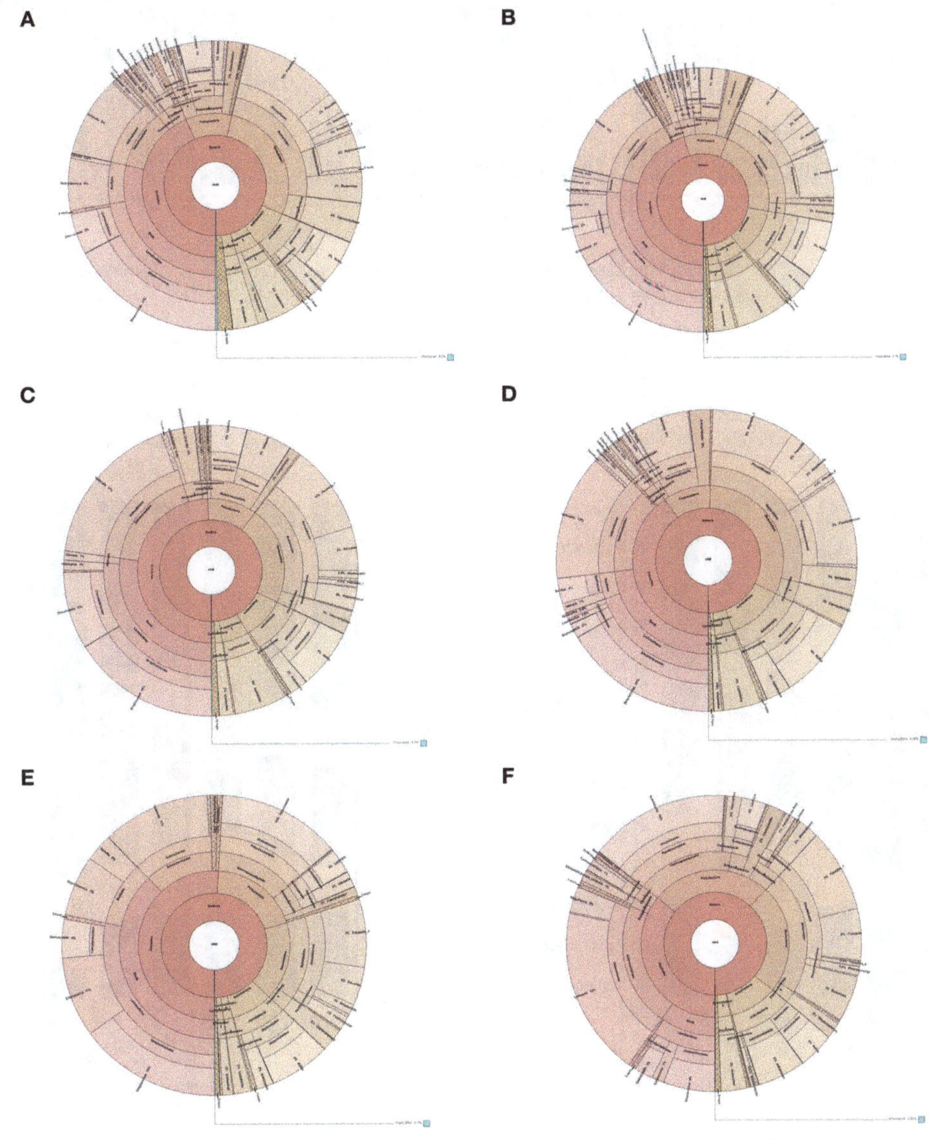

FIGURE 1 | Species distribution of each group. Krona is taxonomy web visualization; circles from inside to outside represent different classification levels, and the area of the sector indicates the proportion of different OTU annotation results. Rings from inside to outside: Contents of various bacteria at the kingdom, phylum, class, order, family, and genus levels. **(A)**: ICS 1 day. **(B)**: SCS 1 day. **(C)**: ICS 7 day. **(D)**: SCS 7 day. **(E)**: ICS 14 day. **(F)**: SCS 14 day.

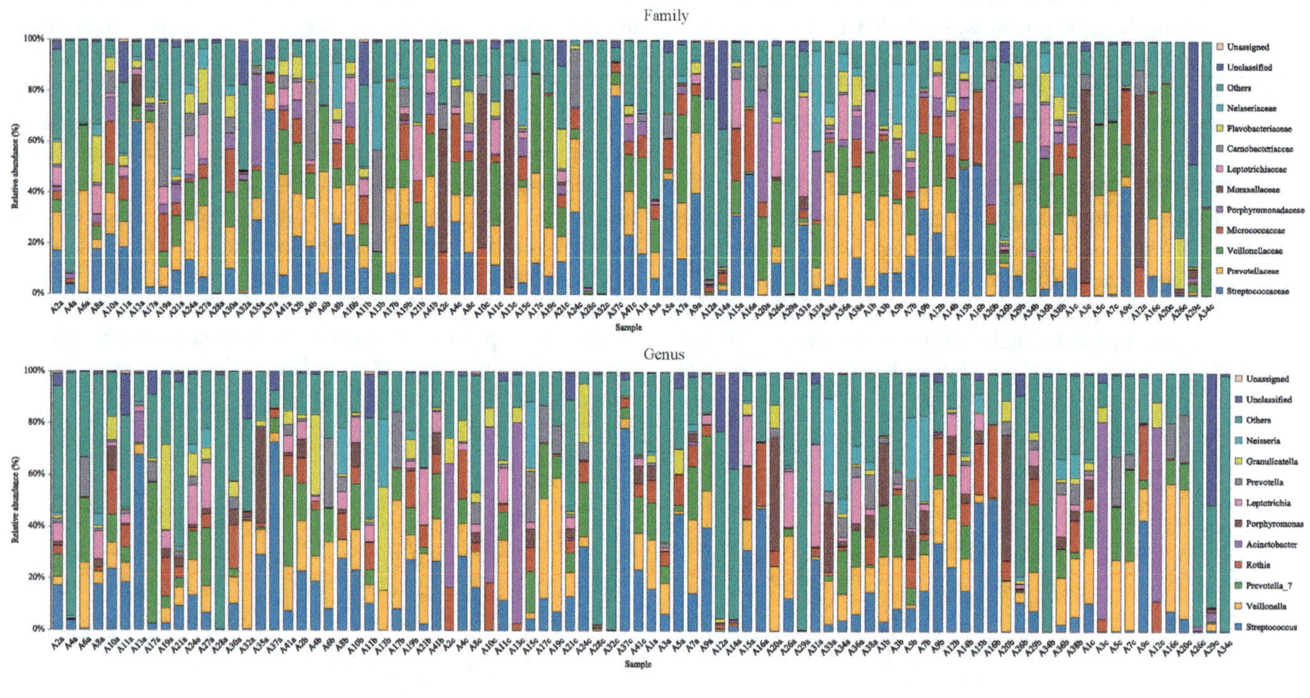

FIGURE 2 | Species distribution of each sample. Species distribution of bacteria in each sample (family and genus level). Community composition based on 16S rRNA gene fragment sequences in sputum samples. Bars represent the relative abundance of the most abundant families (>5% in one sample). The remaining families are subsumed as others.

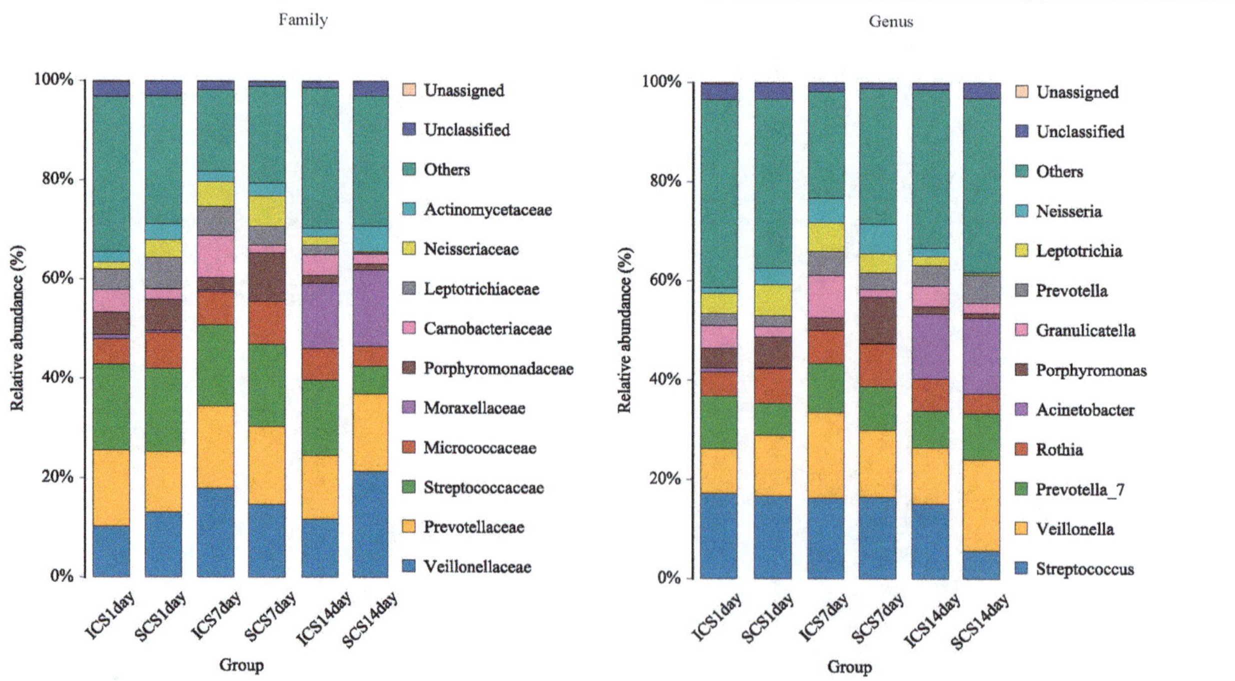

FIGURE 3 | Species distribution of each group. Species distribution of bacteria in each group (family and genus level). Community composition based on 16S rRNA gene fragment sequences in sputum samples. Bars represent the relative abundances of the most abundant families (>5% in one group). The remaining families are subsumed as others.

were computed using mothur software (version 1.30) and R (version 3.5.1), beta diversity estimates were computed using QIIME1 (v1.8.0) software, and non-metric multidimensional scaling (NMDS) based on Bray-Curtis dissimilarity was used to visualize potential clustering patterns among samples based on the estimated beta diversity and its relationship with dominant taxa. BugBase was used to predict bacterial composition based on the sequencing results.

To determine the differentially expressed OTUs between samples, the R package pheatmap was used to construct a heatmap for the OTU expression profile. Spearman rank correlation analysis was used to screen the bacteria demonstrating correlations (family level, HR > 0.1 and p < 0.05), and the microbial network was constructed by Python.

RESULTS

Patient Characteristics

Eighteen ICS patients and 18 SCS patients were enrolled and eligible for this research study. There were no significant differences in basic clinical characteristics between the two groups (age, smoking status, BMI, lung function, CAT, WBC, NEU, Sex, P > 0.05), as shown in **Table 1**.

Comparison of the Effects of ICS and SCS on Lung Bacterial Load in Patients With AECOPD

The species annotation of each group was visualized by using KRONA (**Figure 1**), and a histogram was generated

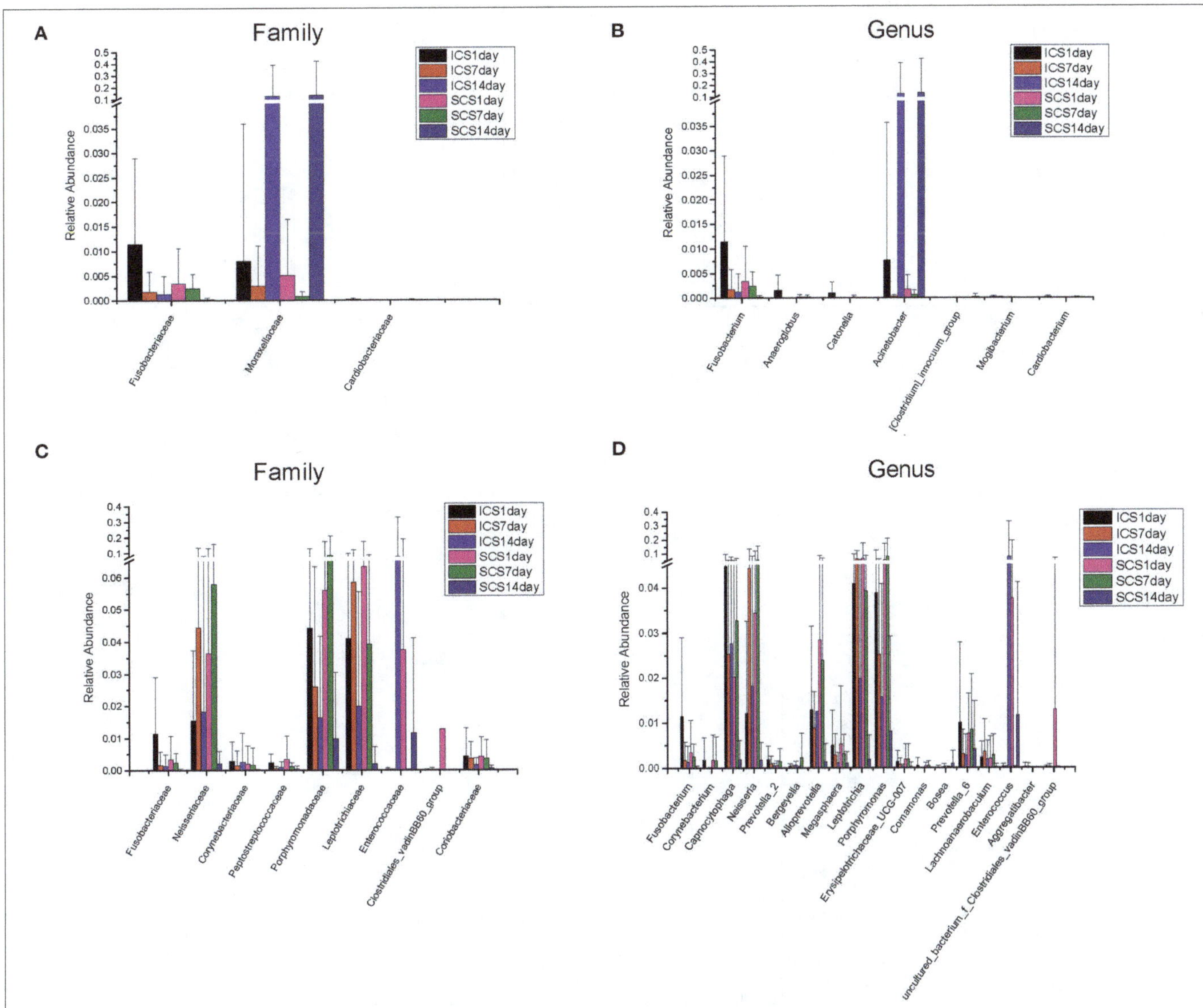

FIGURE 4 | Colonies with different abundances. **(A,B)** Colonies with different abundances in each group. Statistical analyses were calculated by one-way analysis of variance by ANOVA (family and genus levels, p < 0.05). **(C,D)** Colonies with different abundances in each group. Statistical analyses were calculated by the Wilcoxon test (family and genus levels, p < 0.05).

to show the species distribution of each sample (**Figure 2**) and each group (**Figure 3**). ANOVA and Wilcoxon tests were used to analyze the effects of ICS and SCS on the lung bacterial load of patients with COPD. An ANOVA test showed that the colonies with different abundances at the family level were *Fusobacteriaceae, Moraxellaceae,* and *Cardiobacteriaceae*, while *Fusobacterium, Anaeroglobus, Catonella, Acinetobacter, [Clostridium]_innocuum_group, Mogibacterium,* and *Cardiobacterium* showed different abundances at the genus level; the Wilcoxon test showed that colonies with different abundances at the family level were *Fusobacteriaceae, Neisseriaceae, Corynebacteriaceae, Peptostreptococcaceae, Porphyromonadaceae, Leptotrichiaceae, Enterococcaceae, Clostridiales_vadinBB60_group,* and *Coriobacteriaceae*, while *Fusobacterium, Corynebacterium, Capnocytophaga, Neisseria, Prevotella_2, Bergeyella, Alloprevotella, Megasphaera, Leptotrichia, Porphyromonas, Erysipelotrichaceae_UCG-007, Comamonas, Bosea, Prevotella_6, Lachnoanaerobaculum, Enterococcus, Aggregatibacter,* and *uncultured_bacterium_f_Clostridiales_vadinBB60_group* showed different abundances at the genus level (**Figure 4**, $p < 0.05$). After 7 days of SCS treatment, the bacterial abundances of *Sorangium, Acidibacter,* and *Fretibacterium* decreased at the genus level (**Figure 5**, $p < 0.05$). After 14 days of SCS treatment, the bacterial abundances of *Prevotella_2, Bergeyella, Corynebacterium_1,* and *Ruminococcaceae_UCG-014* decreased

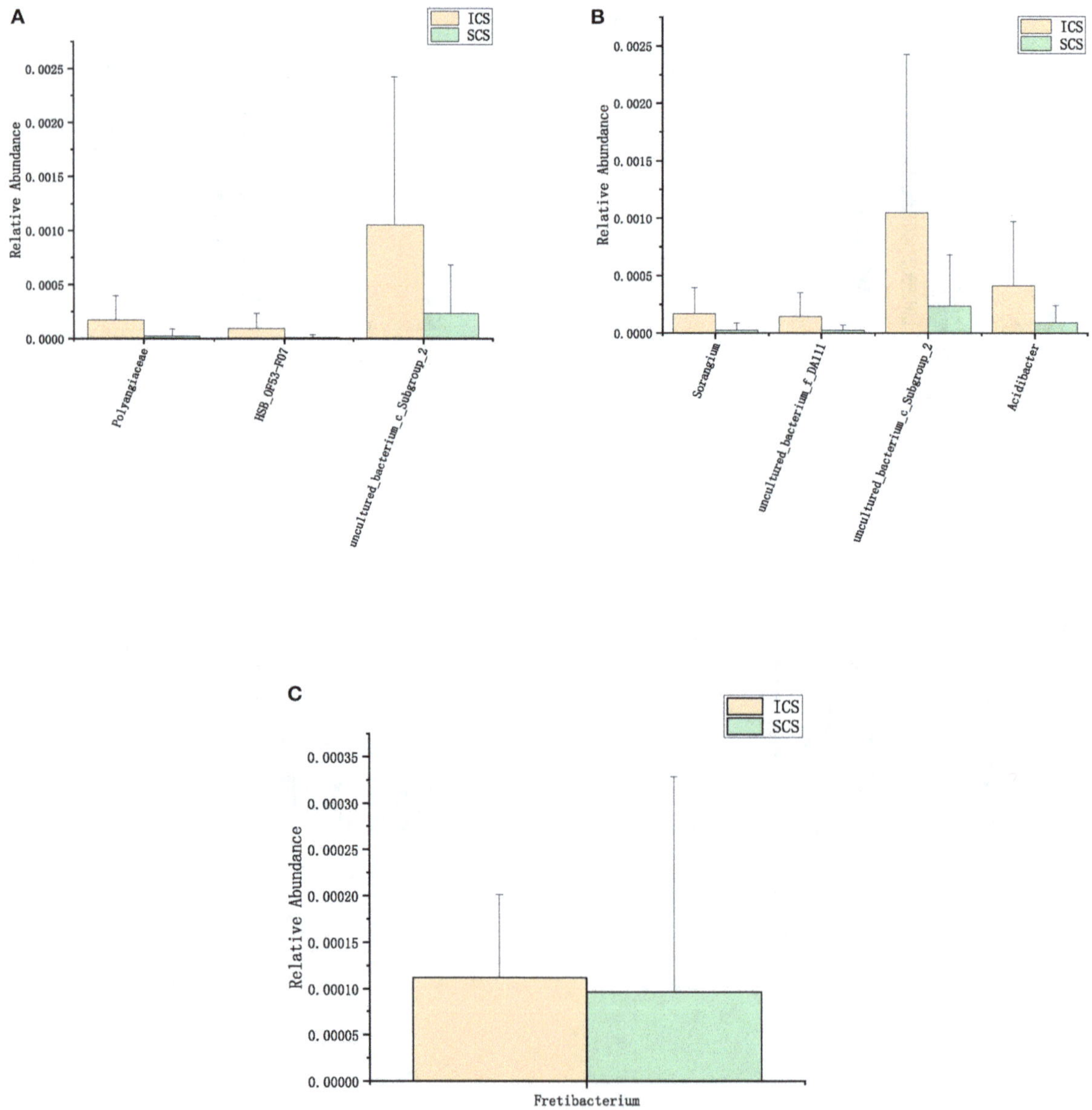

FIGURE 5 | Colonies with different abundances after 7 days of treatment. **(A)** One-way analysis of variance (ANOVA) at the family level. **(B)** Calculated by ANOVA at the genus level. **(C)** Calculated by Wilcoxon test at the genus level ($p < 0.05$).

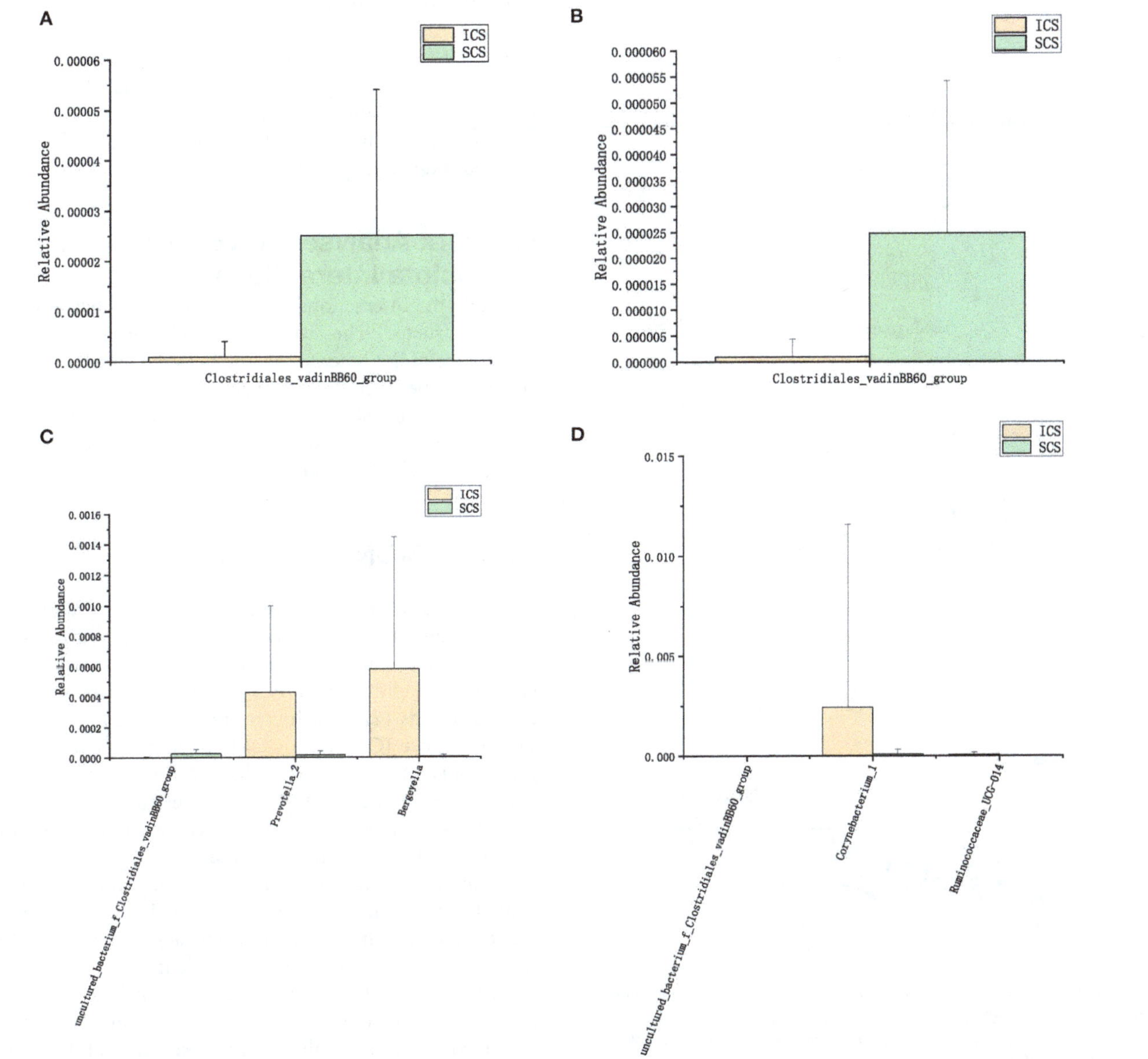

FIGURE 6 | Colonies with different abundances after 14 days of treatment. **(A)**: One-way analysis of variance by ANOVA at the family level. **(B)**: Calculated by Wilcoxon test at the family level. **(C)**: One-way analysis of variance (ANOVA) at the genus level. **(D)**: Calculated by Wilcoxon test at the genus level. ($p < 0.05$).

at the genus level, and an increase in the bacterial abundance of Clostridiales_vadinBB60_group was observed at the family level (**Figure 6**, $p < 0.05$).

Differential taxonomic features between the ICS and SCS were calculated by linear discriminant analysis effect size (LefSe), and the results showed no difference in abundance between the two groups after treatment for 7 days (**Figure 7A**, $p < 0.05$). After treatment for 14 days, *Sphingobacterium* increased after treatment with SCS, and Corynebacterium_1 (genus level), Bacillales (order level), and Lactobacillales (order level) decreased following treatment with ICS (**Figures 7B,C**; $p < 0.05$). However, the content of bacteria with different abundances between the two groups was <1% in each group (**Figure 1**).

The Influence of ICS and SCS on Lung Microecological Diversity in Patients With AECOPD

Alpha diversity analysis results showed that after 14 days of treatment, the ACE index of the SCS group was significantly lower than the first day of treatment, and the Shannon index of the SCS group was significantly lower than the 7th day after treatment. It was also observed that the Shannon index of the ICS group was significantly lower than the first day of treatment. No differences were found between the two groups at the same treatment time (**Figure 8**, $p < 0.05$).

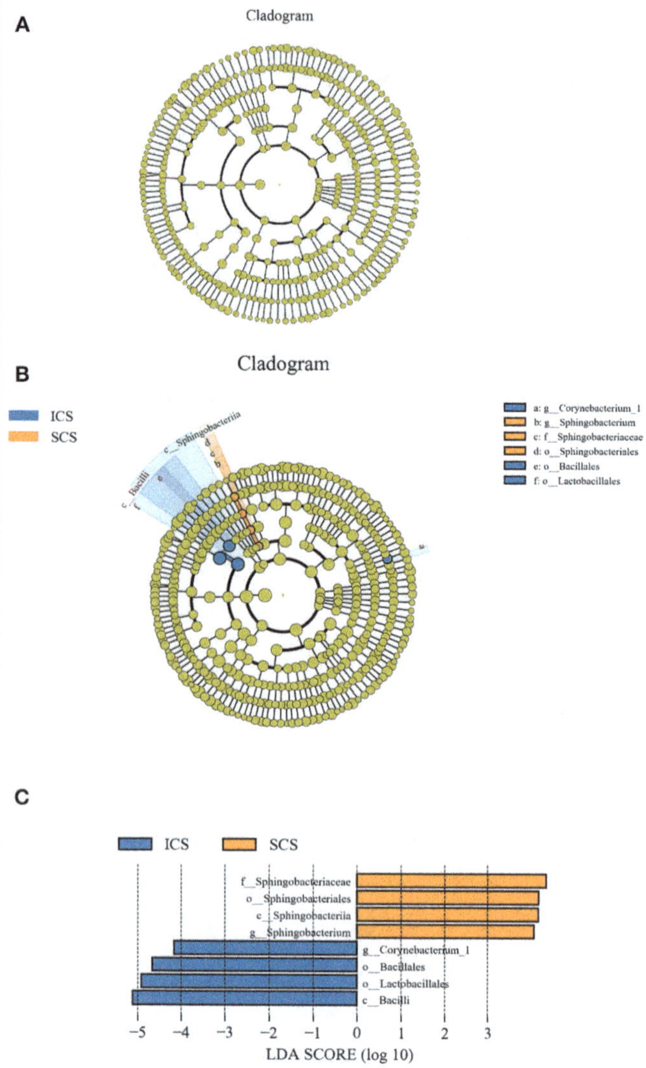

FIGURE 7 | Differential bacterial abundance analyzed by linear discriminant analysis effect size (LEfSe). **(A)** Colonies with different abundances after treatment for 7 days. Our results showed no difference in abundance between the two groups. **(B,C)** Colonies with different abundances after treatment for 14 days, *Sphingobacterium* increased after treatment with SCS, and abundances of Corynebacterium_1 (genus level), Bacillales (order level), and Lactobacillales (order level) were decreased by ICS treatment ($p < 0.05$).

In the beta diversity analysis, PCA, PcoA, and nonmetric multidimensional scaling (NMDS) analyze of bacteria showed no significant divisions into groups (**Figure 9**); Anosim and PERMANOVA statistical analyses showed there was no significant difference in bacterial diversity among the groups and therefore, no significant difference in beta diversity between the two groups (**Figure 10**, $p < 0.05$).

The Influence of ICS and SCS on Microbiome Characteristics

BugBase predicted the bacterial composition of each group (**Figure 11**). After 14 days of treatment, the mobile genetic element (MGE) content in sputum samples of SCS patients was decreased significantly compared with that in patients using ICS. ICS and SCS had the same effects on aerobes, anaerobes, potentially pathogenic bacteria, bacteria related to biofilm formation, gram-negative bacteria, gram-positive bacteria, facultative anaerobes, and oxidative stress-tolerant bacteria (**Figure 12**; $p < 0.05$).

Network Analyses Reveal Potential Microbiota Interactions

To study the interactions between bacteria, a bacterial network was constructed. The size of the circle represents the average abundance of the species; the line between circles represents the correlation between the two species, and the thicker the line, the stronger the correlation; finally, regarding the color of the line, orange represents a positive correlation, and green represents a negative correlation (**Figure 13**).

DISCUSSION

In this study, we observed the effects of corticosteroids on the pulmonary microbiology in patients with AECOPD. Corticosteroids are the main anti-inflammatory drugs for COPD, although most COPD patients have a poor response to corticosteroids (27, 28). Increasing evidence has demonstrated that high-dose ICS use in COPD patients increases the risk of pneumonia (29, 30). Studies have shown that the longer the course of SCS in AECOPD, the higher the risk of pneumonia (31). These studies suggest that glucocorticoids have an impact on lung microbiology in the treatment of COPD. However, the effect of ICS on airway microbiology in acute exacerbation of COPD remains unclear. To our knowledge, our research is the first to study the difference in the efficacy of ICS and SCS on the sputum microbiome of AECOPD patients.

We analyzed the bacterial 16S rRNA *via* bioinformatics methods, and the results showed that the frequently amplified families in the induced sputum of these patients were Streptococcaceae, Veillonellaceae, Prevotellaceae, Micrococcaceae, Moraxellaceae, Porphyromonadaceae, Carnobacteriaceae, Neisseriaceae, Leptotrichia, and Actinomycetaceae; at the genus level, they were *Streptococcus, Veillonella, Prevotella_7, Rothia, Actinomyces, Porphyromonas, Granulicatella, Prevotella, Leptotrichia,* and *Neisseria.* Zhang's research showed that Moraxella, Streptococcus, and Actinobacteria were the major taxonomic groups in the lung microbiome of COPD patients at both the phylum and genus levels (1). The abundance of Moraxella is considered to have a significant positive correlation with the percentage of sputum neutrophils (1). High proportions of Prevotella, Veillonella, and Actinomyces species have been observed in COPD and healthy people, but the difference is not significant (3, 32); our research is consistent with this finding. The occurrence of COPD exacerbation events may be related to the reduction in microbiome diversity and increased proportion of *Proteobacteria* (33, 34).

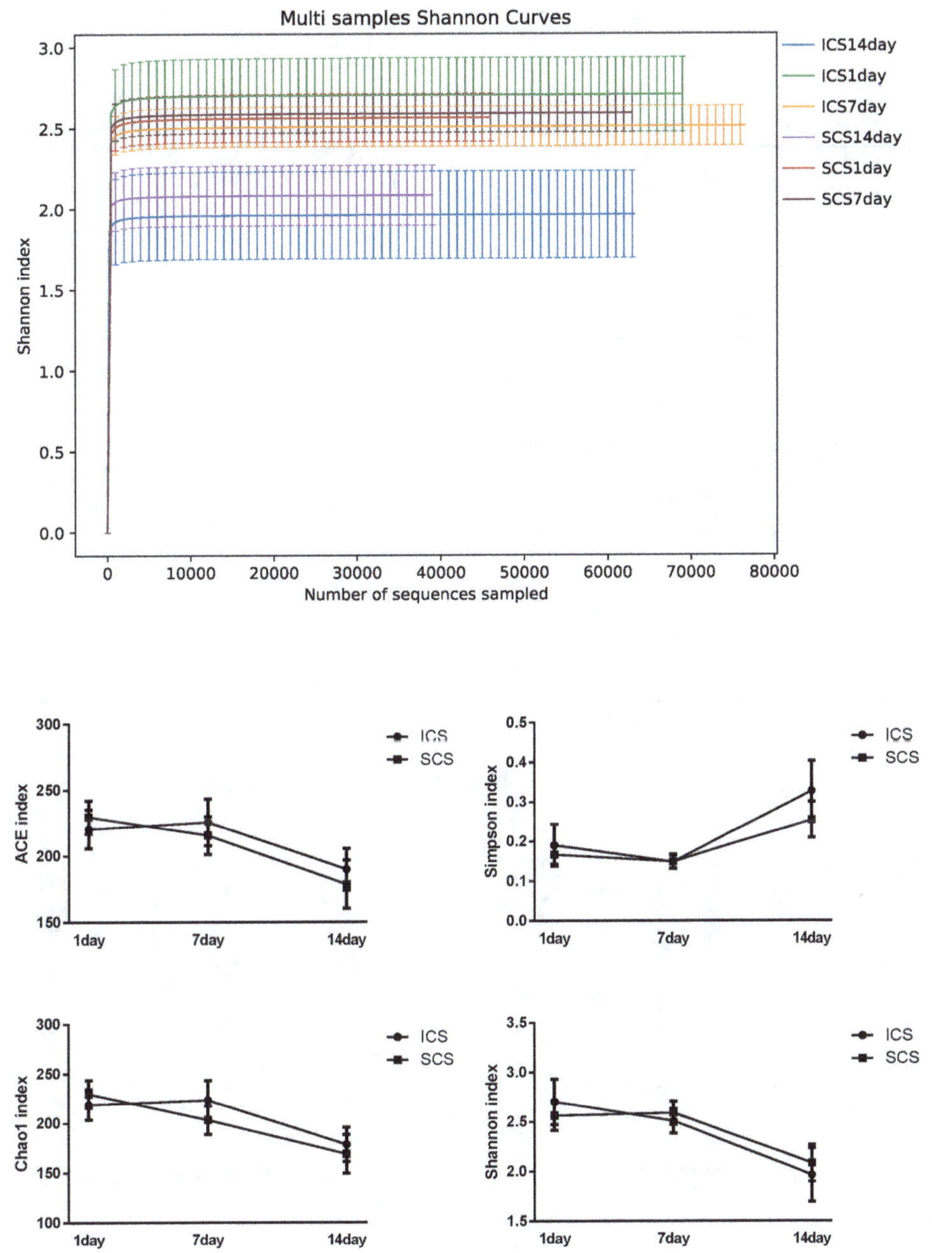

FIGURE 8 | Alpha diversity in ICS vs. SCS. Shannon index of each group and statistical analysis of the ACE index, Chao1 index, Shannon index, and Simpson index ($p < 0.05$). After 14 days of treatment, the ACE index of the SCS group was significantly lower than the first day of treatment, and the Shannon index of the SCS group was significantly lower than the first day of treatment. The Shannon index of the ICS group was also significantly lower than the first day of treatment. No differences were found between the two groups at the same treatment time ($p < 0.05$).

After 7 days of SCS treatment, the bacterial abundance of *Sorangium, Acidibacter,* and *Fretibacterium* decreased at the genus level. After 14 days of SCS treatment, the bacterial abundances of *Prevotella_2, Bergeyella, Corynebacterium_1,* and *Ruminococcaceae_UCG-014* were decreased at the genus level, and an increase in the bacterial abundance of the Clostridiales_vadinBB60_group was observed at the family level. The linear discriminant analysis effect size (LEfSe) algorithm showed that after treatment for 14 days, *Sphingobacterium* increased in the SCS group, and Corynebacterium_1 (genus level), Bacillales (order level), and Lactobacillales (order level) decreased in the ICS group. *Prevotella* and *Corynebacterium* spp. are considered to be common colonizers of healthy airways (35, 36). Other bacteria that differ in relative abundance have not been found to be associated with lung infections to date. In addition, the levels of the abovementioned bacteria with different abundances were <1% in each group of samples. Therefore, we consider that the ICS and

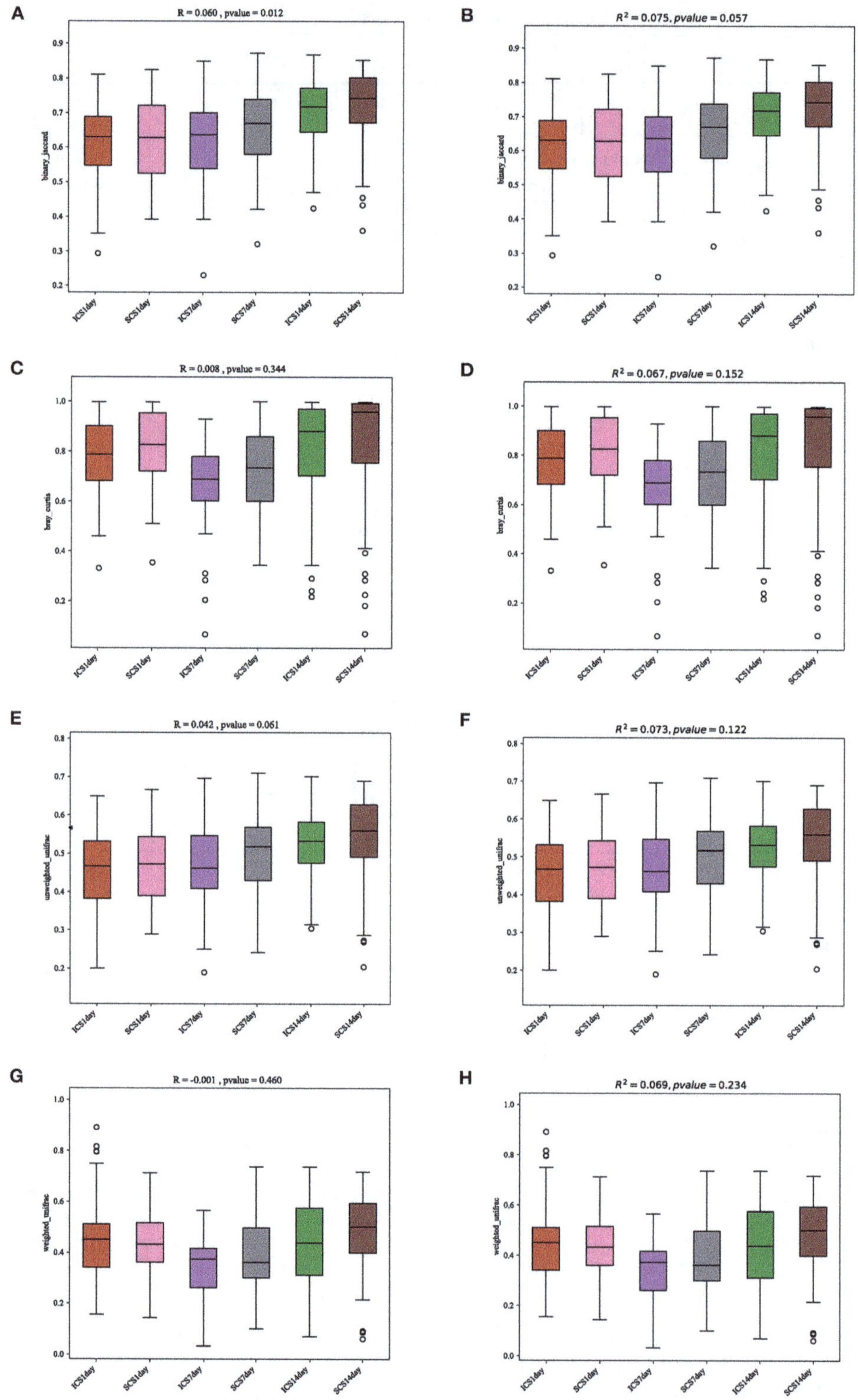

FIGURE 9 | Statistical analysis results for PCA and PcoA. **(A)** Anosim statistical analysis of the results, analyzed by the binary Jaccard algorithm. **(B)** PERMANOVA statistical analysis of the results, analyzed by the binary Jaccard algorithm. **(C)** Anosim statistical analysis of the results, analyzed by the Bray-Curtis algorithm. **(D)** PERMANOVA statistical analysis of the results, analyzed by the Bray-Curtis algorithm. **(E)** Anosim statistical analysis of the results, analyzed by the unweighted UniFrac algorithm. **(F)** PERMANOVA statistical analysis of the results, analyzed by the unweighted UniFrac algorithm. **(G)** Anosim statistical analysis of the results, analyzed by the weighted UniFrac algorithm. **(H)** PERMANOVA statistical analysis of the results, analyzed by the weighted UniFrac algorithm. The results showed no differences between the two groups, and there was no significant difference before or after treatment.

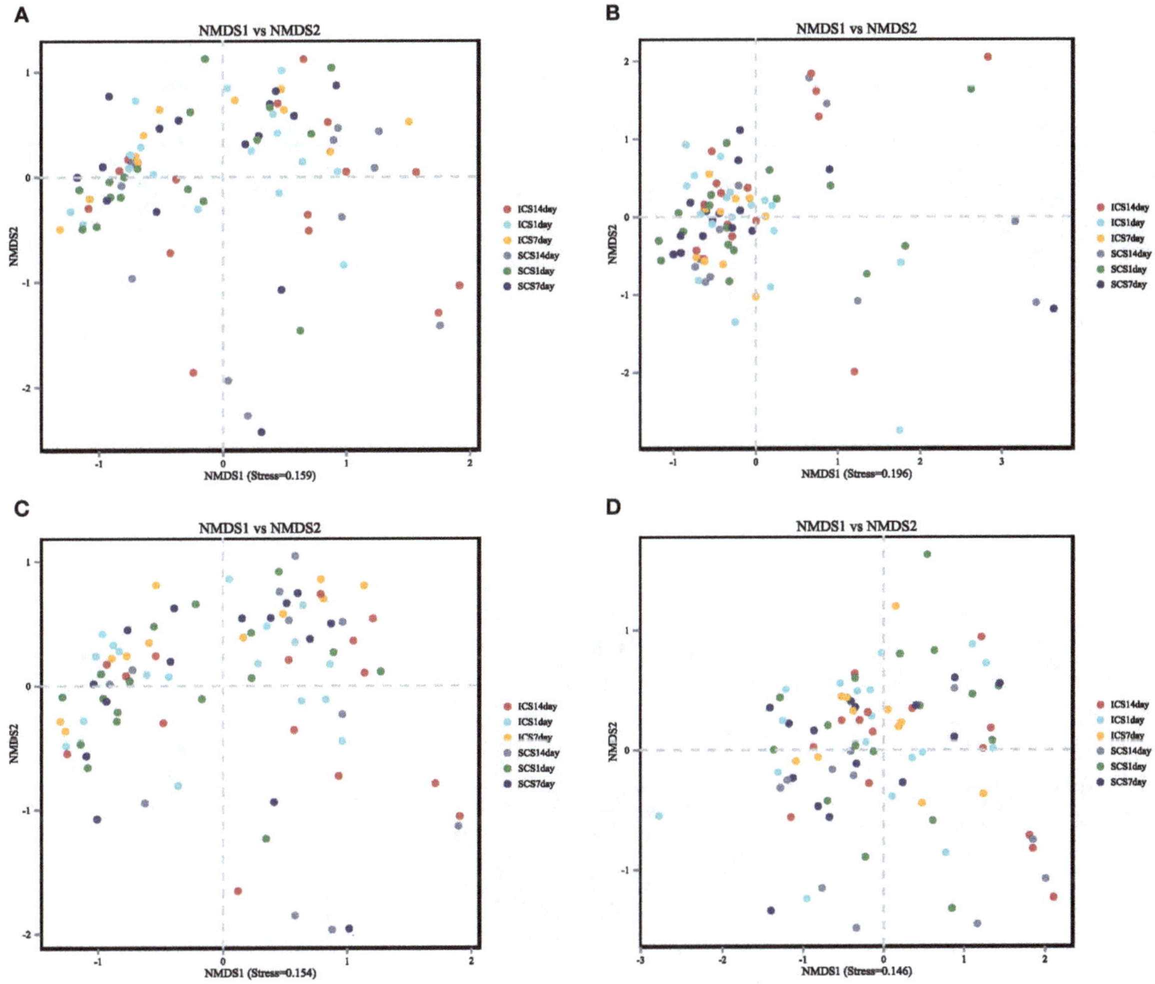

FIGURE 10 | Non-metric multidimensional scaling (NMDS) was used to analyze the colony diversity with the ICS and SCS treatments. The results of NMDS showed that there was no significant difference in bacterial diversity among groups, and ICS and SCS had the same effect on colony diversity via NMDS. Stress < 0.2 in this figure, suggesting that the NMDS analysis is reliable.

SCS will have similar effects on the relative abundance of lung bacteria.

We further analyzed the impact of the two different medication routes on microbial diversity, and the alpha diversity results showed that there were no differences in bacterial abundance between these two treatments at 7 and 14 days. Furthermore, we analyzed the effects of two different glucocorticoid usages on the beta diversity of the microbiome in patients with COPD, including PCA, PCOA, ANOSIM statistical, PERMANOVA statistical, and NMDS analyses. Our results showed that the bacterial abundance of each group was not significantly different in terms of beta diversity. Microbial diversity in the sputum of patients was decreased when acute COPD was exacerbated (1, 34), and lower values of microbial diversity of sputum with COPD were related to increasing 1-year mortality and may be used to predict the poor prognosis of hospitalized patients (14). Our results showed no significant difference between these two methods of glucocorticoid use in terms of the diversity of the microbiome in patients with COPD after 7 or 14 days of treatment. Therefore, we speculate that ICS and SCS may have similar effects on the prognosis of COPD patients. In addition, long-term use of ICS in stable COPD patients will increase the risk of pneumonia (13, 29), which may be due to lung microbiome changes (1). Our research shows that AECOPD patients' lung microbiome is similar before and after treatment with ICS; therefore, we speculate that the use of ICS in AECOPD patients may not increase the risk of pneumonia, and this speculation needs further clinical study for validation.

BugBase is a microbiome characteristics prediction tool that can make predictions based on six phenotype categories: Gram staining, oxygen tolerance, ability to form biofilms, mobile element content, pathogenicity, and oxidative stress tolerance (37). The bacterial composition predicted by BugBase demonstrated that after 14 days of treatment, the mobile genetic element (MGE) content in the sputum of SCS patients was decreased significantly compared with that in patients using ICS. MGEs are considered to be closely related to bacterial antimicrobial resistance (38, 39); thus, the relationship between

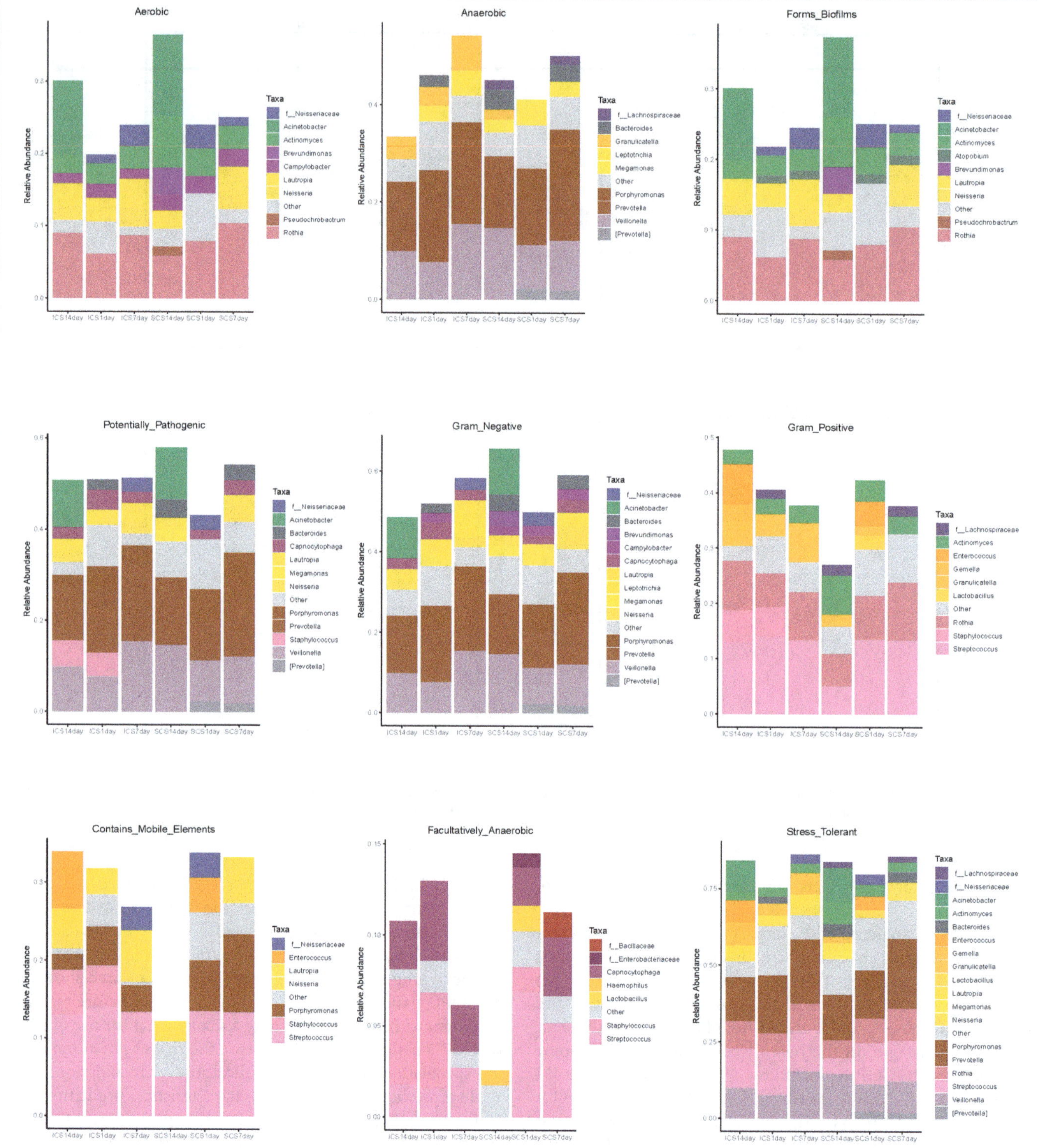

FIGURE 11 | Bacterial composition of each group predicted by BugBase. Bacterial composition of each group, including Gram Positive, Gram Negative, Biofilm Forming, Pathogenic Potential, Mobile Element Containing, Oxygen Utilizing, and Oxidative Stress Tolerant.

ICS and resistant bacteria in COPD patients still needs further clinical research. In the treatment of AECOPD, ICS, and SCS have the same effect on aerobes, anaerobes, potentially pathogenic bacteria, bacteria related to biofilm formation, gram-negative bacteria, gram-positive bacteria, facultative anaerobes, and oxidative stress-tolerant bacteria. Our results show that ICS

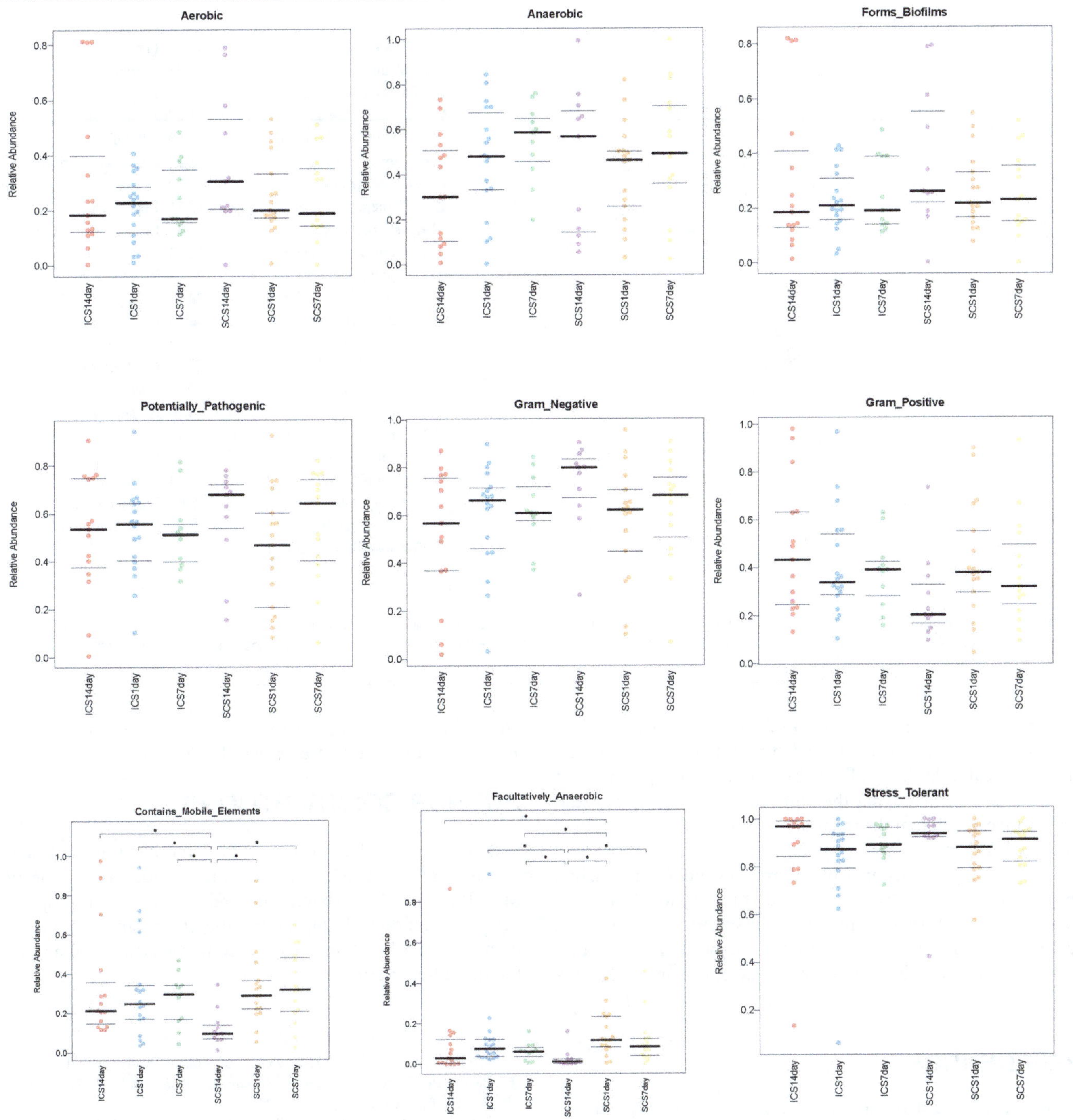

FIGURE 12 | Compared the bacterial composition predicted by BugBase in two groups. Significant differences can be found in facultatively anaerobic content and mobile elements ($p < 0.05$). After treatment for 14 days, the levels of mobile element genes were decreased in the SCS group compared with the ICS group. ICS and SCS have the same effect on aerobes, anaerobes, potentially pathogenic bacteria, bacteria related to biofilm formation, gram-negative bacteria, gram-positive bacteria, facultative anaerobes, and oxidative stress-tolerant bacteria. The data were summarized as the quartile and mean.

and SCS have the same effect on 8 phenotypic categories of bacteria; however, the results are based on BugBase predictions and need to be verified by experiments.

There are also limitations to our study. First, the sample size of this study was small, and it is necessary to increase the sample size and perform further investigation with properly designed studies. Second, the bacterial load of samples and the level of inflammatory factors in induced sputum were not detected because the induced sputum volume was insufficient. Third, there is a close relationship between COPD exacerbation

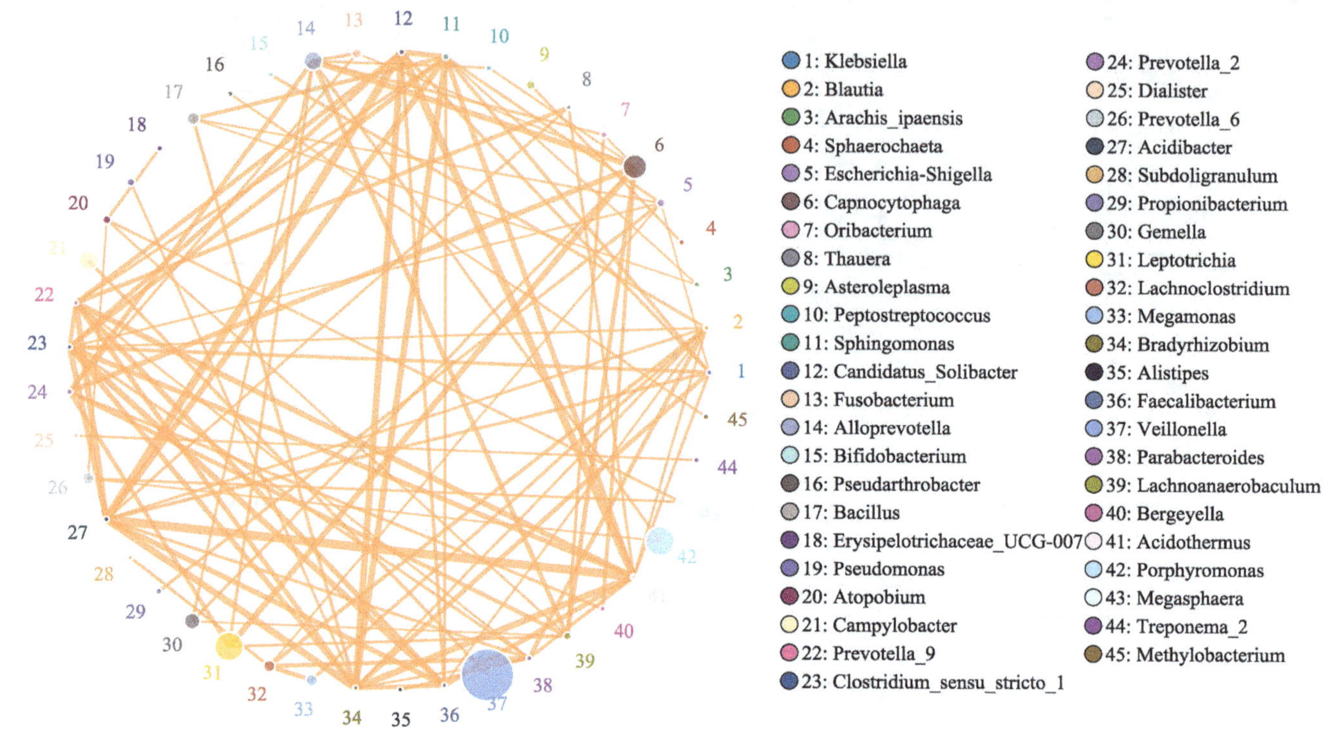

FIGURE 13 | Network of Bacteria. Analyzed by Spearman rank correlation analysis. The size of the circle represents the average abundance of the species; the line represents the correlation between the two species; the thickness of the line represents the strength of the correlation; and regarding the color of the line, orange represents a positive correlation.

and respiratory virus infection (40), and our study failed to analyze the effect of glucocorticoids on virus infection. Finally, the bronchoalveolar lavage fluid (BALF) microbiology has great significance when studying the lung microbiome (12, 41), and further investigation of the microbiome via analysis of AECOPD patients' BALF is needed.

In conclusion, by using a bioinformatics method to analyze 16S data from AECOPD patients, our study showed that there were similar effects of ICS and SCS on the sputum microbiome in patients with AECOPD, and their effects on bacterial abundance and microecological diversity were similar. Additionally, ICS has little effect on the lung microbiome of AECOPD, it may be an advantage of ICS in the treatment of AECOPD.

AUTHOR CONTRIBUTIONS

NM was responsible for part of data analysis and article writing. YQ and XL was responsible for data collection. ML, JB, and JD reviewed and edited the manuscript. ZH designed, conducted, supervised the study, and reviewed the manuscript. All authors contributed to the article and approved the submitted version.

REFERENCES

1. Wang Z, Bafadhel M, Haldar K, Spivak A, Mayhew D, Miller BE, et al. Lung microbiome dynamics in COPD exacerbations. *Eur Resp J.* (2016) 47:1082–92. doi: 10.1183/13993003.01406-2015
2. Sethi S, Mahler DA, Marcus P, Owen CA, Yawn B, Rennard S. Inflammation in COPD: implications for management. *Am J Med.* (2012) 125:1162–70. doi: 10.1016/j.amjmed.2012.06.024
3. Haldar K, George L, Wang Z, Mistry V, Ramsheh MY, Free RC, et al. The sputum microbiome is distinct between COPD and health, independent of smoking history. *Respir Res.* (2020) 21:183. doi: 10.1186/s12931-020-01448-3
4. Pragman AA, Kim HB, Reilly CS, Wendt C, Isaacson RE. The lung microbiome in moderate and severe chronic obstructive pulmonary disease. *PloS ONE.* (2012) 7:e47305. doi: 10.1371/journal.pone.0047305
5. Vogelmeier CF, Criner GJ, Martinez FJ, Anzueto A, Barnes PJ, Bourbeau J, et al. Global strategy for the diagnosis, management, and prevention of chronic obstructive lung disease 2017 report. GOLD executive summary *Am J Respir Crit Care Med.* (2017) 195:557–82. doi: 10.1164/rccm.201701-0218PP
6. Barnes PJ. Glucocorticosteroids. *Handb Exp Pharmacol.* (2017) 237:93–115. doi: 10.1007/164_2016_62
7. O'Donnell DE, Sciurba F, Celli B, Mahler DA, Webb KA, Kalberg CJ, et al. Effect of fluticasone propionate/salmeterol on lung hyperinflation and exercise endurance in COPD. *Chest.* (2006) 130:647–56. doi: 10.1378/chest.130.3.647
8. Celli BR, Thomas NE, Anderson JA, Ferguson GT, Jenkins CR, Jones PW, et al. Effect of pharmacotherapy on rate of decline of lung function in chronic obstructive pulmonary disease - results from the TORCH study. *Am J Respir Crit Care Med.* (2008) 178:332–8. doi: 10.1164/rccm.200712-1869OC
9. Singh D, Agusti A, Anzueto A, Barnes PJ, Bourbeau J, Celli BR, et al. Global strategy for the diagnosis, management, and prevention of chronic obstructive lung disease: the GOLD science committee report 2019. *Eur Respir J.* (2019) 53:1900164. doi: 10.1183/13993003.00164-2019
10. Ding Z, Li X, Lu Y, Rong G, Yang R, Zhang R, et al. A randomized, controlled multicentric study of inhaled budesonide and intravenous

methylprednisolone in the treatment on acute exacerbation of chronic obstructive pulmonary disease. *Respir Med.* (2016) 121:39–47. doi: 10.1016/j.rmed.2016.10.013

11. Sun X, He Z, Zhang J, Deng J, Bai J, Li M, et al. Compare the efficacy of inhaled budesonide and systemic methylprednisolone on systemic inflammation of AECOPD. *Pulm Pharmacol Ther.* (2015) 31:111–6. doi: 10.1016/j.pupt.2014.09.004
12. Dy R, Sethi S. The lung microbiome and exacerbations of COPD. *Curr Opin Pulm Med.* (2016) 22:196–202. doi: 10.1097/MCP.0000000000000268
13. Cantoli M, Pauletti A, Rossi MR, Spanevello A, Casolari P, Marcellini A, et al. Long-term effects of inhaled corticosteroids on sputum bacterial and viral loads in COPD. *Eur Resp J.* (2017) 50:10. doi: 10.1183/13993003.00451-2017
14. Leitao Filho FS, Alotaibi NM, Ngan D, Tam S, Yang J, Hollander Z, et al. Sputum microbiome is associated with 1-year mortality after chronic obstructive pulmonary disease hospitalizations. *Am J Respir Crit Care Med.* (2019) 199:1205–13. doi: 10.1164/rccm.201806-1135OC
15. Tangedal S, Nielsen R, Aanerud M, Persson LJ, Wiker HG, Bakke PS, et al. Sputum microbiota and inflammation at stable state and during exacerbations in a cohort of chronic obstructive pulmonary disease (COPD) patients. *PloS ONE.* (2019) 14:e0222449. doi: 10.1371/journal.pone.0222449
16. Pragman AA, Knutson KA, Gould TJ, Isaacson RE, Reilly CS, Wendt CH. Chronic obstructive pulmonary disease upper airway microbiota alpha diversity is associated with exacerbation phenotype: a case-control observational study. *Respir Res.* (2019) 20:114. doi: 10.1186/s12931-019-1080-4
17. Vogelmeier CF, Criner GJ, Martinez FJ, Anzueto A, Barnes PJ, Bourbeau J, et al. Global strategy for the diagnosis, management, and prevention of chronic obstructive lung disease 2017 report: GOLD executive summary. *Respirology.* (2017) 22:575–601. doi: 10.1111/resp.13012
18. Qi YJ, Sun XJ, Wang Z, Bin YF, Li YH, Zhong XN, et al. Richness of sputum microbiome in acute exacerbations of eosinophilic chronic obstructive pulmonary disease. *Chin Med J.* (2020) 133:542–51. doi: 10.1097/CM9.0000000000000677
19. Westcott SL, Schloss PD. De novo clustering methods outperform reference-based methods for assigning 16S rRNA gene sequences to operational taxonomic units. *PeerJ.* (2015) 3:23. doi: 10.7717/peerj.1487
20. Edgar RC. Search and clustering orders of magnitude faster than BLAST. *Bioinformatics.* (2010) 26:2460–1. doi: 10.1093/bioinformatics/btq461
21. Edgar RC. UPARSE: highly accurate OTU sequences from microbial amplicon reads. *Nat Methods.* (2013) 10:996–8. doi: 10.1038/nmeth.2604
22. Awasthi MK, Zhang ZQ, Wang Q, Shen F, Li RH, Li DS, et al. New insight with the effects of biochar amendment on bacterial diversity as indicators of biomarkers support the thermophilic phase during sewage sludge composting. *Bioresour Technol.* (2017) 238:589–601. doi: 10.1016/j.biortech.2017.04.100
23. White JR, Nagarajan N, Pop M. Statistical methods for detecting differentially abundant features in clinical metagenomic samples. *PLoS Comput Biol.* (2009) 5:11. doi: 10.1371/journal.pcbi.1000352
24. Chumpitazi BP, Cope JL, Hollister EB, Tsai CM, McMeans AR, Luna RA, et al. Randomised clinical trial: gut microbiome biomarkers are associated with clinical response to a low FODMAP diet in children with the irritable bowel syndrome. *Aliment Pharmacol Ther.* (2015) 42:418–27. doi: 10.1111/apt.13286
25. Boon N, De Windt W, Verstraete W, Top EM. Evaluation of nested PCR-DGGE (denaturing gradient gel electrophoresis) with group-specific 16S rRNA primers for the analysis of bacterial communities from different wastewater treatment plants. *FEMS Microbiol Ecol.* (2002) 39:101–12. doi: 10.1016/S0168-6496(01)00198-2
26. Taur Y, Xavier JB, Lipuma L, Ubeda C, Goldberg J, Gobourne A, et al. Intestinal domination and the risk of bacteremia in patients undergoing allogeneic hematopoietic stem cell transplantation. *Clin Infect Dis.* (2012) 55:905–14. doi: 10.1093/cid/cis580
27. Barnes PJ, Bonini S, Seeger W, Belvisi MG, Ward B, Holmes A. Barriers to new drug development in respiratory disease. *Eur Respir J.* (2015) 45:1197–207. doi: 10.1183/09031936.00007915
28. Obeidat M, Faiz A, Li XA, van den Berge M, Hansel NN, Joubert P, et al. The pharmacogenomics of inhaled corticosteroids and lung function decline in COPD. *Eur Resp J.* (2019) 54:12. doi: 10.1164/ajrccm-conference.2019.199.1_MeetingAbstracts.A3786
29. Suissa S, Patenaude V, Lapi F, Ernst P. Inhaled corticosteroids in COPD and the risk of serious pneumonia. *Thorax.* (2013) 68:1029–36. doi: 10.1136/thoraxjnl-2012-202872
30. Agusti A, Fabbri LM, Singh D, Vestbo J, Celli B, Franssen FME, et al. Inhaled corticosteroids in COPD: friend or foe? *Eur Resp J.* (2018) 52:14. doi: 10.1183/13993003.01219-2018
31. Sivapalan P, Ingebrigtsen TS, Rasmussen DB, Sorensen R, Rasmussen CM, Jensen CB, et al. COPD exacerbations: the impact of long versus short courses of oral corticosteroids on mortality and pneumonia: nationwide data on 67 000 patients with COPD followed for 12 months. *BMJ Open Respir Res.* (2019) 6:e000407. doi: 10.1136/bmjresp-2019-000407
32. Einarsson GG, Comer DM, McIlreavey L, Parkhill J, Ennis M, Tunney MM, et al. Community dynamics and the lower airway microbiota in stable chronic obstructive pulmonary disease, smokers, and healthy non-smokers. *Thorax.* (2016) 71:795–803. doi: 10.1136/thoraxjnl-2015-207235
33. Huang YJ, Sethi S, Murphy T, Nariya S, Boushey HA, Lynch SV. Airway microbiome dynamics in exacerbations of chronic obstructive pulmonary disease. *J Clin Microbiol.* (2014) 52:2813–23. doi: 10.1128/JCM.00035-14
34. Millares L, Ferrari R, Gallego M, Garcia-Nunez M, Perez-Brocal V, Espasa M, et al. Bronchial microbiome of severe COPD patients colonised by Pseudomonas aeruginosa. *Eur J Clin Microbiol Infect Dis.* (2014) 33:1101–11. doi: 10.1007/s10096-013-2044-0
35. Yadava K, Pattaroni C, Sichelstiel AK, Trompette A, Gollwitzer ES, Salami O, et al. Microbiota promotes chronic pulmonary inflammation by enhancing IL-17A and autoantibodies. *Am J Respir Crit Care Med.* (2016) 193:975–87. doi: 10.1164/rccm.201504-0779OC
36. Shariff M, Aditi A, Beri K. Corynebacterium striatum: an emerging respiratory pathogen. *J Infect Dev Ctries.* (2018) 12:581–6. doi: 10.3855/jidc.10406
37. Gao X, Zhang M, Xue J, Huang J, Zhuang R, Zhou X, et al. Body mass index differences in the gut microbiota are gender specific. *Front Microbiol.* (2018) 9:1250. doi: 10.3389/fmicb.2018.01250
38. Lam MMC, Wick RR, Wyres KL, Gorrie CL, Judd LM, Jenney AWJ, et al. Genetic diversity, mobilisation, and spread of the yersiniabactin-encoding mobile element ICEKp in Klebsiella pneumoniae populations. *Microbial Genomics.* (2018) 4:e000196. doi: 10.1099/mgen.0.000196
39. Zhou K, Xie L, Han L, Guo X, Wang Y, Sun J. ICESag37, a novel integrative and conjugative element carrying antimicrobial resistance genes and potential virulence factors in streptococcus agalactiae. *Front Microbiol.* (2017) 8:1921. doi: 10.3389/fmicb.2017.01921
40. Dickson RP, Martinez FJ, Huffnagle GB. The role of the microbiome in exacerbations of chronic lung diseases. *Lancet.* (2014) 384:691–702. doi: 10.1016/S0140-6736(14)61136-3
41. Ditz B, Christenson S, Rossen J, Brightling C, Kerstjens HAM, van den Berge M, et al. Sputum microbiome profiling in COPD: beyond singular pathogen detection. *Thorax.* (2020) 75:338–44. doi: 10.1136/thoraxjnl-2019-214168

3

Dysregulated Cell Signaling in Pulmonary Emphysema

Chih-Ru Lin[1,2], *Karim Bahmed*[2,3] *and Beata Kosmider*[1,2*]

[1] *Department of Microbiology, Immunology, and Inflammation, Temple University, Philadelphia, PA, United States,* [2] *Center for Inflammation and Lung Research, Temple University, Philadelphia, PA, United States,* [3] *Department of Thoracic Medicine and Surgery, Temple University, Philadelphia, PA, United States*

Correspondence:
Beata Kosmider
beata.kosmider@temple.edu

Pulmonary emphysema is characterized by the destruction of alveolar septa and irreversible airflow limitation. Cigarette smoking is the primary cause of this disease development. It induces oxidative stress and disturbs lung physiology and tissue homeostasis. Alveolar type II (ATII) cells have stem cell potential and can repair the denuded epithelium after injury; however, their dysfunction is evident in emphysema. There is no effective treatment available for this disease. Challenges in this field involve the large complexity of lung pathophysiological processes and gaps in our knowledge on the mechanisms of emphysema progression. It implicates dysregulation of various signaling pathways, including aberrant inflammatory and oxidative responses, defective antioxidant defense system, surfactant dysfunction, altered proteostasis, disrupted circadian rhythms, mitochondrial damage, increased cell senescence, apoptosis, and abnormal proliferation and differentiation. Also, genetic predispositions are involved in this disease development. Here, we comprehensively review studies regarding dysregulated cell signaling, especially in ATII cells, and their contribution to alveolar wall destruction in emphysema. Relevant preclinical and clinical interventions are also described.

Keywords: lung, alveolar epithelium, alveolar type II cells, emphysema, oxidative stress, tissue homeostasis

INTRODUCTION

Over 300 million people suffer from chronic obstructive pulmonary disease (COPD) worldwide (1). It is the third leading cause of death, resulting in ~3 million deaths every year, according to World Health Organization (WHO) (2). COPD includes lung parenchymal destruction (emphysema) and airway disease (chronic bronchitis). The extent of lung tissue damage in emphysema is measured by chest computed tomography (CT) density. Emphysema is a progressive and irreversible disease with limited therapeutic strategies. Lung volume reduction surgery and lung transplantation represent promising options for end-stage disease (3). At the cellular level, emphysema is characterized by alveolar epithelial cell death and impaired re-epithelialization (**Figure 1**), which causes alveolar wall destruction and decreased surface area in the lung parenchyma for gas exchange (4). Pulmonary vasculature is linked to alveolar architectures and function, whereas endothelial dysfunction and vascular abnormalities were observed in emphysema (5, 6). Furthermore, extracellular matrix (ECM), including elastin, collagen, and proteoglycans, tethers the parenchymal compartments to the airway and affects the tissue mechanics and airway smooth muscle contraction. The process of mechanotransduction provides mechanical cues of the microenvironment to control many cellular events such as proliferation and differentiation and maintain tissue integrity (7). Changes in ECM composition in emphysema may impact

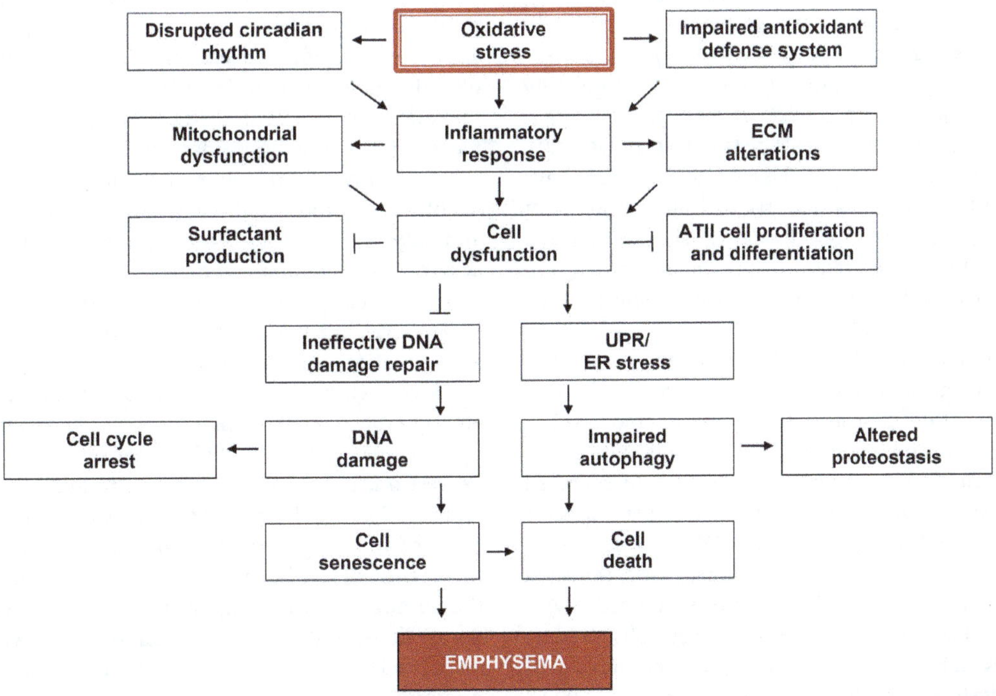

FIGURE 1 | Multiple dysregulated signaling pathways in the pathogenesis of emphysema. Oxidative stress is the major contributor to emphysema. Reactive oxygen species (ROS) and related species disturb cell signaling and impair cell functions, while the antioxidant defense system is overwhelmed. These components are dynamically and progressively interactive over time, and their alterations can lead to emphysema development.

airway smooth muscle cells function, including hypertrophy and hyperplasia, resulting in airway remodeling and obstruction. Also, the loss of elastic recoil leads to airspace enlargements and irreversibly weakens respiratory airflow (8). Increased lung volume, gas trapping, and reduced alveolar units are observed in emphysema patients compared to controls (4).

Environmental irritants, especially cigarette smoke, are the main risk factors of emphysema development. Cigarette smoke contains thousands of chemicals and oxidants that can induce oxidative stress and modify biomolecules, including proteins, lipids, nucleic acids, or carbohydrates, thus affecting lung physiology and tissue homeostasis (9). Surfactant is essential for alveoli and smoking has adverse effects on its function and composition through oxidation and altered proteostasis (10). For instance, Takamiya et al. showed that cigarette smoke extract and its component acrolein modified the surfactant protein (SP)-A in the alveolar epithelium (11). The ability of SP-A to inhibit bacterial growth and macrophage phagocytosis *in vitro* was attenuated due to its conformational changes. The antioxidant defense systems can protect from damage, whereas they are overwhelmed by persisting oxidative stress (9). Cigarette smoke-induced reactive oxygen species (ROS) disturb cell signaling and impair cell functions, including inflammatory responses and protease-antiprotease balance, resulting in ECM destruction and alveolar epithelial cell injury and death (12). Furthermore, emerging senescent cells and vascular dysfunction in the lungs fail the microenvironment for alveolar re-epithelialization.

Besides environmental factors, genetic susceptibility has a significant impact on the morbidity of COPD, such as alpha-1 antitrypsin (AAT) deficiency (13). Studies have identified multiple genetic loci related to this disease susceptibility, e.g., *HHIP, FAM13A, IREB2, MMP12, MMP1, RAGE, SFTPD, FBLN5* in humans and mice (14). These genes are associated with surfactant function, tissue growth, remodeling, and homeostasis. The large complexity of lung pathophysiological processes implicated in emphysema contributes to its heterogeneity. Genetic susceptibility, age, sex, and race-dependent differences may also contribute to this disease development.

DYSREGULATION OF CELL SIGNALING IN EMPHYSEMA DEVELOPMENT

Oxidative Stress

Cigarette smoke-induced oxidative stress and redox imbalance are major contributors to emphysema (15). ROS and related species act as second messengers in cell signal transduction and participate in cellular physiological responses, including the inflammatory immune system and mitochondrial respiration. Oxidative stress refers to high ROS levels that overwhelm the antioxidant defense system. It can alter the activities and functions of redox-sensitive molecules and metabolic enzymes such as p53, NRF2, NF-κB, JNK, MAPK, protein tyrosine phosphatases, glutathione, thioredoxin, peroxiredoxins, and histone deacetylase (15, 16). High oxidative stress and the defective antioxidant defense system were detected in the lungs and alveolar type II (ATII) cells in emphysema patients (15, 17). Especially reduced NRF2 (18) and FOXO3 (19) levels were observed, which are important transcription factors regulating multiple antioxidant genes such as *HO-1*, *NQO1*, and *GPX1*. Also, NF-E2 was downregulated in ATII cells in this disease (20). Several NRF2 activators and different classes of antioxidants have been developed and tested in clinical trials, however, without promising results (15). Increasing evidence shows that the small redox protein thioredoxin relieved animal emphysema and pulmonary inflammation through multiple mechanisms (21). Its therapeutic potential was recently proposed.

We have demonstrated that DJ-1 protein modulates the NRF2-mediated antioxidant defense system in human primary ATII cells after exposure to cigarette smoke (22). Altered DJ-1 function, its overoxidation to sulfonate form ($-SO_3^-$) at the cysteine-106 and ubiquitination, were reported in the pathophysiological response to oxidative damage and emphysema patients (17). Of note, DJ-1 oxidation to sulfinate form ($-SO_2^-$) was detected in smokers, which reflected its cytoprotective activity. Oxidative stress-induced DJ-1 overoxidation and cleavage in mitochondria were observed in A549 cells treated with hydrogen peroxide. DJ-1 ablation resulted in mitochondrial dysfunction. We also showed impaired S100A8 function in ATII cells in emphysema (23). S100A8 belongs to the S100 protein family and responds to oxidative stress. ATII cell death in this disease correlated with decreased S100A8 sulfination (24). Furthermore, the cytoprotective function of S100A8 compensated for the absence of DJ-1 *in vitro* and *in vivo*. Targeting redox regulation appears to be an ideal approach to this disease yet challenging, possibly due to delicate redox balance, disparities between animal models and human diseases, species differences, compound bioavailability, and other variables.

Pro-inflammatory Response

Environmental irritants can promote the recruitment of inflammatory cells into the lungs. The pro-inflammatory and immune responses are evident in emphysema pathophysiology. Glucocorticoids and bronchodilators are commonly used to treat COPD, although both have many side effects, including immunosuppression (21). The PDE4 inhibitor roflumilast is an approved drug that selectively inhibits PDE4 and increases cAMP levels, leading to an anti-inflammatory response. Numerous PDE inhibitors are in clinical testing. Dual PDE3/4 inhibitors such as RPL554 have gained interest in enhanced efficacy as PDE3 is expressed in vascular smooth muscle cells, and its inhibitor induces bronchodilation (25). Similarly, drug combinations may have a synergistic effect over mono-components. For example, combination of PDE4 and PI3Kδ inhibitors significantly increased protection against cigarette smoke extract-induced apoptosis of lung epithelial cells and reduced inflammatory responses of neutrophils and macrophages *in vitro*.

Under normal conditions, the immune cells balance lung defense, tolerance, or tissue repair. Particularly, alveolar macrophages (AM) interact with pulmonary surfactants in the innate immune responses. AM are potent phagocytes, regulate adaptive immunity and recruit neutrophils and monocytes into the lungs. They secrete inflammatory mediators and proteases such as ECM degrading enzymes and cathepsins upon activation, resulting in elastolysis, alveolar tissue damage, and remodeling of alveoli (8, 12). AM show plasticity based on the microenvironment. Lechner et al. indicated that M2-like macrophages and bone marrow-derived monocytes constitute a regenerative ATII cell niche component, modulating their proliferation and differentiation (26). Using knockout mice and adoptive transfer studies, they found that macrophages accumulated in the lung *via* the CCL2-CCR2 chemokine recruitment axis during lung regeneration after pneumonectomy. F4/80+ M2-like macrophage and ATII cell co-culture supported the formation of pneumospheres.

Nevertheless, high inflammation in smokers correlated with emphysema development (8, 27). Inflammatory responses downregulated *SFTPB, SFTPD, SCNN1A*, and *SCNN1B* gene expression, related to surfactant production and alveolar fluid clearance in ATII cells (28). Decreased SP-D expression was detected in the lungs of emphysema patients (29), indicating the defects in ATII cell function and innate immunity. Especially the number of AM is negatively related to alveolar parenchymal tissue density (27), and impaired phagocytosis is positively associated with the severity of emphysema (30). Increased microRNA (miR)-155 expression was recently identified in the smokers' lungs and in AM of mice exposed to cigarette smoke (31), contributing to inflammation and this disease development. ATII cells isolated from subjects with this disease showed high oxidative stress (17, 32) and ECM degradation with the elevation of matrix metalloproteinase (MMP) 9, CD147, and cathepsin B (20). Other proteases elevated in patients with emphysema include neutrophil elastase, dipeptidyl peptidase-4, proteinase-3, MMPs 1, 8, 12, and 13, cathepsins C, D, E, G, K, and S, and caspases 1, 3, 7, 8, 9, and 11 (33). Several studies have shown the efficacy of antiprotease therapy in emphysema; however, without promising results in clinical trials (21). On the other hand, ADAM8 belongs to a disintegrin and metalloproteinase family. It was reported as a protective proteinase negatively related to emphysema development (34). ADAM8 levels were decreased in macrophages and alveolar epithelial cells in patients with this disease and mice exposed to cigarette smoke. Moreover, ADAM8 knockout mice displayed higher inflammatory and oxidative stress levels, mucus cell metaplasia, alveolar septal cell death, and reduced ATII cell proliferation and repair, contributing to the lung destruction caused by cigarette smoke exposure. Accordingly, pro-inflammatory mediators, oxidative stress, protease-antiprotease imbalance, and impaired pathogen phagocytosis contribute to the destruction of lung tissue and this disease progression (12). Many anti-inflammatory drugs have been developed but have limited efficacy (21). Further studies of immune responses and homeostasis can provide a clue for therapeutic interventions and lung regeneration.

Increasing evidence indicates that the nuclear hormone receptor PPARγ, a regulator of lipid metabolism, adipogenesis, and inflammation, represents a potential therapeutic target for emphysema. It was downregulated in antigen-presenting cells (APCs) isolated from the lungs of patients with this disease and mice exposed to cigarette smoke, thus directing Th1 and Th17 cell differentiation (35, 36). Also, overexpression of dominant-negative PPARγ in murine ATII cells induced emphysema with increased inflammatory cytokines, MMPs, and accumulation of myeloid-derived suppressor cells (MDSCs) in the lungs and circulation system (37). As expected, treatment with a PPARγ agonist ciglitazone inhibited pathogenic lung APCs *in vitro* in humans and mice. Further, it attenuated cigarette smoke-induced emphysema in mice (35, 36). Thiazolidinediones (TZDs), including ciglitazone, pioglitazone, rosiglitazone, and troglitazone, are valuable drugs for type 2 diabetes and have shown anti-inflammatory effects through selective stimulation of PPARγ. Their application to emphysema needs to be further evaluated.

Chronic Inflammation

Chronic inflammation can increase susceptibility to lung infection. Cigarette smoke-induced emphysema in animals was challenged with bacterial or viral infections to study the mechanism of this disease exacerbation (38). H3N1 influenza A virus infection caused higher virus titers in the lung, inflammation around bronchi and in the parenchyma, and mucus exudates in the airways in cigarette smoke-exposed mice compared to the influenza virus alone (39). Also, *Pseudomonas aeruginosa* infection resulted in impaired autophagy with an increased number of aggresomes, cell senescence, and alveolar space enlargement in mice exposed to cigarette smoke compared to controls (40). Cysteamine, an antioxidant drug with autophagy-inducing properties, alleviated these changes. *Nippostrongylus brasiliensis,* a nematode in rodents, was used to develop a mouse model of progressive emphysema (38). This infection induced a long-lasting Th2 immune response and alternatively activated M2 macrophages accompanied by substantially upregulated MMP12 expression, resulting in alveolar wall destruction and airspace enlargement. Increasing evidence shows the formation of autoimmune components, including autoantibodies and key mediators (such as BAFF and IL-17A), increased B cell counts, and B cell-rich lymphoid follicles in emphysema patients, which were associated with this disease severity (41, 42). Zhou et al. exposed mice to 150–180 mg/m^3 cigarette smoke for 2 weeks followed by 2 weeks of rest before the elastin challenge to study the autoimmunity in emphysema development (43). MMP12-generated elastin fragments are self-antigens that induce monocyte chemotactic activity and contribute to this disease pathology. Exposure to cigarette smoke sensitized mice to elastin and elicited IL17A-predominant autoimmune processes leading to neutrophilic airway inflammation, mucus hyperproduction, airspace enlargement, and lung function decline. Of note, elastin-specific T cell response was also observed in COPD patients. The correlation of B cell adaptive immune responses with late-stage emphysema introduces opportunities for new therapeutic interventions. However, the crucial role of B cells in the defense against pathogenic infections and immune-regulatory activities limits anti-B cell therapies. Further characterization of B cell subsets and their contribution to disease progression are needed.

Altered Cellular Homeostasis

Cigarette smoke-induced oxidative stress increases protein misfolding (44), thus altering lung homeostasis. It induces endoplasmic reticulum (ER) stress and unfolded protein response (UPR), leading to inflammation and cell apoptosis. ER stress was observed in emphysema patients and animals (45). Activation of UPR with the upregulation of GRP78 was detected in human small airway epithelial cells and ATII cells obtained from smokers (46). The aggresome formation, involved in the cellular response to misfolded proteins and their clearance, was also observed in the lungs of smokers, emphysema patients, mice exposed to cigarette smoke, and aged mice (40). Specifically, the levels of aggresome correlated with smoking history and emphysema severity in humans. Cigarette smoke increased aggresome formation by accumulating ubiquitinated proteins and autophagy proteins p62 and valosin-containing protein (VCP) in murine lungs, indicating aberrant autophagy (40). Intraperitoneal administration with the autophagy-inducing drug cysteamine reduced cigarette smoke-induced aggresome formation in the lungs, inflammatory responses in bronchoalveolar lavage fluid (BALF), and emphysematous changes in mice. Similarly, inhibition of ER stress by treatment with 4-phenylbutyric acid reduced cigarette smoke-induced inflammatory response, alveolar cell apoptosis, and airspace enlargement in mice (47). Therefore, the ER stress-autophagy pathway represents a potential therapeutic intervention.

Several studies have pointed out the deleterious impact of ceramides or lactosylceramides accumulation in the human lung in emphysema progression (48), likely due to impaired autophagy resulting in sphingolipids imbalance. They were accumulated in different cell types, including alveolar epithelial and endothelial cells and macrophages in patients with this disease (49). Ceramides are components of sphingolipids and serve as second messenger lipids. Their upregulation leads to inflammatory responses, which can cause alveolar epithelial cell apoptosis and emphysema development in animal models (49). Cigarette smoke promoted the activation of membrane-localized acid sphingomyelinase, which catalyzes the hydrolysis of sphingomyelin to ceramide. This thereupon increased membrane and intracellular ceramide accumulation in aggresomes (48). Cysteamine reduced cigarette smoke-induced ceramide accumulation in Beas2b cells (48). It improved efferocytosis, cell viability, and decreased cell senescence. Also, intraperitoneal injection of autophagy-inducer gemfibrozil significantly reduced ceramide accumulation in murine lungs after cigarette smoke exposure.

Circadian Rhythm Disruption

The human respiratory system functions with a daily circadian rhythm, affecting airway resistance, ventilatory controls, and immune function, yet it changes with age and smoking (50, 51). Smokers have marked diurnal changes in pulmonary function tests compared to non-smokers (51). The lungs' molecular clock is also altered in response to environmental factors, including allergens, pollutions, pathogens, infections, oxidative stress, hypoxia/hyperoxia, jet lag, and shift work (52). Importantly, circadian gene expression positively connects to cell cycle and immune regulation in mice and humans (53). Increasing evidence shows a link between circadian rhythm disruption and susceptibility to lung infection (54) and inflammatory diseases (55), including asthma and COPD with severe symptoms in the early morning, which correlated with disease exacerbations.

Pekovic-Vaughan et al. have demonstrated the circadian regulation of the NRF2 pathway in the murine lung, mainly in the bronchial and alveolar epithelium (56). The loss of NRF2-dependent antioxidant defense system and reduced-glutathione levels increased oxidative damage in the lungs of Clock$^{\Delta 19}$ mutant mice compared to wild-type mice. SIRT-1 functions as NAD^{+}-dependent protein deacetylases and regulates many pathophysiological processes. It controls the circadian clock through binding with CLOCK-BMAL1 complexes and promoting the deacetylation and degradation of PER2 proteins (57). In the lungs of mice exposed to cigarette smoke, altered rhythms of SIRT-1 protein and core clock genes including *Bmal1*, *Clock*, *Per1*, *Per2*, *Cry1*, *Cry2*, *Nr1d1*, *Nr1d2*, and *Rora* were observed in a circadian manner, increasing the susceptibility to inflammation and emphysema development (58). Similarly, BMAL1 protein was down-regulated in the lungs of smokers and individuals with this disease (58). BMAL1 deficiency accelerated senescence and caused age-associated shrinkage of major organs, including lungs, in 40-week-old mice, which correlated with increased ROS levels and inflammation (59). Melatonin, a natural hormone that regulates sleep-wake cycles, has shown beneficial effects on lung diseases through anti-oxidation and anti-inflammaton (60). It increased SIRT-1 expression *in vitro* and *in vivo* (61, 62). Intraperitoneal injection with melatonin decreased inflammatory response in BALF, and the lungs of mice challenged with cigarette smoke and lipopolysaccharide (61). It also reduced ER stress and bronchial and alveolar epithelial cell apoptosis, and protected alveolar architecture in a rat model of emphysema (62). The daily rhythm of SP-A, SP-B, and SP-C gene expression in the rat lungs was reported (63). This indicates the critical role of circadian rhythm in ATII cell function; however, its alterations in lung pathophysiology are still poorly understood.

Cellular Senescence

Cigarette smoke can cause DNA damage, while the impairment of double-strand DNA break repair in ATII cells was shown in emphysema patients (32). Oxidative stress and persistent DNA damage are associated with stress-induced premature senescence (SIPS) (64). SIPS induces irreversible cell cycle arrest, chromatin changes, and resistance to apoptosis. It also drives a senescence-associated secretory phenotype (SASP) in cells, including secretion of inflammatory cytokines IL-6 and IL-8 and remodeling factors, thereby affecting tissue microenvironment and promoting senescence in an autocrine and paracrine manner (65). DNA damage response (DDR) is required for SASP, including cell cycle regulatory protein NBS1 and checkpoint kinases ATM and CHK2 (66). Transient exposure to SASP promoted stem cell function and tissue regeneration, whereas prolonged exposure had an opposite effect in mice (67). Mice with GFP-expressing ATII cells (CBA/Ca × C57BL6J) exposed to cigarette smoke for over 3 months displayed airspace enlargement and alveolar epithelial cell apoptosis (68). The surviving ATII cells showed higher resistance to apoptosis, which was likely related to circadian rhythm. This suggests the contribution of ATII cell senescence and the circadian clock's regulation to emphysema development. Reduced anti-aging protein SIRT-1 levels were found in the lungs of smokers and patients with emphysema, including AM, airway, and alveolar epithelium (69, 70). Particularly, oxidative stress-induced miR-34a expression was detected in lung tissue in these patients leading to suppression of SIRT-1 and SIRT-6 expression *via* the PI3K pathway (70). Furthermore, increased lipofuscin levels, a marker of senescence, and cell cycle inhibitors p16 and p21 were mainly detected in ATII cells and endothelial cells in emphysema patients compared to controls (71). Telomere signal intensity in these cells was lower in smokers and emphysema than in controls. A negative correlation between p16 and proliferation cell nuclear antigen (PCNA) was also reported. Similarly, other cells displayed characteristics of cellular senescence, including airway epithelial cells, fibroblasts, and immune cells (72). Their accumulation indicates the loss of tissue homeostasis and an altered environment for alveolar re-epithelialization in emphysema. Senotherapies are effective in animal models, including SIRT-1 activators and inhibitors of mTOR, JAK, FOXO4, and anti-apoptotic proteins (72). Drugs targeting anti-apoptotic proteins in senescent cells such as dasatinib and quercetin were well-tolerated in patients with age-related diseases. Senotherapy seems promising since the mechanism of cellular senescence is likely shared between different diseases.

Furthermore, mitochondria generate ATP for cell metabolism, and their dysfunction has been linked to age-related lung diseases. Several mitochondria-targeted antioxidants, including mitoQ, mito-TEMPO, pyrroloquinoline quinone, and SkQl are in clinical trials for other age-related diseases (72). Increased mitochondrial (mt)DNA copy number has been detected in the blood of patients with COPD along with a positive correlation to the number of pack-years smoking (73). It was also found in urine and was associated with respiratory symptoms and emphysema severity (74). Importantly, elevated mitochondrial ROS levels, low mitochondrial amount, accumulation of mtDNA damage, and mitochondrial dysfunction were detected in human ATII cells in this disease progression (75). It has been shown that electronic (e)-cigarette aerosols containing nicotine caused airway hyperreactivity, alveolar destruction, reduced lung function, and emphysematous changes in mice (76). Nicotine altered calcium levels and mitochondrial membrane potential in human primary ATII cells with DJ-1 knockdown (77). Dysregulation of mitochondrial oxidative phosphorylation (OXPHOS) complexes was observed in the lungs of DJ-1 knockout mice exposed to aerosolized nicotine, which disrupted the nuclear/mitochondrial stoichiometry resulting in mitochondrial dysfunction. This was associated with increased AM number and ATII cell apoptosis. Both ER stress and mitochondrial dysfunction were detected in emphysema, however, with unknown integration. It was recently demonstrated that ER stress led to mitochondrial UPR in an ATF4-dependent manner in MLE-12 cells (78). Mitochondrial

UPR has contributed to different disease pathogenesis (79), although its activation is also known to lifespan extension in both *Caenorhabditis elegans* and mice (80). Improving our understanding of the mitochondrial role in cellular senescence can greatly benefit treating emphysema.

Apoptosis

The correlation of alveolar cell apoptosis and decreased lung surface area have been shown in emphysema (81). Intratracheal instillation of active caspase-3 protein led to alveolar epithelial cell apoptosis and this disease development in mice (82). Increased active caspase 3 levels were detected in ATII cells in smokers and individuals with emphysema (24). Histone deacetylase inhibition altered chromatin remodeling leading to ATII cell apoptosis and alveolar structure destruction in trichostatin A-treated rats through increased miR34a, p53, cleaved caspase 3, and microtubule-associated protein-1 light chain 3 (LC3) levels (83). Decreased hypoxia-inducible factor-1α (HIF-1α), vascular endothelial growth factor (VEGF), lysyl oxidase, and collagen expression in this animal model pointed out the involvement of angiogenic factors in the alveolar structure. Subcutaneous injection of VEGF receptor (VEGFR) blocker led to emphysema without the infiltration of inflammatory cells in rats (84). Treatments targeting VEGF signaling have beneficial effects against emphysema development in animal models (85–87). Alveolar and endothelial cells can sense microenvironment changes; therefore, they serve as niches for regulating lung repair and integrity. Angiogenesis impairment by subcutaneous injection of sodium glutamate enhanced lung inflammation and emphysema in mice induced by intratracheal instillation of cigarette smoke extract, which was related to insufficient migration of pericytes and smooth muscle cells in lung tissue (88). Surprisingly, intravenous administration of healthy lung endothelial cells ameliorated emphysematous phenotype and lung function in an elastase-induced mouse model (89). It was recently reported that endothelial cells released angiocrine sphingosine-1-phosphate (S1P) after *Pseudomonas aeruginosa* infection in mice which promoted alveolar re-epithelialization *via* S1PR2-YAP signaling (90). Supplementation of S1P prevented alveolar cell apoptosis in VEGFR blockade-induced emphysema in mice (91). This suggests that sphingolipid balance is important for the maintenance of alveolar septal integrity.

Smooth Muscle Cell Proliferation

In addition to endothelial dysfunction, pulmonary vascular remodeling characterized by increased smooth muscle cell proliferation and narrowing of the vascular lumen has been shown in smokers and to precede airspace enlargement in animal models of emphysema (92). It can subsequently lead to vascular wall thickening, pulmonary hypertension, and right heart failure. Bronchodilators that target the smooth muscles were beneficial in reducing COPD exacerbation risk vs. placebo in large-scale randomized trials (93). Significant improvements in forced expiratory volume (FVC) were reported after bronchodilator administration in subjects with emphysema (95, 96). Treatment with complementary bronchodilators or a combination of inhaled corticosteroids with bronchodilators was more effective than monotherapy (94). Pharmacological lung volume reduction through bronchodilator therapy is an important goal in these patients.

Smooth muscle cells are the mechanical sculptor of the epithelium (97). Nitric oxide (NO) production by nitric oxide synthase (NOS) regulates the degree of contraction of vascular smooth muscle cells and their proliferation. ATII cells express constitutive NOS as well as inducible NOS (iNOS) during inflammatory states, suggesting their interaction with vascular smooth muscle cells. The absence of SP-D in mice displayed iNOS-related chronic inflammation, alterations of surfactant homeostasis, and emphysematous changes. This elucidates the contribution of immune responses to NO/iNOS regulation (98). iNOS inactivation by genetic deficiency and pharmacological inhibition prevented cigarette smoke-induced pulmonary hypertension and emphysema, including structural and functional alterations of the lung vasculature and alveoli in mice (99). In clinical studies, elevated alveolar NO has been associated with COPD severity (100). These patients have higher numbers of $iNOS^{+}$ ATII cells related to increased protein nitration and decreased lung function (101). Especially, the lung tissue from patients with emphysema has a higher ratio of the number of alveoli/vessels and an increased degree of vessel muscularization. Nitrated proteins in vasculature and alveoli were increased in these patients (99). NO can be toxic through combination with superoxide to generate peroxynitrites leading to nitration of biomolecules, altering their structure and function. Further, peroxynitrites induced alveolar epithelial and endothelial cell apoptosis (99). However, chronic exposure to the NOS inhibitor N^{ω}-nitro-L-arginine methyl ester resulted in vascular senescence, hypertension, and emphysema development in mice (102). This emphasizes the importance of NO/NOS balance in vascular health and alveolar structure.

Chronic hypoxia in emphysema induces pulmonary artery smooth muscle cells proliferation and JAK2/STAT3 activation. JAK2 deficiency attenuated pulmonary vascular remodeling and smooth muscle hyperplasia in mice (103). Furthermore, HIF-1α promotes vascular smooth muscle cell proliferation under hypoxic conditions. Its increased expression was detected by immunohistochemistry in the lungs of emphysema patients, indicating vascular remodeling in this disease. Especially, HIF-1α was positively associated with disease severity (104). With oxygen treatment, the HIF-1α and erythropoietin decreased in COPD (105). It has been demonstrated that HIF-1α signaling in ATII cells promoted their proliferation after acute lung injury in mice induced by lipopolysaccharide or hydrochloric acid (106). ATII cell-specific HIF-1α deletion caused higher mortality in these mice. Also, HIF-1α is activated in the ATII to alveolar type I (ATI) cell transitional state (107). Together, these data show the intimate relationship between alveolar epithelium and smooth muscle cells for alveolar architecture and function.

Dysregulated Alveolar Re-epithelialization

ATII cells are progenitors in alveoli. Various ATII niches, mediators, and signaling support their functions for alveolar epithelial cell homeostasis and re-epithelialization. The interactions between signaling molecules arising from and acting on the alveolar epithelium, vasculature, mesenchyme, ECM, and immune cells institute ATII cell niches. Dynamic organization of WNT/β-catenin, TGF-β, YAP/TAZ, NOTCH, and TP53 signaling pathways participate in ATII cell growth and differentiation to ATI cells (108). The importance of WNT/β-catenin, YAP/TAZ, and TGF-β signaling in emphysema development has been demonstrated in animal models. Specifically, *TGF-β2* was identified as a significant emphysema-associated genetic variant by human genome-wide association studies (GWAS) (109). TGF-β regulates multiple context-dependent cellular processes associated with tissue remodeling and is crucial for epithelial-mesenchymal interactions. It includes the regulation of cell polarity, ECM turnover, ATII to ATI cell transdifferentiation, and differentiation of lung fibroblasts to myofibroblasts positive for α-smooth muscle actin (α-SMA). Leucine-rich α-2-glycoprotein-1 (LRG1), known to regulate TGF-β signaling, was increased in endothelial cells in patients with emphysema and correlated to its severity (89). Elevated YAP protein levels were detected in the lungs of patients with this disease compared to healthy donors (110). In contrast, reduced WNT/β-catenin pathway in ATII cells was observed in emphysema patients (111, 112) while the non-canonical WNT pathway was upregulated (113, 114). These data suggest signaling imbalance and ATII cell dysfunction in the emphysematous lung. It is known that WNT/β-catenin and anti-inflammatory PPARγ signaling pathways are integrated, and they work in opposition, highlighting the relationship between immune response and ATII cell fate. Feller et al. demonstrated that a non-canonical WNT ligand WNT5a and pro-inflammatory cytokines can be transported through extracellular vesicles, leading to systemic inflammation in COPD patients (115). This further points out the importance of the interactive signaling and microenvironment in the pathogenesis of this disease.

HHIP is a component of hedgehog signaling, which is important in many developmental processes (116). It is a genetic locus associated with emphysema susceptibility in humans and mice. Sonic hedgehog signaling is required for myofibroblast differentiation and mesenchymal proliferation during alveologenesis, while it maintains quiescence in the adult murine lung (117). A broad population of hedgehog-receptive mesenchymal cells surrounding airways and alveoli was identified in the murine lung (118). The transgenic activation of the hedgehog in the mesenchyme disrupted the alveolar niche. This impaired ATII cell proliferation, increased airspace, and emphysematous changes. Single-cell transcriptome analysis of the human lung shows that mesenchymal subsets are conserved across species. The intermediate mesenchymal subset was involved in cholesterol metabolism, suggesting its role in surfactant biosynthesis of the alveolar epithelium. In addition, Kato et al. demonstrated that the paracrine signaling capabilities of pericytes, specialized mesenchymal cells surrounding the capillary, are crucial for alveologenesis. Loss of pericyte-specific YAP/TAZ reduced endothelial and ATII cell proliferation through paracrine regulation, resulting in defective alveolarization and a severe emphysema-like morphology in mice (119). It changed the growth factor expression profiles of these cells in the lungs, including reduced *Angpt1*, *Tgfb2*, *Wnt11*, *Bmp4*, and *Hgf* (119). Treatments targeting ATII cell proliferation and differentiation to ATI cells have not been developed owing to plenty of unknowns regarding the mechanism of alveolar re-epithelialization.

Signaling Interplay

Oxidative stress, ER stress response, and inflammation are key contributors to emphysema development. Their interactive relationships have been reported (120). ROS provide an oxidizing environment and affect molecular chaperones and enzymes in the ER. In response to ER stress, the UPR helps cells adapt to and survive the stress condition by transcriptional and translational reprogramming. In contrast, programmed cell death signaling is activated when protein homeostasis cannot be achieved. UPR signaling is initiated by ER membrane-bound transducers: IRE1, ATF6, and PERK. Particularly, IRE1α regulates many cell functions, including metabolism, immunity, inflammatory cytokine production, cell differentiation, and apoptosis, through the RIDD mechanism, which induces the degradation of certain mRNAs or miRNAs. Of note, the IRE1α-mediated XBP1 pathway is essential for optimal expression of inflammatory cytokines and proangiogenic factors in human aortic endothelial cells (121, 122). Under chronic or severe ER stress, PERK-mediated phosphorylation of eIF2α induces expression of ATF4 and a proapoptotic factor CHOP/GADD153, resulting in ER stress-induced apoptosis. ATF4 can also induce growth arrest and DNA damage-inducible protein GADD34. Furthermore, ER and mitochondria are physically and functionally connected through mitochondria-associated ER membranes, which contain major calcium channels IP3R and VDAC. ROS can target ER calcium channels, leading to ER calcium release. It subsequently stimulates mitochondrial metabolism and ROS production. The delicate balance between different cell signaling can be the key to therapeutic benefit.

Given that ROS is involved in various physiological processes, the interplay between signaling potentially causes a cascade of cell dysfunction and imbalance under pathological stimuli, leading to tissue damage. Sirtuins (SIRT1-7) maintain cellular redox balance and are an important defense mechanism against oxidative stress according to the different subcellular localization of each sirtuin. Specifically, the ability of SIRT1 to intersect with different signaling, including the circadian clock, inflammation, cell cycle, and senescence, makes it a lucrative target for therapeutics. SIRT1 activators include baicalin, exendin-4, ginkgolide-B, pitavastatin, quercetin, SRT2104, and vitamin D. These medications are in clinical trials for other diseases. Of note, exendin-4 is a licensed medicine for patients with type 2 diabetes. Exendin-4 treatment improved lung function, mortality, and clinical appearance in mice with lipopolysaccharides-induced emphysema, possibly through bronchodilatory effects (123). The mechanistic links between diabetes and COPD imply the applicability of this medicine (124).

CONCLUSION

Despite numerous investigations, therapeutic strategies for pulmonary emphysema remain limited mainly due to the complexity and heterogeneity of disease manifestation. Multiple dysregulated signaling pathways affect physiological processes in emphysema development (**Figure 1**). Its pathological features include high inflammatory and immune response, oxidative stress, defective antioxidant defense system, altered protein homeostasis, cellular senescence, and apoptosis. Circadian rhythm disruption leads to abnormal cell cycle and immune dysregulation, which points out a poor lung repair in this disease. These components are dynamically and progressively interactive over time. Individual differences and genetic variations in surfactant function, tissue growth, remodeling, and homeostasis can also contribute to this disease development. Targeting the cellular processes to decrease alveolar injury and increase alveolar re-epithelialization may restore lung function. Various factors and signaling are interdependent in complex pathophysiology. Therefore, desired outcomes could be achieved by targeting multiple pathways. More systematic and comprehensive studies regarding interactions between different cell types, organelles, and signaling pathways are warranted to uncover new therapeutic strategies.

AUTHOR CONTRIBUTIONS

C-RL performed the literature search, prepared the figures, and wrote the manuscript. KB and BK provided significant works of literature, interpretations, and revision. All authors contributed to the article and approved the submitted version.

REFERENCES

1. Ruvuna L, Sood A. Epidemiology of chronic obstructive pulmonary disease. *Clin Chest Med.* (2020) 41:315–27. doi: 10.1016/j.ccm.2020.05.002
2. World Health Organization. *The Top 10 Causes of Death.* Geneva: World Health Organization (2020).
3. Marchetti N, Criner GJ. Surgical approaches to treating emphysema: lung volume reduction surgery, bullectomy, and lung transplantation. *Semin Respir Crit Care Med.* (2015) 36:592–608. doi: 10.1055/s-0035-1556064
4. Tuder RM. Bringing light to chronic obstructive pulmonary disease pathogenesis and resilience. *Ann Am Thorac Soc.* (2018) 15:S227–33. doi: 10.1513/AnnalsATS.201808-583MG
5. Peinado VI, Barbera JA, Ramirez J, Gomez FP, Roca J, Jover L, et al. Endothelial dysfunction in pulmonary arteries of patients with mild COPD. *Am J Physiol.* (1998) 274:L908–13. doi: 10.1152/ajplung.1998.274.6.L908
6. Estepar RSJ, Kinney GL, Black-Shinn JL, Bowler RP, Kindlmann GL, Ross JC, et al. Computed tomographic measures of pulmonary vascular morphology in smokers and their clinical implications. *Am J Resp Crit Care.* (2013) 188:231–9. doi: 10.1164/rccm.201301-0162OC
7. Bidan CM, Veldsink AC, Meurs H, Gosens R. Airway and extracellular matrix mechanics in COPD. *Front Physiol.* (2015) 6:346. doi: 10.3389/fphys.2015.00346
8. Saetta M, Turato G, Maestrelli P, Mapp CE, Fabbri LM. Cellular and structural bases of chronic obstructive pulmonary disease. *Am J Respir Crit Care Med.* (2001) 163:1304–9. doi: 10.1164/ajrccm.163.6.2009116
9. Birben E, Sahiner UM, Sackesen C, Erzurum S, Kalayci O. Oxidative stress and antioxidant defense. *World Allergy Organ J.* (2012) 5:9–19. doi: 10.1097/WOX.0b013e3182439613
10. Stenger PC, Alonso C, Zasadzinski JA, Waring AJ, Jung CL, Pinkerton KE. Environmental tobacco smoke effects on lung surfactant film organization. *Biochim Biophys Acta.* (2009) 1788:358–70. doi: 10.1016/j.bbamem.2008.11.021
11. Takamiya R, Uchida K, Shibata T, Maeno T, Kato M, Yamaguchi Y, et al. Disruption of the structural and functional features of surfactant protein A by acrolein in cigarette smoke. *Sci Rep.* (2017) 7:8304. doi: 10.1038/s41598-017-08588-5
12. Kapellos TS, Bassler K, Aschenbrenner AC, Fujii W, Schultze JL. Dysregulated functions of lung macrophage populations in COPD. *J Immunol Res.* (2018) 2018:2349045. doi: 10.1155/2018/2349045
13. Lowe KE, Regan EA, Anzueto A, Austin E, Austin JHM, Beaty TH, et al. COPDGene((R)) 2019: redefining the diagnosis of chronic obstructive pulmonary disease. *Chronic Obstr Pulm Dis.* (2019) 6:384–99. doi: 10.15326/jcopdf.6.5.2019.0149
14. Silverman EK. Genetics of COPD. *Annu Rev Physiol.* (2020) 82:413–31. doi: 10.1146/annurev-physiol-021317-121224
15. Barnes PJ. Oxidative stress-based therapeutics in COPD. *Redox Biol.* (2020) 33:101544. doi: 10.1016/j.redox.2020.101544
16. Pennington JD, Wang TJ, Nguyen P, Sun L, Bisht K, Smart D, et al. Redox-sensitive signaling factors as a novel molecular targets for cancer therapy. *Drug Resist Updat.* (2005) 8:322–30. doi: 10.1016/j.drup.2005.09.002
17. Bahmed K, Boukhenouna S, Karim L, Andrews T, Lin J, Powers R, et al. The effect of cysteine oxidation on DJ-1 cytoprotective function in human alveolar type II cells. *Cell Death Dis.* (2019) 10:638. doi: 10.1038/s41419-019-1833-5
18. Malhotra D, Thimmulappa R, Navas-Acien A, Sandford A, Elliott M, Singh A, et al. Decline in NRF2-regulated antioxidants in chronic obstructive pulmonary disease lungs due to loss of its positive regulator, DJ-1. *Am J Respir Crit Care Med.* (2008) 178:592–604. doi: 10.1164/rccm.200803-380OC
19. Hwang JW, Rajendrasozhan S, Yao H, Chung S, Sundar IK, Huyck HL, et al. FOXO3 deficiency leads to increased susceptibility to cigarette smoke-induced inflammation, airspace enlargement, and chronic obstructive pulmonary disease. *J Immunol.* (2011) 187:987–98. doi: 10.4049/jimmunol.1001861
20. Tan LH, Bahmed K, Lin CR, Marchetti N, Bolla S, Criner GJ, et al. The cytoprotective role of DJ-1 and p45 NFE2 against human primary alveolar type II cell injury and emphysema. *Sci Rep.* (2018) 8:3555. doi: 10.1038/s41598-018-21790-3
21. Wang C, Zhou J, Wang J, Li S, Fukunaga A, Yodoi J, et al. Progress in the mechanism and targeted drug therapy for COPD. *Signal Transduct Target Ther.* (2020) 5:248. doi: 10.1038/s41392-020-00345-x
22. Bahmed K, Messier EM, Zhou W, Tuder RM, Freed CR, Chu HW, et al. DJ-1 modulates nuclear erythroid 2-related factor-2-mediated protection in human primary alveolar type II cells in smokers. *Am J Respir Cell Mol Biol.* (2016) 55:439–49. doi: 10.1165/rcmb.2015-0304OC
23. Lin CR, Bahmed K, Criner GJ, Marchetti N, Tuder RM, Kelsen S, et al. S100A8 protects human primary alveolar type II cells against injury and emphysema. *Am J Respir Cell Mol Biol.* (2019) 60:299–307. doi: 10.1165/rcmb.2018-0144OC
24. Lin CR, Bahmed K, Tomar D, Marchetti N, Criner GJ, Bolla S, et al. The relationship between DJ-1 and S100A8 in human primary alveolar type II cells in emphysema. *Am J Physiol Lung Cell Mol Physiol.* (2019) 317:L791–804. doi: 10.1152/ajplung.00494.2018
25. Lakshmi SP, Reddy AT, Reddy RC. Emerging pharmaceutical therapies for COPD. *Int J Chron Obstruct Pulmon Dis.* (2017) 12:2141–56. doi: 10.2147/COPD.S121416
26. Lechner AJ, Driver IH, Lee J, Conroy CM, Nagle A, Locksley RM, et al. Recruited monocytes and type 2 immunity promote lung regeneration following pneumonectomy. *Cell Stem Cell.* (2017) 21:120–34 e7. doi: 10.1016/j.stem.2017.03.024

27. Finkelstein R, Fraser RS, Ghezzo H, Cosio MG. Alveolar inflammation and its relation to emphysema in smokers. *Am J Respir Crit Care Med.* (1995) 152:1666–72. doi: 10.1164/ajrccm.152.5.7582312
28. Schwede M, Wilfong EM, Zemans RL, Lee PJ, Dos Santos C, Fang X, et al. Effects of bone marrow-derived mesenchymal stromal cells on gene expression in human alveolar type II cells exposed to TNF-alpha, IL-1beta, and IFN-gamma. *Physiol Rep.* (2018) 6:e13831. doi: 10.14814/phy2.13831
29. Cornwell WD, Kim C, Lastra AC, Dass C, Bolla S, Wang H, et al. Inflammatory signature in lung tissues in patients with combined pulmonary fibrosis and emphysema. *Biomarkers.* (2019) 24:232–9. doi: 10.1080/1354750X.2018.1542458
30. Berenson CS, Kruzel RL, Eberhardt E, Sethi S. Phagocytic dysfunction of human alveolar macrophages and severity of chronic obstructive pulmonary disease. *J Infect Dis.* (2013) 208:2036–45. doi: 10.1093/infdis/jit400
31. De Smet EG, Van Eeckhoutte HP, Avila Cobos F, Blomme E, Verhamme FM, Provoost S, et al. The role of miR-155 in cigarette smoke-induced pulmonary inflammation and COPD. *Mucosal Immunol.* (2020) 13:423–36. doi: 10.1038/s41385-019-0241-6
32. Kosmider B, Lin CR, Vlasenko L, Marchetti N, Bolla S, Criner GJ, et al. Impaired non-homologous end joining in human primary alveolar type II cells in emphysema. *Sci Rep.* (2019) 9:920. doi: 10.1038/s41598-018-37000-z
33. Dey T, Kalita J, Weldon S, Taggart CC. Proteases and their inhibitors in chronic obstructive pulmonary disease. *J Clin Med.* (2018) 7:90244. doi: 10.3390/jcm7090244
34. Polverino F, Rojas-Quintero J, Wang X, Petersen H, Zhang L, Gai X, et al. A disintegrin and metalloproteinase domain-8: a novel protective proteinase in chronic obstructive pulmonary disease. *Am J Respir Crit Care Med.* (2018) 198:1254–67. doi: 10.1164/rccm.201707-1331OC
35. Shan M, You R, Yuan XY, Frazier MV, Porter P, Seryshev A, et al. Agonistic induction of PPAR gamma reverses cigarette smoke-induced emphysema. *J Clin Investig.* (2014) 124:1371–81. doi: 10.1172/JCI70587
36. Shan M, Cheng HF, Song LZ, Roberts L, Green L, Hacken-Bitar J, et al. Lung myeloid dendritic cells coordinately induce TH1 and TH17 responses in human emphysema. *Sci Transl Med.* (2009) 1:4ra10. doi: 10.1126/scitranlsmed.3000154
37. Wu LY, Wang GX, Qu P, Yan C, Du H. Overexpression of dominant negative peroxisome proliferator-activated receptor-gamma (PPAR gamma) in alveolar type II epithelial cells causes inflammation and T-cell suppression in the lung. *Am J Pathol.* (2011) 178:2191–204. doi: 10.1016/j.ajpath.2011.01.046
38. Craig JM, Scott AL, Mitzner W. Immune-mediated inflammation in the pathogenesis of emphysema: insights from mouse models. *Cell Tissue Res.* (2017) 367:591–605. doi: 10.1007/s00441-016-2567-7
39. Gualano RC, Hansen MJ, Vlahos R, Jones JE, Park-Jones RA, Deliyannis G, et al. Cigarette smoke worsens lung inflammation and impairs resolution of influenza infection in mice. *Respir Res.* (2008) 9:53. doi: 10.1186/1465-9921-9-53
40. Vij N, Chandramani-Shivalingappa P, Van Westphal C, Hole R, Bodas M. Cigarette smoke-induced autophagy impairment accelerates lung aging, COPD-emphysema exacerbations and pathogenesis. *Am J Physiol Cell Physiol.* (2018) 314:C73–87. doi: 10.1152/ajpcell.00110.2016
41. Sullivan JL, Bagevalu B, Glass C, Sholl L, Kraft M, Martinez FD, et al. B cell-adaptive immune profile in emphysema-predominant chronic obstructive pulmonary disease. *Am J Respir Crit Care Med.* (2019) 200:1434–9. doi: 10.1164/rccm.201903-0632LE
42. Polverino F, Seys LJ, Bracke KR, Owen CA. B cells in chronic obstructive pulmonary disease: moving to center stage. *Am J Physiol Lung Cell Mol Physiol.* (2016) 311:L687–95. doi: 10.1152/ajplung.00304.2016
43. Zhou JS, Li ZY, Xu XC, Zhao Y, Wang Y, Chen HP, et al. Cigarette smoke-initiated autoimmunity facilitates sensitisation to elastin-induced COPD-like pathologies in mice. *Eur Respir J.* (2020) 56:2020. doi: 10.1183/13993003.00404-2020
44. Kelsen SG. The unfolded protein response in chronic obstructive pulmonary disease. *Ann Am Thorac Soc.* (2016) 13:S138–45. doi: 10.1513/AnnalsATS.201506-320KV
45. Aggarwal S, Ahmad I, Lam A, Carlisle MA, Li C, Wells JM, et al. Heme scavenging reduces pulmonary endoplasmic reticulum stress, fibrosis, and emphysema. *JCI Insight.* (2018) 3:120694. doi: 10.1172/jci.insight.120694
46. Kelsen SG. Respiratory epithelial cell responses to cigarette smoke: the unfolded protein response. *Pulm Pharmacol Ther.* (2012) 25:447–52. doi: 10.1016/j.pupt.2012.07.005
47. Wang Y, Wu ZZ, Wang W. Inhibition of endoplasmic reticulum stress alleviates cigarette smoke-induced airway inflammation and emphysema. *Oncotarget.* (2017) 8:77685–95. doi: 10.18632/oncotarget.20768
48. Bodas M, Pehote G, Silverberg D, Gulbins E, Vij N. Autophagy augmentation alleviates cigarette smoke-induced CFTR-dysfunction, ceramide-accumulation and COPD-emphysema pathogenesis. *Free Radic Biol Med.* (2019) 131:81–97. doi: 10.1016/j.freeradbiomed.2018.11.023
49. Petrache I, Natarajan V, Zhen L, Medler TR, Richter AT, Cho C, et al. Ceramide upregulation causes pulmonary cell apoptosis and emphysema-like disease in mice. *Nat Med.* (2005) 11:491–8. doi: 10.1038/nm1238
50. Nosal C, Ehlers A, Haspel JA. Why lungs keep time: circadian rhythms and lung immunity. *Annu Rev Physiol.* (2020) 82:391–412. doi: 10.1146/annurev-physiol-021119-034602
51. Borsboom GJ, van Pelt W, van Houwelingen HC, van Vianen BG, Schouten JP, Quanjer PH. Diurnal variation in lung function in subgroups from two Dutch populations: consequences for longitudinal analysis. *Am J Respir Crit Care Med.* (1999) 159:1163–71. doi: 10.1164/ajrccm.159.4.9703106
52. Sundar IK, Yao H, Sellix MT, Rahman I. Circadian molecular clock in lung pathophysiology. *Am J Physiol Lung Cell Mol Physiol.* (2015) 309:L1056–75. doi: 10.1152/ajplung.00152.2015
53. Anafi RC, Francey LJ, Hogenesch JB, Kim J. CYCLOPS reveals human transcriptional rhythms in health and disease. *Proc Natl Acad Sci USA.* (2017) 114:5312–7. doi: 10.1073/pnas.1619320114
54. Sengupta S, Tang SY, Devine JC, Anderson ST, Nayak S, Zhang SL, et al. Circadian control of lung inflammation in influenza infection. *Nat Commun.* (2019) 10:4107. doi: 10.1038/s41467-019-11400-9
55. Krakowiak K, Durrington HJ. The role of the body clock in asthma and COPD: implication for treatment. *Pulm Ther.* (2018) 4:29–43. doi: 10.1007/s41030-018-0058-6
56. Pekovic-Vaughan V, Gibbs J, Yoshitane H, Yang N, Pathiranage D, Guo B, et al. The circadian clock regulates rhythmic activation of the NRF2/glutathione-mediated antioxidant defense pathway to modulate pulmonary fibrosis. *Genes Dev.* (2014) 28:548–60. doi: 10.1101/gad.237081.113
57. Asher G, Gatfield D, Stratmann M, Reinke H, Dibner C, Kreppel F, et al. SIRT1 regulates circadian clock gene expression through PER2 deacetylation. *Cell.* (2008) 134:317–28. doi: 10.1016/j.cell.2008.06.050
58. Hwang JW, Sundar IK, Yao H, Sellix MT, Rahman I. Circadian clock function is disrupted by environmental tobacco/cigarette smoke, leading to lung inflammation and injury *via* a SIRT1-BMAL1 pathway. *FASEB J.* (2014) 28:176–94. doi: 10.1096/fj.13-232629
59. Kondratov RV, Kondratova AA, Gorbacheva VY, Vykhovanets OV, Antoch MP. Early aging and age-related pathologies in mice deficient in BMAL1, the core componentof the circadian clock. *Genes Dev.* (2006) 20:1868–73. doi: 10.1101/gad.1432206
60. Wang W, Gao J. Effects of melatonin on protecting against lung injury. *Exp Ther Med.* (2021) 21:228. doi: 10.3892/etm.2021.9659
61. Shin NR, Ko JW, Kim JC, Park G, Kim SH, Kim MS, et al. Role of melatonin as an SIRT1 enhancer in chronic obstructive pulmonary disease induced by cigarette smoke. *J Cell Mol Med.* (2020) 24:1151–6. doi: 10.1111/jcmm.14816
62. He BM, Zhang WX, Qiao JF, Peng ZY, Chai XP. Melatonin protects against COPD by attenuating apoptosis and endoplasmic reticulum stress via upregulating SIRT1 expression in rats. *Can J Physiol Pharm.* (2019) 97:386–91. doi: 10.1139/cjpp-2018-0529
63. Kim CM, Sohn JW, Yoon HJ, Shin DH, Park SS. Circadian rhythm of surfactant protein A, B and C mRNA in rats. *Korean J Intern Med.* (2003) 18:76–82. doi: 10.3904/kjim.2003.18.2.76
64. Park HY, Sin DD. Stress-induced premature senescence: another mechanism involved in the process of accelerated aging in chronic obstructive pulmonary disease. *Inflam Adv Age Nutr Res Clin Interv.* (2014) 2:193–202. doi: 10.1016/B978-0-12-397803-5.00016-2
65. Kumari R, Jat P. Mechanisms of cellular senescence: cell cycle arrest and senescence associated secretory phenotype. *Front Cell Dev Biol.* (2021) 9:645593. doi: 10.3389/fcell.2021.645593

66. Rodier F, Coppe JP, Patil CK, Hoeijmakers WA, Munoz DP, Raza SR, et al. Persistent DNA damage signalling triggers senescence-associated inflammatory cytokine secretion. *Nat Cell Biol.* (2009) 11:973–9. doi: 10.1038/ncb1909
67. Ritschka B, Storer M, Mas A, Heinzmann F, Ortells MC, Morton JP, et al. The senescence-associated secretory phenotype induces cellular plasticity and tissue regeneration. *Genes Dev.* (2017) 31:172–83. doi: 10.1101/gad.290635.116
68. Tsutsumi A, Ozaki M, Chubachi S, Irie H, Sato M, Kameyama N, et al. Exposure to cigarette smoke enhances the stemness of alveolar type 2 cells. *Am J Respir Cell Mol Biol.* (2020) 63:293–305. doi: 10.1165/rcmb.2019-0188OC
69. Rajendrasozhan S, Yang SR, Kinnula VL, Rahman I. SIRT1, an antiinflammatory and antiaging protein, is decreased in lungs of patients with chronic obstructive pulmonary disease. *Am J Respir Crit Care Med.* (2008) 177:861–70. doi: 10.1164/rccm.200708-1269OC
70. Baker JR, Vuppusetty C, Colley T, Papaioannou AI, Fenwick P, Donnelly L, et al. Oxidative stress dependent microRNA-34a activation *via* PI3Kalpha reduces the expression of sirtuin-1 and sirtuin-6 in epithelial cells. *Sci Rep.* (2016) 6:35871. doi: 10.1038/srep35871
71. Tsuji T, Aoshiba K, Nagai A. Alveolar cell senescence in patients with pulmonary emphysema. *Am J Respir Crit Care Med.* (2006) 174:886–93. doi: 10.1164/rccm.200509-1374OC
72. Baker JR, Donnelly LE, Barnes PJ. Senotherapy: a new horizon for COPD therapy. *Chest.* (2020) 158:562–70. doi: 10.1016/j.chest.2020.01.027
73. Carpagnano GE, Lacedonia D, Malerba M, Palmiotti GA, Cotugno G, Carone M, et al. Analysis of mitochondrial DNA alteration in new phenotype ACOS. *BMC Pulm Med.* (2016) 16:31. doi: 10.1186/s12890-016-0192-6
74. Zhang WZ, Rice MC, Hoffman KL, Oromendia C, Barjaktarevic IZ, Wells JM, et al. Association of urine mitochondrial DNA with clinical measures of COPD in the SPIROMICS cohort. *JCI Insight.* (2020) 5:133984. doi: 10.1172/jci.insight.133984
75. Kosmider B, Lin CR, Karim L, Tomar D, Vlasenko L, Marchetti N, et al. Mitochondrial dysfunction in human primary alveolar type II cells in emphysema. *EBioMedicine.* (2019) 46:305–16. doi: 10.1016/j.ebiom.2019.07.063
76. Garcia-Arcos I, Geraghty P, Baumlin N, Campos M, Dabo AJ, Jundi B, et al. Chronic electronic cigarette exposure in mice induces features of COPD in a nicotine-dependent manner. *Thorax.* (2016) 71:1119–29. doi: 10.1136/thoraxjnl-2015-208039
77. Bahmed K, Lin CR, Simborio H, Karim L, Aksoy M, Kelsen S, et al. The role of DJ-1 in human primary alveolar type II cell injury induced by e-cigarette aerosol. *Am J Physiol Lung Cell Mol Physiol.* (2019) 317:L475–85. doi: 10.1152/ajplung.00567.2018
78. Jiang D, Cui H, Xie N, Banerjee S, Liu RM Dai H, Thannickal VJ, et al. ATF4 mediates mitochondrial unfolded protein response in alveolar epithelial cells. *Am J Respir Cell Mol Biol.* (2020) 63:478–89. doi: 10.1165/rcmb.2020-0107OC
79. Sorrentino V, Menzies KJ, Auwerx J. Repairing mitochondrial dysfunction in disease. *Annu Rev Pharmacol Toxicol.* (2018) 58:353–89. doi: 10.1146/annurev-pharmtox-010716-104908
80. Houtkooper RH, Mouchiroud L, Ryu D, Moullan N, Katsyuba E, Knott G, et al. Mitonuclear protein imbalance as a conserved longevity mechanism. *Nature.* (2013) 497:451. doi: 10.1038/nature12188
81. Imai K, Mercer BA, Schulman LL, Sonett JR, D'Armiento JM. Correlation of lung surface area to apoptosis and proliferation in human emphysema. *Eur Respir J.* (2005) 25:250–8. doi: 10.1183/09031936.05.00023704
82. Aoshiba K, Yokohori N, Nagai A. Alveolar wall apoptosis causes lung destruction and emphysematous changes. *Am J Respir Cell Mol Biol.* (2003) 28:555–62. doi: 10.1165/rcmb.2002-0090OC
83. Mizuno S, Yasuo M, Bogaard HJ, Kraskauskas D, Natarajan R, Voelkel NF. Inhibition of histone deacetylase causes emphysema. *Am J Physiol Lung Cell Mol Physiol.* (2011) 300:L402–13. doi: 10.1152/ajplung.00207.2010
84. Tuder RM, Zhen L, Cho CY, Taraseviciene-Stewart L, Kasahara Y, Salvemini D, et al. Oxidative stress and apoptosis interact and cause emphysema due to vascular endothelial growth factor receptor blockade. *Am J Respir Cell Mol Biol.* (2003) 29:88–97. doi: 10.1165/rcmb.2002-0228OC
85. Adini A, Wu H, Dao DT, Ko VH, Yu LJ, Pan A, et al. PR1P stabilizes VEGF and upregulates its signaling to reduce elastase-induced murine emphysema. *Am J Resp Cell Mol.* (2020) 63:452–63. doi: 10.1165/rcmb.2019-0434OC
86. Dhapare S, Sakagami M. Salvianolic acid B as an anti-emphysema agent I: *in vitro* stimulation of lung cell proliferation and migration, and protection against lung cell death, and *in vivo* lung STAT3 activation and VEGF elevation. *Pulm Pharmacol Ther.* (2018) 53:107–15. doi: 10.1016/j.pupt.2018.10.001
87. Truong TM Li H, Dhapare S, Desai UR, Voelkel NF, Sakagami M. Sulfated dehydropolymer of caffeic acid: *in vitro* anti-lung cell death activity and *in vivo* intervention in emphysema induced by VEGF receptor blockade. *Pulm Pharmacol Ther.* (2017) 45:181–90. doi: 10.1016/j.pupt.2017.06.007
88. Pakhomova AV, Pershina OV, Ermakova NN, Krupin VA, Pan ES, Putrova OD, et al. Pericytes and smooth muscle cells circulating in the blood as markers of impaired angiogenesis during combined metabolic impairments and lung emphysema. *B Exp Biol Med.* (2020) 168:334–40. doi: 10.1007/s10517-020-04703-1
89. Hisata S, Racanelli AC, Kermani P, Schreiner R, Houghton S, Palikuqi B, et al. Reversal of emphysema by restoration of pulmonary endothelial cells. *J Exp Med.* (2021) 2021:218. doi: 10.1084/jem.20200938
90. Chen Q, Rehman J, Chan MW, Fu PF, Dudek SM, Natarajan V, et al. Angiocrine sphingosine-1-phosphate activation of S1PR2-YAP signaling axis in alveolar type II cells is essential for lung repair. *Cell Rep.* (2020) 31:107828. doi: 10.1016/j.celrep.2020.107828
91. Diab KJ, Adamowicz JJ, Kamocki K, Rush NI, Garrison J, Gu Y, et al. Stimulation of sphingosine 1-phosphate signaling as an alveolar cell survival strategy in emphysema. *Am J Resp Crit Care.* (2010) 181:344–52. doi: 10.1164/rccm.200906-0826OC
92. Weissmann N. Chronic obstructive pulmonary disease and pulmonary vascular disease. A comorbidity? *Ann Am Thorac Soc.* (2018) 15:S278–81. doi: 10.1513/AnnalsATS.201808-532MG
93. Halpin DM, Miravitlles M, Metzdorf N, Celli B. Impact and prevention of severe exacerbations of COPD: a review of the evidence. *Int J Chron Obstruct Pulmon Dis.* (2017) 12:2891–908. doi: 10.2147/COPD.S139470
94. Beeh KM. The role of bronchodilators in preventing exacerbations of chronic obstructive pulmonary disease. *Tuberc Respir Dis.* (2016) 79:241–7. doi: 10.4046/trd.2016.79.4.241
95. O'Donnell DE, Forkert L, Webb KA. Evaluation of bronchodilator responses in patients with "irreversible" emphysema. *Eu Respirat J.* (2001) 18:914–20. doi: 10.1183/09031936.01.00216501
96. Han MK, Wise R, Mumford J, Sciurba F, Criner GJ, Curtis JL, et al. Prevalence and clinical correlates of bronchoreversibility in severe emphysema. *Eur Respir J.* (2010) 35:1048–56. doi: 10.1183/09031936.00052509
97. Oczypok EA, Perkins TN, Oury TD. Alveolar epithelial cell-derived mediators: potential direct regulators of large airway and vascular responses. *Am J Resp Cell Mol.* (2017) 56:694–9. doi: 10.1165/rcmb.2016-0151PS
98. Knudsen L, Atochina-Vasserman EN, Guo CJ, Scott PA, Haenni B, Beers MF, et al. NOS2 is critical to the development of emphysema in Sftpd deficient mice but does not affect surfactant homeostasis. *PLoS ONE.* (2014) 9:85722. doi: 10.1371/journal.pone.0085722
99. Seimetz M, Parajuli N, Pichl A, Veit F, Kwapiszewska G, Weisel FC, et al. Inducible NOS inhibition reverses tobacco-smoke-induced emphysema and pulmonary hypertension in mice. *Cell.* (2011) 147:293–305. doi: 10.1016/j.cell.2011.08.035
100. Brindicci C, Ito K, Resta O, Pride NB, Barnes PJ, Kharitonov SA. Exhaled nitric oxide from lung periphery is increased in COPD. *Eur Respirat J.* (2005) 26:52–9. doi: 10.1183/09031936.04.00125304
101. Maestrelli P, Paska C, Saetta M, Turato G, Nowicki Y, Monti S, et al. Decreased haem oxygenase-1 and increased inducible nitric oxide synthase in the lung of severe COPD patients. *Eur Respir J.* (2003) 21:971–6. doi: 10.1183/09031936.03.00098203
102. Boe AE, Eren M, Morales-Nebreda L, Murphy SB, Budinger GR, Mutlu GM, et al. Nitric oxide prevents alveolar senescence and emphysema in a mouse model. *PLoS ONE.* (2015) 10:e0116504. doi: 10.1371/journal.pone.0116504
103. Zhang L, Wang Y, Wu GR, Rao LZ, Wei YQ, Yue HH, et al. Blockade of JAK2 protects mice against hypoxia-induced pulmonary arterial hypertension by repressing pulmonary arterial smooth muscle cell proliferation. *Cell Proliferat.* (2020) 53:12742. doi: 10.1111/cpr.12742

104. Fu X, Zhang F. Role of the HIF-1 signaling pathway in chronic obstructive pulmonary disease. *Exp Ther Med.* (2018) 16:4553–61. doi: 10.3892/etm.2018.6785
105. Fernandez-Plata R, Thirion-Romero I, Nava-Quiroz KJ, Perez-Rubio G, Rodriguez-Llamazares S, Perez-Kawabe M, et al. Clinical markers of chronic hypoxemia in respiratory patients residing at moderate altitude. *Life-Basel.* (2021) 11:50428. doi: 10.3390/life11050428
106. McClendon J, Jansing NL, Redente EF, Gandjeva A, Ito Y, Colgan SP, et al. Hypoxia-inducible factor 1alpha signaling promotes repair of the alveolar epithelium after acute lung injury. *Am J Pathol.* (2017) 187:1772–86. doi: 10.1016/j.ajpath.2017.04.012
107. Kobayashi Y, Tata A, Konkimalla A, Katsura H, Lee RF, Ou JH, et al. Persistence of a regeneration-associated, transitional alveolar epithelial cell state in pulmonary fibrosis. *Nat Cell Biol.* (2020) 22:934. doi: 10.1038/s41556-020-0542-8
108. Aspal M, Zemans RL. Mechanisms of ATII-to-ATI cell differentiation during lung regeneration. *Int J Mol Sci.* (2020) 21:93188. doi: 10.3390/ijms21093188
109. Parker MM, Hao Y, Guo F, Pham B, Chase R, Platig J, et al. Identification of an emphysema-associated genetic variant near TGFB2 with regulatory effects in lung fibroblasts. *Elife.* (2019) 8:42720. doi: 10.7554/eLife.42720
110. Gokey JJ, Sridharan A, Xu Y, Green J, Carraro G, Stripp BR, et al. Active epithelial Hippo signaling in idiopathic pulmonary fibrosis. *JCI Insight.* (2018) 3:98738. doi: 10.1172/jci.insight.98738
111. Kneidinger N, Yildirim AO, Callegari J, Takenaka S, Stein MM, Dumitrascu R, et al. Activation of the WNT/beta-catenin pathway attenuates experimental emphysema. *Am J Respir Crit Care Med.* (2011) 183:723–33. doi: 10.1164/rccm.200910-1560OC
112. Skronska-Wasek W, Mutze K, Baarsma HA, Bracke KR, Alsafadi HN, Lehmann M, et al. Reduced frizzled receptor 4 expression prevents WNT/beta-catenin-driven alveolar lung repair in chronic obstructive pulmonary disease. *Am J Respir Crit Care Med.* (2017) 196:172–85. doi: 10.1164/rccm.201605-0904OC
113. Heijink IH, de Bruin HG, Dennebos R, Jonker MR, Noordhoek JA, Brandsma CA, et al. Cigarette smoke-induced epithelial expression of WNT-5B: implications for COPD. *Eur Respir J.* (2016) 48:504–15. doi: 10.1183/13993003.01541-2015
114. Baarsma HA, Skronska-Wasek W, Mutze K, Ciolek F, Wagner DE, John-Schuster G, et al. Noncanonical WNT-5A signaling impairs endogenous lung repair in COPD. *J Exp Med.* (2017) 214:143–63. doi: 10.1084/jem.20160675
115. Feller D, Kun J, Ruzsics I, Rapp J, Sarosi V, Kvell K, et al. Cigarette smoke-induced pulmonary inflammation becomes systemic by circulating extracellular vesicles containing Wnt5a and inflammatory cytokines. *Front Immunol.* (2018) 9:1724. doi: 10.3389/fimmu.2018.01724
116. Zheng Y, Pan D. The Hippo signaling pathway in development and disease. *Dev Cell.* (2019) 50:264–82. doi: 10.1016/j.devcel.2019.06.003
117. Kugler MC, Loomis CA, Zhao Z, Cushman JC, Liu L, Munger JS. Sonic hedgehog signaling regulates myofibroblast function during alveolar septum formation in murine postnatal lung. *Am J Respir Cell Mol Biol.* (2017) 57:280–93. doi: 10.1165/rcmb.2016-0268OC
118. Wang C, de Mochel NSR, Christenson SA, Cassandras M, Moon R, Brumwell AN, et al. Expansion of hedgehog disrupts mesenchymal identity and induces emphysema phenotype. *J Clin Invest.* (2018) 128:4343–58. doi: 10.1172/JCI99435
119. Kato K, Dieguez-Hurtado R, Park DY, Hong SP, Kato-Azuma S, Adams S, et al. Pulmonary pericytes regulate lung morphogenesis. *Nat Commun.* (2018) 9:2448. doi: 10.1038/s41467-018-04913-2
120. Dandekar A, Mendez R, Zhang KZ. Cross talk between er stress, oxidative stress, and inflammation in health and disease. *Stress Responses.* (2015) 1292:205–14. doi: 10.1007/978-1-4939-2522-3_15
121. Gargalovic PS, Gharavi NM, Clark MJ, Pagnon J, Yang WP, He AQ, et al. The unfolded protein response is an important regulator of inflammatory genes in endothelial cells. *Arterioscl Throm Vas.* (2006) 26:2490–6. doi: 10.1161/01.ATV.0000242903.41158.a1
122. Pereira ER, Liao N, Neale GA, Hendershot LM. Transcriptional and post-transcriptional regulation of proangiogenic factors by the unfolded protein response. *PLoS ONE.* (2010) 5:12521. doi: 10.1371/journal.pone.0012521
123. Viby NE, Isidor MS, Buggeskov KB, Poulsen SS, Hansen JB, Kissow H. Glucagon-like peptide-1 (GLP-1) reduces mortality and improves lung function in a model of experimental obstructive lung disease in female mice. *Endocrinology.* (2013) 154:4503–11. doi: 10.1210/en.2013-1666
124. Cazzola M, Rogliani P, Calzetta L, Lauro D, Page C, Matera MG. Targeting mechanisms linking COPD to type 2 diabetes mellitus. *Trends Pharmacol Sci.* (2017) 38:940–51. doi: 10.1016/j.tips.2017.07.003

4

Respiratory *Aspergillus* Colonization was Associated with Relapse of Acute Exacerbation in Patients with Chronic Obstructive Pulmonary Disease

Yi-xing Wu [1†], *Yi-hui Zuo* [1†], *Qi-jian Cheng* [2], *Yi Huang* [3], *Zhi-yao Bao* [4], *Xiao-yan Jin* [5], *Xi-wen Gao* [6], *Chun-lin Tu* [7], *Wei-ping Hu* [1], *Jing-qing Hang* [8], *Wei-qin Wang* [5], *Feng-ying Zhang* [8] and *Jing Zhang* [1*]

[1] Department of Pulmonary and Critical Care Medicine, Zhongshan Hospital, Fudan University, Shanghai, China, [2] Department of Respiratory Medicine, Ruijin North Hospital, School of Medicine, Shanghai Jiao Tong University, Shanghai, China, [3] Department of Pulmonary and Critical Care Medicine, Changhai Hospital of Shanghai, Second Military Medical University, Shanghai, China, [4] Department of Respiratory Medicine, Ruijin Hospital, School of Medicine, Shanghai Jiao Tong University, Shanghai, China, [5] Department of Respiratory Medicine, Tongren Hospital, School of Medicine, Shanghai Jiao Tong University, Shanghai, China, [6] Department of Respiratory Medicine, Central Hospital of Minhang District, Shanghai, Fudan University, Shanghai, China, [7] Department of Respiratory Medicine, Central Hospital of Jiading District, Shanghai, Fudan University, Shanghai, China, [8] Department of Respiratory Medicine, Shanghai Putuo District People's Hospital, Shanghai, China

***Correspondence:**
Jing Zhang
huxizhangjing@foxmail.com

† These authors share first authorship

Background: Patients with chronic obstructive pulmonary disease (COPD) are more susceptible to *Aspergillus* colonization or infection. Several studies have demonstrated that invasive pulmonary Aspergillosis (IPA) and *Aspergillus* hypersensitivity (AH) have a detrimental effect on COPD. However, it remains to be clarified whether *Aspergillus* colonization is associated with acute exacerbation of COPD (AECOPD). This study aimed to explore the impact of *Aspergillus* colonization in the lower respiratory tract on AECOPD.

Method: Patients with *Aspergillus* colonization were identified from a retrospective cohort of hospitalized AECOPD from 2011 to 2016 in eight centers in Shanghai, China. The demographic information, conditions of the stable stage, clinical characteristics during hospitalization, and 1-year follow-up information after discharge were collected and compared to participants without fungi colonization.

Result: Twenty-six hospitalized AECOPD patients with *Aspergillus* colonization and 72 controls were included in the final analysis after excluding patients with other fungi isolation and matching. The rates of recurrence of acute exacerbation within 90 days and 180 days after discharge in the patients with *Aspergillus* colonization were both significantly higher than that in the fungi negative patients (90 days: 19.2 vs. 4.2%, $p = 0.029$; 180 days: 23.1 vs. 4.2%, $p = 0.010$), and the all-cause mortality within 1 year was also higher (11.5 vs. 0.0%, $p = 0.017$). Multivariate logistic regression analysis showed that *Aspergillus* colonization was an independent risk factor for the recurrence of acute exacerbation within 90 days and 180 days (90 days: OR = 8.661, 95% CI: 1.496-50.159, $p = 0.016$; 180 days: OR =10.723, 95% CI: 1.936-59.394, $p = 0.007$).

Conclusion: *Aspergillus* colonization may predict poor prognosis of AECOPD while leading to an increased risk of recurrent AECOPD in a short period.

Keywords: chronic obstructive pulmonary disease, acute exacerbation, *Aspergillus*, prognosis, recurrence of AECOPD

INTRODUCTION

Chronic obstructive pulmonary disease (COPD) is a common chronic respiratory disease characterized by progressive and irreversible airflow limitation. Due to the aging population, the expanding epidemic of cigarette smoking, and other reasons, COPD's prevalence and mortality are among the highest worldwide while causing significant economic and social burden (1). Acute exacerbation of chronic obstructive pulmonary disease (AECOPD) refers to the deterioration of respiratory symptoms in a short period and requiring additional treatment. Exacerbation is the primary factor of poor outcomes of this disease, including loss of working capacity, a decline in lung function, hospitalization, and sometimes even death (2–4). AECOPD is mainly induced by pathogenic microorganisms and environmental factors. Bacteria and viruses are considered as the usual triggers for acute exacerbations rather than fungi.

Aspergillus is an airborne fungal pathogen that spreads all over the world. The conidia can reach the pulmonary parenchyma through the airway as its diameter is only 2-3 μm. Meanwhile, chronic airway inflammation in COPD results in damage to the epithelium of the lower respiratory tract (LRT) and further weakens the defense of the airways. As a result, COPD patients are susceptible to *Aspergillus* colonization or infection (5). *Aspergillus* usually colonize the airways without generating infection. It is reported that the prevalence of *Aspergillus* colonization in COPD patients is from 8.33 (6) to 16.6% (7). According to the host immune response, *Aspergillus* can cause invasive pulmonary aspergillosis (IPA), allergic bronchopulmonary aspergillosis (ABPA), or other clinical syndromes (8). Growing evidence support that COPD is the risk factor of IPA, which carries an abysmal prognosis (5, 9). A study between COPD patients and healthy volunteers demonstrated that COPD might predispose *Aspergillus* hypersensitivity (AH) and ABPA (10). It has been reported that allergy and AH are associated with severe symptoms and reduction of lung function in COPD patients (11, 12).

It is necessary to find out the significance of *Aspergillus* colonization in COPD patients for clinical decision making. But the effect of *Aspergillus* colonization in COPD remains to be studied and clarified, especially on the prognosis. Therefore, we carried out this study to investigate the impact of LRT *Aspergillus* colonization on the prognosis of patients hospitalized for AECOPD, which might help with the management strategies.

PATIENTS AND METHODS

Study Design

This multicenter retrospective cohort study was initiated by the Department of Pulmonary and Critical Care Medicine, Zhongshan Hospital, Fudan University in Shanghai, China. We collected patients hospitalized with AECOPD from January 2011 to December 2016 in eight hospitals in Shanghai. From the cohort, those with LRT *Aspergillus* colonization were identified (*Aspergillus* positive group) and those without evidence of *Aspergillus* colonization were classified as controls (*Aspergillus* negative group). The LRT *Aspergillus* colonization was defined as culture positive for *Aspergillus* from samples including sputum, endotracheal suction, bronchoscopic flushing, and/or lavage fluid (BALF), and had no clinical presentation of fungal infection during hospitalization. Propensity score matching was applied if there was a significant difference in baseline characteristics between the two groups. The ethics committee of Zhongshan Hospital of Fudan University approved this study (Approval notice number: B2015-119R).

Culture of *Aspergillus*

The microbiologic findings of LRT samples were carried out in the following way. After obtaining the sample from the patient, it was quickly sent to the microbiology laboratory at room temperature, and processed on the same day. About 10 μl samples were pipetted directly from the submitted specimen and inoculated onto sabouraud dextrose agar (SDA) containing chloramphenicol and incubated at 28°C~35°C for 7 days. The eight units that performed the *Aspergillus* culture were all under the quality control of Shanghai Center For Clinical Laboratory, and the examiners had all received professional training.

Inclusion Criteria

Those with all the following criteria were enrolled: (1) Age over 18 years old. (2) The hospitalized patient met the diagnostic criteria for COPD and acute exacerbations in the 2017 GOLD report. (3) The patients' LRT samples had been detected for *Aspergillus*.

Exclusion Criteria

Those who met any of the following items were excluded: (1) Chest CT findings suggested chronic pulmonary aspergillosis (CPA), IPA or ABPA. (2) A positive result of serum or BALF galactomannan determination. (3) Treatment of anti-fungal therapy. (4) A positive culture of other fungi except for *Aspergillus* from LRT specimens. (5) Sputum smears showed spores indicating *Candida*. (6) Patients with mental diseases that made themselves unable to cooperate in data collection. (7) Combined with other underlying lung diseases, such as lung cancer, bronchiectasis, interstitial pulmonary diseases, lung abscess, and tuberculosis. (8) Patients with immunocompromised diseases.

Data Collection

The patients' clinical data who met the inclusion criteria through their hospitals' electronic and paper medical records were collected and put into the Epidata system (The EpiData Association, Odense, Denmark). An independent investigator would check the collected data. If inconsistent data were found, the examiner would correct it after checking the original case history.

The information to be collected was as follows: basic patient characteristics (sex, age, smoking history, etc.), CAT and mMRC scores, treatment during the stable stage, complications, lung function, microbiologic findings of LRT samples, chest CT findings, laboratory test results, length of hospitalization or ICU stay, hospitalization expense, mortality during hospitalization, recurrent exacerbations within 90 days, 180 days, 1 year, and the mortality within 1 year. As for smoking history, we collected the information on whether the patient had smoked, how much he/she smoked, and how long he/she had smoked. Smoking history was defined as over 10 pack-years, regardless of current smoking status.

Statistical Analysis

Statistical analysis was performed on Stata 14 (StataCorp., College Station, TX).

Categorical variables were presented as absolute numbers and rates or percentages. Chi-square test or Fisher's exact test was used for comparison. The Shapiro-Wilk test would evaluate the normality of continuous variables. The continuous variables with normal distribution were presented as means and standard deviations, and the Student t-test was performed in comparison. The non-normally distributed continuous variables were presented as medians and quartiles, and the difference between the two groups was compared using Mann-Whitney U-test. Logistic regression was applied to explore possible risk factors for *Aspergillus* colonization and the recurrence of exacerbations. Variables with $p < 0.10$ in the univariate analysis would enter the multivariate analysis. All tests were two-tailed, and $p < 0.05$ was considered statistically significant.

RESULTS

A total of 1,116 patients hospitalized for AECOPD in the retrospective cohort were screened, and 626 patients met the inclusion and exclusion criteria. Thirty-one patients with *Aspergillus* and no other fungi identified in their LRT samples and 459 with no LRT fungi were kept in the remaining cases. As the baseline characteristics were significantly different in these two groups (shown in **Table 1**), we adopted propensity score matching at a ratio of 1:3 (caliper = 0.05). Finally, 26 cases were included in the positive group and 72 cases in the negative group for the final analysis.

Baseline Characteristics Before and After Matching

Table 1 showed the baseline data of the *Aspergillus* positive group and *Aspergillus* negative group, including the age, gender, smoking history, and the CAT scores and mMRC scores before exacerbation, which were used to assess the patients' symptom burden during the stable stage.

Before applying propensity score matching, the age in the positive group was considerably lower than that of the negative group (69 vs. 78, $p = 0.003$), and the percentage of patients with smoking history was also dramatically lower (32 vs. 83%, $p < 0.001$). The CAT scores of the positive group were notably higher compared with the negative group (27.5 vs. 22, $p = 0.001$), which presented that COPD patients with *Aspergillus* colonization had a higher symptom burden.

The baseline characteristics of the two groups were controlled at a similar level after matching of age, gender, smoking history, and CAT score and mMRC score of stable stage, which was more conducive for us to assess the clinical characteristics and prognosis of AECOPD patients based on *Aspergillus* colonization.

Corticosteroids Use Was Related to *Aspergillus* Colonization

Inhaled corticosteroids use in patients with positive *Aspergillus* culture during the stable phase was distinctly higher than that of negative patients (65.4 vs. 27.8%, $p = 0.001$, **Table 2**). Univariate logistic regression analysis indicated that inhaled corticosteroids use was a risk factor for *Aspergillus* colonization (OR = 4.911, 95% CI: 1.883-12.807, $p = 0.001$). In terms of other drugs and treatment methods, we found no statistical differences. There was no remarkable difference in the prevalence of comorbidities, either.

The airflow limitation was assessed by forced expiratory volume in one second (FEV_1)% predicted and forced expiratory volume in one second/forced vital capacity (FEV_1/FVC) post-bronchodilators recorded in stable stage. FEV_1% predicted and FEV_1/FVC values of the two groups after matching showed no difference. The FEV_1/FVC values were <70%, which met the diagnostic criteria of COPD and both groups had severe airflow obstruction.

Table 3 summarized the examination results of AECOPD patients on admission. Laboratory test results showed a difference between patients with LRT *Aspergillus* colonization and controls in the number and percentage of eosinophils (Eosinophil count: 33.21 vs. 70.4, $p = 0.030$; Eosinophils%: 0.3 vs. 0.7, $p = 0.019$). Accordingly, there was a trend of an increase in neutrophil counts and percentage in the *Aspergillus* colonization group on admission, which could be explained by the bacterial infection which served as the trigger of exacerbations. No significant difference was identified in other clinical characteristics. No laboratory results on admission were found to be a risk factor or protective factor of LRT *Aspergillus* colonization.

TABLE 1 | Baseline characteristics of hospitalized COPD patients with and without lower respiratory *Aspergillus* colonization before and after propensity score matching.

	Before matching		*P*-value	After matching		*P*-value
	Patients with *Aspergillus* colonization ($n = 31$)	Controls ($n = 459$)		*Aspergillus* colonization ($n = 26$)	Controls ($n = 72$)	
Age	69 (61, 80)	78 (69, 84)	0.003	70 (63, 82)	71.5 (64, 82.5)	0.545
Gender (male)	25 (80.6)	388 (84.5)	0.608	20 (76.9)	52 (72.2)	0.642
Smoking history (≥10 pack-years)	10 (32.3)	379 (82.6)	<0.001	9 (34.6)	34 (47.2)	0.267
CAT score	27.5 (21, 35)	22 (15, 27)	0.001	26 (20, 34)	25.5 (22, 29)	0.721
mMRC score			0.547			0.141
1	2 (6.5)	23 (5)		2 (7.7)	0 (0)	
2	6 (19.4)	121 (26.4)		6 (23.1)	12 (16.7)	
3	14 (45.2)	178 (38.8)		11 (42.3)	41 (56.9)	
4	3 (9.7)	23 (5)		2 (7.7)	3 (4.2)	
Lost	6 (19.4)	114 (24.8)		5 (19.2)	16 (22.2)	

Data are presented as medians (1st quartile, 3rd quartile) or absolute numbers (%) as appropriate. COPD, chronic obstructive pulmonary disease; CAT, COPD assessment test; mMRC, modified British research council.

Patients With *Aspergillus* Colonization Were at a High Risk of Relapse of AECOPD

Table 4 presented the clinical outcomes of the patients during hospitalization and within 1 year after discharge. We did not find notable differences in length of hospitalization, length of ICU stays, hospitalization costs, and in-hospital mortality. Compared with those *Aspergillus* cultured-negative, the rate of recurrent exacerbation within 90 days of the *Aspergillus* positive group was significantly higher (19.2 vs. 4.2%, $p = 0.029$). The recurrence rate within 180 days was obviously higher, too (23.1 vs. 4.2%, $p = 0.010$). There was no considerable difference in the rate of recurrence of AECOPD within 1 year. The all-cause 1-year mortality was higher in *Aspergillus* positive group than the negative group (11.5 vs. 0.0%, $p = 0.017$).

Tables 5, 6 manifested the results of logistic regression analysis. Univariate analysis proved that *Aspergillus* colonization was a risk factor for relapse of acute exacerbation within 90 days and 180 days (90 days: OR = 5.476, 95% CI: 1.207-24.849, $p = 0.028$; 180 days: OR = 6.9, 95% CI: 1.582-30.087, $p = 0.010$). Besides, pleural effusion in chest CT findings was also a risk factor of recurrent exacerbations in COPD patients (90 days: OR = 5.4, 95% CI: 1.103-26.438, $p = 0.037$; 180 days: OR = 4.444, 95% CI: 0.945-20.893, $p = 0.059$). Multivariate analysis agreed with the results of univariate analysis. Variables associated with the relapse of acute exacerbation were *Aspergillus* colonization (90 days: OR = 8.661, 95% CI: 1.496-50.159, $p = 0.016$; 180 days: OR =10.723, 95% CI: 1.936-59.394, $p = 0.007$) and pleural effusion (90 days: OR = 9.793, 95% CI: 1.470-65.237, $p = 0.018$; 180 days: OR = 8.791, 95% CI: 1.317-58.689, $p = 0.025$).

DISCUSSION

Aspergillus Colonization Predict Poor Outcomes of AECOPD

We investigated a large sample of more than 1,000 patients with severe exacerbation of COPD from eight centers and collected abundant information on the stable stage, acute exacerbation stage, clinical outcomes, and prognosis. While other researchers focused on the risk factors and clinical manifestations of COPD patients colonized or infected by *Aspergillus*, we were the first to concentrate on the prognosis of COPD patients after hospitalization discharge. We established three follow-up periods of 90 days, 180 days, and 1 year to observe the short-term and long-term prognosis, which was a new attempt in similar researches. The results of this study suggested that *Aspergillus* colonization is associated with poor clinical outcomes of hospitalized AECOPD, including higher acute exacerbation rates within 90 days, 180 days, and higher mortality within 1 year after discharge.

We speculated that the worse prognosis is attributed to AH. Firstly, COPD patients are more likely to have an allergic reaction to *Aspergillus* than those without the disease. A prospective multicenter study demonstrated that COPD had a high frequency of sensitization in various allergens, including *Aspergillus* (13). Agarwal et al. found AH in 8.5% (17 in 200) COPD patients, while none in healthy volunteers (10). Secondly, COPD patients with *Aspergillus* were at higher levels of specific-IgE (14), related to AH. A study of *Aspergillus* sensitization and asthma's relationships indicated that *Aspergillus*'s long-term colonization is related to sensitization (15). For COPD patients, it is also possible that persistent *Aspergillus* colonization has a stimulating effect on AH. Thirdly, AH can lead to decreased lung function and severe respiratory symptoms (11, 12). Tiew et al. found that fungal sensitization was associated with the frequency of exacerbations (13). Moreover, another study suggested that the cluster characterized by *Aspergillus*, *Curvularia*, and *Penicillium* had increased exacerbations and higher mortality than another cluster with *Saccharomyces* (14). These findings are consistent with ours, indicating that it is long-term colonization of *Aspergillus* in the airways of COPD patients that cause sensitization and make patients more susceptible to acute exacerbations under specific stimulation.

TABLE 2 | Treatment during the stable stage, comorbidities, and airflow limitation of hospitalized COPD patients with or without *Aspergillus* colonization.

	Patients with *Aspergillus* colonization ($n = 26$)	Controls ($n = 72$)	*P*-value
Treatment during stable stage			
SABA	13 (50)	26 (36.1)	0.215
SAMA	3 (11.5)	11 (15.3)	0.754
LABA	0 (0)	3 (4.2)	0.563
LAMA	6 (23.1)	20 (27.8)	0.642
Inhaled corticosteroids (including ICS/LABA and ICS/LABA + LAMA)	17 (65.4)	20 (27.8)	0.001
Oral corticosteroids	1 (3.8)	1 (1.4)	0.452
Theophylline	4 (15.4)	16 (22.2)	0.458
Mucolytics	4 (15.4)	4 (5.6)	0.203
Home oxygen therapy	7 (26.9)	27 (37.5)	0.331
Home ventilator	1 (3.8)	11 (15.3)	0.173
Comorbidities			
Patients with complications	17 (65.4)	35 (48.6)	0.142
OSAS	1 (3.8)	1 (1.4)	0.462
Hypertension	14 (53.8)	26 (36.1)	0.115
Left ventricular dysfunction	3 (11.5)	11 (15.3)	0.754
Coronary artery disease	4 (15.4)	17 (23.6)	0.481
Cerebral apoplexy	1 (3.8)	1 (1.4)	0.462
Diabetes	2 (7.7)	12 (16.7)	0.342
Post-bronchodilator spirometry			
FEV_1% pred (%)	32.05 (25.2, 58.15)	42.3 (26.8, 52.4)	0.817
FEV_1/FVC (%)	48.63 ± 12.65	51.72 ± 10.51	0.460

Data are presented as means ± SD, medians (1st quartile, 3rd quartile), or absolute numbers (%) as appropriate. COPD: chronic obstructive pulmonary disease; SABA, short-acting beta$_2$-agonists; SAMA, short-acting muscarinic antagonists; LABA, long-acting beta$_2$-agonists; LAMA, long-acting muscarinic antagonists; OSAS, obstructive sleep apnea syndrome; ICS, inhaled corticosteroids; FEV_1, forced expiratory volume in one second; FEV_1/FVC, forced expiratory volume in one second/forced vital capacity.

Furthermore, researchers found that sensitization to recombinant antigens of *Aspergillus* increases the risk for bronchiectasis in COPD patients (16). And a study published recently identified that the number of fungal interactions is increased in COPD patients with very frequent exacerbations (exacerbate more than three times per year) (14). To some extent, these findings support our conclusion that *Aspergillus* causes a worse prognosis in COPD patients.

However, the molecular mechanism of the effects of *Aspergillus* on acute exacerbation remains unclear. The reason for no statistical difference in 1-year mortality is also waiting to explore. Would the intensity of AH fluctuate over time and result in the difference between short-term and long-term outcomes? Is it possible to determine which COPD patients are susceptible to AH based on specific characteristics? Is it able to help with treatment strategies by measuring total-IgE or specific-IgE? These are the keys to future study.

TABLE 3 | Clinical characteristics and treatments of COPD patients on admission with or without *Aspergillus* colonization.

	Patients with *Aspergillus* colonization ($n = 26$)	Controls ($n = 72$)	*P*-value
Laboratory findings			
Leucocyte count ($\times 10^9$/L)	7.66 (5.6, 11.19)	7.89 (5.8, 9.94)	0.964
Neutrophil count ($\times 10^9$/L)	6018 (4250, 9466)	5700 (4087, 8159)	0.525
Neutrophils% (%)	81.55 (72.7, 85.5)	75 (65, 82.9)	0.069
Eosinophil count ($\times 10^9$/L)	33.21 (0, 42.6)	70.4 (10.8, 188.6)	0.030
Eosinophils% (%)	0.3 (0, 0.71)	0.7 (0.1, 2.6)	0.019
CRP (mg/dL)	16.85 (11.6, 34)	12.4 (3.3, 51.5)	0.326
Confirmed bacterial infection	4 (15.4)	10 (13.9)	1.000
Chest CT findings			
Patients with imaging findings	16 (61.5)	42 (58.3)	0.776
Consolidation	2 (7.7)	3 (4.2)	0.606
Patchy shadows	13 (50)	33 (45.8)	0.715
Multilobar lesions	6 (23.1)	15 (20.8)	0.811
Bilateral lesions	7 (26.9)	35 (48.6)	0.055
Pleural effusion	2 (7.7)	10 (13.9)	0.507
Treatment during hospitalization			
Mechanical ventilation	6 (23.1)	25 (34.7)	0.274
Invasive mechanical ventilation	5 (19.2)	23 (31.9)	0.219
Non-invasive mechanical ventilation	1 (3.8)	3 (4.2)	1.000

Data are presented as medians (1st quartile, 3rd quartile) or absolute numbers (%) as appropriate. COPD, chronic obstructive pulmonary disease; CRP, C-reactive protein.

TABLE 4 | Prognosis of hospitalized COPD patients with or without *Aspergillus* colonization.

	Patients with *Aspergillus* colonization ($n = 26$)	Controls ($n = 72$)	*P*-value
Length of hospital stay (days)	12 (7,22)	13 (10,15)	0.759
ICU admission	2 (7.7)	9 (12.5)	0.722
Hospitalization expense (RMB)	17,290 (12,601, 23,049)	17,110 (13,204, 21,348)	0.728
Mortality during hospitalization	1 (3.8)	1 (1.4)	0.462
Recurrent exacerbations within 90 days	5 (19.2)	3 (4.2)	0.029
Recurrent exacerbations within 180 days	6 (23.1)	3 (4.2)	0.010
Recurrent exacerbations within 1 year	9 (34.6)	39 (54.2)	0.087
Mortality within 1 year	3 (11.5)	0 (0)	0.017

Data are presented as medians (1st quartile, 3rd quartile) or absolute numbers (%) as appropriate. COPD, chronic obstructive pulmonary disease; ICU, intensive care unit.

Also, we found that the eosinophil count and eosinophils% on admission in *Aspergillus* positive group were lower than those in the control group, which might be explained

TABLE 5 | Univariate and multivariate logistic analysis for relapse of acute exacerbation in COPD patients within 90 days after discharge.

	Univariate logistic analysis			Multivariate logistic analysis		
	OR	95% CI	*P*-value	OR	95% CI	*P*-value
Aspergillus colonization	5.476	1.207-24.849	0.028	8.661	1.496-50.159	0.016
FEV1% pred (%)	0.928	0.783-1.101	0.391			
FEV_1/FVC (%)	0.945	0.769-1.162	0.592			
Neutrophils% (%)	1.022	0.955-1.094	0.527			
Eosinophils% (%)	0.715	0.369-1.387	0.321			
Patients with imaging findings	2.192	0.419-11.462	0.352			
Consolidation	3.071	0.301-31.341	0.344			
Patchy shadows	1.992	0.449-8.840	0.365			
Multilobar lesions	0.500	0.058-4.307	0.528			
Bilateral lesions	0.785	0.177-3.484	0.750			
Pleural effusion	5.4	1.103-26.438	0.037	9.793	1.470-65.237	0.018
Length of hospital stay	1	0.898-1.114	1.000			

COPD, chronic obstructive pulmonary disease; FEV_1, forced expiratory volume in one second; FEV_1/FVC, forced expiratory volume in one second/forced vital capacity.

TABLE 6 | Univariate and multivariate logistic analysis for relapse of acute exacerbation in COPD patients within 180 days after discharge.

	Univariate logistic analysis			Multivariate logistic analysis		
	OR	95% CI	*P*-value	OR	95% CI	*P*-value
Aspergillus colonization	6.9	1.582-30.087	0.010	10.723	1.936-59.394	0.007
FEV1% pred (%)	0.844	0.687-1.037	0.107			
FEV_1/FVC (%)	0.852	0.702-1.034	0.106			
Neutrophils% (%)	1.010	0.950-1.075	0.741			
Eosinophils (%)	0.656	0.328-1.310	0.232			
Patients with imaging findings	2.608	0.513-13.265	0.248			
Consolidation	2.656	0.264-26.709	0.407			
Patchy shadows	2.45	0.576-10.418	0.225			
Multilobar lesions	0.431	0.051-3.657	0.441			
Bilateral lesions	1.074	0.270-4.269	0.920			
Pleural effusion	4.444	0.945-20.893	0.059	8.791	1.317-58.689	0.025
Length of hospital stay	0.962	0.855-1.081	0.513			

COPD, chronic obstructive pulmonary disease; FEV_1, forced expiratory volume in one second; FEV_1/FVC, forced expiratory volume in one second/forced vital capacity.

by the bacterial infection which served as the trigger of exacerbations.

The Risk Factors of *Aspergillus* Colonization

We observed that *Aspergillus* was more likely to colonize in patients treated with inhaled corticosteroids during the stable stage. This observation is consistent with the study of Tong et al. (6), who found that the proportion of patients who inhale high doses of corticosteroids during the stable stage in the *Aspergillus* colonization group was higher than that in the control group. Another study also indicated that patients with *Aspergillus* cultured positive had a higher inhaled corticosteroid dose during the stable stage compared with those cultured negative (12). The use of corticosteroids reduces the anti-fungal capacity of macrophages in the airways, inhibits the production of proinflammatory cytokine and chemokine (17, 18). In general, corticosteroids inhibit the ability of immune systems to eliminate *Aspergillus* conidia and promote the growth of *Aspergillus* (19). So, the use of inhaled corticosteroids is responsible for *Aspergillus* colonization.

The study of Tong et al. suggested that smoking history should be a risk factor for *Aspergillus* colonization (6). Chronic tobacco smoke can damage the function of cilia, reduce the removal rate of *Aspergillus* in the airways, and adjust the microbial environment to be suitable for *Aspergillus*'s growth. In our baseline data before matching, the lower percentage of smokers in the *Aspergillus* positive group should be due to selection bias.

The genetic factor is also a possible risk factor for *Aspergillus* colonization. It is showed that genetic mutations could affect protein levels in the extracellular matrix and promote the adhesion of *Aspergillus* conidia. Moreover, affected by genetic factors, some patients might show a stronger inflammatory response to the conidia of *Aspergillus* (20).

Strengths and Limitations

This study was the first retrospective multicenter study on the impact of LRT *Aspergillus* colonization on the early relapse long-term prognosis of AECOPD. Another strength is propensity score matching. By matching control age, sex, smoking history, and severity of symptoms before acute exacerbation, this study minimized the individual differences in patients and obtained the data of impacts of *Aspergillus* colonization on the prognosis.

However, our study had several limitations. Firstly, this was a retrospective study. We could not confirm whether *Aspergillus* colonization was acquired during the stable stage or after the onset of the exacerbation. We only proved the relationship between the LRT *Aspergillus* colonization and outcome variables, like other available studies on this topic (6). Secondly, the positivity rate of *Aspergillus* culture was quite low (6%, 31/490), as we excluded the patients who received antifungal therapy, who should have positive results of *Aspergillus* culture. We didn't process the sputum samples to obtain homogenized sputum or sputum plugs, and we didn't use high-volume culture or quantitative real-time polymerase chain reaction to detect *Aspergillus*, which might be responsible for the low positive rate (21–23). We plan to perform a prospective study and adopt more sensitive methods to detect *Aspergillus*. Thirdly, data collected from medical records could not help us screen out the patients with AH through hypersensitivity skin testing or IgE determination. We intend to verify the causal relationship and explore the impacts of AH in the prospective study. Besides, we do not have a comprehensive microbiological test result, which may have some influence on the conclusion. It is reported that changes in the microbiome of COPD patients' airways may be related to the risk of exacerbations (14, 24). After various stimulations induce an inflammatory response, the airway environment would be conducive to the growth of certain microorganisms. This leads to the disturbance and imbalance of the airway microbiome homeostasis, causing further airway inflammation and forming a vicious circle (25, 26). For instance, several studies have confirmed that COPD patients who are positive for *Pseudomonas aeruginosa* culture have a higher risk of acute exacerbations and higher mortality (27, 28). More comprehensive detection of the microbiome in the airway will be taken in our future prospective study.

In conclusion, we presented that *Aspergillus* colonization would lead to the relapse of exacerbation in hospitalized AECOPD patients in a short period. We should pay attention to the *Aspergillus* cultured in LRT samples. But the mechanisms and the adjustment of clinical strategies still require further studies.

AUTHOR CONTRIBUTIONS

Y-xW collected and analyzed the data and wrote the manuscript. Y-hZ screened the patients and checked the data. Q-jC, YH, Z-yB, X-yJ, X-wG, C-lT, W-pH, J-qH, W-qW, and F-yZ contributed to the data collection. JZ designed, supervised the study, and revised the manuscript. All authors contributed to the manuscript, read, and approved the submitted version.

ACKNOWLEDGMENTS

The authors would like to thank all the patients who cooperated with the collection of follow-up information and all the staff in the centers who helped with the study.

REFERENCES

1. Global Initiative for Chronic Obstructive Lung Disease. *Global Strategy for the Diagnosis, Management, and Prevention of Chronic Obstructive Pulmonary Disease (2021 report).* (2020). Available online at: https://goldcopd.org/2021-gold-reports/ (accessed November 24, 2018).
2. Dransfield MT, Kunisaki KM, Strand MJ, Anzueto A, Bhatt SP, Bowler RP, et al. Acute exacerbations and lung function loss in smokers with and without chronic obstructive pulmonary disease. *Am J Respir Crit Care Med.* (2017) 195:324–30. doi: 10.1164/rccm.201605-1014OC
3. Groenewegen KH, Schols AM, Wouters EF. Mortality and mortality-related factors after hospitalization for acute exacerbation of COPD. *Chest.* (2003) 124:459–67. doi: 10.1378/chest.124.2.459
4. Kim V, Aaron SD. What is a COPD exacerbation? Current definitions, pitfalls, challenges and opportunities for improvement. *Eur Respir J.* (2018) 52:1801261. doi: 10.1183/13993003.01261-2018
5. Bulpa P, Dive A, Sibille Y. Invasive pulmonary aspergillosis in patient with chronic obstructive pulmonary disease. *Eur Respir J.* (2007) 30:782–800. doi: 10.1183/09031936.00062206
6. Tong X, Cheng A, Xu H, Jin J, Yang Y, Zhu S, et al. *Aspergillus fumigatus* during COPD exacerbation: a pair-matched retrospective study. *BMC Pulm Med.* (2018) 18:55. doi: 10.1186/s12890-018-0611-y
7. Huerta A, Soler N, Esperatti M, Guerrero M, Menendez R, Gimeno A, et al. Importance of *Aspergillus* spp. isolation in acute exacerbations of severe COPD: prevalence, factors and follow-up: the FUNGI-COPD study. *Respir Res.* (2014) 15:17. doi: 10.1186/1465-9921-15-17
8. Connell D, Shah A. The contribution of *Aspergillus fumigatus* to COPD exacerbations: a "sensitive" topic. *Eur Respir J.* (2020) 56:2002223. doi: 10.1183/13993003.02223-2020
9. Guinea J, Torres-Narbona M, Gijón P, Muñoz P, Pozo F, Peláez T, et al. Pulmonary aspergillosis in patients with chronic obstructive pulmonary disease: incidence, risk factors, and outcome. *Clin Microbiol Infect.* (2010) 16:870–7. doi: 10.1111/j.1469-0691.2009.03015.x
10. Agarwal R, Hazarika B, Gupta D, Aggarwal AN, Chakrabarti A, Jindal SK. *Aspergillus* hypersensitivity in patients with chronic obstructive pulmonary disease: COPD as a risk factor for ABPA? *Med Mycol.* (2010) 48:988–94. doi: 10.3109/13693781003743148
11. Jin J, Liu X, Sun Y. The prevalence of increased serum IgE and *Aspergillus* sensitization in patients with COPD and their association with symptoms and lung function. *Respir Res.* (2014) 15:130. doi: 10.1186/s12931-014-0130-1
12. Bafadhel M, McKenna S, Agbetile J, Fairs A, Desai D, Mistry V, et al. *Aspergillus fumigatus* during stable state and exacerbations of COPD. *Eur Respir J.* (2014) 43:64–71. doi: 10.1183/09031936.00162912
13. Tiew PY, Ko FWS, Pang SL, Matta SA, Sio YY, Poh ME, et al. Environmental fungal sensitisation associates with poorer clinical outcomes in COPD. *Eur Respir J.* (2020) 56:2000418. doi: 10.1183/13993003.00418-2020

14. Tiew PY, Dicker AJ, Keir HR, Poh ME, Pang SL, Mac Aogáin M, et al. A high-risk airway mycobiome is associated with frequent exacerbation and mortality in COPD. *Eur Respir J.* (2020) 57:2002050. doi: 10.1183/13993003.02050-2020
15. Fairs A, Agbetile J, Hargadon B, Bourne M, Monteiro WR, Brightling CE, et al. IgE sensitization to *Aspergillus fumigatus* is associated with reduced lung function in asthma. *Am J Respir Crit Care Med.* (2010) 182:1362–8. doi: 10.1164/rccm.201001-0087OC
16. Everaerts S, Lagrou K, Dubbeldam A, Lorent N, Vermeersch K, Hoeyveld EV, et al. Sensitization to *Aspergillus fumigatus* as a risk factor for bronchiectasis in COPD. *Int J Chron Obstruct Pulmon Dis.* (2017) 12:2629–38. doi: 10.2147/COPD.S141695
17. Brummer E, Kamberi M, Stevens DA. Regulation by granulocyte-macrophage colony-stimulating factor and/or steroids given in vivo of proinflammatory cytokine and chemokine production by bronchoalveolar macrophages in response to *Aspergillus* conidia. *J Infect Dis.* (2003) 187:705–9. doi: 10.1086/368383
18. Duong M, Ouellet N, Simard M, Bergeron Y, Olivier M, Bergeron MG. Kinetic study of host defense and inflammatory response to *Aspergillus fumigatus* in steroid-induced immunosuppressed mice. *J Infect Dis.* (1998) 178:1472–82. doi: 10.1086/314425
19. Ng TT, Robson GD, Denning DW. Hydrocortisone-enhanced growth of *Aspergillus spp.*: implications for pathogenesis. *Microbiology (Reading).* (1994) 140:2475–9. doi: 10.1099/13500872-140-9-2475
20. Gago S, Overton NLD, Ben-ghazzi N, Novak-Frazer L, Read ND, Denning DW, et al. Lung colonization by *Aspergillus fumigatus* is controlled by ZNF77. *Nat Commun.* (2018) 9:3835. doi: 10.1038/s41467-018-06148-7
21. Fraczek MG, Kirwan MB, Moore CB, Morris J, Denning DW, Richardson MD. Volume dependency for culture of fungi from respiratory secretions and increased sensitivity of *Aspergillus* quantitative PCR. *Mycoses.* (2014) 57:69–78. doi: 10.1111/myc.12103
22. Pashley CH, Fairs A, Morley JP, Tailor S, Agbetile J, Bafadhel M, et al. Routine processing procedures for isolating filamentous fungi from respiratory sputum samples may underestimate fungal prevalence. *Med Mycol.* (2012) 50:433–8. doi: 10.3109/13693786.2011.615762
23. Vergidis P, Moore CB, Novak-Frazer L, Rautemaa-Richardson R, Walker A, Denning DW, et al. High-volume culture and quantitative real-time PCR for the detection of *Aspergillus* in sputum. Clin *Microbiol Infect.* (2020) 26:935–40. doi: 10.1016/j.cmi.2019.11.019
24. Han MK, Huang YJ, Lipuma JJ, Boushey HA, Boucher RC, Cookson WO, et al. Significance of the microbiome in obstructive lung disease. *Thorax.* (2012) 67:456–63. doi: 10.1136/thoraxjnl-2011-201183
25. Dickson RP, Martinez FJ, Huffnagle GB. The role of the microbiome in exacerbations of chronic lung diseases. *Lancet.* (2014) 384:691–702. doi: 10.1016/S0140-6736(14)61136-3
26. Dima E, Kyriakoudi A, Kaponi M, Vasileiadis I, Stamou P, Koutsoukou A, et al. The lung microbiome dynamics between stability and exacerbation in chronic obstructive pulmonary disease (COPD): current perspectives. *Respir Med.* (2019) 157:1–6. doi: 10.1016/j.rmed.2019.08.012
27. Jacobs DM, Ochs-Balcom HM, Noyes K, Zhao J, Leung WY, Pu CY, et al. Impact of *Pseudomonas aeruginosa* isolation on mortality and outcomes in an outpatient chronic obstructive pulmonary disease cohort. *Open Forum Infect Dis.* (2020) 7:ofz546. doi: 10.1093/ofid/ofz546
28. Eklöf J, Sørensen R, Ingebrigtsen TS, Sivapalan P, Achir I, Boel JB, et al. *Pseudomonas aeruginosa* and risk of death and exacerbations in patients with chronic obstructive pulmonary disease: an observational cohort study of 22 053 patients. *Clin Microbiol Infect.* (2020) 26:227–34. doi: 10.1016/j.cmi.2019.06.011

5

Effects of Exercise Intervention on Peripheral Skeletal Muscle in Stable Patients with COPD

Peijun Li[1], Jian Li[1], Yingqi Wang[1], Jun Xia[1*] and Xiaodan Liu[2,3*]

[1] Department of Sports Rehabilitation, Shanghai University of Sport, Shanghai, China, [2] School of Rehabilitation Science, Shanghai University of Traditional Chinese Medicine, Shanghai, China, [3] Institute of Rehabilitation Medicine, Shanghai University of Traditional Chinese Medicine, Shanghai, China

***Correspondence:**
Xiaodan Liu
hzhp403@126.com
Jun Xia
dx00122@163.com

Objectives: Peripheral skeletal muscle dysfunction is an important extrapulmonary manifestation of chronic obstructive pulmonary disease (COPD) that can be counteracted by exercise training. This study aimed to review the effect of three major exercise training modalities, which are used in pulmonary rehabilitation to improve on skeletal muscle mass, function, and exercise capacity in COPD.

Methods: PubMed, Embase, EBSCO, Web of Science, and the PEDro database were searched on April 25, 2020. Only randomized controlled studies published in English evaluating the effects of exercise interventions on peripheral skeletal muscle mass, strength, and exercise capacity in stable COPD patients were included. The quality of included studies was evaluated using the PEDro scale. The mean difference (MD) or the standardized mean difference (SMD) with 95% CI was calculated to summarize the results. Subgroup meta-analysis was used to investigate the effects of different exercise training modalities and different outcome measures. The Grading of Recommendations Assessment, Development, and Evaluation guidelines were used to rate evidence quality.

Results: A total of 30 randomized controlled trials involving 1,317 participants were included. Data from trials investigating endurance exercise (EE), resistance exercise (RE), and combined aerobic and resistance exercise (CE) were pooled into a meta-analysis, and the differences compared with the non-exercising COPD control were improvement in the muscle strength and exercise capacity in stable COPD patients. Subgroup meta-analysis for different exercise training modalities showed that RE significantly improved muscle strength (SMD = 0.6, 95% CI 0.35–0.84, I^2 = 61%), EE and CE significantly increased VO_{2peak} (EE: MD = 3.5, 95% CI 1.1–5.91, I^2 = 92%; CE: MD = 1.66, 95% CI 0.22–3.1, I^2 = 1%). Subgroup meta-analysis for different outcome measures showed that only isotonic strength was improved after exercise interventions (SMD = 0.89, 95% CI 0.51–1.26, I^2 = 71%).

Conclusion: Moderate evidence supports that exercise training in stable COPD patients has meaningful and beneficial effects on peripheral skeletal muscle strength and exercise capacity. Peripheral skeletal muscle shows a higher response to RE, and the isotonic test is relatively sensitive in reflecting muscle strength changes. The proportion of aerobic and resistance exercise components in a combined exercise program still needs exploration.

Systematic Review Registration: The review was registered with the PROSPERO: (The website is https://www.crd.york.ac.uk/PROSPERO/, and the ID is CRD42020164868).

Keywords: chronic obstructive pulmonary disease, exercise training, meta-analysis, skeletal muscle dysfunction, exercise capacity

INTRODUCTION

Chronic obstructive pulmonary disease (COPD) is a common disease characterized by persistent respiratory symptoms and expiratory flow limitation (1). Furthermore, many patients with COPD experience systematic symptoms, including impaired cardiopulmonary and skeletal muscle function (2, 3). Skeletal muscle dysfunction is one of the significant systemic manifestations of COPD, characterized by the loss of muscle mass, a transition of the fiber type proportion, a decrease in the capillary to fiber ratio, and muscle strength and endurance (4, 5). In most patients with COPD, the observed decrease in muscle strength is proportional to muscle mass loss, suggesting that the onset of skeletal muscle dysfunction is caused by paralleled chronic inactivity and muscle deconditioning rather than myopathy (6). The existence of dyspnea in COPD decreases physical activity, and the decrease in physical activity induces and accelerates skeletal muscle dysfunction, worsening the dyspnea in patients, forming a vicious cycle that causes further deconditioning on COPD (7). Recently, lower limb muscle function has been associated with exercise capacity in COPD (8). Previous studies have confirmed that skeletal muscle dysfunction is an additional important contributor to COPD exercise restriction and function impairments (9, 10), and it is closely related to the quality of life, readmission rate, and mortality (11, 12).

Pulmonary rehabilitation is a comprehensive management program designed for COPD and has significant clinical effects in improving dyspnea, quality of life, and exercise capacity (1). As the cornerstone of pulmonary rehabilitation, exercise training can effectively reverse or at least stabilize the loss of skeletal muscle mass and strength in patients with COPD, and it is considered currently the most effective non-pharmaceutical intervention for COPD skeletal muscle dysfunction (13). The American Thoracic Society/European Respiratory Society (ATS/ERS) statement provided a short overview of the effects of exercise interventions on the muscle function and mass in COPD, showing that exercise interventions can improve the morphology and function of COPD skeletal muscle (12), but the included literatures are extensive and heterogeneous. Another international guideline described and analyzed the effects of different exercise modalities in COPD skeletal muscle dysfunction and provided a GRADE scale for evidence quality (4). In 2018, a review included 70 English language literature to be analyzed and concluded that exercise intervention could improve COPD skeletal muscle strength, endurance, and mass, despite the fact that intervention programs and outcome measures were heterogeneous (14). Therefore, although previous international guidelines and recent reviews have consistently concluded that exercise training improves COPD skeletal muscle dysfunction, it is still difficult to clarify the degree of real benefit due to the diversity and heterogeneity of exercise intervention programs and outcome measures. Previous meta-analysis of exercise in COPD explored the effects of resistance exercise (RE) on exercise capacity (15), endurance exercise (EE) vs. RE (16), and combined aerobic and resistance exercise (CE) vs. EE on lower limb muscle strength and exercise capacity (17). However, these studies focused on the effects of single exercise modality or the compared effects of two exercise modalities. There is still a lack of comprehensive quantitative effect of exercise on peripheral skeletal muscle mass, strength, and exercise capacity in COPD.

In this systematic review and meta-analysis, the effects of exercise interventions on peripheral skeletal muscle mass, strength, and exercise capacity in COPD were determined. The characteristics of different exercise modalities were further discussed to provide a theoretical reference for developing a targeted COPD exercise rehabilitation program.

METHODS

Search Strategy and Selection Criteria

This systematic review and meta-analysis was registered (PROSPERO registration number: CRD42020164868) and conducted according to the preferred reporting items for systematic reviews and meta-analysis (PRISMA) recommendations (18). According to the principle of population intervention comparison outcomes, the inclusion criteria were as follows: (a) participants diagnosed with stable COPD, and without gender and age restrictions; (b) EE and or RE was used for intervention; (c) a comparable control group applied with other treatments, including health education and sham training;

Abbreviations: 6MWD, 6-min walking distance; ATS/ERS, the American Thoracic Society/European Respiratory Society; BMI, body mass index; CE, combined aerobic and resistance exercise; COPD, chronic obstructive pulmonary disease; CPET, cardiopulmonary exercise test; CSA, cross-sectional area; EE, endurance exercise; FEV_1, forced expiratory volume in 1 s; FFM, fat-free mass index; GOLD, Global strategy for the diagnosis, management, and prevention of chronic obstructive pulmonary disease; GRADE, the Grading of Recommendations Assessment, Development and Evaluation; MD, mean difference; MeSH, medical subject headings; OR, odds ratio; PEDro, the Physiotherapy Evidence Database; PRISMA, the Preferred Reporting Items for Systematic Reviews and Meta-Analysis; RE, resistance exercise; SMD, standardized mean difference; VO_{2peak}, peak oxygen consumption.

(d) outcomes including skeletal muscle mass related parameters (body mass index, BMI; fat-free mass index, FFM; and cross-sectional area, CSA), strength-related parameters (isometric, isotonic, and isokinetic strength), endurance exercise capacity (6-min walking distance, 6MWD), and peak exercise capacity (peak oxygen consumption, VO_{2peak}); and (e) randomized controlled study published in English. The exclusion criteria were as follows: (a) the immediate response to a single exercise test or exercise session was studied; (b) the follow-up effects of previous exercise program were studied; (c) traditional Chinese exercise and yoga were used for interventions; (d) animal trials, observational trials, expert opinions, literature reviews, comments, and letters were involved; (e) regular exercise programs were utilized in control groups (e.g., breath training, ≥twice a week); and (f) data could not be extracted.

Electronic searches of PubMed, Embase, EBSCO, Web of Science, and PEDro database were conducted from inception to April 25, 2020 using Medical Subject Headings (MeSH) terms and free-text keywords. In addition to the PEDro database, the following search terms were used: (COPD OR chronic obstructive pulmonary disease OR chronic obstructive lung disease OR chronic obstructive airway disease) AND (exercise OR exercise training OR rehabilitation OR pulmonary rehabilitation OR aerobic exercise OR endurance exercise OR resistance exercise OR strength training OR combined exercise) AND (muscle OR skeletal muscle). Search filters were applied, including article type (randomized controlled trials), species (humans), and language (English). In the PEDro database, the search terms were as follows: topic (chronic respiratory disease), method (clinical trial), therapy (fitness training), and abstract and title (COPD). Searches were supplemented by reviewing the reference lists of the included studies, previous review, meta-analysis, and guidelines.

To determine the eligibility of identified studies, two investigators independently conducted the process of study selection. Cohen's kappa was used to quantify the interrater agreement. Discrepancies of opinion between authors about study eligibility were resolved through discussions with a third investigator.

Data Analysis

Two investigators independently extracted data on study design, sample characteristics, intervention programs, and effects of exercise from included studies. Discrepancies were resolved through discussions with a third investigator. The studies were described in terms of study design (sample size, and PEDro score), sample characteristics (age, sex, FEV1%pred for forced expiratory volume in 1 s, and BMI), intervention programs (site, exercise modality, intensity, frequency, and duration), effects of exercise (outcome measures and change data), and adherence to the program. For trials with more than one exercise intervention group, the effects of each exercise intervention were evaluated. For trials with more than one outcome measures, the data of each outcome measures was included and analyzed. For trials with multiple time points, only the pre-intervention and post-intervention outcomes were extracted.

Predetermined primary outcomes included skeletal muscle mass (BMI, FFM, and CSA), strength (isometric, isotonic, and isokinetic strength), endurance exercise capacity (6MWD), and peak exercise capacity (VO_{2peak}). Secondary outcomes were attrition rate and severe adverse events. The change in mean and SD were calculated for each outcome and used to estimate the effects of the exercise. Summary measures for continuous outcomes were mean difference (MD) or standard mean difference (SMD) with 95% CI, and odds ratio (OR) with 95% CI for the attrition rate.

Review Manager (version 5.3) provided by Cochrane was used for meta-analysis. Random-effects model was used for analyzing. The I^2 statistic, representing the percentage of variation across studies due to heterogeneity, was used to assess heterogeneity between studies. Planned subgroup analyses were conducted in terms of exercise modalities (EE, RE, and CE) and outcome measures (isometric, isotonic, and isokinetic strength test). Sensitivity analyses were performed to check the heterogeneity source based on the intervention program and characteristics of the participants when subgroup analysis could not determine the source of substantial heterogeneity. Visual inspection of funnel plots and Egger's test were undertaken in Stata (version 15) to assess publication bias. Trim and fill method was used when there was a publication bias. The methodological quality of randomized controlled trial (RCTs) was assessed using the physiotherapy evidence database (PEDro) scale. When available, the PEDro rating and score were obtained from the PEDro database. Otherwise, two investigators independently rated and scored the publications; discrepancies were resolved through discussions with a third investigator. The PEDro scale includes 11 items with 10 scores, and a higher score means better quality (19). It should be noted that the eligibility criteria item does not contribute to the total score. PEDro scale 9–10 was considered high quality, 6–8 was generally high quality, 4–5 was moderate quality, and <4 was low quality. The quality of evidence was assessed according to the Grading of Recommendations Assessment, Development, and Evaluation (GRADE) recommendations (limitation of study design, inconsistency, indirectness, imprecision, and publication bias) (20).

RESULTS

A total of 2,665 records were identified, and 30 RCTs were included in the quantitative analysis (**Figure 1**). A strong agreement was observed with respect to the interrater reliability of study selection (kappa $= 0.89$, $P < 0.001$). The PEDro scale of all included studies is 5.7 ± 1.4 (**Supplementary Table S1**), and the characteristics of participants of each included study are reported in **Table 1**. A total of 1,317 participants with stable COPD (age range from 46 to 79.8 years) were included, and 675 (51%) participants accepted exercise intervention. According to the criteria of Global strategy for the diagnosis, management, and prevention of COPD (GOLD), majority of the participants showed moderate to severe airflow restriction (30% ≤ FEV1%pred ≤ 80%), and four studies did not provide the

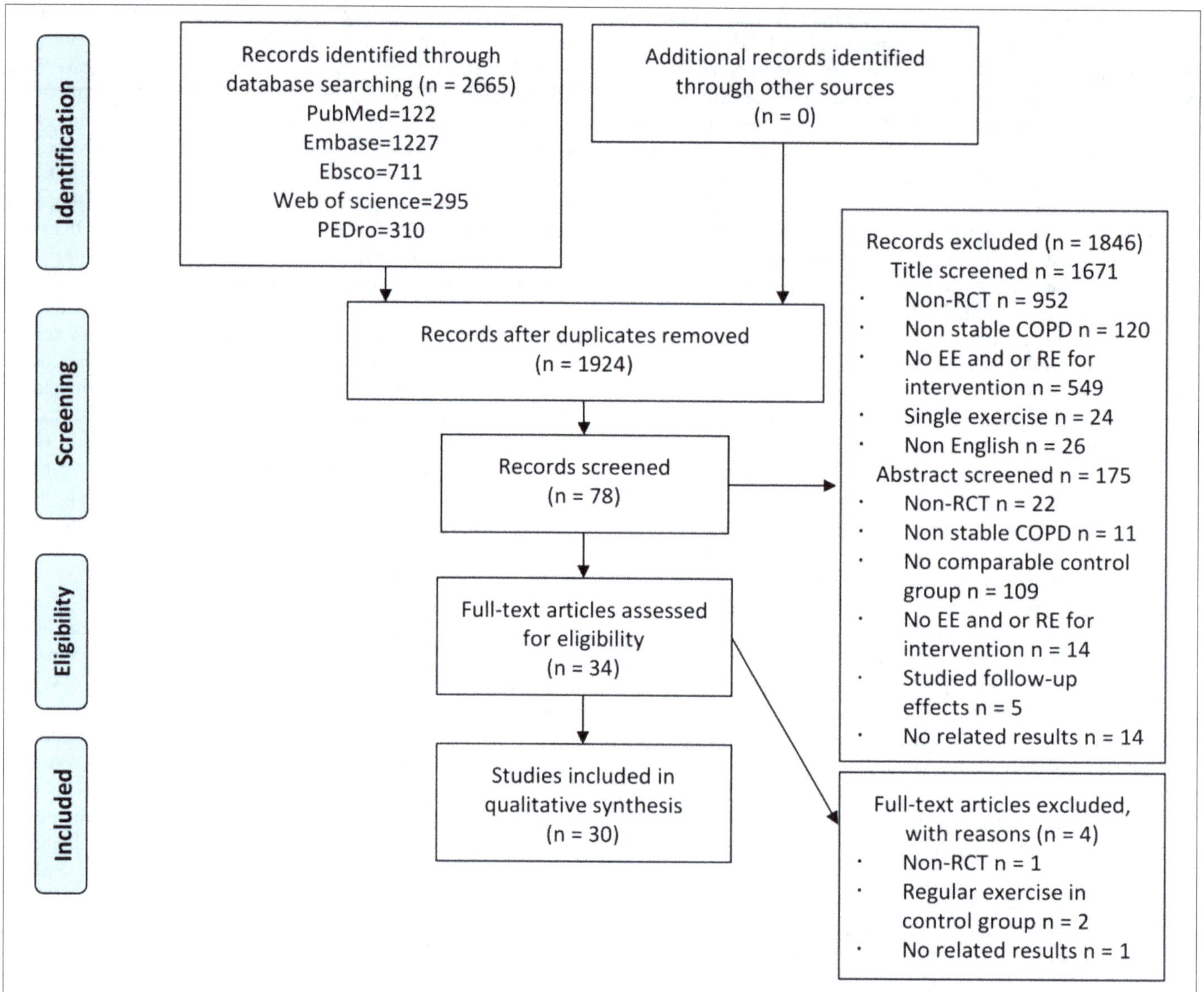

FIGURE 1 | Study flow diagram. COPD, chronic obstructive pulmonary disease; EE, endurance exercise; RCT, randomized controlled trial; RE, resistance exercise.

baseline data of FEV1%pred (27, 30, 38, 41). Most participants were normal to overweight (BMI: 18.5–29.9 kg/cm^2), while five studies did not provide this data (27, 38, 39, 42, 49). In addition, exercise intervention programs of all the included studies are presented in **Table 2**. Most trials were conducted in a hospital, at home, or at both the places, while six studies did not report a place (31, 35, 38, 40, 45, 50). Most studies applied exercise program duration ranges from 6 to 12 weeks, while some studies applied 14 weeks (22), 16 weeks (47), and 24 weeks (38). EE was mainly performed in the form of treadmill, cycling, or walking with a moderate to vigorous exercise intensity (Borg 4–6, even exhaustion, despite indexes used to assess were various) for two to three sessions per week. RE was mainly performed on weight machines, free weights, and elastic bands through the movements of the upper and lower limbs. One study performed RE only through the upper limbs (35) and three studies conducted RE only through the lower limbs (31, 33, 34). Exercise intensity of RE ranged from 50 to 85% 1-repetition maximum (1RM) or Borg 4–6, and exercise frequency was two to three sessions per week. The performance of CE was consistent with EE and RE. The exercise intensity of EE was Borg 4–6, while the exercise intensity of RE was often unclear. The characteristics of muscle strength testing relative to the variety of muscle strength testing methods and programs are summarized in **Table 3**.

Five studies (21, 31, 32, 34, 47) provided data on skeletal muscle mass, assessed by mid-thigh CSA, BMI, FFMI, and total lean mass. In the meta-analysis, the estimated results showed that exercise intervention did not have a significant effect on changes in BMI (MD = −0.11, 95% CI: 1.13–0.91, I^2 = 84%, **Figure 2**). Considering the high heterogeneity detected, we excluded studies with PEDro < 6, and found a significant improvement in BMI (MD = 0.26, 95% CI 0.23–0.29, I^2 = 0%). In addition, a CE

TABLE 1 | Characteristics of included studies.

Author, Country	I/C sample size/Male%	Age	FEV1%pred	BMI	Outcome			Attrition number*	PEDro
					Mass	Strength	Exercise capacity		
Endurance exercise									
Alcazar et al. (21), Spain	14(79%)/ 15(87%)	77.7 ± 7.9/ 79.8 ± 6.4	47.4 ± 18.1/ 58.7 ± 15.2	28.8 ± 3/ 32.5 ± 5.9	Mid-thigh CSA	Leg press	6MWD VO_{2peak}	5/1*	4
Barakat et al. (22), France	40(85%)/ 40(83%)	63.7 ± 11.9/ 65.9 ± 10.3	41.9 ± 2.6/ 43.33 ± 3.6	24.2 ± 6.4/ 25.6 ± 4.3	/	/	6MWD	5/4*	6
Borghi-silva et al. (23), USA	20(65%)/ 14(86%)	67 ± 10/ 67 ± 10	33 ± 9/ 35 ± 11	25 ± 4/ 24 ± 5	/	/	6MWD VO_{2peak}	0/6	5
Borghi-silva et al. (24), USA	10(70%)/ 10(50%)	67 ± 7/ 66 ± 10	32 ± 11/ 35 ± 12	23.4 ± 4.4/ 27.2 ± 4.7	/	/	6MWD VO_{2peak}	7/5	5
de Souto Araujo et al. (25), Brazil	13(62%)/ 11(73%)	56.9 ± 7.9/ 71.1 ± 10.1	39.2 ± 11.4/ 45.1 ± 12.6	30 ± 10.1/ 24.4 ± 6.7	/	/	6MWD	1/3	4
Gallo-Silva et al. (26), Brazil	10/9	66.3 ± 6.5/ 66.5 ± 9.5	47.9 ± 20.5/ 47.8 ± 26.2	23.2 ± 2.6/ 25.7 ± 6.1	/	/	6MWD	2/3	6
Mehri et al. (27), Iran	20(55%)/ 18(39%)	52.1 ± 10.7/ 52.17 ± 11.6	/	/	/	/	VO_{2peak}	0/0	5
Petersen et al. (28), Denmark	9(22%)/ 10(40%)	67 ± 3/ 66 ± 3	33 ± 5/ 30 ± 4	23 ± 2/ 26 ± 2	/	/	VO_2 max	0/4	5
Pradella et al. (29), Brazil	29(79%)/ 15(87%)	62.4 ± 10.7/ 65.3 ± 8	43.9 ± 16.2/ 54 ± 22.2	25.2 ± 5/ 26.7 ± 5.3	/	/	6MWD	3/3	5
Wiyono et al. (30), Indonesia	27(93%)/ 29(96%)	64.3 ± 6.3/ 67.2 ± 4.5	/	19.7 ± 8.5/ 20.2 ± 6.4	/	/	6MWD VO_2 max	3/1	5
Resistance exercise									
Casaburi et al. (31), USA	12 (100%)/ 12(100%)	68.9 ± 9.8/ 67.7 ± 8.7	35.9 ± 9.2/ 38.6 ± 12.1	27.57/ 26.31	Total lean mass	Leg press	VO_{2peak}	1/1	5
Clark et al. (32), Scotland	26(58%)/ 17(59%)	51 ± 10/ 46 ± 11	76 ± 23/ 79 ± 23	26 ± 4/ 26 ± 4	BMI	Quadriceps	VO_2 max		5
Chen et al. (33), China	25(88%)/ 22(68%)	69.04 ± 8.07/ 64.95 ± 11.59	54.49 ± 23.62/ 54.93 ± 25.58	23.86 ± 3.9/ 24.15 ± 3.93	/	Quadriceps	6MWD	4/4	6
Hoff et al. (34), USA	6(67%)/ 6(67%)	62.8 ± 1.4/ 60.6 ± 3	32.9 ± 3.3/ 39.5 ± 6.4	26.27/ 26.65	BMI	Leg press	VO_{2peak}	0/0	6
Janaudis-Ferreira et al. (35), Canada	17(53%)/ 19(37%)	67 ± 11/ 67 ± 11	37.8 ± 16.2/ 32.5 ± 14.1	27.9 ± 7.9/ 25.7 ± 8.2	/	Biceps Triceps Anterior Middle deltoids	/	4/1*	9
Nyberg et al. (36), Sweden	22(55%)/ 22(50%)	69 ± 5/ 68 ± 6	59 ± 11/ 55 ± 15	26 ± 4/ 25 ± 5	/	Shoulder flexion Knee extension	6MWD	2/2*	8
O'shea et al. (37), Australia	27/27	66.9 ± 7/ 68.4 ± 9.9	49 ± 25/ 52 ± 22	25.5 ± 5.1/ 27.8 ± 7.9	/	Knee extension Hip abduction Shoulder horizontal flexion Shoulder flexion	6MWD	7/3*	7
Thabitha et al. (38), India	30	/	/	/	/	/	6MWD VO_{2peak}	/	4
Simpson et al. (39), Canada	14(35%)/ 14(71%)	73 ± 4.8/ 70 ± 5.7	39.5 ± 18.96/ 39.2 ± 21.39	/	/	Elbow flexion Quadriceps Leg press	6MWD VO_2 max	3/3	6
Zambom-Ferraresi et al. (40), Spain	14(100%)/ 8(100%)	68 ± 7/ 69 ± 5	48 ± 12/ 39.7 ± 5	28.5 ± 3.9/ 25.7 ± 4.6	/	Leg press Chest press	6MWD VO_{2peak}	1/1	7
Combined exercise									
Cameron-Tucker et al. (41), Australia	43(53%)/ 41(54%)	64.5 ± 9.3/ 67.1 ± 9.41	/	28.4 ± 7.63/ 29.7 ± 6.5	/	/	6MWD	5/10*	6
Emery et al. (42), USA	30(50%)/ 24(42%)	65.4 ± 6.4/ 67.4 ± 5.9	43 ± 18/ 43 ± 18	/	/	/	VO_2 max	4/2*	6

(Continued)

TABLE 1 | Continued

Author, Country	I/C sample size/Male%	Age	FEV1%pred	BMI	Outcome			Attrition number*	PEDro
					Mass	Strength	Exercise capacity		
Lahham et al. (43), Australia	29(59%)/ 29(59%)	68 ± 9/ 67 ± 10	90 ± 8/ 92 ± 7	28 ± 4.5/ 28 ± 4.3	/	/	6MWD	3/4*	8
Mendes et al. (44), Brazil	23(83%)/ 29(66%)	71.3 ± 6.7/ 70.8 ± 8.7	51.5 ± 23.9/ 41.4 ± 18.4	23.5 ± 4.2/ 24.6 ± 6.3	/	/	6MWD	23/0	4
Nakamura et al. (45), Japan	10/ 10	69 ± 8.7/ 69.9 ± 7.1	53.2 ± 15.1/ 48.2 ± 20.1	21.9 ± 3.5/ 21.6 ± 3	/	HGF	6MWD VO_{2peak}	/	5
Tsai et al. (46), Australia	19(63%)/ 17(35%)	78 ± 3/ 75 ± 9	60 ± 23/ 68 ± 19	28 ± 4/ 28 ± 5	/	/	6MWD	1/0	8
van Wetering et al. (47), Netherlands	102(71%)/ 97(71%)	65.9 ± 8.8 / 67.2 ± 8.9	58 ± 17/ 60 ± 15	26.1 ± 4.4/ 27.3 ± 4.7	BMI FFMI	HGF Quadriceps	6MWD	15/9*	7
Wadell et al. (48), Canada	17(53%)/ 24(54%)	68 ± 6/ 66 ± 7	48 ± 12/ 48 ± 19	26.7 ± 4.9/ 28.9 ± 4.3	/	Knee extension	6MWD	3/ 4*	6
Wadell et al. (49), Sweden	15(33%)/ 13(54%)	65 ± 7/ 63 ± 7	53 ± 12/ 49 ± 12	/	/	/	VO_{2peak}	1/ 1*	6
Weiner et al. (50), Israel	18/ 5	63.2 ± 2.3/ 60.1 ± 2.8	35 ± 2.2/ 36 ± 1.9	23.84/ 24.84	/	/	6MWD	1/1*	5
Zambom-Ferraresi et al. (40), Spain	14(100%)/ 8(100%)	68 ± 7/ 69 ± 5	44.3 ± 11.9/ 39.7 ± 5	29.3 ± 6.4/ 25.7 ± 4.6	/	Leg press Chest press	6MWD VO_{2peak}	2/1	7

6MWD, 6-min walking distance; HGF, Handgrip force; I/C, Intervention group/Control group; RM, Repetition maximum; VO_2, Oxygen uptake.
*/Not accessible; *Attrition number is included in the sample size.*

program significantly improved FFMI (P = 0.01) (47), an EE program significantly improved the mid-thigh CSA (+4.5%, P < 0.05) of elderly patients with COPD (age: 77.7 ± 7.9 years old) (21), an RE program only found an increasing trend in the total lean mass (31). A total of 13 studies (21, 31–37, 39, 40, 45, 47, 48) with 27 data on skeletal muscle strength were provided, demonstrating a significant improvement after exercise intervention (SMD = 0.58, 95% CI 0.21–0.95, I^2 = 89%). Considering the high heterogeneity detected, we first excluded studies with PEDro < 6, and found a consistent result with high heterogeneity (SMD = 0.62, 95% CI 0.19–1.05, I^2 = 91%). Then, we only pooled data in kilograms unit, and found a consistent result (MD = 0.78, 95% CI 0.64–0.92, I^2 = 0%) besides the isometric strength test. Finally, subgroup analysis for different exercise modalities (**Figure 3**), muscle strength measures (**Figure 4**), and upper or lower limbs muscle strength found that RE provided significant benefits (SMD = 0.6, 95% CI 0.35–0.84, I^2 = 61%), isometric strength significantly improved (SMD = 0.89, 95% CI 0.51–1.26, I^2 =71%), and both upper and lower limbs muscle strength significantly improved (SMD = 0.78, 95% CI 0.4–1.17, I^2 = 79%; SMD = 0.67, 95% CI 0.12–1.22, I^2 = 91%).

A total of 22 studies (21–26, 29, 30, 33, 36–41, 43–48, 50) provided data on endurance exercise capacity, demonstrating a significant improvement in 6MWD after exercise intervention (MD = 26.64, 95% CI 15.38–37.91, I^2 = 77%). Subgroup analysis for different exercise modalities showed a consistent result, namely that all EE, RE, and CE can improve 6MWD significantly (EE: MD = 40.99, 95% CI 34.65–47.32, I^2 = 0%; RE: MD = 22.32, 95% CI 6.76–37.89, I^2 = 0%; CE: MD=11.89, 95% CI 10.81–12.97, I^2 = 0%, **Figure 5**). A total of 13 studies (21, 23, 27, 28, 30, 32, 34, 36, 38, 40, 42, 45, 49) provided data on the peak exercise capacity, demonstrating a significant improvement in VO_{2peak} after exercise intervention (MD = 1.82, 95% CI 0.62–3.02, I^2 =77%). Subgroup analysis for different exercise modalities showed that EE and CE can improve VO_{2peak} significantly (EE: MD = 3.5, 95% CI 1.1–5.91, I^2 =92%; CE: MD = 1.66, 95% CI 0.22–3.1, I^2 =1%, **Figure 5**). Considering that the methodological quality of included studies in EE was relatively low (PEDro < 6), the results need to be carefully considered.

There was no difference of attrition number between exercise and control group (OR = 1.12, 95% CI 0.75–1.67, I^2 = 15%, **Supplementary Figure S1**). The reasons for attrition in the exercise and control groups were similar (**Supplementary Table S2**).

Funnel plots are presented in **Supplementary Figure S2**. The results of Egger's test showed a significant publication bias in the results of skeletal muscle strength and 6MWD (P = 0.031 and P = 0.018, respectively). Then, the trim and fill method was used to adjust the impact of publication bias, and the results showed 0 missing studies for skeletal muscle strength results, and five missing studies for 6MWD results were merged to diminish the publication bias (**Supplementary Figure S3**). The certainty of the evidence for endurance and peak exercise capacity was deemed moderate, for skeletal muscle strength was deemed low, and for BMI was deemed very low (**Table 4**).

DISCUSSION

This systematic review and meta-analysis confirmed that regular exercise intervention for more than 6 weeks can effectively

TABLE 2 | Characteristics of intervention protocols.

Author,Country	Setting	Intervention contents	Intervention intensity	Intervention duration/ frequency	Control group
Endurance exercise					
Alcazar et al. (21), Spain	Outpatient	First 3 weeks: HIIT (5 sets of 90 s at light intensity plus 30 s at heavy intensity) + power training (2–3 sets of 8–12 reps) Week 4–12: HIIT (10stes) + 3sets of 8reps with the optimal load	First 3 weeks: HIIT (heavy-80%W_{peak}, light-40% W_{peak}) + power training (50–60% 1RM) Week 4–12: HIIT (augmented) + power training (optimal load)	2 sessions/week, 12 weeks	Usual care
Barakat et al. (22), France	Outpatient	30 min cycling + 30 min aerobic activity (5 min warm-up, 10 min aerobic activity, 15 min cool-down)	Cycle: 80%VO_2 max	3 sessions/week, 14 weeks	Routine outpatient attendance
Borghi-Silva et al. (23), USA	Outpatient	30 min stretching + treadmill ambulation	70% of the maximal speed	3 sessions/week, 6 weeks	Usual care
Borghi-Silva et al. (24), USA	Outpatient	5 min warm-up + 30 min treadmill	70% of the peak speed/Borg 4	3 sessions/week, 12 weeks	Respiratory therapy, 1session/week
de Sauto Araujo et al. (25), Brazil	Outpatient	15 min callisthenic activities + 30 min unsupported upper limb exercise using weights + 30 min bicycle + 15 min cool-down	Upper: 50% of the maximum load; Lower: Borg 5	3 sessions/week, 8 weeks	No exercise
Gallo-Silva et al. (26), Brazil	Laboratory	60 min water aerobic interval exercise (10 min warm-up, 20–40min aerobic exercise, 10 min cool-down)	Borg 4–6	3 sessions/week, 8 weeks	Usual care
Mehri et al. (27), Iran	Outpatient	Treadmill exercise training with gradually increased speed	Exhaustion	2 sessions/week, 8 weeks	No exercise
Petersen et al. (28), Denmark	Outpatient	Walking with 85% maximal speed + progressive ergometer cycling	Exhaustion	2 sessions/week, 7 weeks	Usual daily activities
Pradella et al. (29), Brazil	Home	40 min walking + 15 min stair exercise + arm exercise with 1 kg load (3 sets of 30 movements)	Walking: 60–70% HR_{max}	3 sessions/week, 8 weeks	No exercise
Wiyono et al. (30), Indonesia	Outpatient	5 min cycling, and gradually increased for 5 min/week	/	3 sessions/week, 6 weeks	Routine outpatient attendance
Resistance exercise					
Casaburi et al. (31), USA	/	First 4 weeks: 3 sets of 12 reps; Week 5–10: 4 sets of 8–10 reps (seated leg press, seated leg curl, seated leg extension, standing calf raise, seated ankle dorsiflexion)	First 4 weeks: 60% 1RM Week 5–10: 80% 1RM	3 sessions/week, 10 weeks	No exercise
Clark et al. (32), Scotland	Outpatient	3 sets of 10 reps weight exercises (bench press/triceps, body squat/quadriceps, squat calf/medial and lateral gastrocnemiius soleus, latissimus/latissimus dorsi/arm curls/biceps, leg press/quadriceps hamstrings gluteals, knee flexion/quadriceps, hamstrings)	70% maximal load	2 sessions/week, 12 weeks	Usual daily activities
Chen et al. (33), China	Home	20–30min, 8–12 reps Thera-band exercise (straight-leg lifting, prone hip extension, thigh abduction, posterior muscle group exercises, anterior muscle group exercises, and standing calf raise)	Borg 5	3 sessions/week, 12 weeks	No exercise
Hoff et al. (34), USA	Laboratory	4 sets of 5 reps concentric contraction of quadriceps	85–90% 1RM	3 sessions/week, 8 weeks	Normal daily living
Janaudis-Ferreira et al. (35), Canada	/	10–12RM using free weights and a multistation gym (biceps brachii, triceps brachii, pectoralis major and minor, latissimus dorsi, deltoids, rhomoboids)	10–12RM	3 sessions/week, 6 weeks	Upper limb flexibility and stretching exercises
Nyberg et al. (36), Sweden	Outpatient	40 min, 2 sets of 25 reps Thera-band exercise (Latissimus row/chest press/leg extension/shoulder flexion/leg curl/elbow flexion/heel-raise/step up)	Borg 4	3 sessions/week, 8 weeks	No exercise

(Continued)

TABLE 2 | Continued

Author, Country	Setting	Intervention contents	Intervention intensity	Intervention duration/ frequency	Control group
O'shea et al. (37), Australia	1 hospital + 2 home	3 sets of 8–12 reps Thera-band exercise (hip abduction in standing, simulated lifting, SST, seated row, lunges, chest press)	12RM and gradually increased	3 sessions/week, 12 weeks	No exercise
Thabitha et al. (38), India	/	15–30min, 1–3 sets of 10 reps using multi exerciser (chest pull-lattismus dorsi, butterfly-pectoralis major muscle, neck press-triceps brachii and deltoid, leg flexion-biceps femoris and gastronemious, leg extension)	10RM and increased by 10%	2 sessions/day, 3 days/week, 24 weeks	No exercise
Simpson et al. (39), Canada	Outpatient	3 sets of 10 reps single limb weight lifting exercise (arm curl/leg extension/leg press)	50–85% 1RM	3 sessions/week, 8 weeks	No exercise
Zambom-Ferraresi et al. (40), Spain	/	90 min, 3–4 sets of 6–12 reps (chest press, seated row, shoulder press, leg press, knee extension and flexion)	50–70% 1RM	2 sessions/week, 12 weeks	Habitual physical activity
Combined exercise					
Cameron-Tucker et al. (41), Australia	Outpatient	1 h combine exercises, individualized for each participant	RPE 3–5	1 sessions/week, 6 weeks	No exercise
Emery et al. (42), USA	Outpatient	First 5 weeks: 45 min combine exercises on Nautilus equipment; Week 6–10: 60–90 min	/	First 5 weeks: every-day; Week 6–10: 3 sessions/week	No exercise
Lahham et al. (43), Australia	Home	Aerobic: 80% of walking speed from 6MWD + 30 min whole-body exercise; Resistance: using equipment available at home (stairs and sealed water bottles)	/	5 sessions/week, 8 weeks	No exercise
Mendes et al. (44), Brazil	Outpatient	Aerobic: 30 min treadmill walking; Resistance: 10 reps (hand weight, elbow flexion, elbow abduction, shoulder abduction, shoulder flexion, hip flexion, knee extension)	Aerobic: 60–80% HR_{max} Resistance: 50% 1RM with an increase of 0.5 kg every 2 weeks	3 sessions/week, 12 weeks	No exercise
Nakamura et al. (45), Japan	/	Aerobic: 20 min walking; Resistance: 30 min, 3 sets of 10 reps using self-weight or elastic bands (push-ups, leg squats, sit-ups, back extension)	Aerobic: Borg 3–5	12 weeks	No exercise
Tsai et al. (46), Australia	Home	Aerobic: 15–20 min cycling + 15–20 min walking Resistance: 3 sets of 10 reps SST and squats exercise	Cycle: 60–80% W_{peak} Walk: 80% of best 6MWD or Aerobic: Borg 3–4	3 sessions/week, 8 weeks	Usual care
van Wetering et al. (47), Netherlands	Community	Aerobic: 30 min cycling/walking Resistance: 4 specific exercises for upper and lower limbs	/	2 sessions/week, 16 weeks	Usual care
Wadell et al. (48), Canada	Outpatient	2.5 h combine exercise	Moderate intensity	3 sessions/week, 8 weeks	Usual care
Wadell et al. (49), Sweden	Outpatient	45 min, (4 min aerobic, 3 min leg resistance, 4 min aerobic, 3 min arm resistance, 4 min aerobic, 3 min torso resistance)	80–100%HR peak or Borg 5 or RPE 15	3 sessions/week, 12 weeks	No exercise
Weiner et al. (50), Israel	/	Aerobic: 30 min cycling; Resistance: 15 min rowing with low resistance +15 min resistance exercises for limbs and abdominal muscles	Aerobic: 50% W_{max}	3 sessions/week, 6 weeks	Sham training
Zambom-Ferraresi et al. (40), Spain	/	Aerobic: 20–35 min cycle Resistance: 90 min, 3–4 sets of 6–12 reps (chest press, seated row, shoulder press, leg press, knee extension and flexion)	Aerobic: 40–85% W_{max} Resistance: 50–70% 1RM	2 sessions/week for each exercise types, 12 weeks	Habitual physical activity

6MWD, 6-min walking distance; HIIT, high intensity interval training; HGF, Handgrip force; HR, Heart rate; reps, repetitions; RM, Repetition maximum; SST, sit to stand; W_{max}, Maximal work rate; VO_2, Oxygen uptake.
/Not accessible.

improve peripheral skeletal muscle strength and exercise capacity of patients with stable COPD. Furthermore, the greatest improvement in peripheral skeletal muscle strength appears in RE, the greatest improvement in endurance exercise capacity (6MWD: 40.99 m) appears in EE, and both EE and CE can significantly improve the peak exercise capacity.

TABLE 3 | Characteristics of skeletal muscle strength tests.

Type	Author, Country	Outcomes	Methods	Apparatus	Site
Isometric test	Alcazar et al. (21), Spain	Leg press (N)	Evaluate two legs performance, test for at least 4s	Force plate	Lower limb
	Chen et al. (33), China	Quadriceps (Nm)	Evaluate the maximal strength of dominant leg	Computerized dynamometer	Lower limb
	Janaudis-Ferreira et al. (35), Canada	Biceps (kg) Triceps (kg) Anterior (kg) Middle deltoids (kg)	Evaluate the dominant side by Micro FET2, the average of the highest 3 measures were used for analysis	Hand-held dynamometer	Upper limb
	Nakamura et al. (45), Japan	HGF (kg)	Evaluate the dominant side	Hand-grip dynamometer	Upper limb
	Wadell et al. (48), Canada	Knee extension (kg)		Fixed dynamometer	Lower limb
	van Wetering et al. (47), Netherlands	HGF (kg) Quadriceps (Nm)		Unknown device	Upper limb Lower limb
Isotonic test	Casaburi et al. (31), USA	Leg press (kg)	Evaluate two legs performance by 1RM test	Pneumatic device	Lower limb
	Clark et al. (32), Scotland	Quadriceps (kg)	1RM test	Multigym	
	Hoff et al. (34), USA	Leg press (kg)	1RM test	Force platform	
	O'shea et al. (37), Australia	Knee extension (kg) Hip abduction (kg) Shoulder horizontal flexion (kg) Shoulder flexion (kg)	Averaged across right and left limbs were used for analysis	Hand-held dynamometry	Lower limb Lower limb Upper limb Upper limb
	Simpson et al. (39), Canada	Elbow flexion (kg) Quadriceps (kg) Leg press (kg)	Unilateral 1RM test	Unknown device	Upper limb Lower limb
	Zambom-Ferraresi et al. (40), Spain	Leg press (kg) Chest press (kg)	1RM test	Force plate	Lower limb Upper limb
Isokinetic test	Chen et al. (33), China	Quadriceps (Nm)	Evaluate the maximal strength of dominant leg	Computerized dynamometer	Lower limb
	Nyberg et al. (36), Sweden	Shoulder flexion (Nm) Knee extension (Nm)	The highest of 5 maximal contractions was used for analysis	Computerized dynamometer	Upper limb Lower limb

Kg, Kilogram; HGF, Handgrip force; N, Newton; RM, Repetition maximum.

Study or Subgroup	Exercise Mean	Exercise SD	Exercise Total	Control Mean	Control SD	Control Total	Weight	Mean Difference IV, Random, 95% CI
Clark 2000	-0.61	1.1	26	0.54	1.4	17	33.7%	-1.15 [-1.94, -0.36]
Hoff 2007	0.7	1.6	6	0	0.56	6	24.2%	0.70 [-0.66, 2.06]
van Wetering 2010	0.28	0.1	102	0.02	0.1	97	42.1%	0.26 [0.23, 0.29]
Total (95% CI)			**134**			**120**	**100.0%**	**-0.11 [-1.13, 0.91]**

Heterogeneity: Tau² = 0.65; Chi² = 12.68, df = 2 (P = 0.002); I² = 84%
Test for overall effect: Z = 0.21 (P = 0.84)

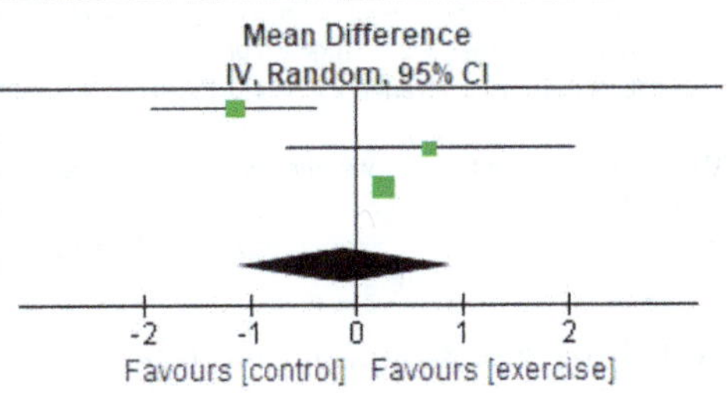

FIGURE 2 | Pooled effect of exercise on BMI in patients with COPD. BMI, body mass index (kg/m²); CI, confidence interval; COPD, chronic obstructive pulmonary disease; SD, standard deviation.

In a previous study, skeletal muscle wasting could occur in the early COPD stages (51), and different exercise modalities could effectively improve lower limb muscle mass in COPD (14). However, in this study, exercise significantly improved the BMI of patients with COPD after excluding studies with PEDro < 6. Through the analysis of literature characteristics, we proposed that exercise improved the BMI of patients with COPD unrelated to exercise modalities, but it was more affected by age and FEV1%pred. That is, the younger the age and better FEV1%pred, the lower the potential for improvement by exercise intervention. A recent meta-analysis of clinical trials has found a negative correlation between the BMI and decline of FEV1 in patients with COPD (52). Age, severity of COPD, and dyspnea degree are closely and clinically related to the loss of skeletal muscle mass and the decline of muscle function in patients with COPD (51). The results from the above-mentioned cross-sectional trials

Study or Subgroup	Exercise Mean	Exercise SD	Exercise Total	Control Mean	Control SD	Control Total	Weight	Std. Mean Difference IV, Random, 95% CI
5.1.1 Endurance exercise versus control								
Alcazar 2019	118	507.43	14	-110.9	309.9	15	3.7%	0.53 [-0.21, 1.28]
Subtotal (95% CI)			**14**			**15**	**3.7%**	**0.53 [-0.21, 1.28]**
Heterogeneity: Not applicable								
Test for overall effect: Z = 1.41 (P = 0.16)								
5.1.2 Resistance exercise versus control								
Casaburi 2004	48	97.1	12	6	64.09	12	3.6%	0.49 [-0.32, 1.31]
Chen 2018	17.1	27.44	25	11.77	42.22	22	3.9%	0.15 [-0.42, 0.72]
Chen 2018	14.31	22.22	25	4.6	33.36	22	3.9%	0.34 [-0.24, 0.92]
Clark 2000	7.6	7.2	26	0.4	4.8	17	3.8%	1.11 [0.45, 1.77]
Hoff 2007	32	19.31	6	-4	23.51	6	2.7%	1.54 [0.18, 2.90]
Janaudis-ferreira 2011	2.2	5.1	17	0.6	3.75	19	3.8%	0.35 [-0.31, 1.01]
Janaudis-ferreira 2011	2	5.41	17	0	5.42	19	3.8%	0.36 [-0.30, 1.02]
Janaudis-ferreira 2011	2.3	5.85	17	-0.2	4.94	19	3.8%	0.45 [-0.21, 1.12]
Janaudis-ferreira 2011	2.1	4.7	17	0.5	4.6	19	3.8%	0.34 [-0.32, 1.00]
Nyberg 2015	5	14.35	22	1	14.35	22	3.9%	0.27 [-0.32, 0.87]
Nyberg 2015	8	33.75	22	-2	32.3	22	3.9%	0.30 [-0.30, 0.89]
Oshea 2007	3.3	10.76	27	2.3	7.66	27	4.0%	0.11 [-0.43, 0.64]
Oshea 2007	5.6	13.84	27	3.8	12.64	27	4.0%	0.13 [-0.40, 0.67]
Oshea 2007	1.9	9.26	27	1.6	8.84	27	4.0%	0.03 [-0.50, 0.57]
Oshea 2007	5.3	13	27	0.3	13.42	27	4.0%	0.37 [-0.17, 0.91]
Simpson 1992	17.2	8.04	14	-3.2	9.74	14	3.3%	2.22 [1.25, 3.19]
Simpson 1992	3.8	1.36	14	0.3	1.41	14	3.3%	2.45 [1.44, 3.47]
Simpson 1992	7.6	3.38	14	2.4	3.5	14	3.5%	1.47 [0.62, 2.32]
Zambom-ferraresi 2015	61.21	77.28	14	-2.85	46.28	8	3.4%	0.91 [-0.01, 1.82]
Zambom-ferraresi 2015	14.29	16.99	14	-1.43	15.61	8	3.4%	0.92 [-0.00, 1.83]
Subtotal (95% CI)			**384**			**365**	**73.7%**	**0.60 [0.35, 0.84]**
Heterogeneity: Tau² = 0.18; Chi² = 48.73, df = 19 (P = 0.0002); I² = 61%								
Test for overall effect: Z = 4.77 (P < 0.00001)								
5.1.3 Combined exercise versus control								
Nakamura 2008	-1.7	5.95	10	-0.6	7.7	10	3.5%	-0.15 [-1.03, 0.73]
van Wetering 2010	-1	2.2	102	2.4	2.3	97	4.2%	-1.51 [-1.82, -1.19]
van Wetering 2010	1.31	0.49	102	0.54	0.54	97	4.2%	1.49 [1.17, 1.80]
Wadell 2013	3	14	20	1	12.51	28	3.9%	0.15 [-0.43, 0.72]
Zambom-ferraresi 2015	49.82	60.11	14	-2.85	46.28	8	3.4%	0.91 [-0.01, 1.83]
Zambom-ferraresi 2015	16.08	15.72	14	-1.43	15.61	8	3.4%	1.07 [0.14, 2.01]
Subtotal (95% CI)			**262**			**248**	**22.6%**	**0.32 [-0.97, 1.60]**
Heterogeneity: Tau² = 2.46; Chi² = 181.79, df = 5 (P < 0.00001); I² = 97%								
Test for overall effect: Z = 0.48 (P = 0.63)								
Total (95% CI)			**660**			**628**	**100.0%**	**0.58 [0.21, 0.95]**
Heterogeneity: Tau² = 0.81; Chi² = 240.76, df = 26 (P < 0.00001); I² = 89%								
Test for overall effect: Z = 3.10 (P = 0.002)								
Test for subgroup differences: Chi² = 0.19, df = 2 (P = 0.91), I² = 0%								

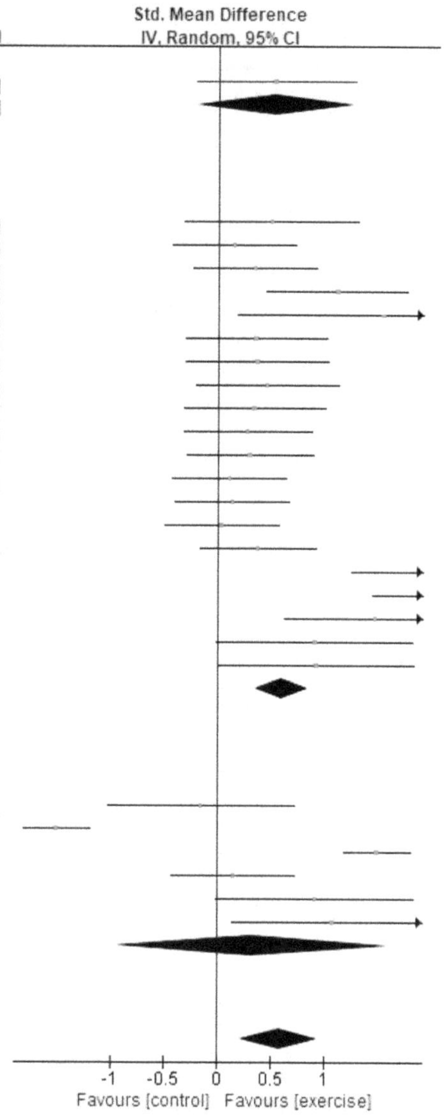

FIGURE 3 | Effects of three types of exercise on skeletal muscle strength in patients with COPD. CI, confidence interval; COPD, chronic obstructive pulmonary disease; SD, standard deviation.

supported the speculation, but the factors that modulated the effects of exercise in COPD skeletal muscle mass still need to be explored due to the small data size in this study. Furthermore, BMI is affected by adipose and connective tissues in the body and may inadequately reflect muscle mass changes. Previous studies have found that RE can significantly improve lower limb lean muscle mass, increase the CSA of the rectus femoris and quadriceps, and decrease the density of muscle fiber (which indicate increased muscle mass per unit area) in COPD (53, 54), but have no effects on the proportion of muscle fiber type and the CSA of different muscle fiber types (an increasing trend only be found in type IIx fibers) (54). Another trial compared the effects of EE and RE on quadriceps muscle morphology and found no significant change in proportion and CSA of type I fibers, intermediate fibers, type IIx fibers, and capillarization (expressed as capillary-to-fiber ratio capillary density) after both exercise modalities, while the proportion of type IIa fibers significantly decreases after EE (55). Consistent with the present study results, both EE and RE have a beneficial effect on the peripheral skeletal muscle mass of patients with COPD, and EE seems to bring more changes in the aerobic metabolism phenotype. The exercise intervention mechanism to improve COPD skeletal muscle mass may be related to inhibiting the level of systemic inflammation, promoting skeletal muscle protein synthesis, muscle hypertrophy and regeneration, and improving the skeletal muscle metabolic enzyme activity (56).

Although there was a high heterogeneity in the methods and programs used to assess muscle strength, the results of this

Study or Subgroup	Exercise Mean	Exercise SD	Exercise Total	Control Mean	Control SD	Control Total	Weight	Std. Mean Difference IV, Random, 95% CI
2.1.1 Isometric strength								
Alcazar 2019	118	507.43	14	-110.9	309.9	15	3.7%	0.53 [-0.21, 1.28]
Chen 2018	17.1	27.44	25	11.77	42.22	22	3.9%	0.15 [-0.42, 0.72]
Janaudis-ferreira 2011	2.2	5.1	17	0.6	3.75	19	3.8%	0.35 [-0.31, 1.01]
Janaudis-ferreira 2011	2.3	5.85	17	-0.2	4.94	19	3.8%	0.45 [-0.21, 1.12]
Janaudis-ferreira 2011	2	5.41	17	0	5.42	19	3.8%	0.36 [-0.30, 1.02]
Janaudis-ferreira 2011	2.1	4.7	17	0.5	4.6	19	3.8%	0.34 [-0.32, 1.00]
Nakamura 2008	-1.7	5.95	10	-0.6	7.7	10	3.5%	-0.15 [-1.03, 0.73]
van Wetering 2010	-1	2.2	102	2.4	2.3	97	4.2%	-1.51 [-1.82, -1.19]
van Wetering 2010	1.31	0.49	102	0.54	0.54	97	4.2%	1.49 [1.17, 1.80]
Wadell 2013	3	14	20	1	12.51	28	3.9%	0.15 [-0.43, 0.72]
Subtotal (95% CI)			**341**			**345**	**38.6%**	**0.22 [-0.54, 0.97]**
Heterogeneity: Tau² = 1.38; Chi² = 178.60, df = 9 (P < 0.00001); I² = 95%								
Test for overall effect: Z = 0.56 (P = 0.58)								
2.1.2 Isotonic strength								
Casaburi 2004	48	97.1	12	6	64.09	12	3.6%	0.49 [-0.32, 1.31]
Clark 2000	7.6	7.2	26	0.4	4.8	17	3.8%	1.11 [0.45, 1.77]
Hoff 2007	32	19.31	6	-4	23.51	6	2.7%	1.54 [0.18, 2.90]
Oshea 2007	3.3	10.76	27	2.3	7.66	27	4.0%	0.11 [-0.43, 0.64]
Oshea 2007	5.6	13.84	27	3.8	12.64	27	4.0%	0.13 [-0.40, 0.67]
Oshea 2007	5.3	13	27	0.3	13.42	27	4.0%	0.37 [-0.17, 0.91]
Oshea 2007	1.9	9.26	27	1.6	8.84	27	4.0%	0.03 [-0.50, 0.57]
Simpson 1992	3.8	1.36	14	0.3	1.41	14	3.3%	2.45 [1.44, 3.47]
Simpson 1992	7.6	3.38	14	2.4	3.5	14	3.5%	1.47 [0.62, 2.32]
Simpson 1992	17.2	8.04	14	-3.2	9.74	14	3.3%	2.22 [1.25, 3.19]
Zambom-ferraresi 2015	14.29	16.99	14	-1.43	15.61	8	3.4%	0.92 [-0.00, 1.83]
Zambom-ferraresi 2015	49.82	60.11	14	-2.85	46.28	8	3.4%	0.91 [-0.01, 1.83]
Zambom-ferraresi 2015	16.08	15.72	14	-1.43	15.61	8	3.4%	1.07 [0.14, 2.01]
Zambom-ferraresi 2015	61.21	77.28	14	-2.85	46.28	8	3.4%	0.91 [-0.01, 1.82]
Subtotal (95% CI)			**250**			**217**	**49.7%**	**0.89 [0.51, 1.26]**
Heterogeneity: Tau² = 0.35; Chi² = 44.83, df = 13 (P < 0.0001); I² = 71%								
Test for overall effect: Z = 4.61 (P < 0.00001)								
2.1.3 Isokinetic strength								
Chen 2018	14.31	22.22	25	4.6	33.36	22	3.9%	0.34 [-0.24, 0.92]
Nyberg 2015	5	14.35	22	1	14.35	22	3.9%	0.27 [-0.32, 0.87]
Nyberg 2015	8	33.75	22	-2	32.3	22	3.9%	0.30 [-0.30, 0.89]
Subtotal (95% CI)			**69**			**66**	**11.7%**	**0.30 [-0.03, 0.64]**
Heterogeneity: Tau² = 0.00; Chi² = 0.03, df = 2 (P = 0.99); I² = 0%								
Test for overall effect: Z = 1.76 (P = 0.08)								
Total (95% CI)			**660**			**628**	**100.0%**	**0.58 [0.21, 0.95]**
Heterogeneity: Tau² = 0.81; Chi² = 240.76, df = 26 (P < 0.00001); I² = 89%								
Test for overall effect: Z = 3.10 (P = 0.002)								
Test for subgroup differences: Chi² = 5.78, df = 2 (P = 0.06), I² = 65.4%								

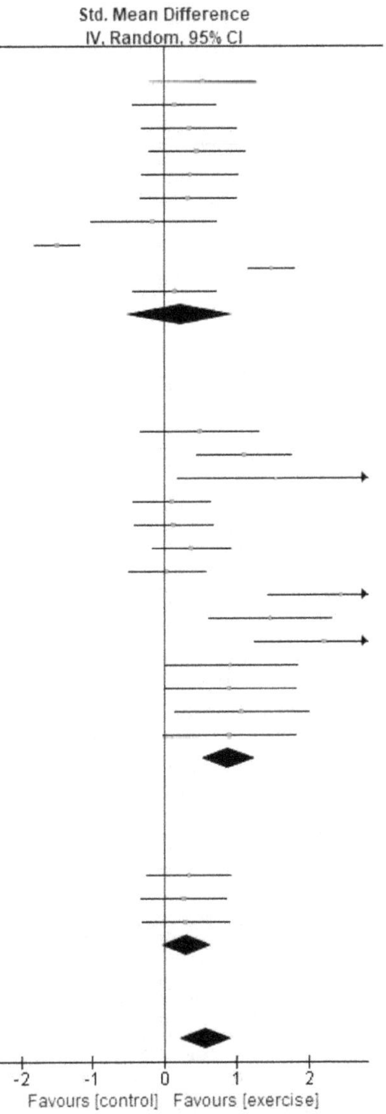

FIGURE 4 | Effects of exercise on skeletal muscle strength evaluated by three types of measurements in patients with COPD. CI, confidence interval; COPD, chronic obstructive pulmonary disease; SD, standard deviation.

study still confirmed the significant positive effect of exercise on improving peripheral skeletal muscle strength in stable COPD. Subgroup analysis for different exercise modalities found that RE showed significant effects. We speculated that RE was designed for specific muscle groups that have less pressure on ventilation load and can effectively improve neuromuscular adaptation (57). Previous studies hypothesized that high-intensity whole/local body EE is sufficient to induce changes in the morphology and function of peripheral skeletal muscles in COPD (14). In the present study, only Alcazar et al. applied a 12-week high-intensity interval training program (high intensity: 80–90% W_{peak} and low intensity: 40–50% W_{peak}) in stable COPD patients and found that the maximum isometric contraction strength and the force development rate of leg press significantly improved (21). Hence, the dose-response relationship between EE intensity and effect still needs to be determined. Also, there was a high heterogeneity in the pooled estimates of CE, and the heterogeneity decreased after a sensitivity analysis excluding the results from van Wetering et al., but still without reaching statistical significance. In the analysis of the literature characteristics, we found that the quadriceps muscle strength of the participants was 92–95% of the normal predicted value (47), which may lead to a small potential for improvement. However, the results are still inconsistent with speculations and previous research results, that is, CE has similar or even greater effects than EE and RE alone (16, 17, 40), which may be attributed to a variety of CE programs included in this meta-analysis. First, the proportion of EE and RE in CE programs. Most programs scheduled EE and RE in one session

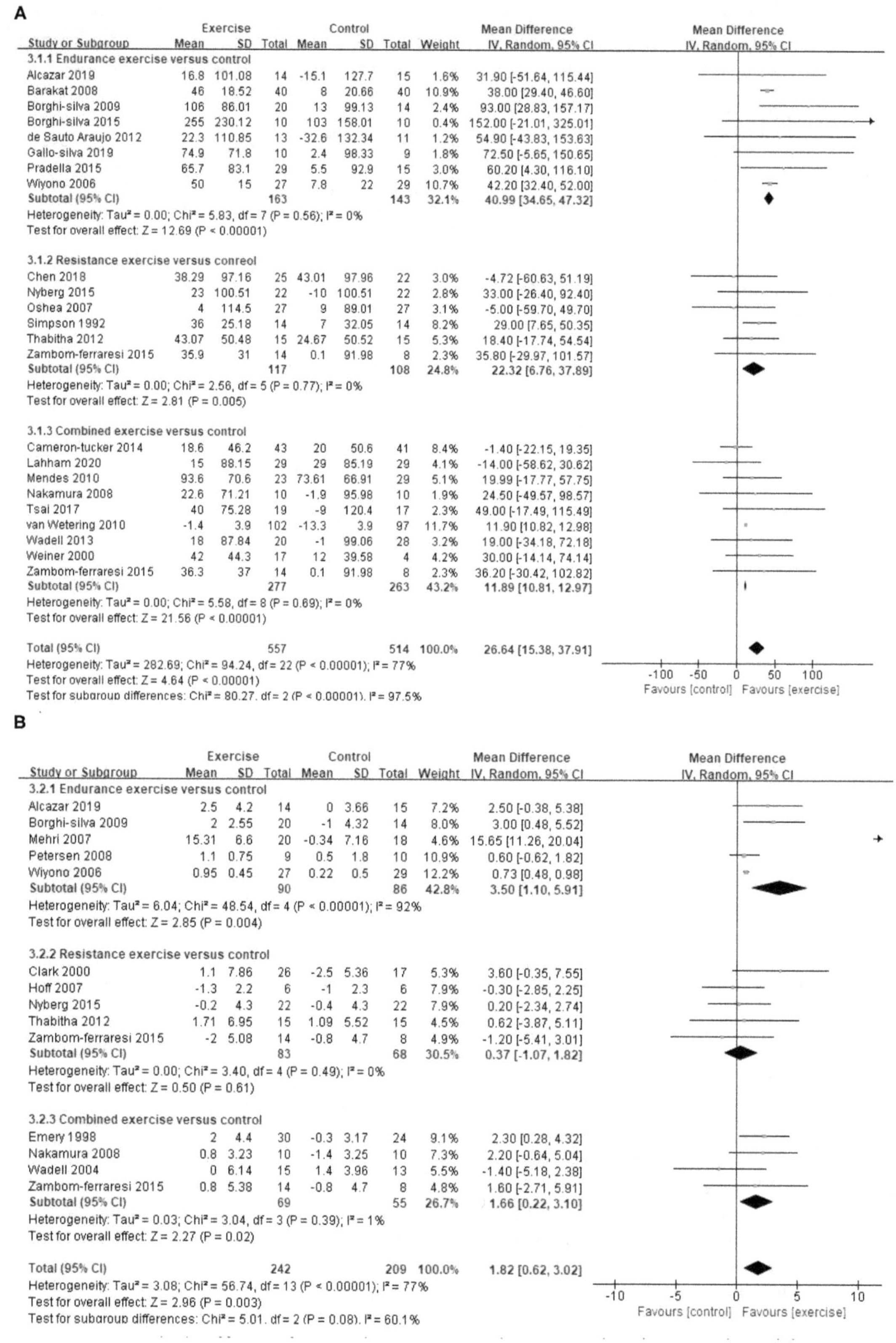

FIGURE 5 | Pooled effect of exercise on exercise capacity in people with COPD. **(A)** 6MWD, **(B)** VO_{2peak}. 6MWD, 6-min walking distance (m); CI, confidence interval; COPD, chronic obstructive pulmonary disease; SD, standard deviation; VO_{2peak}, peak oxygen consumption (ml/kg/min).

TABLE 4 | Grading of recommendations assessment, development, and evaluation summary of findings.

	Certainty Assessment							No. of Patients		Effect		Certainty
Outcomes	**No. of Studies**	**Study design**	**Risk of bias**	**Inconsistency**	**Indirectness**	**Imprecision**	**Other considerations**	**EG**	**CG**	**Relative (95% CI)**	**Absolute (95% CI)**	
BMI	3	Randomized trials	Serious[a]	Serious[b]	Not serious	Serious[c]	None	134	120	–	MD 0.11 lower (1.13 lower to 0.91 higher)	⊕○○○ Very low
Skeletal muscle strength	13	Randomized trials	Serious[a]	Serious[b]	Not serious	Not serious	None	660	628	–	SMD 3.48 higher (1.81 to 5.15 higher)	⊕⊕○○ Low
6MWD	22	Randomized trials	Serious[a]	Not serious	Not serious	Not serious	None	557	514	–	MD 12.76 higher (11.69 to 13.82 higher)	⊕⊕⊕○ Moderate
VO_{2peak}	13	Randomized trials	Serious[a]	Not serious	Not serious	Not serious	None	242	209	–	MD 1.82 higher (0.62 to 3.02 higher)	⊕⊕⊕○ Moderate

[a]*Most of the studies are without allocation concealment, subject blinded and intention-to-treatment analysis.*
[b]*There was a substantial heterogeneity among the three studies according to the heterogeneity test.*
[c]*Only three studies were included in the analysis, and the sample size was relatively low.*

and two to three sessions a week, respectively, apart from the program in Zambom-Ferraresi et al. (scheduled EE in one session and RE in another session, only two sessions a week). Second, the range of exercise intensity was relatively extensive, which may play a role in maintenance but not in improvement. Therefore, in the CE program for improving COPD's skeletal muscle strength, the different proportions and intensities of EE and RE might have different effects, and it is still necessary to explore the best program.

Subgroup analysis for different muscle strength testing methods found that exercise can only significantly improve isotonic muscle strength. We speculated that the isotonic muscle strength test is more familiar to the participants and has a higher correlation with daily life than other tests (58). Considering that different strength units may be the source of heterogeneity, we pooled data units in kilograms and found that exercise significantly improved isometric muscle strength. Although the data of isokinetic muscle strength showed an increasing trend after exercise (33, 36), many studies are still needed to determine the degree of response. We also conducted subgroup analysis to determine the effects of exercise on upper limbs and lower limbs muscle strength and found that exercise can improve the muscle strength of both upper and lower limbs. Although subgroup analysis was performed, high heterogeneity still existed, and the source of heterogeneity was unclear. A standard and clinically feasible measurement program is needed to quantitatively evaluate the damage of peripheral skeletal muscle strength and the response to exercise in COPD.

Consistent with previous meta-analysis (15, 59), this study found that exercise can significantly improve 6MWD (26.64 m) in patients with COPD. However, only the EE improvement reached the minimal clinical important difference of 30 m (60), which may be attributed to EE bringing more aerobic metabolism changes and greater improvements in ventilation capacity; the relatively low proportion of EE in the CE program cannot bring significant improvement. The peak exercise capacity is often evaluated using a cardiopulmonary exercise test (CPET), which is considered the gold standard to assess the exercise capacity and closely related to COPD's prognosis (61, 62). A progressive incremental exercise protocol in a treadmill or cycle ergometer is often used for CPET, and the results can provide abundant physiological information related to exercise restriction, including the heart (e.g., heart rate, VO_{2peak}, and oxygen pulse), lung (e.g., inspiratory capacity, gas exchange, and dynamic inflation), muscle (e.g., power and lactic acid), dyspnea (Borg), and exercise initiative (62). A Cochrane review conducted in 2015 showed that pulmonary rehabilitation (at least 4 weeks of exercise training) is beneficial in improving maximal exercise capacity (measured by W_{max}) in patients with COPD, and the effect size exceeds the minimal clinically important difference (4 W) (63). Although a different outcome was used in this present study, the effect of exercise is confirmed. The comparison results of the effects of different modalities exercise showed no significant differences between RE vs. the control group (15, 64), RE vs. EE (16), and CE vs. EE (64) in improving the peak exercise capacity (VO_{2peak}, W_{peak}) of patients with COPD. It seems that a contradictory deduction

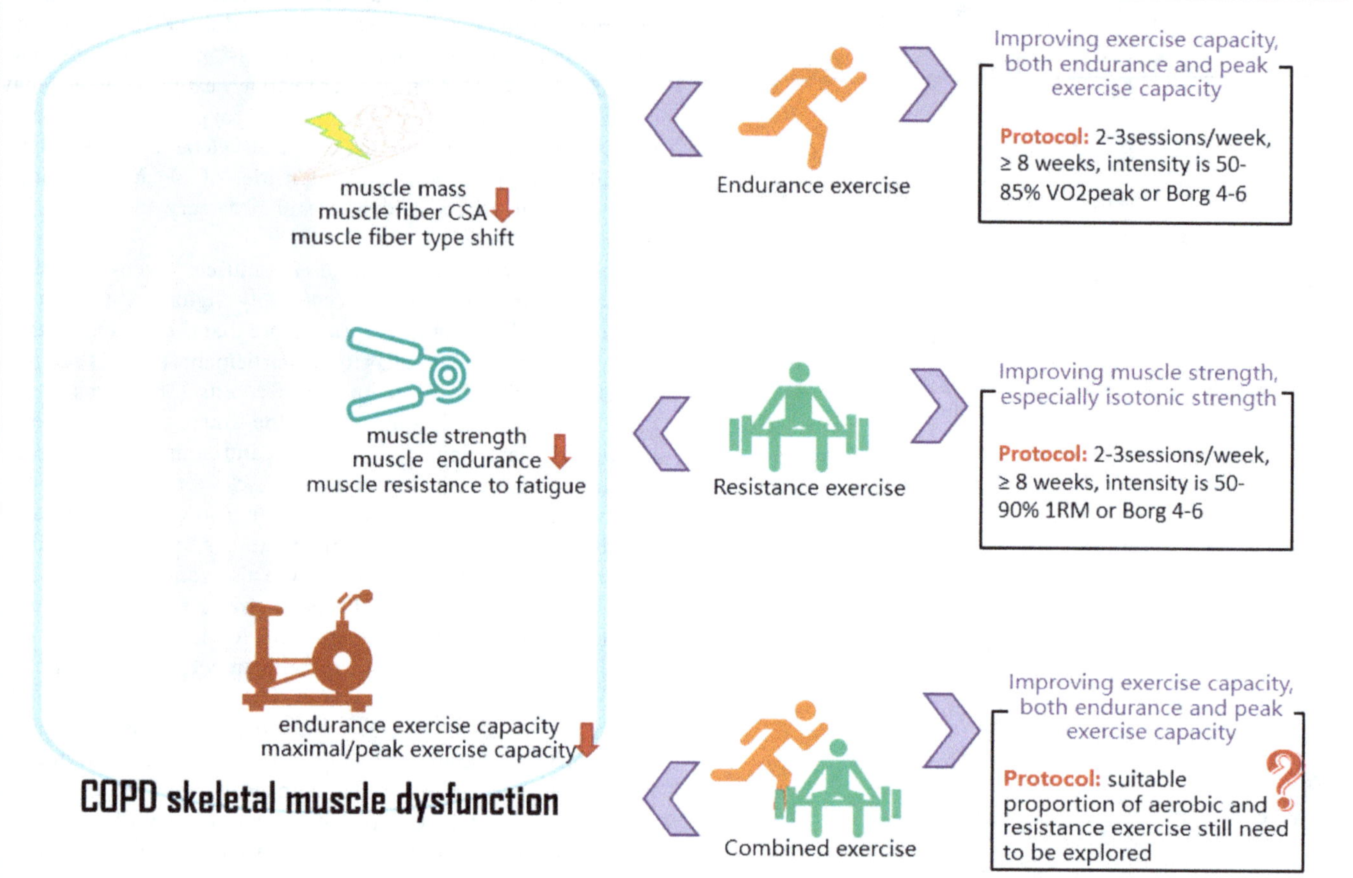

FIGURE 6 | COPD skeletal muscle dysfunction and the effects of exercise on it. COPD, chronic obstructive pulmonary disease; CSA, cross-sectional area; RM, repetition maximum; VO_{2peak}, peak oxygen consumption.

might be concluded that exercise does not have a significant positive effect on peak exercise capacity of patients with COPD. Based on the primary pathophysiological mechanisms of exercise limitation in patients with COPD undergoing CPET, including ventilatory abnormalities, pulmonary gas exchange abnormalities, and skeletal muscle dysfunction (61), exercise with different modalities seems beneficial in improving peak exercise capacity in patients with COPD. Consistent with the hypothesis, this meta-analysis showed that exercise could significantly improve COPD's peak exercise capacity (1.82 ml/kg/min), and both EE and CE have positive effects.

This systematic review and meta-analysis had some limitations. First, there were flaws in methodological quality of the original studies, namely the lack of subject blinding and evaluator blinding in exercise intervention trials. Second, one of the included literatures had an apparently large sample size, which may have had an impact on the research results. Sensitivity analysis was performed to reduce the impact when high heterogeneity was found. Third, we only analyzed the effects of exercise on skeletal muscle strength and still needed to explore the effects of exercise on skeletal muscle endurance and power. Fourth, the outcomes of skeletal muscle function were not assessed comprehensively in most of the included studies, which may cause a limitation. Fifth, trial designs were heterogeneous. For high heterogeneity, we used a random-effects model and subgroup analysis to analyse the source of heterogeneity, and the results were consistent.

CONCLUSIONS

Exercise with different modalities seems effective in improving peripheral skeletal muscle strength and exercise capacity in patients with stable COPD. Specifically, EE shows a greater improvement in endurance and peak exercise capacity, and RE shows a greater improvement in peripheral skeletal muscle strength, and the isotonic test is relatively sensitive in reflecting muscle strength changes. Therefore, for patients with COPD whose exercise limitation is caused by a decreased cardiorespiratory capacity, EE might be a suitable choice. EE can be conducted in cycling, running, and walking, with an intensity of 50–85% VO_{2peak}, 2–3 times/week, for at least 8 weeks. For patients with COPD whose exercise limitation is caused by an impaired peripheral skeletal muscle function, RE might be a preferable intervention. RE can be conducted in weight machines, free weights, and elastic bands, with an intensity of 50–90% 1RM, 2–3 times/week, for at least 8 weeks. The proportion of EE and RE in CE programs still needs to be explored and analyzed (**Figure 6**). High methodological quality RCTs with a large sample size are still needed to verify the present study results because of the relatively small inclusion of literature on the peripheral skeletal muscle structure and function in patients with COPD. It is also necessary to explore the effect of exercise intervention on peripheral skeletal muscle in AECOPD or patients with COPD with different severity.

AUTHOR CONTRIBUTIONS

XL and JX conceived of the idea for this review. JL and YW did the literature search. PL and YW collected the data. PL and JL did the quality assessment. PL did the statistical analyses and wrote the first draft of the manuscript. All authors analyzed and interpreted the data and revised and approved the final manuscript for submission.

REFERENCES

1. Global Initiative for Chronic Obstructive Lung Disease-GOLD. *Global Strategy for the Diagnosis, Management, and Prevention of Chronic Obstructive Pulmonary Disease (2019 report)*. Available online at: https://goldcopd.org/2019 (accessed December 5, 2018).
2. Decramer M, Janssens W, Miravitlles M. Chronic obstructive pulmonary disease. *Lancet.* (2012) 379:1341–51. doi: 10.1016/S0140-6736(11)60968-9
3. Rabe KF, Watz H. Chronic obstructive pulmonary disease. *Lancet.* (2017) 389:1931–40. doi: 10.1016/S0140-6736(17)31222-9
4. Barreiro E, Bustamante V, Cejudo P, Gáldiz JB, Gea J, de Lucas P, et al. Guidelines for the evaluation and treatment of muscle dysfunction in patients with chronic obstructive pulmonary disease. *Arch Bronconeumol.* (2015) 51:384–95. doi: 10.1016/j.arbres.2015.04.011
5. Rabinovich R, Vilaro J. Structural and functional changes of peripheral muscles in chronic obstructive pulmonary disease patients. *Curr Opin Pulm Med.* (2010) 16:123–33. doi: 10.1097/MCP.0b013e328336438d
6. Bernard S, LeBlanc P, Whittom F, Carrier G, Jobin J, Belleau R, et al. Peripheral muscle weakness in patients with chronic obstructive pulmonary disease. *Am J Respir Crit Care Med.* (1998) 158:629–34. doi: 10.1164/ajrccm.158.2.9711023
7. Corhay JL, Dang DN, Van Cauwenberge H, Louis R. Pulmonary rehabilitation and COPD: providing patients a good environment for optimizing therapy. *Int J Chron Obstruct Pulmon Dis.* (2014) 9:27–39. doi: 10.2147/COPD.S52012
8. Li P, Wang Z, Lu Y, Li N, Xiao L, Su J, et al. Assessment of knee extensor and flexor function using isokinetic test in COPD: impact on exercise capacity. *Int J Tuberc Lung Dis.* (2020) 24:776–81. doi: 10.5588/ijtld.19.0588
9. Saey D, Debigare R, LeBlanc P, Mador MJ, Cote CH, Jobin J, et al. Contractile leg fatigue after cycle exercise: a factor limiting exercise in patients with chronic obstructive pulmonary disease. *Am J Respir Crit Care Med.* (2003) 168:425–30. doi: 10.1164/rccm.200208-856OC
10. Gagnon P, Saey D, Vivodtzev I, Laviolette L, Mainguy V, Milot J, et al. Impact of preinduced quadriceps fatigue on exercise response in chronic obstructive pulmonary disease and healthy subjects. *J Appl Physiol (1985).* (2009) 107:832–40. doi: 10.1152/japplphysiol.91546.2008
11. Nyberg A, Carvalho J, Bui KL, Saey D, Maltais F. Adaptations in limb muscle function following pulmonary rehabilitation in patients with COPD—a review. *Rev Port Pneumol (2006).* (2016) 22:342–50. doi: 10.1016/j.rppnen.2016.06.007
12. Maltais F, Decramer M, Casaburi R, Barreiro E, Burelle Y, Debigaré R, et al. An official American Thoracic Society/European Respiratory Society statement: update on limb muscle dysfunction in chronic obstructive pulmonary disease. *Am J Respir Crit Care Med.* (2014) 189:e15–62. doi: 10.1164/rccm.201402-0373ST
13. Jaitovich A, Barreiro E. Skeletal muscle dysfunction in chronic obstructive pulmonary disease (COPD): what we know and can do for our patients. *Am J Respir Crit Care Med.* (2018) 198:175–86. doi: 10.1164/rccm.201710-2140CI
14. De Brandt J, Spruit MA, Hansen D, Franssen FM, Derave W, Sillen MJ, et al. Changes in lower limb muscle function and muscle mass following exercise-based interventions in patients with chronic obstructive pulmonary disease: a review of the English-language literature. *Chron Respir Dis.* (2018) 15:182–219. doi: 10.1177/1479972317709642
15. Li N, Li P, Lu Y, Wang Z, Li J, Liu X, et al. Effects of resistance training on exercise capacity in elderly patients with chronic obstructive pulmonary disease: a meta-analysis and systematic review. *Aging Clin Exp Res.* (2019) 32:1911–22. doi: 10.1007/s40520-019-01339-8
16. Iepsen UW, Jørgensen KJ, Ringbaek T, Hansen H, Skrubbeltrang C, Lange P, et al. Systematic review of resistance training vs. endurance training in COPD. *J Cardiopulm Rehabil Prev.* (2015) 35:163–72. doi: 10.1097/HCR.0000000000000105
17. Iepsen UW, Jørgensen KJ, Ringbæk T, Hansen H, Skrubbeltrang C, Lange P, et al. combination of resistance and endurance training increases leg muscle strength in COPD: an evidence-based recommendation based on systematic review with meta-analyses. *Chron Respir Dis.* (2015) 12:132–45. doi: 10.1177/1479972315575318
18. Moher D, Liberati A, Tetzlaff J, Altman D, PRISMA Group. Preferred reporting items for systematic reviews and meta-analyses: the PRISMA statement. *PLoS Med.* (2009) 6:e1000097. doi: 10.1371/journal.pmed.1000097
19. Maher CG, Sherrington C, Herbert RD, Moseley AM, Elkins M. Reliability of the PEDro scale for rating quality of randomized controlled trials. *Phys Ther.* (2003) 83:713–21. doi: 10.1093/ptj/83.8.713
20. Guyatt GH, Oxman AD, Vist GE, Kunz R, Falck-Ytter Y, Alonso-Coello P, et al. GRADE: an emerging consensus on rating quality of evidence and strength of recommendations. *BMJ.* (2008) 336:924–6. doi: 10.1136/bmj.39489.470347.AD
21. Alcazar J, Losa-Reyna J, Rodriguez-Lopez C, Navarro-Cruz R, Alfaro-Acha A, Ara I, et al. Effects of concurrent exercise training on muscle dysfunction and systemic oxidative stress in older people with COPD. *Scand J Med Sci Sports.* (2019) 29:1591–603. doi: 10.1111/sms.13494
22. Barakat S, Michele G, George P, Nicole V, Guy A. Outpatient pulmonary rehabilitation in patients with chronic obstructive pulmonary disease. *Int J Chron Obstruct Pulmon Dis.* (2008) 3:155–62. doi: 10.2147/COPD.S2126
23. Borghi-Silva A, Arena R, Castello V, Simões RP, Martins LE, Catai AM, et al. Aerobic exercise training improves autonomic nervous control in patients with COPD. *Respir Med.* (2009) 103:1503–10. doi: 10.1016/j.rmed.2009.04.015
24. Borghi-Silva A, Mendes RG, Trimer R, Oliveira CR, Fregonezi GA, Resqueti VR, et al. Potential effect of 6 vs. 12-weeks of physical training on cardiac autonomic function and exercise capacity in chronic obstructive pulmonary disease. *Eur J Phys Rehabil Med.* (2015) 51:211–21. Available online at: https://pubmed.ncbi.nlm.nih.gov/24594853/
25. de Souto Araujo ZT, de Miranda Silva Nogueira PA, Cabral EE, de Paula Dos Santos L, da Silva IS, Ferreira GM. Effectiveness of low-intensity aquatic exercise on COPD: a randomized clinical trial. *Respir Med.* (2012) 106:1535–43. doi: 10.1016/j.rmed.2012.06.022
26. Gallo-Silva B, Cerezer-Silva V, Ferreira DG, Sakabe DI, Kel-Souza LD, Bertholo VC, et al. Effects of water-based aerobic interval training in patients with COPD: a randomized controlled trial. *J Cardiopulm Rehabil Prev.* (2019) 39:105–11. doi: 10.1097/HCR.0000000000000352
27. Mehri SN, Khoshnevis MA, Zarrehbinan F, Hafezi S, Ghasemi A, Ebadi A. Effects of treadmill exercise training on VO2 peak in chronic obstructive pulmonary disease. *Natl Res Inst Tuberc Lung Dis.* (2007) 6:18–24. Available online at: https://scholar.google.com/scholar_lookup?title=Effect+of+treadmill+exercise+training+on+VO2+peak+in+chronic+obstructive+pulmonary+disease+&author=SN+Mehri&author=MA+Khoshnevis&author=F+Zarrehbinan&author=S+Hafezi&author=A+Ghasemi&author=A+Ebadi&publication_year=2007&hl=en
28. Petersen AM, Mittendorfer B, Magkos F, Iversen M, Pedersen BK. Physical activity counteracts increased whole-body protein breakdown in chronic obstructive pulmonary disease patients. *Scand J Med Sci Sports.* (2008) 18:557–64. doi: 10.1111/j.1600-0838.2007.00727.x

29. Pradella CO, Belmonte GM, Maia MN, Delgado CS, Luise AP, Nascimento OA, et al. Home-based pulmonary rehabilitation for subjects with COPD: a randomized study. *Respir Care.* (2015) 60:526–32. doi: 10.4187/respcare.02994
30. Wiyono WH, Riyadi J, Yunus F, Ratnawati A, Prasetyo S. The benefit of pulmonary rehabilitation against quality of life alteration and functional capacity of chronic obstructive pulmonary disease (COPD) patient assessed using St George's respiratory questionnaire (SGRQ) and 6 minutes walking distance test (6MWD). *Med J Indones.* (2006) 15:165–72. doi: 10.13181/mji.v15i3.232
31. Casaburi R, Bhasin S, Cosentino L, Porszasz J, Somfay A, Lewis MI, et al. Effects of testosterone and resistance training in men with chronic obstructive pulmonary disease. *Am J Respir Crit Care Med.* (2004) 170:870–8. doi: 10.1164/rccm.200305-617OC
32. Clark C, Cochrane L, Mackay E, Paton B. Skeletal muscle strength and endurance in patients with mild COPD and the effects of weight training. *Eur Respir J.* (2000) 15:92–7. doi: 10.1183/09031936.00.15109200
33. Chen Y, Niu M, Zhang X, Qian H, Xie A, Wang X. Effects of home-based lower limb resistance training on muscle strength and functional status in stable chronic obstructive pulmonary disease patients. *J Clin Nurs.* (2018) 27:e1022–e37. doi: 10.1111/jocn.14131
34. Hoff J, Tjønna AE, Steinshamn S, Høydal M, Richardson RS, Helgerud J. Maximal strength training of the legs in COPD: a therapy for mechanical inefficiency. *Med Sci Sports Exerc.* (2007) 39:220–6. doi: 10.1249/01.mss.0000246989.48729.39
35. Janaudis-Ferreira T, Hill K, Goldstein RS, Robles-Ribeiro P, Beauchamp MK, Dolmage TE, et al. Resistance arm training in patients with COPD: a randomized controlled trial. *Chest.* (2011) 139:151–8. doi: 10.1378/chest.10-1292
36. Nyberg A, Lindstrom B, Rickenlund A, Wadell K. Low-load/high-repetition elastic band resistance training in patients with COPD: a randomized, controlled, multicenter trial. *Clin Respir J.* (2015) 9:278–88. doi: 10.1111/crj.12141
37. O'Shea S, Taylor N, Paratz J, A. predominantly home-based progressive resistance exercise program increases knee extensor strength in the short-term in people with chronic obstructive pulmonary disease: a randomised controlled trial. *Aust J Physiother.* (2007) 53:229–37. doi: 10.1016/S0004-9514(07)70003-X
38. Thabitha P, Madhavi K, Charan K. Jyothi KA. Effect of peripheral muscle strength training on exercise capacity in subjects with chronic obstructive pulmonary disease. *Indian J Physiother Occup Ther.* (2012) 6:91–5. Available online at: https://search.pedro.org.au/search-results/record-detail/31163
39. Simpson K, Killian K, McCartney N, Stubbing DG, Jones NL. Randomised controlled trial of weightlifting exercise in patients with chronic airflow limitation. *Thorax.* (1992) 47:70–5. doi: 10.1136/thx.47.2.70
40. Zambom-Ferraresi F, Cebollero P, Gorostiaga EM, Hernández M, Hueto J, Cascante J, et al. Effects of combined resistance and endurance training vs. resistance training alone on strength, exercise capacity, and quality of life in patients with COPD. *J Cardiopulm Rehabil Prev.* (2015) 35:446–53. doi: 10.1097/HCR.0000000000000132
41. Cameron-Tucker HL, Wood-Baker R, Owen C, Joseph L, Walters EH. Chronic disease self-management and exercise in COPD as pulmonary rehabilitation: a randomized controlled trial. *Int J Chron Obstruct Pulmon Dis.* (2014) 9:513–23. doi: 10.2147/COPD.S58478
42. Emery CF, Schein RL, Hauck ER, MacIntyre NR. Psychological and cognitive outcomes of a randomized trial of exercise among patients with chronic obstructive pulmonary disease. *Health Psychol.* (1998) 17:232–40. doi: 10.1037/0278-6133.17.3.232
43. Lahham A, McDonald CF, Moore R, Cox NS, Rawlings S, Nichols A, et al. The impact of home-based pulmonary rehabilitation on people with mild chronic obstructive pulmonary disease: a randomised controlled trial. *Clin RespirJ.* (2020) 14:335–44. doi: 10.1111/crj.13138
44. Mendes de. Oliveira JC, Studart Leitão Filho FS, Malosa Sampaio LM, Negrinho de Oliveira AC, Hirata RP, Costa D, et al. Outpatient vs home-based pulmonary rehabilitation in COPD: a randomized controlled trial. *Multidiscip Respir Med.* (2010) 5:401–8. doi: 10.1186/2049-6958-5-6-401
45. Nakamura Y, Tanaka K, Shigematsu R, Nakagaichi M, Lnoue M, Homma T. Effects of aerobic training and recreational activities in patients with chronic obstructive pulmonary disease. *In J Rehabil Res.* (2008) 31:275–83. doi: 10.1097/MRR.0b013e3282fc0f81
46. Tsai LL, McNamara RJ, Moddel C, Alison JA, McKenzie DK, McKeough ZJ. Home-based telerehabilitation *via* real-time videoconferencing improves endurance exercise capacity in patients with COPD: The randomized controlled TeleR Study. *Respirology.* (2017) 22:699–707. doi: 10.1111/resp.12966
47. van Wetering CR, Hoogendoorn M, Mol SJM. Rutten-van Mölken MPMH, Schols AM. Short- and long-term efficacy of a community-based COPD management programme in less advanced COPD: a randomised controlled trial. *Thorax.* (2010) 65:7–13. doi: 10.1136/thx.2009.118620
48. Wadell K, Webb KA, Preston ME, Amornputtisathaporn N, Samis L, Patelli J, et al. Impact of pulmonary rehabilitation on the major dimensions of dyspnea in COPD. *COPD.* (2013) 10:425–35. doi: 10.3109/15412555.2012.758696
49. Wadell K, Sundelin G, Henriksson-Larsén K, Lundgren R. High intensity physical group training in water—an effective training modality for patients with COPD. *Respir Med.* (2004) 98:428–38. doi: 10.1016/j.rmed.2003.11.010
50. Weiner P, Magadle R, Berar-Yanay N, Davidovich A, Weiner M. The cumulative effect of long-acting bronchodilators, exercise, and inspiratory muscle training on the perception of dyspnea in patients with advanced COPD. *Chest.* (2000) 118:672–8. doi: 10.1378/chest.118.3.672
51. Benz E, Trajanoska K, Lahousse L, Schoufour JD, Terzikhan N, De Roos E, et al. Sarcopenia in COPD: a systematic review and meta-analysis. *Eur Respir Rev.* (2019) 28:190049. doi: 10.1183/16000617.0049-2019
52. Sun Y, Milne S, Jaw JE, Yang CX, Xu F, Li X, et al. BMI is associated with FEV_1 decline in chronic obstructive pulmonary disease: a meta-analysis of clinical trials. *Respir Res.* (2019) 20:236. doi: 10.1186/s12931-019-1209-5
53. Menon MK, Houchen L, Harrison S, Singh SJ, Morgan MD, Steiner MC. Ultrasound assessment of lower limb muscle mass in response to resistance training in COPD. *Respir Res.* (2012) 13:119. doi: 10.1186/1465-9921-13-119
54. Lewis MI, Fournier M, Storer TW, Bhasin S, Porszasz J, Ren SG, et al. Skeletal muscle adaptations to testosterone and resistance training in men with COPD. *J Appl Physiol (1985).* (2007) 103: 1299–310. doi: 10.1152/japplphysiol.00150.2007
55. Iepsen UW, Munch GD, Rugbjerg M, Rinnov AR, Zacho M, Mortensen SP. et.al. Effect of endurance vs. resistance training on quadriceps muscle dysfunction in COPD: a pilot study. *Int J Chron Obstruct Pulmon Dis.* (2016) 11:2659–69. doi: 10.2147/COPD.S114351
56. Nasis I, Kortianou EA, Clini E, Koulouris NG, Vogiatzis I. Effect of rehabilitative exercise training on peripheral muscle remodelling in patients with COPD: targeting beyond the lungs. *Curr Drug Targets.* (2013) 14:262–73. doi: 10.2174/1389450111314020011
57. Spruit MA, Singh SJ, Garvey C, ZuWallack R, Nici L, Rochester C. et.al. An official American Thoracic Society/European Respiratory Society statement: key concepts and advances in pulmonary rehabilitation. *Am J Respir Crit Care Med.* (2013) 188:e13–64. doi: 10.1164/rccm.201309-1634ST
58. Marklund S, Bui KL, Nyberg A. Measuring and monitoring skeletal muscle function in COPD: current perspectives. *Int J Chron Obstruct Pulmon Dis.* (2019) 14:1825–38. doi: 10.2147/COPD.S178948
59. Paneroni M, Simonelli C, Vitacca M, Ambrosino N. Aerobic exercise training in very severe chronic obstructive pulmonary disease: a systematic review and meta-analysis. *Am J Phys Med Rehabil.* (2017) 96:541–8. doi: 10.1097/PHM.0000000000000667
60. Holland AE, Spruit MA, Troosters T, Puhan MA, Pepin V, Saey D, et al. An official European Respiratory Society/American Thoracic Society technical standard: field walking tests in chronic respiratory disease. *Eur Respir J.* (2014) 44:1428–46. doi: 10.1183/09031936.00150314
61. Ferrazza AM, Martolini D, Valli G, Palange P. Cardiopulmonary exercise testing in the functional and prognostic evaluation of patients with pulmonary diseases. *Respiration.* (2009) 77:3–17. doi: 10.1159/000186694
62. Stringer W, Marciniuk D. The role of cardiopulmonary exercise testing (CPET) in pulmonary rehabilitation (PR) of chronic obstructive pulmonary disease (COPD) patients. *COPD.* (2018) 15:621–31. doi: 10.1080/15412555.2018.1550476
63. McCarthy B, Casey D, Devane D, Murphy K, Murphy E, Lacasse Y. Pulmonary rehabilitation for chronic obstructive pulmonary disease. *Cochrane Database Syst Rev.* (2015) CD003793:1–188. doi: 10.1002/14651858.CD003793.pub3

6

COVID-19, COPD and AECOPD: Immunological, Epidemiological and Clinical Aspects

Francesca Polverino [1*] *and Farrah Kheradmand* [2]

[1] *Asthma and Airway Disease Research Center, University of Arizona, Tucson, AZ, United States,* [2] *Baylor College of Medicine, Houston, TX, United States*

***Correspondence:**
Francesca Polverino
fpolverino@copdnet.org

The newly identified severe acute respiratory syndrome Coronavirus 2 (SARS-CoV-2) causes several heterogeneous clinical conditions collectively known as Coronavirus disease-19 (COVID-19). Older patients with significant cardiovascular conditions and chronic obstructive pulmonary disease (COPD) are predisposed to a more severe disease complicated with acute respiratory distress syndrome (ARDS), which is associated with high morbidity and mortality. COPD is associated with increased susceptibility to respiratory infections, and viruses are among the top causes of acute exacerbations of COPD (AECOPD). Thus, COVID-19 could represent the ultimate cause of AECOPD. This review will examine the pathobiological processes underlying SARS-CoV-2 infection, including the effects of cigarette smoke and COPD on the immune system and vascular endothelium, and the known effects of cigarette smoke on the onset and progression of COVID-19. We will also review the epidemiological data on COVID-19 prevalence and outcome in patients with COPD and analyze the pathobiological and clinical features of SARS-CoV-2 infection in the context of other known viral causes of AECOPD. Overall, SARS-CoV-2 shares common pathobiological and clinical features with other viral agents responsible for increased morbidity, thus representing a novel cause of AECOPD with the potential for a more long-term adverse impact. Longitudinal studies aimed at COPD patients surviving COVID-19 are needed to identify therapeutic targets for SARS-CoV2 and prevent the disease's burden in this vulnerable population.

Keywords: COPD, COVID-19, SARS-CoV-2, cigarette smoke (CS), therapy, endothelium

INTRODUCTION

COVID-19: Coronavirus disease-19 (COVID-19) is an acute and heterogeneous clinical condition caused by the newly identified severe acute respiratory syndrome Coronavirus 2 (SARS-CoV-2). In most cases, the disease is characterized by a mild presentation of respiratory symptoms and/or other extra-pulmonary conditions such as anosmia, gastrointestinal distress, and malaise. When severe, the disease can lead to acute lung injury (ALI) and acute respiratory distress syndrome (ARDS) which carry high morbidity and mortality. Despite the tremendous worldwide burden, our understanding of the pathophysiology and treatment of SARS-CoV-2 illnesses remains limited.

The elderly and those with comorbidities (mainly cardio/respiratory diseases, diabetes, and kidney failure) carry the highest risk of poor prognosis and death (1–5). Chronic Obstructive Pulmonary Disease (COPD) is one of the most frequent chronic respiratory conditions affecting millions worldwide, and is mainly caused by exposure to cigarette smoke. COPD predominantly affects smokers in their sixth or seventh decade of life, and leads to deconditioning with frequent comorbid conditions. Because of off-target immune responses (6), COPD is associated with increased susceptibility to infections, including respiratory viral diseases that are among the leading causes of acute exacerbations of COPD (AECOPD) (7). Therefore, predictably SARS-CoV2 pandemic has critically impacted COPD patients (8).

Here, we discuss the epidemiology of COVID-19 in the COPD population, the clinical and therapeutic implications of COVID-19 as the ultimate cause of AECOPD, and the pathological and immunological factors that play key roles in ever smokers with and without COPD affecting SARS-CoV2 infection and COVID-19 outcome.

COVID-19 AND COPD: EPIDEMIOLOGY

The majority of COPD patients are older, and have frequent comorbid conditions, making those diagnosed with COVID-19 display with worse outcomes, including a higher incidence of hospitalization, Intensive Care Unit (ICU) admission, and mortality (9, 10). However, it remains to be determined how pre-existing chronic inflammatory airway diseases, such as COPD, and their treatment might modify the risk for SARS-CoV-2 infection and development of COVID-19.

In mainland China and worldwide, several cohort studies showed a lower prevalence of active smokers than expected gender and age-adjusted prevalence among COVID-19 patients (1–4, 11–13). Whether this is caused by incomplete or incorrect information about smoking patterns due to significant methodological limitations, including small sample sizes and ascertainment bias, remains unclear. Similarly, the data on COPD among COVID-19 patients revealed a wide-ranging prevalence (1.1–38%) of COPD among patients hospitalized with COVID-19. To estimate the COPD patient excess risk for contracting COVID-19 has been challenging since reporting has concentrated on hospitalized and ICU patients rather than on milder (e.g., outpatient settings) cases. Further, not all the COPD patients with COVID-19 sought medical treatment in a hospital setting because of overburdened hospitals at the peak of pandemic. Thus, COVID-19 related AECOPD may have contributed to the mortality statistics without having affected the hospitalization or ICU-related statistics (14). Understandably, pulmonary function tests are not performed in COVID-19 patients before or after hospitalization, and thus, airflow limitation might have been underestimated.

A meta-analysis of 15 studies where the presence of COPD was assessed among 2,473 confirmed COVID-19 patients revealed that the pooled prevalence of COPD diagnosis in COVID-19 patients was relatively low [2% [95% CI, 1%–3%]]. Whether this observed effect is due to self-isolation of COPD patients resulting in lower representations in some of the COVID cohorts, remains less clear. However, COPD patients were at a higher risk of more severe disease burden, and significantly higher risk of mortality, compared to controls (calculated RR, 1.88) (8). Another cohort study with covariate adjustment using multivariate logistic regression revealed no significant differences in the rate of SARS-CoV-2 positivity between COPD and non-COPD patients. However, significantly higher rates of hospitalization [adjusted odds ratio [OR]of 1.36], ICU admissions (adjusted OR of 1.20), and invasive mechanical ventilation (adjusted OR of 1.49) were observed in COPD patients infected with the virus when compared with non-COPD patients (15).

Taken together, if, on the one hand, published studies show a diverse prevalence of COPD among COVID-19 patients, on the other hand, they consistently show a worse clinical outcome in the same population. Further studies are needed to rule out potential ascertainment biases in profiling the COPD COVID-19 population and establishing whether the graver outcome in COPD patients is due to their underlying lung disease, the nature of the immune responses, the underlying pharmacologic COPD treatment (e.g., chronic steroid use), or a combination thereof.

AECOPD AND COVID-19

Coronaviruses are seasonal causes of AECOPD. Several factors can play a role in the increased susceptibility to develop severe SARS-CoV-2 infection in COPD patients. First, COPD patients often use many metered dose inhalant medications such as corticosteroids (ICS). The study by Attaway et al. (15) showed that COPD patients who tested positive for SARS-CoV-2 were 2.4 times less likely to have used corticosteroids at the time of testing than those who tested negative. Notwithstanding a few significant methodological limitations, such as proper control for confounding factors including treatment indication and disease severity, they raise a question about corticosteroids' role in COVID-19. ICS and long-acting bronchodilators are first-line therapies for AECOPD. When appropriate, AECOPD can be managed with antibiotics and oral corticosteroids (OCS). AECOPD directly related to SARS-CoV-2 infection should be treated with OCS such as dexamethasone, especially if they require supplemental oxygenation or invasive mechanical ventilation.

Further, in a randomized study of patients hospitalized with COVID-19, dexamethasone use resulted in lower 28-day mortality among those requiring either invasive mechanical ventilation or oxygen alone but not among those not requiring supplemental oxygen (16). On the other hand, long-term treatment with systemic corticosteroids is immunosuppressive, increasing the risk and severity of viral infections. Chronic impairment of the innate and acquired antiviral immune responses results in delayed viral clearance, enhanced mucus production, impaired antimicrobial peptide secretion, and increased pulmonary bacterial load during virus-induced exacerbations (17). Thus, the use of ICS during this pandemic has been called into question (18). Notably, a recent meta-analysis on COVID-19 outcomes in patients with chronic respiratory diseases using ICS concluded that there is currently no evidence on benefits or harms in COVID-19 in patients with underlying chronic respiratory illnesses (19). Consistently, an observational study using the OpenSafely platform that assessed more than 140,000 COPD patients, did not find a protective role for regular ICS use against COVID-19-related death in

COPD patients (20). The Global Initiative for Obstructive Lung Disease (GOLD) recommendations recently released a statement confirming the lack of scientific evidence to support that ICS or OCS should be avoided in patients with COPD during the COVID-19 epidemic (www.goldcopd.org). Research efforts should focus on profiling the characteristics of COVID-19, who could have more benefit from the use of ICS than potential complications.

COPD, ACE2, AND SARS-COV2: MATTERS OF DEBATE

COPD emerges from a complex interaction between genetic predisposition and environmental factors, while cigarette smoke remains the leading environmental cause of COPD. Between 15% and 50% of smokers develop COPD, 80–90% of COPD patients are smokers or ex-smokers (21, 22). To date, no definitive evidence on whether ever-smokers are at an increased risk of SARS-CoV-2 infection exists.

There are several possible ways cigarette smoke and COPD could affect SARS-CoV-2 entry and COVID-19 development (see **Figure 1**). SARS-CoV-2 uses the angiotensin-converting enzyme 2 (ACE2) as the host cell entry receptor (23). High-sensitivity RNA *in situ* mappings revealed the highest ACE2 expression in the nasal epithelium (24) with decreasing expression throughout the lower respiratory tract. Similarly, *in vitro* studies showed a striking gradient of SARS-CoV-2 infection in proximal (high) vs. distal (low) pulmonary epithelial cultures (24). Additionally, the expression of ACE2 in the lower respiratory tract and the upper respiratory tract is under different regulation (25). ACE2 gene in the peripheral lung has been found mainly expressed in goblet cells in smokers and club cells and alveolar type 2 (AT-II) cells in never smokers (23, 26).

Interestingly, cigarette smoke remodels cells in the bronchial epithelium inducing mucous cell metaplasia with a loss of club cells and apoptosis of alveolar septal cells (particularly AT-II cells) (27, 28), but this does not necessarily translate into higher SARS-CoV-2 infectivity. Notably, *in vitro* studies have shown that, whereas the ciliated cells are infected with SARS-CoV-2 and become extruded, the MUC5B+ club cells, or MUC5AC+ metaplastic goblet cells in the airway lumen, express high levels of ACE2 but are not easily infected (24). When conflated with features of attributable COVID-19 lung morbidity, these studies show quite persuasively that lung ACE2 expression is a suboptimal marker of SARS-CoV-2 infection and COVID-19 disease expression and morbidity.

Most of the studies published so far have implied that increases in lung ACE2 observed in ever smokers with and/or without COPD indicate greater susceptibility to SARS-CoV-2 infection and its expected complications (13, 26, 29, 30). However, there are several conflicting factors to consider when assessing the effects of cigarette smoke on ACE2 and SARS-CoV-2 infection. First, if, on the one hand, cigarette smoke and COPD have been associated with elevated pulmonary ACE2 levels (26), it is unclear whether this translates into higher SARS-CoV-2 infectivity and worse disease. A pivotal study published by Imai et al. (31) showed that ACE2 protects mice from severe ALI induced by acid aspiration or sepsis, and loss of ACE2 resulted in increased pulmonary inflammation and vascular permeability, causing worsening of the ARDS. Second, nicotine interacts with many components of the renin-angiotensin system (RAS) in multiple organ systems. In the ACE/Angiotensin II (AT-II) / Angiotensin$_1$ Receptor (AT_1R) arm, nicotine increases the expression and/or activity of renin, ACE, and AT_1R, whereas, in the compensatory ACE2/Angiotensin-(1–7) arm, nicotine downregulates the expression and/or activity of ACE2 and Angiotensin II Receptor (32–34). Third, cigarette smoke [both via activation of nicotinic acetylcholine receptors abundant in the bronchial epithelium (35), and via upregulation of macrophages] (36) can lead to enhanced activity of proteinases that can cleave SARS-CoV-2 S protein leading to viral entry into the host cells (37), and cause ACE2 shedding thus increasing viral uptake (38, 39). Fourth, soluble ACE2 can be released from the epithelial surface into the airways via cleavage by sheddases (38, 39). The release of soluble ACE2 is a dynamic process, occurring both constitutively and in response to various stimuli, possibly cigarette smoke and COPD. This process may activate off-targeted innate and adaptive immune responses and play a role in SARS-CoV-2 infection, as described below.

THE IMMUNE SYSTEM IN COPD: IMPLICATIONS DURING SARS-COV-2 INFECTION

COPD patients have blunted protective immune responses (6), affecting the mucociliary clearance and the activity of alveolar macrophages (40), dendritic cells (41), cytotoxic and regulatory T cells (42, 43), B cells and mucosal antibody production (44–46). Importantly, anti-viral immune responses such as Irf-7, IFN-α, factors contribute to the and IFN-β are significantly compromised in the lungs of active smokers (17, 47, 48). These factors contribute to the increased susceptibility to infections, and viral infections are one of the main causes of AECOPD.

Cigarette smoke compromises cellular anti-viral defenses via several mechanisms that involve both innate and adaptive immune responses. For example, exposure to cigarette smoke increases the numbers of alveolar macrophages in COPD. However, their phagocytic ability, anti-viral mediator expression, and clearance of apoptotic cells are reduced in COPD (36, 49–51). In particular, some of the macrophage-derived proteinases (e.g., A Disintegrin and A Metalloproteinase 17; ADAM17) can shed both SARS-CoV-2 S protein, inducing viral entry into the host cells (37), and ACE2 (38, 39) releasing it from the epithelial surface into the airways. Further, IFN-β, a critical cytokine required to inhibit coronavirus replication (52), is significantly reduced in lung epithelium and alveolar macrophages of COPD patients (47). Similarly, cigarette smoke stimulates specific serine phosphorylation-dependent ubiquitination and degradation of a type I IFN receptor subunit leading to attenuation of IFN signaling and decreased resistance to viral infection (53).

Cigarette smoke exposure also affects the adaptive immune system by inducing off-targeted T and B cell responses (42,

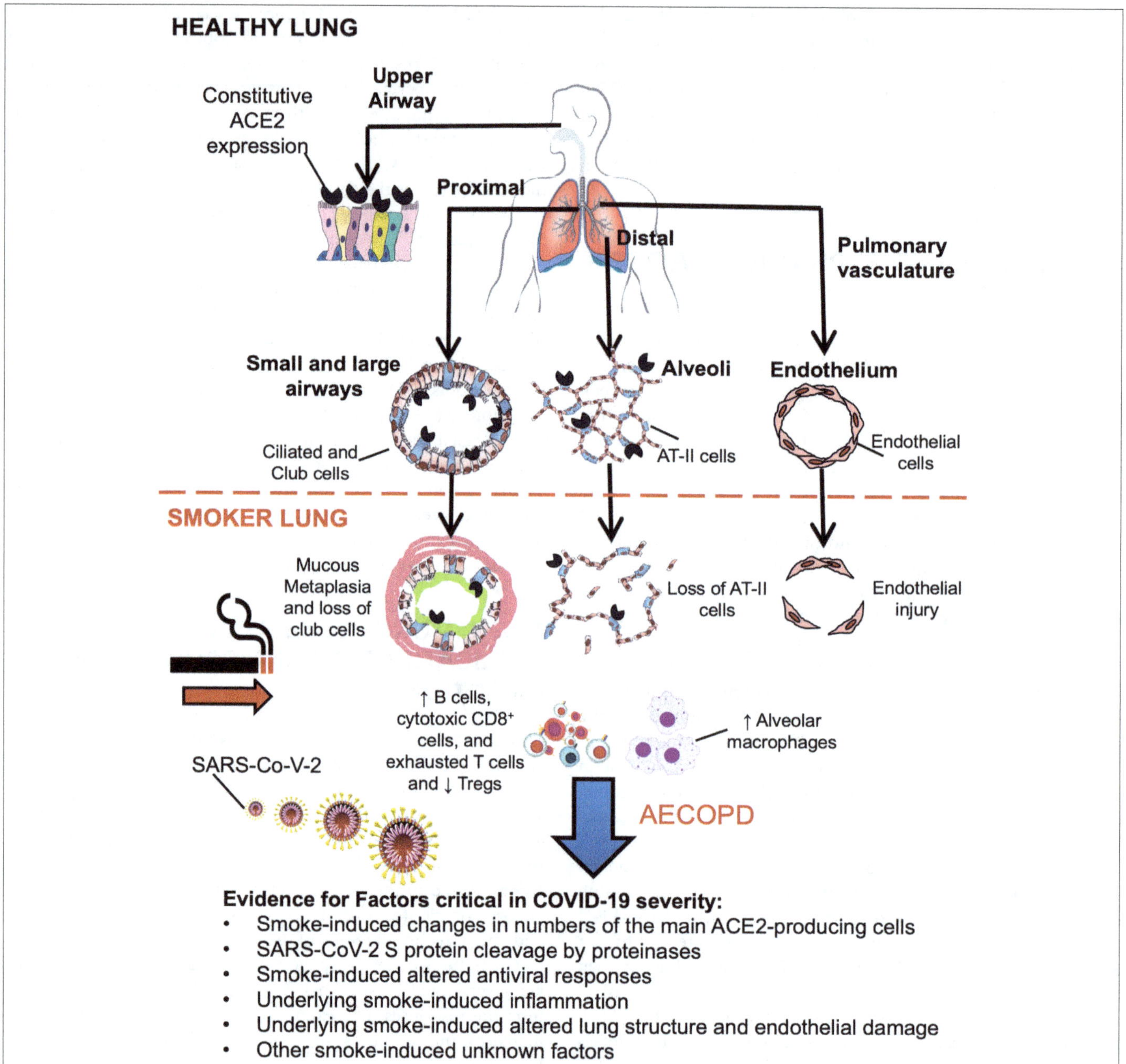

FIGURE 1 | There is a gradient of ACE2 expression throughout the respiratory tract. The highest ACE2 expression is found in the nasal epithelium followed by the larger airway epithelium, waning in the more distal bronchiolar and alveolar lung regions, in particular ciliated and secretory club cells, and alveolar type II (AT-II) cells. Cigarette smoke induces a loss of club cells and AT-II cells and extensive hyperplasia of goblet cells, but whether this is associated with increased susceptibility to SARS-CoV-2 infection is unclear. Additionally, cigarette smoke induces increases in the numbers of alveolar macrophages, that are the main cells expressing proteinases, and upregulates B cells, cytotoxic $CD8^+$ T cells often with an exhausted phenotype, while downregulating the T regulatory cell compartment. This chronic impairment of the innate and acquired immune responses results in delayed viral clearance, enhanced mucus production, impaired antimicrobial peptide secretion, and increased pulmonary bacterial load during virus-induced exacerbations and possibly during SARS-CoV-2 infection.

54, 55) that could contribute to worsening of SARS-CoV-2 infection and clinical outcome. B cells are critical players in the mucosal adaptive immune responses, leading to soluble IgA (sIgA) production against microbial and/or self-antigens (56, 57). There is a downregulation of the epithelial polymeric immunoglobulin receptor (pIgR, essential for the generation of mucosal sIgA) (58), thus causing an impaired viral clearance in COPD. Further in the emphysematous phenotype, there is an abundance of memory B cells that is not common in the lungs of subjects without COPD (54). The T cell compartment is also affected by the presence of COPD. T cells in the COPD lung tend to express an exhausted phenotype with reduced cytotoxicity and upregulation of programmed cell death protein-1 (PD-1) expression, which renders immunosuppressive actions on $CD8^+$ cells (59), paralleled by an expansion of oligoclonal $CD4^+$ T cells in lung tissue from COPD patients (60). Additionally, COPD patients have decreased numbers of circulating and pulmonary Treg cells, and reduced levels of FoxP3 mRNA and lung interleukin 10 (IL-10) secretion compared with never and ever smokers without COPD (42, 46).

The pathogenesis of COVID-19 has some immune features in common with COPD. CD4 T and CD8 T cell numbers are substantially decreased, whereas the Th17 and CD8 cytotoxic T cell populations are significantly grown in the peripheral blood from COVID-19 patients with ARDS (61). Instead, the SARS-CoV-2 infected pulmonary tissue's main changes include increases in natural killer (NK) cell, macrophage (mainly type I macrophage), B cell, and dendritic cell numbers, which contribute to the activation of CD8 and CD4 T cells (61). Simultaneously, the presence of exhausted T cells and a decrease in a blunted T regulatory compartment has been described in both blood and lung from COVID-19 patients (62, 63), likely contributing to the inflammatory storm and the pulmonary tissue damage observed in severe COVID-19. Also, a shift of the B cell compartment toward "atypical" memory B cells (lacking CD27 and low CD21 expression, unlike classical B cells that are $CD27^+$ $CD21^+$), described in other viral infections such as HIV, HBV, or HCV, have been described in COVID-19 patients (64), but the exact role of these atypical B cells needs to be clarified.

Overall, while it is unclear whether ever smokers with and/or without COPD may be at higher risk of SARS-CoV-2-infection (e.g., due to cigarette smoke -induced changes in numbers of the main ACE2-producing cells in the lung and/or increased SARS-CoV-2 S protein cleavage) if infected, they may be more severe due to underlying pulmonary inflammation and altered lung structure due to remodeling. Additional studies, both targeting cigarette smoke -exposed animals and *in vitro* models, are needed to shed light on the mechanisms by which cigarette smoke and COPD affect SARS-CoV-2 entry in the host cells and cause pulmonary disease.

ENDOTHELIAL DYSFUNCTION: A COMMON CULPRIT IN COPD AND COVID-19

In addition to the lungs, chronic cigarette smoke has been linked to dysfunction in multiple organs including the kidney, and systemic vascular endothelial dysfunction or injury (65, 66). Cigarette smoke-induced endothelial dysfunction can manifest as arterial hypertension (~70% of COPD patients), atherosclerosis, systemic inflammation, pulmonary arterial hypertension, cor-pulmonale, venous thromboembolism, and microalbuminuria (67).

A number of mechanisms underlie endothelial injury/dysfunction in COPD which include: (1) direct toxic effects of cigarette smoke on endothelial cells; (2) generation of auto-antibodies directed against endothelial cells; (3) vascular inflammation and oxidative stress, with reduced activation of the anti-oxidant pathways in endothelial cells; (4) increase in endothelial cell release of mediators with vasoconstrictor, pro-inflammatory, and remodeling activities (endothelin-1) and reduced endothelial cell expression of mediators that promote vasodilation and homeostasis of endothelial cells, such as nitric oxide and prostacyclin; 5) increased endoplasmic reticular stress and the unfolded protein response in endothelial cells; and (6) decreased expression of Vascular Endothelial Growth Factor (VEGF) associated with reduced hypoxia inducible factor- 1, a transcription factor that drives the expression of genes involved in endothelial function (66, 68).

Notably, some of the same pathological mechanisms in cigarette smoke-mediated endothelial dysfunction are hallmarks of respiratory viral infections, including SARS-CoV-2 infection. Clinically, coronavirus-infected patients show hypercoagulable state with thrombosis, with fibrin clots being one of the most common histopathological findings in the lungs and other organs from COVID-19 patients (69).

SARS-CoV-2 infection triggers an inflammatory cascade with increased IL-6, C-reactive protein, erythrocyte sedimentation rate, and elevated fibrinogen at presentation (70). Some patients appear to have a more pronounced inflammatory response to infection with SARS-CoV-2, such as seen with systemic inflammatory response syndrome or cytokine storm. Importantly, increased IL-6 levels correlate with increased fibrinogen, further supportin a strong link between inflammation and procoagulant changes (71). Together, the pulmonary and systemic effects of cigarette smoke could further potentiate SARS-CoV-2-induced endothelial dysfunction and the systemic inflammation in COPD patients. The mechanisms underlying this potential synergy, remains elusive. Nicotine interacts with many components of the renin-angiotensin system in multiple organ systems by decreasing ACE2 levels, thus indirectly regulating the vascular tone (34), but it is unknown whether cigarette smoke and/or COPD directly decrease ACE2 expression in the endothelial cells. Similarly, it is unclear whether cigarette smoke and/or COPD exacerbate inflammation in COVID-19 patients, since previous studies point at both inflammatory and anti-inflammatory effects of cigarette smoke (72). Further studies are needed in order to elucidate the direct effects of cigarette smoke and COPD on endothelial cells in the context of SARS-CoV-2 infection.

CONCLUSIONS

Overall, the effect of cigarette smoke on initial sites of SARS-CoV-2 infection, the mechanisms that seed infection distally in the lungs, and the virus-host interactions that attenuate or augment intra-regional virus growth in the cigarette smoke -exposed lung to produce severe disease are unclear (**Figure 1**). We suggest that *in vivo* and *in vitro* models aimed at testing the effects of cigarette smoke on SARS-CoV-2 infection could shed light needed insight.

Some of the unmet needs and knowledge gaps identified as follows:

- How does SARS-CoV-2 infection affect different types of COPD endotypes (e.g., emphysema-predominant, chronic bronchitis, eosinophilic-predominant, frequent exacerbators)?; what is/are the long-term effect/s of COVID-19 on their systemic and respiratory outcome?
- Should the gold standard recommendations for treating COPD and AECOPD (bronchodilators + corticosteroids) be applicable in COVID-19? Or should they be personalized according to the underlying COPD phenotype?
- How broadly should we expand the current therapeutic, radiological, and clinical follow-up of COPD patients post-COVID-19 infection to better understand its impact on disease progression?
- Are ever smokers with and/or without COPD at increased risk of getting infected with SARS-CoV-2? Moreover, if infected, are they at increased risk of developing severe COVID-19 outcomes?
- How do the innate and adaptive immune systems, and the anatomic changes associated with cigarette smoke exposure that play a significant role in the pathogenesis of COPD, affect the COVID-19 outcome in ever smokers with and/or without COPD?
- How does cigarette smoke and COPD affect the endothelium in COVID-19 patients? Do they exacerbate the endothelial dysfunction known to be key in the pathogenesis of COVID-19?

AUTHOR CONTRIBUTIONS

All authors listed have made a substantial, direct and intellectual contribution to the work, and approved it for publication.

REFERENCES

1. Reynolds HR, Adhikari S, Pulgarin C, Troxel AB, Iturrate E, Johnson SB, et al. Renin-angiotensin-aldosterone system inhibitors and Risk of Covid-19. *N Engl J Med.* (2020) 382:2441–8. doi: 10.1056/NEJMoa2008975
2. Richardson S, Hirsch JS, Narasimhan M, Crawford JM, McGinn T, Davidson KW, et al. Presenting characteristics, comorbidities, and outcomes among 5700 patients hospitalized with COVID-19 in the new york city area. *JAMA.* (2020) 323:2052–9. doi: 10.1001/jama.2020.6775
3. Zhou F, Yu T, Du R, Fan G, Liu Y, Liu Z, et al. Clinical course and risk factors for mortality of adult inpatients with COVID-19 in Wuhan, China: a retrospective cohort study. *Lancet.* (2020) 395:1054–62. doi: 10.1016/S0140-6736(20)30566-3
4. de Lusignan S, Dorward J, Correa A, Jones N, Akinyemi O, Amirthalingam G, et al. Risk factors for sars-cov-2 among patients in the oxford royal college of general practitioners research and surveillance centre primary care network: a cross-sectional study. *Lancet Infect Dis.* (2020) 20:1034–42. doi: 10.1016/S1473-3099(20)30371-6
5. Polverino F, Stern DA, Ruocco G, Balestro E, Bassetti M, Candelli M, et al. Comorbidities, cardiovascular therapies, and COVID-19 mortality: a nationwide, italian observational Study (ItaliCO). *Front Cardiovasc Med.* (2020) 7:585866. doi: 10.3389/fcvm.2020.585866
6. Mallia P, Message SD, Gielen V, Contoli M, Gray K, Kebadze T, et al. Experimental rhinovirus infection as a human model of chronic obstructive pulmonary disease exacerbation. *Am J Respir Crit Care Med.* (2011) 183:734–742. doi: 10.1164/rccm.201006-0833OC
7. Polverino F, Celli B. The challenge of controlling the copd epidemic: unmet needs. *Am J Med.* (2018) 131:1–6. doi: 10.1016/j.amjmed.2018.05.001
8. Alqahtani JS, Oyelade T, Aldhahir AM, Alghamdi SM, Almehmadi M, Alqahtani AS, et al. Prevalence, severity and mortality associated with COPD and Smoking in patients with COVID-19: a rapid systematic review and meta-analysis. *PLoS ONE.* (2020) 15:e0233147. doi: 10.1371/journal.pone.0233147
9. Wu Z, McGoogan JM. Characteristics of and important lessons from the coronavirus disease 2019. (COVID-19) Outbreak in China: Summary of a Report of 72314 Cases From the Chinese Center for Disease Control and Prevention. *JAMA.* (2020). 323:1239–42. doi: 10.1001/jama.2020.2648
10. Lippi G, Henry BM. Chronic obstructive pulmonary disease is associated with severe coronavirus disease (2019). (COVID-19). *Respir Med.* (2020). 167: 105941. doi: 10.1016/j.rmed.2020.105941
11. Farsalinos K, Angelopoulou A, Alexandris N, Poulas K. COVID-19 and the nicotinic cholinergic system. *Eur Respir J.* (2020) 56:2001589. doi: 10.1183/13993003.01589-2020
12. Guan WJ, Ni ZY, Hu Y, Liang WH, Ou CQ, He JX, et al. Clinical characteristics of coronavirus disease 2019 in China. *N Engl J Med.* (2020) 382:1708–1720. doi: 10.1056/NEJMoa2002032
13. Zhang H, Rostami MR, Leopold PL, Mezey JG, O'Beirne SL, Strulovici-Barel Y, et al. Expression of the SARS-CoV-2 ACE2 receptor in the human airway epithelium. *Am J Respir Crit Care Med.* (2020) 202:219–29. doi: 10.1164/rccm.202003-0541OC
14. Michelozzi P, de'Donato F, Scortichini M, De Sario M, Noccioli F, Rossi P, et al. Mortality impacts of the coronavirus disease (COVID-19) outbreak by sex and age: rapid mortality surveillance system, Italy, 1 February to 18 April (2020). *Euro Surveill.* (2020) 25:30506. doi: 10.2807/1560-7917.ES.2020.25.19.2000620
15. Attaway AA, Zein J, Hatipoglu US. SARS-CoV-2 infection in the COPD population is associated with increased healthcare utilization: An analysis of Cleveland clinic's COVID-19 registry. *EClinicalMedicine.* (2020) 26:100515. doi: 10.1016/j.eclinm.2020.100515
16. Group RC, Horby P, Lim WS, Emberson JR, Mafham M, Bell JL, et al. Dexamethasone in hospitalized patients with Covid-19 - preliminary report. *N Engl J Med.* (2020).
17. Singanayagam A, Glanville N, Girkin JL, Ching YM, Marcellini A, Porter JD, et al. Corticosteroid suppression of antiviral immunity increases bacterial loads and mucus production in COPD exacerbations. *Nat Commun.* (2018) 9:2229. doi: 10.1038/s41467-018-04574-1
18. Maes T, Bracke K, Brusselle GG. COVID-19, asthma, and inhaled corticosteroids: another beneficial effect of inhaled corticosteroids? *Am J Respir Crit Care Med.* (2020) 202:8. doi: 10.1164/rccm.202005-1651ED
19. Halpin DMG, Singh D, Hadfield RM. Inhaled corticosteroids and COVID-19: a systematic review and clinical perspective. *Eur Respir J.* (2020) 55:2001009. doi: 10.1183/13993003.01009-2020
20. Schultze A, Walker AJ, MacKenna B, Morton CE, Bhaskaran K, Brown JP, et al. Risk of COVID-19-related death among patients with chronic obstructive pulmonary disease or asthma prescribed inhaled corticosteroids: an observational cohort study using the OpenSAFELY platform. *Lancet Respir Med.* (2020) 8:1106–20. doi: 10.1016/S2213-2600(20)30415-X
21. Lokke A, Lange P, Scharling H, Fabricius P, Vestbo J. Developing COPD: a 25 year follow up study of the general population. *Thorax.* (2006) 61:935–9. doi: 10.1136/thx.2006.062802

22. Kim EJ, Yoon SJ, Kim YE, Go DS, Jung Y. Effects of aging and smoking duration on cigarette smoke-induced COPD severity. *J Korean Med Sci.* (2019) 34:e90. doi: 10.3346/jkms.2019.34.e90
23. Hoffmann M, Kleine-Weber H, Schroeder S, Kruger N, Herrler T, Erichsen S, et al. SARS-CoV-2 cell entry depends on ACE2 and TMPRSS2 and is blocked by a clinically proven protease inhibitor. *Cell.* (2020) 181:271–280 e278. doi: 10.1016/j.cell.2020.02.052
24. Hou YJ, Okuda K, Edwards CE, Martinez DR, Asakura T, Dinnon KH, et al. SARS-CoV-2 reverse genetics reveals a variable infection gradient in the respiratory tract. *Cell.* (2020) 182:429–46 e414. doi: 10.1016/j.cell.2020.05.042
25. Bunyavanich S DA, Vicencio A. Nasal gene expression of angiotensin-converting enzyme 2 in children and adults. *JAMA.* (2020) 323:2427–9. doi: 10.1001/jama.2020.8707
26. Cai G, Bosse Y, Xiao F, Kheradmand F, Amos CI. Tobacco smoking increases the lung gene expression of ACE2, the receptor of SARS-CoV-2. *Am J Respir Crit Care Med.* (2020) 201:1557–9. doi: 10.1164/rccm.202003-0693LE
27. Laucho-Contreras ME, Polverino F, Gupta K, Taylor KL, Kelly E, Pinto-Plata V, et al. Protective role for club cell secretory protein-16 (CC16) in the development of COPD. *Eur Respir J.* (2015) 45:1544–56. doi: 10.1183/09031936.00134214
28. Mebratu YA, Schwalm K, Smith KR, Schuyler M, Tesfaigzi Y. Cigarette smoke suppresses Bik to cause epithelial cell hyperplasia and mucous cell metaplasia. *Am J Respir Crit Care Med.* (2011) 183:1531–8. doi: 10.1164/rccm.201011-1930OC
29. Jacobs M, Van Eeckhoutte HP, Wijnant SRA, Janssens W, Joos GF, Brusselle GG, et al. Increased expression of ACE2, the SARS-CoV-2 entry receptor, in alveolar and bronchial epithelium of smokers and COPD subjects. *Eur Respir J.* (2020) 56:2002378. doi: 10.1101/2020.05.27.20114298
30. Leung JM, Yang CX, Tam A, Shaipanich T, Hackett TL, Singhera GK, et al. ACE-2 expression in the small airway epithelia of smokers and COPD patients: implications for COVID-19. *Eur Respir J.* (2020) 55:2000688. doi: 10.1183/13993003.00688-2020
31. Imai Y, Kuba K, Rao S, Huan Y, Guo F, Guan B, et al. Angiotensin-converting enzyme 2 protects from severe acute lung failure. *Nature.* (2005) 436:112–116. doi: 10.1038/nature03712
32. Ferrari MF, Raizada MK, Fior-Chadi DR. Differential regulation of the renin-angiotensin system by nicotine in WKY and SHR glia. *J Mol Neurosci.* (2008) 35:151–60. doi: 10.1007/s12031-007-9025-7
33. Ferrari MF, Raizada MK, Fior-Chadi DR. Nicotine modulates the renin-angiotensin system of cultured neurons and glial cells from cardiovascular brain areas of Wistar Kyoto and spontaneously hypertensive rats. *J Mol Neurosci.* (2007) 33:284–93. doi: 10.1007/s12031-007-9006-x
34. Oakes JM, Fuchs RM, Gardner JD, Lazartigues E, Yue X. Nicotine and the renin-angiotensin system. *Am J Physiol Regul Integr Comp Physiol.* (2018) 315:R895–R906. doi: 10.1152/ajpregu.00099.2018
35. Lam DC, Luo SY, Fu KH, Lui MM, Chan KH, Wistuba, et al. Nicotinic acetylcholine receptor expression in human airway correlates with lung function. *Am J Physiol Lung Cell Mol Physiol.* (2016) 310:L232–9. doi: 10.1152/ajplung.00101.2015
36. Polverino F, Rojas-Quintero J, Wang X, Petersen H, Zhang L, Gai X, et al. A disintegrin and metalloproteinase domain-8: a novel protective proteinase in chronic obstructive pulmonary disease. *Am J Respir Crit Care Med.* (2018) 198:1254–67. doi: 10.1164/rccm.201707-1331OC
37. Hoffmann M, Kleine-Weber H, Pohlmann S. A multibasic cleavage site in the spike protein of sars-cov-2 is essential for infection of human lung cells. *Mol Cell.* (2020) 78:779–84 e775. doi: 10.1016/j.molcel.2020.04.022
38. Jia HP, Look DC, Tan P, Shi L, Hickey M, Gakhar L, Chappell MC, Wohlford-Lenane C, McCray PB, Jr. Ectodomain shedding of angiotensin converting enzyme 2 in human airway epithelia. *Am J Physiol Lung Cell Mol Physiol.* (2009). 297: L84-96. doi: 10.1152/ajplung.00071.2009
39. Lambert DW, Yarski M, Warner FJ, Thornhill P, Parkin ET, Smith AI, et al. Tumor necrosis factor-alpha convertase (ADAM17) mediates regulated ectodomain shedding of the severe-acute respiratory syndrome-coronavirus (SARS-CoV) receptor, angiotensin-converting enzyme-2 (ACE2). *J Biol Chem.* (2005) 280:30113–30119. doi: 10.1074/jbc.M505111200
40. Barnes PJ. Alveolar macrophages in chronic obstructive pulmonary disease (COPD). *Cell Mol Biol (Noisy -le-grand).* (2004) 50 Online Pub: OL627-OL637.
41. Freeman CM, Curtis JL. Lung dendritic cells: shaping immune responses throughout chronic obstructive pulmonary disease progression. *Am J Respir Cell Mol Biol.* (2017) 56:152–9. doi: 10.1165/rcmb.2016-0272TR
42. Barcelo B, Pons J, Ferrer JM, Sauleda J, Fuster A, Agusti AG. Phenotypic characterisation of T-lymphocytes in COPD: abnormal CD4+CD25+ regulatory T-lymphocyte response to tobacco smoking. *Eur Respir J.* (2008) 31:555–62. doi: 10.1183/09031936.00010407
43. Barcelo B, Pons J, Fuster A, Sauleda J, Noguera A, Ferrer JM, et al. Intracellular cytokine profile of T lymphocytes in patients with chronic obstructive pulmonary disease. *Clin Exp Immunol.* (2006) 145:474–9. doi: 10.1111/j.1365-2249.2006.03167.x
44. Polverino F, Cosio BG, Pons J, Laucho-Contreras M, Tejera P, Iglesias A, et al. B Cell-Activating Factor. An orchestrator of lymphoid follicles in severe chronic obstructive Pulmonary disease. *Am J Respir Crit Care Med.* (2015) 192:695–705. doi: 10.1164/rccm.201501-0107OC
45. Ladjemi MZ, Lecocq M, Weynand B, Bowen H, Gould HJ, Van SJ, et al. Increased IgA production by B-cells in COPD via lung epithelial interleukin-6 and TACI pathways. *Eur Respir J.* (2015) 45:980–93. doi: 10.1183/09031936.00063914
46. Lee SH, Goswami S, Grudo A, Song LZ, Bandi V, Goodnight-White S, et al. Antielastin autoimmunity in tobacco smoking-induced emphysema. *Nat Med.* (2007) 13:567–9. doi: 10.1038/nm1583
47. Garcia-Valero J, Olloquequi J, Montes JF, Rodriguez E, Martin-Satue M, Texido L, et al. Deficient pulmonary IFN-beta expression in COPD patients. *PLoS One.* (2019) 14:e0217803. doi: 10.1371/journal.pone.0217803
48. Singanayagam A, Loo SL, Calderazzo M, Finney LJ, Trujillo Torralbo MB, Bakhsoliani E, et al. Antiviral immunity is impaired in COPD patients with frequent exacerbations. *Am J Physiol Lung Cell Mol Physiol.* (2019) 317:L893–L903. doi: 10.1152/ajplung.00253.2019
49. Berenson CS, Wrona CT, Grove LJ, Maloney J, Garlipp MA, Wallace PK, et al. Impaired alveolar macrophage response to Haemophilus antigens in chronic obstructive lung disease. *Am J Respir Crit Care Med.* (2006) 174:31–40. doi: 10.1164/rccm.200509-1461OC
50. Wang X, Polverino F, Rojas-Quintero J, Zhang D, Sanchez J, Yambayev I, et al. A disintegrin and a metalloproteinase-9 (adam9): a novel proteinase culprit with multifarious contributions to COPD. *Am J Respir Crit Care Med.* (2018) 198:1500–18. doi: 10.1164/rccm.201711-2300OC
51. Retamales I, Elliott WM, Meshi B, Coxson HO, Pare PD, Sciurba FC, et al. Amplification of inflammation in emphysema and its association with latent adenoviral infection. *Am J Respir Crit Care Med.* (2001) 164:469–73. doi: 10.1164/ajrccm.164.3.2007149
52. Sainz B, Jr., Mossel EC, Peters CJ, Garry RF. Interferon-beta and interferon-gamma synergistically inhibit the replication of severe acute respiratory syndrome-associated coronavirus (SARS-CoV). *Virology.* (2004) 329:11–7. doi: 10.1016/j.virol.2004.08.011
53. HuangFu WC, Liu J, Harty RN, Fuchs SY. Cigarette smoking products suppress anti-viral effects of Type I interferon via phosphorylation-dependent downregulation of its receptor. *FEBS Lett.* (2008) 582:3206–10. doi: 10.1016/j.febslet.2008.08.013
54. Sullivan JL, Bagevalu B, Glass C, Sholl L, Kraft M, Martinez FD, et al. B Cell Adaptive Immune Profile in Emphysema-Predominant COPD. *Am J Respir Crit Care Med.* (2019) 200:1434–9. doi: 10.1164/rccm.201903-0632LE
55. Pons J, Sauleda J, Ferrer JM, Barcelo B, Fuster A, Regueiro V, et al. Blunted gamma delta T-lymphocyte response in chronic obstructive pulmonary disease. *Eur Respir J.* (2005) 25:441–6. doi: 10.1183/09031936.05.00069304
56. Ladjemi MZ, Martin C, Lecocq M, Detry B, Aboubakar Nana F, Moulin C, et al. Increased IgA Expression in Lung Lymphoid Follicles in Severe COPD. *Am J Respir Crit Care Med.* (2019) 199:592–602. doi: 10.1164/rccm.201802-0352OC
57. Polverino F, Baraldo S, Bazzan E, Agostini S, Turato G, Lunardi F, et al. A novel insight into adaptive immunity in chronic obstructive pulmonary disease: B cell activating factor belonging to the tumor necrosis factor family. *Am J Respir Crit Care Med.* (2010) 182:1011–9. doi: 10.1164/rccm.200911-1700OC
58. Gohy ST, Detry BR, Lecocq M, Bouzin C, Weynand BA, Amatngalim GD, et al. Polymeric immunoglobulin receptor down-regulation in chronic obstructive pulmonary disease. Persistence in the cultured epithelium and

role of transforming growth factor-beta. *Am J Respir Crit Care Med.* (2014) 190:509–21. doi: 10.1164/rccm.201311-1971OC
59. McKendry RT, Spalluto CM, Burke H, Nicholas B, Cellura D, Al-Shamkhani A, et al. Dysregulation of Antiviral Function of CD8(+) T Cells in the Chronic Obstructive Pulmonary Disease Lung. Role of the PD-1-PD-L1. *Axis. Am J Respir Crit Care Med.* (2016) 193:642–51. doi: 10.1164/rccm.201504-0782OC
60. Sullivan AK, Simonian PL, Falta MT, Mitchell JD, Cosgrove GP, Brown KK, et al. Oligoclonal CD4+ T cells in the lungs of patients with severe emphysema. *Am J Respir Crit Care Med.* (2005) 172:590–6. doi: 10.1164/rccm.200410-1332OC
61. Xu Z, Shi L, Wang Y, Zhang J, Huang L, Zhang C, et al. Pathological findings of COVID-19 associated with acute respiratory distress syndrome. *Lancet Respir Med.* (2020) 8:420–2. doi: 10.1016/S2213-2600(20)30076-X
62. Tan L, Wang Q, Zhang D, Ding J, Huang Q, Tang YQ, et al. Lymphopenia predicts disease severity of COVID-19: a descriptive and predictive study. *Signal Transduct Target Ther.* (2020) 5:33. doi: 10.1038/s41392-020-0159-1
63. Chen Z, John Wherry E. T cell responses in patients with COVID-19. *Nat Rev Immunol.* (2020) 20:529–536. doi: 10.1038/s41577-020-0402-6
64. Oliviero B, Varchetta S, Mele D, Mantovani S, Cerino A, Perotti CG, et al. Expansion of atypical memory B cells is a prominent feature of COVID-19. *Cell Mol Immunol.* (2020) 17:1101–3. doi: 10.1038/s41423-020-00542-2
65. Polverino F, Laucho-Contreras ME, Petersen H, Bijol V, Sholl LM, Choi ME, et al. A Pilot Study Linking Endothelial Injury in Lungs and Kidneys in COPD. *Am J Respir Crit Care Med.* (2017) 195:1464–76. doi: 10.1164/rccm.201609-1765OC
66. Polverino F, Celli BR, Owen CA. COPD as an endothelial disorder: endothelial injury linking lesions in the lungs and other organs? (2017 Grover Conference Series). *Pulmonary circulation.* (2018). 8: 2045894018758528. doi: 10.1177/2045894018758528
67. Divo MJ, Casanova C, Marin JM, Pinto-Plata VM, de-Torres JP, Zulueta JJ, et al. COPD comorbidities network. *Eur Respir J.* (2015) 46:640–50. doi: 10.1183/09031936.00171614
68. Yasuo M, Mizuno S, Kraskauskas D, Bogaard HJ, Natarajan R, Cool CD, et al. Hypoxia inducible factor-1alpha in human emphysema lung tissue. *Eur Respir J.* (2011) 37:775–83. doi: 10.1183/09031936.00022910
69. Connors JM, Levy JH. COVID-19 and its implications for thrombosis and anticoagulation. *Blood.* (2020) 135:2033–40. doi: 10.1182/blood.2020006000
70. Chen G, Wu D, Guo W, Cao Y, Huang D, Wang H, et al. Clinical and immunological features of severe and moderate coronavirus disease (2019). *J Clin Invest.* (2020) 130:2620–9. doi: 10.1172/JCI137244
71. Ranucci M, Ballotta A, Di Dedda U, Bayshnikova E, Dei Poli M, Resta M, et al. The procoagulant pattern of patients with COVID-19 acute respiratory distress syndrome. *J Thromb Haemost.* (2020) 18:1747–51. doi: 10.1111/jth.14854
72. Chen H, Cowan MJ, Hasday JD, Vogel SN, Medvedev AE. Tobacco smoking inhibits expression of proinflammatory cytokines and activation of IL-1R-associated kinase, p38, and NF-kappaB in alveolar macrophages stimulated with TLR2 and TLR4 agonists. *J Immunol.* (2007) 179:6097–6106. doi: 10.4049/jimmunol.179.9.6097

7

Ketogenic Diet is Associated with Improvements in Chronic Obstructive Pulmonary Disease

Nicholas G. Norwitz[1*], *Russell Winwood*[2], *Brianna J. Stubbs*[3], *Dominic P. D'Agostino*[4,5] *and Peter J. Barnes*[6]

[1] *Department of Nutrition, Harvard Medical School, Boston, MA, United States,* [2] *Respiratory Network, Ministry of Health Agency for Clinical Innovation, St Leonards, NSW, Australia,* [3] *Buck Institute for Research on Aging, Novato, CA, United States,* [4] *Morsani College of Medicine, University of South Florida, Tampa, FL, United States,* [5] *Institute for Human and Machine Cognition, Pensacola, FL, United States,* [6] *National Heart and Lung Institute, Imperial College, London, United Kingdom*

Correspondence:
Nicholas G. Norwitz
nicholas_norwitz@hms.harvard.edu

Chronic Obstructive Pulmonary Disease (COPD) is a debilitating inflammatory respiratory condition that presents with worsening breathing difficulties and it is assumed to be progressive and incurable. As an inflammatory disease, COPD is associated with recruitment of immune cells to lung tissue and increased levels of pro-inflammatory cytokines, including TNF-α, IL-1β, IL-6, IL-8, and GM-CSF. Low-carbohydrate ketogenic diets have anti-inflammatory properties that could, in theory, improve COPD symptoms and progression. Herein, we report on a 54-year-old patient (C.A.) with COPD who adopted a ketogenic diet (70% calories from fat). Subsequently, C.A. experienced a reduction in inflammatory markers in association with a meaningful improvement in lung function. His inflammatory markers decreased into the normal range and his forced expiratory volume increased by 37.5% relative to its pre-ketogenic diet value. Future research should explore nutritional ketosis and ketogenic diets as possible therapeutic options for individuals with COPD.

Keywords: chronic objective pulmonary disease, ketogenic diet, forced expiratory volume 1, inflammation, case report

INTRODUCTION

Chronic Obstructive Pulmonary Disease (COPD) affects over 300 million patients worldwide and is currently the third ranked cause of death globally (1). COPD is characterized by slowly progressive airflow limitation as a result of peripheral airway obstruction (chronic bronchiolitis) and lung parenchymal destruction (emphysema), which lead to increasing shortness of breath on exertion (2). COPD is further associated with inflammation of the lung, including the recruitment of macrophages, neutrophils and lymphocytes and the secretion of multiple inflammatory mediators, including cytokines such as TNF-α, IL-1β, IL-6, IL-8, and GM-CSF (3). This pulmonary inflammation is not reduced by the mainstay of current therapy, inhaled long-acting bronchodilators, and is also largely resistant to corticosteroids (4). Targeting of individual cytokines has been unsuccessful, reflecting the fact that many mediators are involved in pathogenesis of the disease (5). Importantly, there are no current therapies that significantly improve disease progression. Therefore, there is a pressing need to find broader spectrum anti-inflammatory treatments for COPD that will improve symptoms, disease progression, and patient quality of life (6).

Ketogenic diets (KD) have a near century long history of being used to treat pediatric epilepsy (7), and newer research is beginning to explore their therapeutic potential in other chronic disease, such as type II diabetes (8, 9), polycystic ovarian syndrome (10), Alzheimer's disease (11), Parkinson's disease (12), cardiovascular risk (13), metabolic syndrome (14), and various mental illnesses (15). Many of these disease have an inflammatory component and, correspondingly, well-formulated ketogenic diets have been shown to improve a broad spectrum of inflammatory markers (16).

The anti-inflammatory effects of KD may be mediated, in part, by the ability of the ketone molecule, β-hydroxybutyrate (βHB), to inhibit the NLRP3 inflammasome (17, 18). NLRP3 is a protein complex that positively regulates the inflammatory response, and inhibition of NLRP3 is a mechanism whereby βHB is thought to mitigate inflammatory conditions such as gout (19). NLRP3 is also elevated in active COPD, as measured by circulating and local levels of NLRP3, Asc, and caspase-1 mRNAs (20). These mechanistic data, along with the clinical data mentioned above, suggest that a KD could have a beneficial effect in COPD patients, possibly by inhibiting NLRP3.

With respect to pulmonary diseases, KD improve symptoms in asthma (21) and trials are ongoing to determine whether KD may protect against severe COVID-19 disease, including lung disease (22). Importantly, a 3-week controlled trial including 60 COPD patients demonstrated a small but significant improvement in forced expiratory volume in 1 s (FEV_1) with a lower carbohydrate group (47% calories from carbohydrates) compared to a higher carbohydrate group (65% calories from carbohydrates) (23). In this study 10% of calories in the lower carbohydrate group were obtained from medium chain triglycerides to induce mild ketosis.

While COPD is an inflammatory disease and KD are known to be anti-inflammatory, there are no reports of KD being used to treat COPD existing in the medical literature. Herein we report on such a case in which an individual with COPD adopted a KD and subsequently observed improvements in inflammatory markers and lung function.

CASE DESCRIPTION

The subject of this study (C.A.) is a 54-year-old male in whom COPD was diagnosed in 2011, at age 45 years. Early in childhood, at age 10, C.A. was diagnosed with asthma. He also smoked cigarettes from age 17 and to 37 (~15 pack-years) and his grandfather died of lung cancer at age 67. C.A.'s only co-morbidity was and remains asthma, and he is free of other common comorbidities of COPD, including diabetes, pre-diabetes, cardiovascular disease, osteoporosis, sleep or mood disorders, metabolic syndrome, or obesity.

Abbreviations: COPD, Chronic obstructive pulmonary disease; FEV_1, forced expiratory volume in 1 second; GM-CSF, granulocyte-macrophage colony stimulating factor; KD, ketogenic diet; IL-1, interleukin; NLRP3, NOD-, LRR- and pyrin domain-containing protein 3; TNF-α, tumor necrosis factor-α; βHB, β-hydroxybutyrate.

In year prior to diagnosis, C.A.'s chief complaints were worsening shortness of breath and more frequent chest infections. In 2011, spirometry showed an FEV_1 of 0.79L (22% predicted normal) with an FEV_1/FVC ratio of 40%. There was an increase in lung volume measured by body plethysmography, with an increase in air trapping, but there was no reduction in gas transfer. There was no significant bronchodilator response to inhaled salbutamol, nor any response to a trial of oral corticosteroids (prednisolone 40 mg od for 4 weeks). A computerized tomography scan showed no evidence of emphysema, indicating that the COPD is due to small airway disease. C.A. was diagnosed with very severe COPD (GOLD stage 4) and was treated with inhaled tiotropium bromide once daily and budesonide-formoterol combination twice daily, which he has continued. He has also taken zinc and vitamin C supplements daily since his diagnosis in 2011.

Over the ensuring 4 years C.A. undertook an aerobic exercise program consisting of daily running, cycling or swimming and ate a "balanced diet" consisting of fats, proteins, and carbohydrates, including fruits, vegetables and whole grains. In association with his daily activity and diet, his BMI decreased (from 29.4 kg/m^2 at time of diagnosis in 2011 to 23.8 kg/m^2 in 2017), his exercise maximal peak capacity increased from 165 to a peak of 193 watts, as measured by cycle ergometer, and his FEV_1 improved only marginally to 0.91L (25% predicted normal).

In 2017, he began a low-carbohydrate, high-fat diet KD. The macronutrient composition of the diet comprised calories from 70% fat, 20% protein, and 10% carbohydrates and C.A. confirmed nutritional ketosis of >0.5 mmol/L daily by fingerstick using an Abbott Optium Neo device that measured blood D-βHB. While on the KD, he lost no more weight, remaining at a BMI of 23.8 kg/m^2 at the time of the 2019 and 2020 measurements listed below.

Prior to starting the KD, baseline plasma TNF-α, IL-1β, IL-6, IL-8, and GM-CSF, concentrations were 16, 4.9, 13.9, 499, and 193.5 pg/mL, respectively, and CRP was 7 mg/L. All measurements were above the upper threshold of normal. In 2019, 2 years into his KD, blood concentrations decreased to 3.4 (TNF-α), 0.6 (IL-1β), 4.2 (IL-6), 2.7 (IL-8), and 21.6 pg/mL (GM-CSF), and CRP was 1 – 2 mg/L (**Figure 1**). These measurements were repeated in 2020, with maintenance of the KD, and results were similar. On both occasions all post-KD inflammatory markers were within the normal range with the singular exception of the 2020 IL-8 (62 pg/mL), although this measure still represented an 8-fold decrease from its pre-KD level. All three cytokine panels were ordered direct to consumer (NutriPath) by C.A. The 2017 baseline test was ordered for interest following his self-study on COPD. At this time, there was no thought of a case report; however, C.A.'s response to dietary change was—in his perspective (below)—so remarkable that, in 2019, he decided he wanted to collect follow-up data to correlate with his improved symptoms and quality of life out of interest. He also ordered the 2020 tests as a replicate.

In conjunction with the improvement in inflammatory blood biomarkers (**Figure 1**), C.A.'s FEV_1 improved to 1.24 (35% predicted) and 1.25L in 2019 and in 2020, respectively, representing an improvement in FEV_1 of 38% relative to

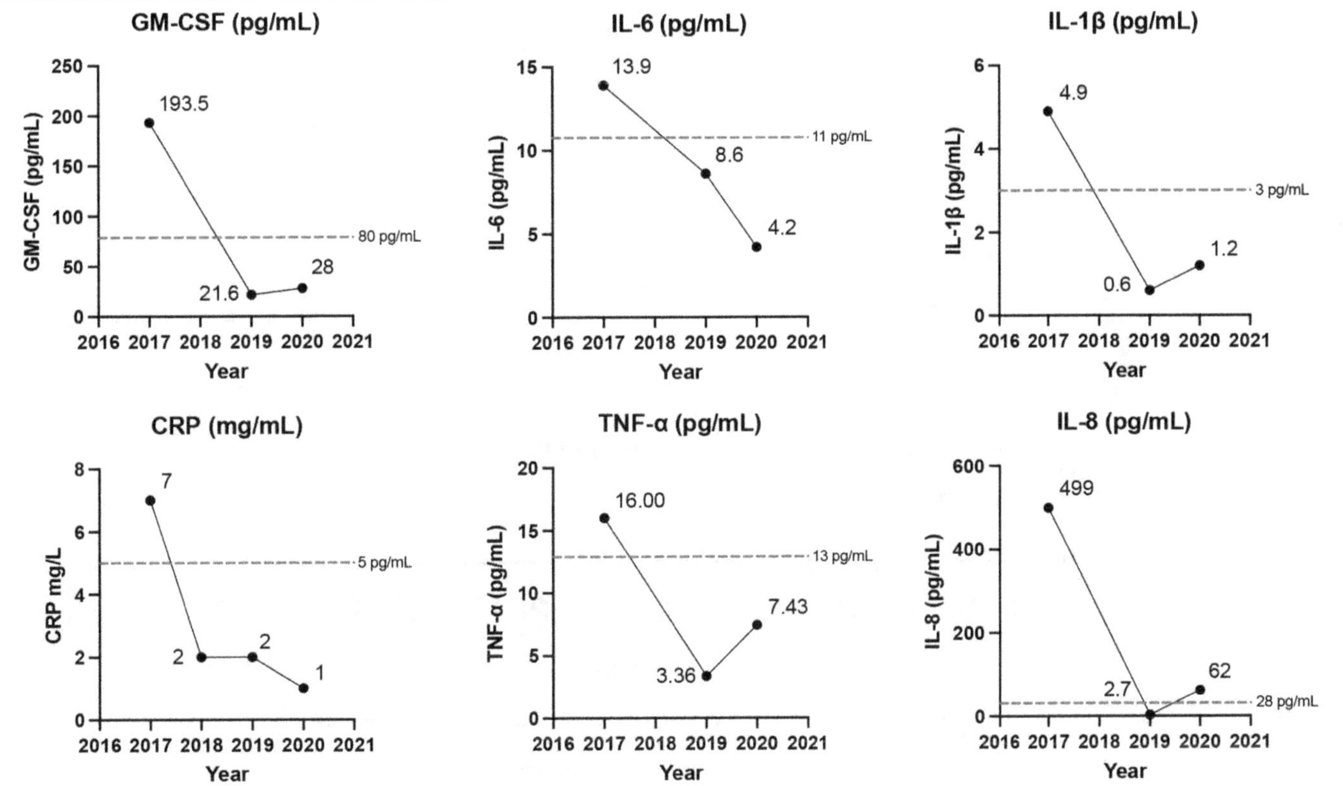

FIGURE 1 | Inflammatory biomarkers. Data represent C.A.'s inflammatory biomarkers prior to starting a ketogenic diet and at two time points, 2019 and 2020, after commencing the diet. Green dotted line represent the threshold of normal range for each biomarker. All markers improved on a ketogenic diet.

pre-KD measurements (**Figure 2**). All lung function tests, including the baseline test, were administered 24 h after stopping bronchodilators. Prior to the diet he suffered from 1 to 2 acute exacerbations/year but reported no exacerbations since taking the KD. He also reported improvement in symptoms and quality of life, with reduced use of rescue salbutamol inhaler from 3 to 4 puffs daily before the KD to only one or less puffs on the diet. His exercise tolerance also improved markedly to the extent that he was able to complete marathons.

DISCUSSION

C.A. suffers from severe COPD, predominantly due to small airway disease and showed only modest improvement in symptoms and lung function with maximal inhaler therapy (inhaled corticosteroid, long-acting muscarinic antagonist and long-acting β_2-agonist), as recommended by current management strategies (24). After switching to a KD, he had reduced symptoms and improved exercise tolerance, used less rescue inhaler and had no further acute exacerbations. His FEV_1 improved by over 35%, relative to baseline, whereas there had previously been no significant improvement with a bronchodilator or a systemic corticosteroid. Furthermore, between 2011 and 2017, his self-prescribed exercise program increased his FEV_1 from 0.79L (22% predicted normal) to FEV_1 from 0.91L (25% predicted normal), in conjunction with a BMI decrease from 29.4 to 23.8 kg/m^2. By comparison, the addition of a KD was associated with a much larger improvement in FEV_1 to 1.24 and 1.25, in 2019 and 2020, respectively (~35% predicted), without any change in weight. As the KD improved C.A.'s exercise tolerance, it's possible that there was a synergy between the KD and exercise, i.e., that the KD acted as a therapeutic adjunct. It is also possible, and perhaps more likely, that the KD had an independent effect.

The clinical improvements C.A. experienced after adopting the KD were accompanied by a marked fall in plasma concentrations of several inflammatory cytokines known to be increased in COPD (TNF-α, IL-1β, IL6, IL-8, GM-CSF, and CRP) that were elevated prior to the diet. While the data on hand do not permit us to draw a causal conclusion that the KD improved C.A.'s COPD, the coincident drop in serum cytokines and improvements in FEV_1, along with prior clinical and non-clinical literature demonstrating anti-inflammatory and therapeutic beneficial effects of a KD in inflammatory disorders, suggest that a KD could have potential for the treatment of COPD. This is an area that deserves more structured investigation.

Several dietary interventions have been evaluated in COPD, mainly with a view to increasing skeletal muscle mass as well as addition of nutraceuticals, such as antioxidant vitamins and vitamin D, but so far there is no convincing evidence for the efficacy of these diets, and they are not recommended in the routine management of COPD patients (25). Since diagnosis in 2011, C.A. only ever reported consuming a zinc and vitamin

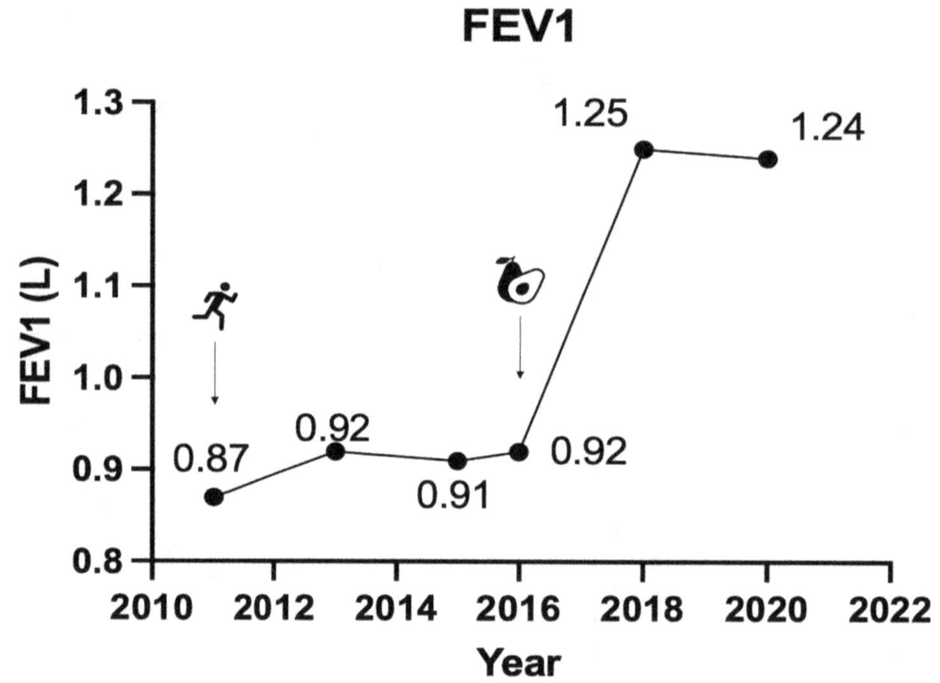

FIGURE 2 | Forced expiratory volume in 1 s. Data represent C.A.'s FEV1 at four time points prior to starting a ketogenic diet and at two time points, 2019 and 2020, after commencing the diet.

C supplement and their dosing did not change upon starting a KD. Dietary interventions may theoretically benefit the lung disease, but also the comorbidities that are commonly seen in COPD patients (26), including diabetes, pre-diabetes, obesity, ad metabolic syndrome, although C.A. presented with none of these conditions nor did the KD cause C.A. to lose weight. Furthermore, dietary interventions may be more acceptable to patients than long-term drug therapies, which have poor adherence in COPD (27). Conversely, despite the common conception that KD are not sustainable for patients, trials show that patients given adequate education and support adhere to and enjoy KD as much as other diets and standard of care (8, 28).

Although a KD has been shown to improve asthma, there are no previous reports of its use in COPD patients. Given the parallel decrease in cytokines and improvement in FEV_1, it is possible, if not likely, that the direct anti-inflammatory effect of the KD mediate part of the therapeutic benefit of the lifestyle in this case. βHB is known to inhibit the NLRP3 inflammasome (17, 18), which plays a pathological role in COPD (20). Ketogenic diets have also been shown to lower a wide range of inflammatory cytokines and have been shown to outperform isocaloric low-fat diets in their ability to lower TNF-α, IL-6, and IL-8 (16) and reverse insulin resistance and metabolic syndrome (14), which are common inflammatory comorbidities associated with COPD (29, 30).

Another possible mechanism for the clinical improvement in COPD may be a change in the gut or lung microbiome. Lung microbiome is abnormal in COPD, and patients with severe COPD commonly have colonization of the lower respiratory tract with bacteria such as *Haemphilus influenzae, Streptococcus pneumoniae*, and *Moraxella cattarhalis* (31, 32). These colonizing bacteria may be important in inducing a chronic inflammatory response, with increases in cytokines TNF-α, IL-1β, IL-6, and IL-8. Correspondingly, mouse data suggest that changes in the microbiome mediate some of the therapeutic effects of ketogenic diet against epilepsy (33) and that KDs can alter the microbiome to protect against activation of Th17 cells and other inflammatory mediators (34).

An obvious limitation of this case study is that the data do not allow us to draw conclusions about the mechanism of action by which a KD improved inflammation and respiratory function in the patient, C.A. We can only note the striking association among the onset and maintenance of KD and concomitant improvements in all measured inflammatory markers and FEV_1. Nevertheless, C.A.'s improvements make mechanistic sense in the context of the broader literature on COPD as an inflammatory disorder and KD as an anti-inflammatory intervention. Future animal model research should focus on exploring the mechanisms of action of KD on COPD and related respiratory conditions with a mind toward providing patients with a lifestyle option to treat disease and improve quality of life.

PATIENT PERSPECTIVE

After my COPD diagnosis, I made a commitment to myself that I would do anything I could to improve my health so took up running, swimming, and cycling. Even though, I wasn't very good, I especially loved distance running. I started listening to podcasts and reading about how nutrition could improve my breathing and endurance running performance. The information I gathered suggested a low-carb ketogenic diet could help burn fat as fuel more efficiently, I thought I'd give it a go. I was surprised to find my breathlessness diminished as soon as I was in ketosis and, 4 months later, I ran my personal best marathon time of 5½ h, which for me was astonishing. I started to notice when I adhered to my diet my breathing was less labored. Encouraged, I started to read more including a paper that showed ketones inhibit the NLRP3 inflammasome. I had also read about the NLRP3 and its role in COPD. I asked a respiratory professional whom I met at a conference, "what if we had a medication to inhibit NLRP3?" He said, "that could represent a remarkable step forward in the treatment and patient care." That sealed it for me. I've been on a ketogenic diet ever since and, combined with my exercise, my respiration appears to be ever improving. It's unlikely I'll ever have completely normal breathing, but I'm so grateful to being trending upward, not downward. I hope my experience will encourage others to try a lifestyle that significantly improved my quality of life.

LIMITATIONS

As with any retrospective $n = 1$ patient case, this report contains limitations that must be acknowledged. (i) First, the duration of time between the initiation of the KD and subsequent FEV_1 and cytokine tests was ~2 years. It is plausible that other changes in the patient's lifestyle during this time contributed to his symptomatic and inflammatory improvements. While the patient attests that "I was surprised to find my breathlessness diminished as soon as I was in ketosis," and that "when I adhered to my diet my breathing was less labored," and that he ran his personal best marathon time 4 months after the initiation of his diet, these data are self-reported and/or subjective and should be taken as such. (ii) Second, and building on the above, there is the possibility of a placebo interaction. As the patient was encouraged about the possibility that a ketogenic diet could improve his athletic performance and symptoms, it is feasible that this optimism changed his exercise confidence, or other aspects of lifestyle, contributing to his improvements. It is also possible that his enthusiasm and optimism led him to order the direct-to-consumer cytokine panels at symptomatically favorable moments when inflammation might have been in a trough. Although he denies this was the case, and it seems unlikely that a placebo interaction could explain the full effect and its consistency (assuming the effect is genuine and due to the diet), it is an important caveat, nonetheless. (iii) Third, the patient represents a highly particular case of COPD, as most patients are not marathon runners and do not engage in intensive physical activities. It would therefore be premature to generalize the findings of this report to a wider COPD population. (iv) Finally, it would have been ideal to not only have more data timepoints but also more functional measures of lung function. Unfortunately, as this is a retrospective case, the data are limited to that which the patients and treating physician had available to us.

SUMMARY

We report on a case in which initiation and continuation of a ketogenic diet was associated with improvements in the lung function and inflammatory markers of a patient with COPD. As ketogenic diets have the potential to be anti-inflammatory diets, COPD is an inflammatory disorder, and ketogenic diets are being explored for an increasing array of inflammatory conditions, this case suggests ketogenic diets could have therapeutic potential in COPD and that more research is needed.

AUTHOR CONTRIBUTIONS

All authors listed have made a substantial, direct and intellectual contribution to the work, and approved it for publication.

REFERENCES

1. Collaboration GCRD. Prevalence and attributable health burden of chronic respiratory diseases, 1990–2017: a systematic analysis for the Global Burden of Disease Study 2017. *Lancet Respirat Med.* (2020) 8:585–96. doi: 10.1016/S2213-2600(20)30105-3
2. Agustí A, Hogg JC. Update on the pathogenesis of chronic obstructive pulmonary disease. *N Engl J Med.* (2019) 381:1248–56. doi: 10.1056/NEJMra1900475
3. Barnes PJ. The cytokine network in COPD. *Am J Respir Cell Mol Biol.* (2009) 41:631–8. doi: 10.1165/rcmb.2009-0220TR
4. GOLD. *Global Initiative for Chronic Obstructive Lung Disease (GOLD): Global Strategy for the Diagnosis, Management and Prevention of COPD.* GOLD. (2021). Available online at: www.goldcopd.com (accessed April 10, 2021).
5. Barnes PJ. Targeting cytokines to treat asthma and chronic obstructive pulmonary disease. *Nat Rev Immunol.* (2018) 18:454–66. doi: 10.1038/s41577-018-0006-6
6. Barnes PJ. New anti-inflammatory treatments for chronic obstructive pulmonary disease. *Nat Rev Drug Discov.* (2013) 12:543–59. doi: 10.1038/nrd4025
7. Sourbron J, Klinkenberg S, van Kuijk SMJ, Lagae L, Lambrechts D, Braakman HMH, et al. Ketogenic diet for the treatment of pediatric epilepsy: review and meta-analysis. *Childs Nerv Syst.* (2020) 36:1099–109. doi: 10.1007/s00381-020-04578-7
8. Athinarayanan SJ, Adams RN, Hallberg SJ, McKenzie AL, Bhanpuri NH, Campbell WW, et al. Long-term effects of a novel continuous remote care intervention including nutritional ketosis for the management of type 2 diabetes: a 2-year non-randomized clinical trial. *Front Endocrinol.* (2019) 10:348. doi: 10.3389/fendo.2019.00348
9. Unwin D, Khalid AA, Unwin J, Crocombe D, Delon C, Martyn K, et al. Insights from a general practice service evaluation supporting a lower carbohydrate diet in patients with type 2 diabetes mellitus and prediabetes: a secondary analysis of routine clinic data including HbA1c, weight and prescribing over 6 years. *BMJ Nutr Prev Health.* (2020) 3:285–94. doi: 10.1136/bmjnph-2020-000072
10. Li J, Bai WP, Jiang B, Bai LR, Gu B, Yan SX, et al. Ketogenic diet in women with polycystic ovary syndrome and liver dysfunction who are obese: a randomized, open-label, parallel-group, controlled pilot trial. *J Obstet Gynaecol Res.* (2021) 47:1145–52. doi: 10.1111/jog.14650
11. Phillips MCL, Deprez LM, Mortimer GMN, Murtagh DKJ, McCoy S, Mylchreest R, et al. Randomized crossover trial of a modified ketogenic diet in Alzheimer's disease. *Alzheimers Res Ther.* (2021) 13:51. doi: 10.1186/s13195-021-00783-x
12. Norwitz NG, Dearlove DJ, Lu M, Clarke K, Dawes H, Hu MT, et al. Ketone ester drink enhances endurance exercise performance in Parkinson's disease. *Front Neurosci.* (2020) 14:584130. doi: 10.3389/fnins.2020.584130

13. Norwitz NG, Loh V, A. Standard lipid panel is insufficient for the care of a patient on a high-fat, low-carbohydrate ketogenic diet. *Front Med.* (2020) 7:97. doi: 10.3389/fmed.2020.00097
14. Hyde PN, Sapper TN, Crabtree CD, LaFountain RA, Bowling ML, Buga A, et al. Dietary carbohydrate restriction improves metabolic syndrome independent of weight loss. *JCI Insight.* (2019) 4:128308. doi: 10.1172/jci.insight.128308
15. Norwitz NG, Dalai SS, Palmer CM. Ketogenic diet as a metabolic treatment for mental illness. *Curr Opin Endocrinol Diabetes Obes.* (2020) 27:269–74. doi: 10.1097/MED.0000000000000564
16. Forsythe CE, Phinney SD, Fernandez ML, Quann EE, Wood RJ, Bibus DM, et al. Comparison of low fat and low carbohydrate diets on circulating fatty acid composition and markers of inflammation. *Lipids.* (2008) 43:65–77. doi: 10.1007/s11745-007-3132-7
17. Youm YH, Nguyen KY, Grant RW, Goldberg EL, Bodogai M, Kim D, et al. The ketone metabolite beta-hydroxybutyrate blocks NLRP3 inflammasome-mediated inflammatory disease. *Nat Med.* (2015) 21:263–9. doi: 10.1038/nm.3804
18. Shippy DC, Wilhelm C, Viharkumar PA, Raife TJ, Ulland TK. β-Hydroxybutyrate inhibits inflammasome activation to attenuate Alzheimer's disease pathology. *J Neuroinflammation.* (2020) 17:280. doi: 10.1186/s12974-020-01948-5
19. Goldberg EL, Asher JL, Molony RD, Shaw AC, Zeiss CJ, Wang C, et al. β-hydroxybutyrate deactivates neutrophil NLRP3 inflammasome to relieve gout flares. *Cell Rep.* (2017) 18:2077–87. doi: 10.1016/j.celrep.2017.02.004
20. Wang H, Lv C, Wang S, Ying H, Weng Y, Yu W. NLRP3 Inflammasome involves in the acute exacerbation of patients with chronic obstructive pulmonary disease. *Inflammation.* (2018) 41:1321–33. doi: 10.1007/s10753-018-0780-0
21. Peshkin MM. Asthma in children. *Am J Dis Child.* (1930) 39:1240–54. doi: 10.1001/archpedi.1930.01930180090008
22. Paoli Aea. *Ketogenic Diet as Protective Factor During COVID-19.* clincaltrials.gov Sponsor of study: University of Padova (2021). Available online at: https://clinicaltrials.gov/ct2/show/NCT04615975
23. Cai B, Zhu Y, Ma Y, Xu Z, Zao Y, Wang J, et al. Effect of supplementing a high-fat, low-carbohydrate enteral formula in COPD patients. *Nutrition.* (2003) 19:229–32. doi: 10.1016/S0899-9007(02)01064-X
24. G. *2021 Global Strategy for Prevention, Diagnosis and Management COPD.* (2021).
25. Scoditti E, Massaro M, Garbarino S, Toraldo DM. Role of diet in chronic obstructive pulmonary disease prevention and treatment. *Nutrients.* (2019) 11:61357. doi: 10.3390/nu11061357
26. Triest FJJ, Franssen FME, Reynaert N, Gaffron S, Spruit MA, Janssen DJA, et al. Disease-specific comorbidity clusters in COPD and accelerated aging. *J Clin Med.* (2019) 8:40511. doi: 10.3390/jcm8040511
27. Cushen B, Sulaiman I, Greene G, MacHale E, Mokoka M, Reilly RB, et al. The clinical impact of different adherence behaviors in patients with severe chronic obstructive pulmonary disease. *Am J Respir Crit Care Med.* (2018) 197:1630–3. doi: 10.1164/rccm.201712-2469LE
28. Landry MJ, Crimarco A, Perelman D, Durand LR, Petlura C, Aronica L, et al. Adherence to ketogenic and mediterranean study diets in a crossover trial: the keto-med randomized trial. *Nutrients.* (2021) 13:30967. doi: 10.3390/nu13030967
29. Machado FVC, Pitta F, Hernandes NA, Bertolini GL. Physiopathological relationship between chronic obstructive pulmonary disease and insulin resistance. *Endocrine.* (2018) 61:17–22. doi: 10.1007/s12020-018-1554-z
30. Naik D, Joshi A, Paul TV, Thomas N. Chronic obstructive pulmonary disease and the metabolic syndrome: consequences of a dual threat. *Indian J Endocrinol Metab.* (2014) 18:608–16. doi: 10.4103/2230-8210.139212
31. Singh R, Mackay AJ, Patel AR, Garcha DS, Kowlessar BS, Brill SE, et al. Inflammatory thresholds and the species-specific effects of colonising bacteria in stable chronic obstructive pulmonary disease. *Respir Res.* (2014) 15:114. doi: 10.1186/s12931-014-0114-1
32. Wang Z, Singh R, Miller BE, Tal-Singer R, Van Horn S, Tomsho L, et al. Sputum microbiome temporal variability and dysbiosis in chronic obstructive pulmonary disease exacerbations: an analysis of the COPDMAP study. *Thorax.* (2018) 73:331–8. doi: 10.1136/thoraxjnl-2017-210741
33. Olson CA, Vuong HE, Yano JM, Liang QY, Nusbaum DJ, Hsiao EY. The gut microbiota mediates the anti-seizure effects of the ketogenic diet. *Cell.* (2018) 173:1728–41.e13. doi: 10.1016/j.cell.2018.04.027
34. Ang QY, Alexander M, Newman JC, Tian Y, Cai J, Upadhyay V, et al. Ketogenic diets alter the gut microbiome resulting in decreased intestinal Th17 cells. *Cell.* (2020) 181:1263–75.e16. doi: 10.1016/j.cell.2020.04.027

8

Development and Validation of Risk Prediction Model for In-Hospital Mortality among Patients Hospitalized with Acute Exacerbation Chronic Obstructive Pulmonary Disease Between 2015 and 2019

Fen Dong[1,2,3,4], *Xiaoxia Ren*[2,3,4], *Ke Huang*[2,3,4], *Yanyan Wang*[5], *Jianjun Jiao*[6] *and Ting Yang*[2,3,4*]

[1] *Institute of Clinical Medical Sciences, China–Japan Friendship Hospital, Beijing, China,* [2] *Department of Pulmonary and Critical Care Medicine, China-Japan Friendship Hospital, Beijing, China,* [3] *National Clinical Research Center for Respiratory Diseases, Beijing, China,* [4] *Institute of Respiratory Medicine, Chinese Academy of Medical Science, Beijing, China,* [5] *Department of Medical Records, China–Japan Friendship Hospital, Beijing, China,* [6] *Department of Medical Administration, China–Japan Friendship Hospital, Beijing, China*

Correspondence:
Ting Yang
dryangting@qq.com

Background: In patients with chronic obstructive pulmonary disease (COPD), acute exacerbations affect patients' health and can lead to death. This study was aimed to develop a prediction model for in-hospital mortality in patients with acute exacerbations of COPD (AECOPD).

Method: A retrospective study was performed in patients hospitalized for AECOPD between 2015 and 2019. Patients admitted between 2015 and 2017 were included to develop model and individuals admitted in the following 2 years were included for external validation. We analyzed variables that were readily available in clinical practice. Given that death was a rare outcome in this study, we fitted Firth penalized logistic regression. C statistic and calibration plot quantified the model performance. Optimism-corrected C statistic and slope were estimated by bootstrapping. Accordingly, the prediction model was adjusted and then transformed into risk score.

Result: Between 2015 and 2017, 1,096 eligible patients were analyzed, with a mean age of 73 years and 67.8% male. The in-hospital mortality was 2.6%. Compared to survivors, non-survivors were older, more admitted from emergency, more frequently concomitant with respiratory failure, pneumothorax, hypoxic-hypercarbic encephalopathy, and had longer length of stay (LOS). Four variables were included into the final model: age, respiratory failure, pneumothorax, and LOS. In internal validation, C statistic was 0.9147, and the calibration slope was 1.0254. Their optimism-corrected values were 0.90887 and 0.9282, respectively, indicating satisfactory discrimination and calibration. When externally validated in 700 AECOPD patients during 2018 and 2019, the model demonstrated good discrimination with a C statistic of 0.8176. Calibration plot illustrated a varying discordance between predicted and observed mortality. It demonstrated good calibration in low-risk patients with predicted mortality rate $\leq$10% ($P = 0.3253$) but overestimated mortality in patients with predicted rate >10% ($P < 0.0001$). The risk score of 20 was regarded as a threshold with an optimal Youden index of 0.7154.

Conclusion: A simple prediction model for AECOPD in-hospital mortality has been developed and externally validated. Based on available data in clinical setting, the model could serve as an easily used instrument for clinical decision-making. Complications emerged as strong predictors, underscoring an important role of disease management in improving patients' prognoses during exacerbation episodes.

Keywords: prediction model, development, validation, in-hospital mortality, acute exacerbation of COPD

INTRODUCTION

Chronic obstructive pulmonary disease (COPD) is a burdensome illness that accounts for 96% chronic respiratory disease deaths in China (1). In COPD progression, acute exacerbations can be easily triggered and affect patients' health. Severe exacerbations always increase the use of health service in hospital and cause great medical costs (2, 3). It may also lead to poor patient outcomes and even early death. Elderly patients are at particularly high risk of poor prognosis. Some co-existing morbidities, including COPD complications and comorbidities that occur during exacerbation episodes might worsen conditions and place patients at high risk of death. Prior studies have demonstrated an increased mortality risk in COPD patients with severe exacerbations (4).

Identifying high-risk patients for mortality during exacerbation episodes can help care providers deliver proper interventions to improve prognosis and avoid early death. Predicting health outcomes by the use of patient characteristics as predictors has been mentioned as a cornerstone in modern clinical medicine (5). An effective risk prediction model needs to incorporate prognostic factors that may influence patients' survival. Substantial efforts have been made to predict mortality in COPD patients, including the DECAF score, BAP-65, and 2008 scores for in-hospital mortality due to exacerbation (6). As health-care systems vary across nations, some predictors in the existing risk scores are not readily available in clinical setting. China has a heavy burden of COPD, with nearly 100 million COPD patients (7). Data routinely collected in clinical practice are seldom utilized for prognosis prediction in patients hospitalized for acute exacerbations of COPD (AECOPD). Studies on prediction models for in-hospital mortality in this subgroup of patients are limited.

Therefore, we developed and validated a risk prediction model for mortality in patients hospitalized with AECOPD. A clinical prediction tool was developed, incorporating easy-to-measure indicators that were readily available in clinical practice, aimed to help decision-making and optimize clinical care for patients in the real-world setting.

MATERIALS AND METHODS

Study Patients

We performed a retrospective study in National Clinical Research Center for Respiratory Diseases, a 354-bed, medical and clinical research center in a tertiary hospital in Beijing, China. Eligible patients were individuals who were diagnosed as AECOPD, aged $\geq$40 years and admitted between January 1, 2015 and December 31, 2019. Patients with primary diagnosis of respiratory failure and secondary diagnosis of AECOPD were also included since their root cause of hospitalization was still AECOPD. All diagnoses in electronic medical records, including primary and secondary diagnoses, were determined by International Classification of Diseases, 10th Revision (ICD10) coding system. COPD was defined as J40-J44 in ICD-10 codes. In the study site, exacerbation was diagnosed when patients experienced at least any two of the following symptoms at clinics or emergency visits: dyspnea, increased sputum purulence and volume, increased cough and wheeze. To ascertain the accuracy of diagnoses, we reviewed medical records to ensure that our study patients were hospitalized due to acute exacerbations. Patients were excluded if they had been hospitalized within recent 30 days, or discharged against medical advice. Index admissions of eligible patients were included for analysis. The index admission was defined as the first admission for AECOPD during the study period.

Potential Predictors and Outcome

We gathered the following information from electronic medical records: demographic characteristics (age, sex, marital status), concomitant diseases of COPD, source of admission (emergency or out-patient department), season and day of week of admission (weekday or weekend), and length of stay (LOS) at index admission. Concomitant diseases were determined by secondary diagnoses and classified into complications and comorbidities of COPD according to guidelines and researches (8–10). In this study, complications included respiratory failure, pulmonary heart diseases, hypoxemia, venous thromboembolism (VTE), pneumothorax, and hypoxic-hypercarbic encephalopathy. Comorbidities were cardio/cerebrovascular diseases, diabetes, respiratory infection, bronchiectasis, gastroesophageal reflux, obstructive sleep apnea syndrome, lung cancer, depression or anxiety, and osteoporosis. LOS was calculated as days by subtracting the admission date from discharge date. If patients were discharged and readmitted on the same day, their readmissions were actually the same hospitalization as the initial one. Their LOS were calculated as the summed days of hospital stay in each consecutive admission. If patients were admitted to the hospital for multiple times but not on the same day as aforementioned, we only analyzed their first admissions during 2015 and 2019. The primary outcome was all-cause mortality during hospitalization.

Statistical Analysis

Data were summarized as number (percentage) for categorical variables and mean ± SD or median (interquartile ranges [IQRs]) for continuous variables where appropriate. *T*-test was adopted for normally distributed continuous variables and Mann–Whitney's test was for non-normally distributed ones. Categorical variables were analyzed using Chi's-square test or Fisher's exact test.

A large sample size can develop a robust model (11). We utilized all data on AECOPD admissions between 2015 and 2017 as a derivation dataset for model development and internal validation. Predictors that have plausible relationship with outcome are recommended as candidate predictors (12). Based on existing knowledge and literature review, we analyzed indicators that were potentially associated with death, including demographics, hospital admission and stay, season at admission, complications, and comorbidities of COPD. Baseline information were compared between patients alive and those who died. Univariable associations between potential predictors and mortality were examined. Indicators that were statistically significant were regarded as candidate predictors, including age, source of admission, LOS, respiratory failure, pneumothorax, and hypoxic-hypercarbic encephalopathy. To minimize potential overfitting, we anticipated a shrinkage factor of at least 0.9, and the shrinkage was 0.1 correspondingly. According to the new guideline on sample size for developing prediction model (11, 13), an estimated number of 510 participants were needed using the six aforementioned candidate predictor parameters and shrinkage factor. As death was a rare event in our study, penalized regression was adopted to avoid the overfitting arising from the low number of outcomes (14). We fitted penalized logistic regression for model selection using the LASSO method. Coefficients of predictors were estimated in Firth's penalized regression, which was an effective approach to overcome overfitting when the outcome was rare (14). A single-model analysis was also performed. The final model was determined by model selection and clinical relevance.

Performance of prediction model was evaluated by discrimination and calibration. C statistic, also known as the area under the curve (AUC), was a metric for the model's discrimination, which referred to the ability to classify patients who died from those alive in this study. Calibration characterized the accurate prediction of absolute death risk, being visually illustrated in a plot by comparing predicted and observed mortality rates at different levels. The curve's slope and intercept were estimated to quantify the calibration performance. Hosmer–Lemeshow test was utilized to examine discordances between the observed and predicted in-hospital mortality rate. In order to obtain a stable and unbiased estimate of discrimination and calibration, we deployed bootstrap to internally validate the performance of prediction model. The bootstrapped resample had the same size as derivation data. The modeling process was repeated in each resampled data. Optimism-corrected C statistic and calibration slope were estimated by bootstrapping 500 resamples according to Transport Reporting of a Multivariable Prediction Model for Individual Prognosis of Diagnosis (TRIPOD) statement (15).

To externally validate the prediction model, we longitudinally collected data on AECOPD patients hospitalized in the following 2 years (2018–2019). Discrimination and calibration of the prediction model were assessed by C statistics and calibration plot, respectively.

To apply this prediction model into clinical practice as a friendly used tool, we further transformed the model into a risk prediction algorithm and calculated risk score for individuals. According to beta coefficients of predictors in final prediction model and values of predictors, we assigned point for each predictor and calculated the total risk points (16). The threshold of risk score for in-hospital mortality was determined by the optimal Youden index. Also, a clinically relevant threshold was determined via visual inspection of an obvious increase in mortality risk. Sensitivity, specificity, and the Youden index were estimated at the thresholds.

This study was approved by China-Japan Friendship Hospital Clinical Research Ethics Committee (approval no. 2018-163-K119). Privacy and confidentiality of all patients' information were maintained. Patient informed consent was not required.

RESULTS

Totally, 1,096 AECOPD patients admitted between 2015 and 2017 were available for model development. The mean ± SD of age was 73 ± 10 years, and 67.8% were male. Most patients were admitted from outpatient department (55.1%) and at weekdays (89.8%). The majority of patients were admitted to respirology department, with only 3.84% admitted into intensive care unit (ICU). Cardio/cerebrovascular diseases were the predominant comorbidities (67.2%), and respiratory failure was the most common complication (26.1%). During hospitalization, 29 (2.6%) patients died. Compared to survivors, the non-survivors were older, more admitted from emergency, more frequently concomitant with respiratory failure, pneumothorax, hypoxic-hypercarbic encephalopathy, and had longer LOS (all $P < 0.05$) (**Table 1**). All these variables were associated with increased risk of mortality (**Supplementary Table 1**). Age, emergency admission, LOS, complications of respiratory failure, pneumothorax, and hypoxic-hypercarbic encephalopathy were determined as candidate predictors for model selection.

TABLE 1 | Characteristics of COPD patients hospitalized for acute exacerbation between 2015 and 2017.

Variables		All $N = 1,096$	Alive $N = 1,067$	Dead $N = 29$	*P*-value*
Demographic characteristics	Age, years**	75 (66, 81)	75 (66, 81)	80 (72, 84)	0.0098
	Male	743 (67.8)	722 (67.7)	21 (72.4)	0.5893
	Married	1,048 (95.6)	1,021 (95.7)	27 (93.1)	0.5020
Admission and hospital stay	Admitted on weekend	112 (10.2)	108 (10.1)	4 (13.8)	0.5284
	Admitted from emergency	491 (44.9)	467 (43.9)	24 (82.8)	<0.0001
	Length of stay, days	11 (8, 15)	11 (8, 15)	22 (10, 31)	0.0002
Season at admission	Mar.–May	281 (25.6)	271 (25.4)	10 (34.5)	0.5387
	Jun.–Aug.	216 (19.7)	209 (19.6)	7 (24.1)	
	Sep.–Nov.	251 (22.9)	246 (23.1)	5 (17.2)	
	Dec.–Feb.	348 (31.8)	341 (32.0)	7 (24.1)	
Complications of COPD	Respiratory failure	286 (26.1)	259 (24.3)	27 (93.1)	<0.0001
	VTE	28 (2.6)	28 (2.6)	0 (0.0)	1.0000
	Pneumothorax	13 (1.2)	10 (0.9)	3 (10.3)	0.0040
	Pulmonary heart disease	225 (20.5)	218 (20.4)	7 (24.1)	0.6258
	Hypoxic-hypercarbic encephalopathy	27 (2.5)	23 (2.2)	4 (13.8)	0.0046
	Hypoxemia	31 (2.8)	31 (2.9)	0 (0.0)	1.0000
Comorbidities of COPD	Cardio/cerebrovascular Diseases	736 (67.2)	719 (67.4)	17 (58.6)	0.3214
	Bronchiectasis	93 (8.5)	90 (8.4)	3 (10.3)	0.7306
	Diabetes	183 (16.7)	181 (17.0)	2 (6.9)	0.2072
	Respiratory infection	137 (12.5)	133 (12.5)	4 (13.8)	0.7762
	Anxiety depression	17 (1.6)	17 (1.6)	0 (0.0)	1.0000
	Lung cancer	22 (2.0)	21 (2.0)	1 (3.4)	0.4489
	Osteoporosis	18 (1.6)	18 (1.7)	0 (0.0)	1.0000
	Reflux esophagitis	66 (6.0)	65 (6.1)	1 (3.4)	1.0000
	OSAS	19 (1.7)	19 (1.8)	0 (0.0)	1.0000

Chi-square or Fisher exact test was performed where appropriate. Age was abnormally distributed in all patients, survivors and non-survivors. They were expressed as median (interquartile range). Their mean ± SD were 73 ± 10, 73 ± 10, and 78 ± 8, respectively.

Model Development and Internal Validation

Using LASSO selection method, a model retaining age and LOS was selected based on schwarz bayesian criterion (SBC). Considering the aim to identify coexisting morbidities that may affect patients' outcome, we also incorporated another two significant predictors in single model analyses: respiratory failure and pneumothorax (**Supplementary Table 2**). Finally, age, LOS, respiratory failure, and pneumothorax were included into Firth's penalized logistic model for coefficient estimation. All the four predictors were statistically significant (all $P < 0.05$) (**Table 2**). The odds ratio (OR) and 95% confidence interval (CI) was 1.05 (1.002–1.09) for age, 27.47 (7.49–100.81) for respiratory failure, 6.71 (1.24–36.40) for pneumothorax and 1.03 (1.005–1.05) for LOS.

In internal validation, C statistic of the prediction model was 0.9147 (95% CI 0.8850, 0.9444). After bootstrapping 500 times with replacement, the optimism was estimated as 0.00582. Optimism-corrected C statistic was 0.90887, indicating excellent discrimination of the prediction model to differentiate alive inpatients from those who died. The model had satisfactory apparent calibration with slope of 1.0254 and intercept of 0.0326. In calibration plot, the curve of observed vs. predicted mortality was closed to the diagonal. The Hosmer–Lemeshow test was insignificant ($P = 0.9556$). After adjustment for optimism, the slope was 0.9282 (**Table 3**, **Figure 1**).

TABLE 2 | Firth's penalized logistic regression for in-hospital mortality between 2015 and 2017.

Variable	β coefficients	*P*-value	OR (95% CI)*
Intercept	−9.5187	<0.0001	–
Age, years	0.045	0.0382	1.05 (1.002, 1.09)
Respiratory failure	3.3131	<0.0001	27.47 (7.49, 100.81)
Pneumothorax	1.9041	0.0273	6.71 (1.24, 36.40)
Length of stay, days	0.0262	0.017	1.03 (1.005, 1.05)

OR, odds ratio; CI, confidence interval.

External Validation

The external validation was performed in 700 AECOPD patients admitted in the following 2 years (2018 and 2019), of whom 12 (1.7%) patients died. Patients were mainly admitted to respirology department, with only 6.14% admitted into ICU. The mean ± SD of age was 72 ± 10 years and 73.1% were male. C

TABLE 3 | Apparent and validation performance of prediction model.

Performance Statistics	Apparent performance in original sample	Internal validation[a]			External validation[b]
		Bootstrap performance	Test performance in original sample	Optimism corrected	
C statistic	0.9147	0.91739	0.91157	0.90887	0.8176
Calibration[c]	Slope: 1.0254 Intercept: 0.0326	Slope: 1.0244 Intercept: 0.0150	Slope: 0.9272 Intercept: −0.1874	Slope: 0.9282	Slope: 0.5986 Intercept: −1.4804

[a] *Prediction model was internally validated in AECOPD patients admitted between 2015 and 2017. The estimates (95% confidence interval) of apparent performance of prediction model in original sample: 0.9147 (0.8850, 0.9444) for C statistic, 1.0254 (0.7276, 1.3233) for calibration slope and 0.0326 (−0.7834, 0.8486) for intercept. The apparent performance in the model derived from bootstrap sample was compared with the test performance obtained when applying the model to the original sample. Differences in apparent and test performances across all models were averaged to estimate the overall optimism for C statistics and slope. The optimism-corrected C statistics and slope were 0.90887 and 0.9282, respectively. The corrected slope (0.9282) was also shrinkage factor to adjust the original prediction model.*

[b] *External validation was performed in AECOPD patients admitted between 2018 and 2019. At external validation, the calibration slope reflects the combined effect of overfitting on the development data (2015–2017) and true differences in effects of predictors. Estimates (95% confidence interval) of prediction model performance were 0.8176 (0.7487, 0.8865) for C statistic, 0.5986 (0.2409, 0.9563) for calibration slope, and −1.4804 (−2.8037, −0.1571) for intercept, respectively.*

[c] *Intercept and slope of calibration plot were estimated in a logistic regression model with in-hosptial death events as outcome and linear predictor as the only independent variable.*

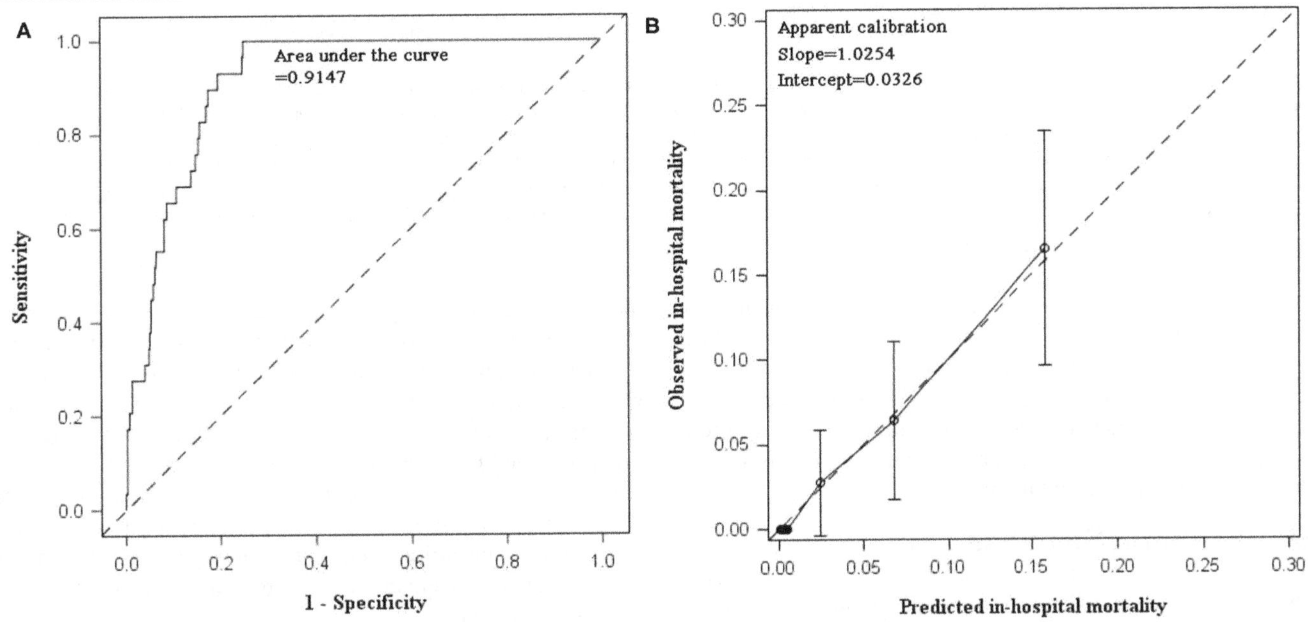

FIGURE 1 | Discimination and calibration of in-hospital mortality prediction model in internal validation using data collected between 2015 and 2017. **(A)** AUC of prediabetes prediction model: the prediction model demonstrated excellent discrimination. The apparent C statistics and optimism-corrected C statistics were 0.9147 and 0.90887, respectively. After recalibration, C statistics remained the same and the estimate (95% CI) was still 0.9147 (0.8850, 0.9444). **(B)** Calibration plot of prediction model: calibration slope was 1.0254 (95% CI: 0.7276, 1.3233) and intercept was 0.0326 (95% CI: −0.7834, 0.8486). Hosmer–Lemeshow test was insignificant (chi-square statistics = 2.6249, df = 8, $P = 0.9556$).

statistics was 0.8176 (0.7487, 0.8865) for mortality prediction. In respect to calibration, we observed that the magnitude of difference between predicted and observed mortality varied along the death risk. The model was well-calibrated in low-risk patients with predicted mortality rate ≤10%, with a fairly large *P*-value in Hosmer–Lemeshow test ($P = 0.3253$). Whereas, mortality was overestimated in patients with predicted rate >10% ($P < 0.0001$). The overall Hosmer–Lemeshow test result was significant ($P = 0.0292$). The slope and intercept deviated from the ideal values of 1 and 0 (**Table 3**, **Figure 2**).

Coefficient Adjustment and Intercept Recalibration

To account for optimism, predictor coefficients in original prediction model were adjusted using a shrinkage factor, which was the optimism-corrected slope of 0.9282 (**Table 3**). To maintain the overall apparent calibration, the intercept was re-estimated as −9.1935. **Supplementary Table 3** demonstrated the final prediction model with shrunken predictor coefficients and recalibrated intercept. Applying the final model to derivation dataset of 2015–2017, there was no substantial change in C

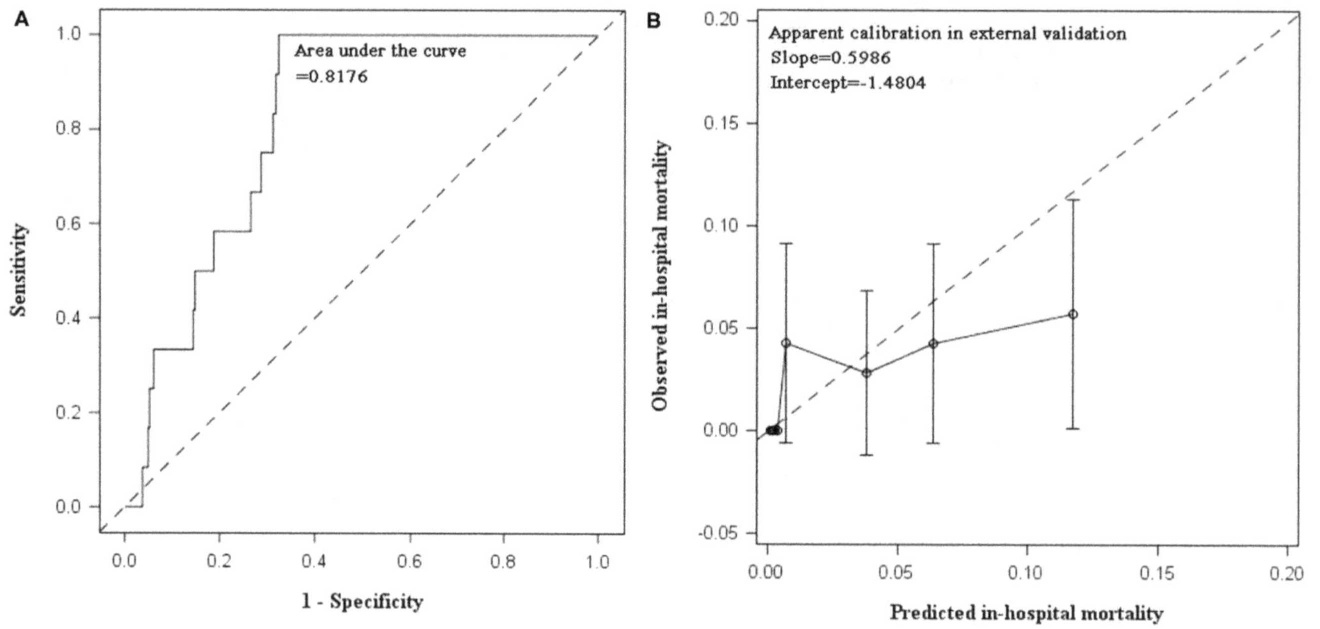

FIGURE 2 | Discrimination and calibration of in-hospital mortality prediction model in external validation using data collected between 2018 and 2019. **(A)** AUC of in-hospital mortality prediction model: C statistic was 0.8176 (95% CI: 0.7487, 0.8865) in patients hospitalized for AECOPD during 2018 and 2019. **(B)** Calibration plot of prediction model: calibration slope was 0.5986 (95% CI: 0.2409, 0.9563) and intercept was −1.4804 (95% CI: −2.8037, −0.1571). Hosmer–Lemeshow test indicated poor calibration of our prediction model in AECOPD inpatients between 2018 and 2019. When stratified by predicted mortality, the prediction model was well-calibrated in low-risk patients with predicted mortality rate ≤10%. The Hosmer–Lemeshow test was insignificant (chi-square = 9.2052, $P = 0.3253$). Whereas, the death risk was overestimated in patients with predicted mortality rate greater than 10% (chi-square = 281.1386, $P < 0.0001$). The overall Hosmer–Lemeshow test result was significant (chi-square = 17.0856, $P = 0.0292$).

statistics since the ordering of predicted probabilities for models with original or shrunk coefficients are identical (17). But the model demonstrated excellent calibration in the derivation data of 2015–2017 with slope of 1.1048 and intercept of 0.43149 (**Supplementary Figure 1A**) and improved calibration with slope and intercept closer to 1 and 0 in the validation data of 2018–2019 (**Supplementary Figure 1B**).

Risk Score and Stratification

After model adjustment with shrunken coefficients and recalibrated intercept, risk point of each predictor and total point were calculated on the basis of beta coefficients in the final model (**Supplementary Table 4**). The actual total risk points in AECOPD patients during 2015 and 2017 ranged from 0 to 35. The risk score of 20 was set as threshold to differentiate alive individuals from non-survivors, with an optimal Youden index of 0.7154, sensitivity 0.9310 (95% CI 0.8388–1.0000), and specificity 0.7844 (95% CI 0.7598–0.8091). The 20-risk score was also the point where both observed and predicted death risk started to increase, with almost all deaths (27/29) occurring in this subgroup of patients. The majority (76.55%) had <20 points (**Figure 3**). Predicted mortality at 20-risk score was 3.9%.

DISCUSSION

A simple risk prediction model was developed using routinely collected data in hospital. The recalibrated prediction model, incorporating demographic and clinical indicators, accurately predict in-hospital mortality in patients with AECOPD, with excellent discriminative and calibration ability in internal validation and good performance in external validation. Among patients experiencing acute exacerbation, advanced age, prolonged hospital stay, and concomitant morbidities were identified as important predictors for mortality. Respiratory failure and pneumothorax were particularly important concomitant morbidities, suggesting the key role of concomitant morbidities management in improvement of outcomes in AECOPD inpatients.

Several predictive models have been proposed for AECOPD mortality. The DECAF score is a well-known instrument for mortality prediction, with information gathered by medical and research staff following standard protocols (18). There exists a high heterogeneity of indicators used for model construction in the existing studies (6, 18, 19). Some indicators are not routinely collected in clinical practice, which might be attributed to disparities in health-care systems across nations. Also, definitions of outcome events and time frame of mortality varies. In a study performed in AECOPD patients visiting emergency, the outcome was short-term mortality, including mortality in hospital and within a week of discharge to home (19).

Consistent with previously reported studies on mortality in AECOPD, advanced age was recognized as a significant predictor for mortality in our study (18, 20). Respiratory failure emerged as a strong risk factor for in-hospital mortality, which

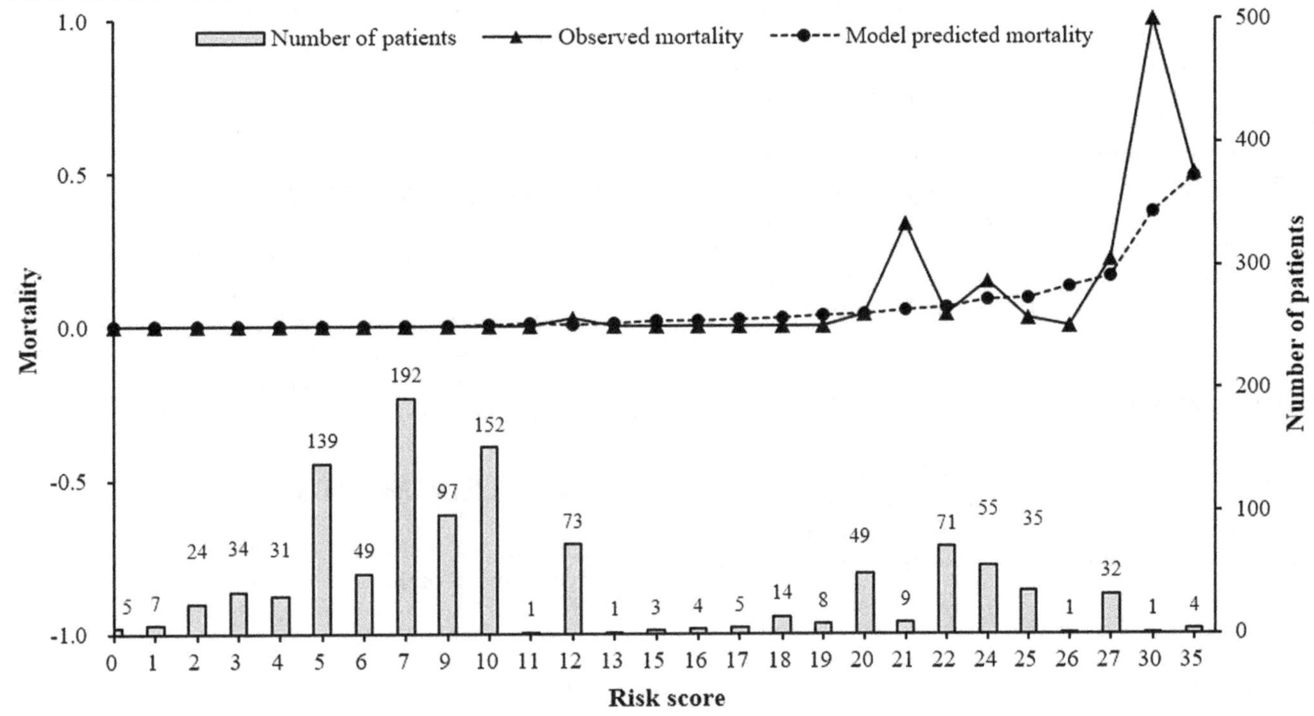

FIGURE 3 | Observed, predicted in-hospital mortality along with risk score and distribution of risk score in AECOPD patients between 2015 and 2017. Model predicted mortality was calculated using our final prediction model: Log(mortality/(1-mortality)) = −9.1935 + 0.0418*age +3.0752*Respiratory failure + 1.7674*Pneumothorax + 0.0243*Length of stay Risk score was the total risk points, which was the sum of each predictor's risk point based on individual values.

is similar to a recent research on hypercapnia during respiratory failure increased the risk of mortality (21, 22). The increase in mortality risk was also observed in patients with respiratory failure in a cohort in Thailand (20). Respiratory failure is a serious complication in severe exacerbations. It reflects disease severity with a manifestation of dramatical drop in lung function. This condition can be modified through early interventions, for example, blood gas and proper management when admitted and utilization of ventilation or supplemental oxygen (20, 23, 24). Co-existing morbidities have been regarded as mortality predicting factors after hospital admission (4, 25, 26). But they were mostly measured as a comprehensive index such as Charlson. Analyses specific to a certain concomitant morbidity were not provided. To identify important prognostic factors for survival and guide clinical decision-making, it's necessary to specify concomitant morbidities that greatly affect the prognosis. Complications identified as mortality predictors in our study are potentially treatable and can be intervened early to curb disease progression, indicating significant clinical implications.

There are several limitations in this study. First, as the study was aimed to predict mortality risk in AECOPD patients, the study population was restricted to patients experiencing severe acute exacerbation that leads to hospital admission. Survival in patients with less severe exacerbations was not analyzed, which might compromise the generalizability of our prediction model. To strengthen the validity of our prediction model, it still needs to be validated in independent populations with diverse disease severity. Second, easy-to-measure indicators in daily clinical practice were used as candidate predictors. Differences in data collection in existing studies resulted in disparities in prognostic factors, making our findings incomparable with the prior ones (6, 18, 19). Third, this study focused on mortality risk during hospitalization, not including post-discharge deaths. It merits further study to address mortality prediction after hospital discharge. Finally, this study was performed in a single hospital center. Temporal validation in this center may limit the broad application of this risk score. There remains a need to validate it prospectively in an independent population from geographically different areas.

In spite of these weaknesses, this study sheds some light on clinical value of the routinely collected data in predicting patients' prognoses. The risk prediction model was built from four readily available indicators in clinical practice, including demographic and complications that commonly occur in AECOPD progression (e.g., respiratory failure and pneumothorax), which implies a straight-forward application of the prediction model in clinical practice. As data were collected in a standard process, the risk algorithm could be readily integrated into hospital information system, which may aid doctors in identifying high-risk individuals in an interactive and real-time way. This could facilitate implementation of tailored interventions to prevent fatal outcomes. Also, the model can be replicated in other hospitals owing to the standard process of data collection. Besides, the prediction model was simple with only four readily available predictors involved. It can save care providers' time in their busy work. Although the model was simple, it had good performance with high discriminative ability and good calibration. All available data were included for modeling by the use of bootstrap, and penalized regression was adopted to minimize potential overfitting arising from low mortality in this study. Our findings showed a shrinkage factor of >0.9, indicating no large overfitting (13). Furthermore, temporal validation was performed to assess external validity of the model, in which model was retrained and recalibrated, and any temporal trends that may affect the prediction could be captured (27).

CONCLUSION

Complications emerged as important predictors for in-hospital mortality in acute exacerbated COPD patients requiring hospitalization. The model's prediction capability was satisfactory in terms of discriminating alive patients from individuals who died and estimating the absolute mortality risk in low-risk patients. This real-world data analysis indicates the potential value of risk algorithms as a toolkit to help doctors identify high-risk patients and adopt appropriate disease management to prevent death during COPD exacerbation.

AUTHOR CONTRIBUTIONS

TY and JJ were involved in conceptualization, funding acquisition and supervision. FD and YW collected data. FD, XR, and KH analyzed and interpreted the data. FD wrote the draft of manuscript. TY, JJ, FD, XR, KH, and YW contributed to writing-review and approved the final manuscript. All authors contributed to the article and approved the submitted version.

ACKNOWLEDGMENTS

We appreciate the staff's help with data collection in medical record departments of the study hospital.

REFERENCES

1. Global Burden of Disease Collaborative Network. *Global Burden of Disease Study 2017 (GBD 2017) Results*. Seattle: Institute for Health Metrics and Evaluation (IHME) (2018). Available online at: http://ghdx.healthdata.org/gbd-results-tool
2. Donaldson GC, Wedzicha JA. COPD exacerbations 1: epidemiology. *Thorax*. (2006) 61 164–8. doi: 10.1136/thx.2005.041806
3. Fang X, Wang X, Bai C. COPD in China: the burden and importance of proper management. *Chest*. (2011) 139:920–9. doi: 10.1378/chest.10-1393
4. Soler-Cataluna JJ. Severe acute exacerbations and mortality in patients with chronic obstructive pulmonary disease. *Thorax*. (2005) 60:925–31. doi: 10.1136/thx.2005.040527
5. Moons KGM, Royston P, Vergouwe Y, Grobbee DE, Altman DG. Prognosis and prognostic research: what, why, and how? *BMJ*. (2009) 338:b375. doi: 10.1136/bmj.b375
6. Yousif M, Rabab A, Wahsh E. Predicting in-hospital mortality in acute exacerbation of COPD: is there a golden score? *Egypt J Chest Dis Tuberc*. (2016). 65:579–84. doi: 10.1016/j.ejcdt.2016.03.003
7. Wang C, Xu J, Yang L, Xu Y, Zhang X, Bai C, et al. Prevalence and risk factors of chronic obstructive pulmonary disease in China (the China Pulmonary Health [CPH] study): a national cross-sectional study. *Lancet*. (2018) 391:1706–17. doi: 10.1016/S0140-6736(18)30841-9
8. García-Olmos L, Alberquilla á, Ayala V, García-Sagredo P, Morales L, Carmona M, et al. Comorbidity in patients with chronic obstructive pulmonary disease in family practice: a cross sectional study. *BMC Family Practice*. (2013) 14:11. doi: 10.1186/1471-2296-14-11
9. Cavailles A, Brinchault-Rabin G, Dixmier A, Goupil F, Gut-Gobert C, Marchand-Adam S, et al. Comorbidities of COPD. *Eur Respir Rev*. (2013) 22:454–75. doi: 10.1183/09059180.00008612
10. Sethi S. Infection as a comorbidity of COPD. *Eur Respir J*. (2010) 35:1209–15. doi: 10.1183/09031936.00081409
11. Riley RD, Ensor J, Snell KIE, Harrell FE Jr, Martin GP, Reitsma JB, et al. Calculating the sample size required for developing a clinical prediction model. *BMJ*. (2020) 368:m441. doi: 10.1136/bmj.m441
12. Grant SW, Collins GS, Nashef SAM. Statistical primer: developing and validating a risk prediction model. *Eur J Cardiothorac Surg*. (2018) 54:203–8. doi: 10.1093/ejcts/ezy180
13. Riley RD, Snell KI, Ensor J, Burke DL, Harrell FE Jr, Moons KG, et al. Minimum sample size for developing a multivariable prediction model: PART II—binary and time-to-event outcomes. *Stat Med*. (2019) 38:1276–96. doi: 10.1002/sim.7992
14. Pavlou M, Ambler G, Seaman SR, Guttmann O, Elliott P, King M, et al. How to develop a more accurate risk prediction model when there are few events. *BMJ*. (2015) 351:h3868. doi: 10.1136/bmj.h3868
15. Moons KGM, Altman DG, Reitsma JB, Ioannidis JPA, Macaskill P, Steyerberg EW, et al. Transparent Reporting of a multivariable prediction model for Individual Prognosis Or Diagnosis (TRIPOD): Explanation and Elaboration. *Ann Intern Med*. (2015). 162:W1–73. doi: 10.7326/M14-0698
16. Sullivan LM, Massaro JM Sr. RBDA. Presentation of multivariate data for clinical use: the Framingham Study risk score functions. *Stat Med*. (2004) 23:1631–60. doi: 10.1002/sim.1742
17. Steyerberg EW, Eijkemans MJC, Habbema JDF. Application of shrinkage techniques in logistic regression analysis: a case study. *Stat Neerl*. (2001) 55:76–88. doi: 10.1111/1467-9574.00157
18. Steer J, Gibson J, Bourke SC. The DECAF Score: predicting hospital mortality in exacerbations of chronic obstructive pulmonary disease. *Thorax*. (2012) 67:970–6. doi: 10.1136/thoraxjnl-2012-202103
19. Quintana JM, Esteban C, Unzurrunzaga A, Garcia-Gutierrez S, Gonzalez N, Barrio I, et al. Predictive score for mortality in patients with COPD exacerbations attending hospital emergency departments. *BMC Med*. (2014) 12:66. doi: 10.1186/1741-7015-12-66
20. Morasert T, Jantarapootirat M, Phinyo P, Patumanond J. Prognostic indicators for in-hospital mortality in COPD with acute exacerbation in Thailand: a retrospective cohort study. *BMJ Open Respir Res*. (2020) 7: e000488. doi: 10.1136/bmjresp-2019-000488
21. Sorge R, Deblieux P. Acute exacerbations of chronic obstructive pulmonary disease: a primer for emergency physicians. *J Emerg Med*. (2020) 59:643–59. doi: 10.1016/j.jemermed.2020.07.001
22. Calverley P MA. Respiratory failure in chronic obstructive pulmonary disease. *Eur Respir J Suppl*. (2003) 47(Suppl. 47):26s—30s. doi: 10.1183/09031936.03.00030103
23. Hartl S, Lopez-Campos JL, Pozo-Rodriguez F, Castro-Acosta A, Studnicka M, Kaiser B, et al. Risk of death and readmission of hospital-admitted COPD exacerbations: European COPD audit. *Eur Respir J*. (2016) 47:113–21. doi: 10.1183/13993003.01391-2014
24. Siela D. Acute respiratory failure and COPD: recognition and care. *Nurs Crit Care*. (2018) 13:28–37. doi: 10.1097/01.CCN.0000525926.13357.c0
25. Fuso L, Incalzi RA, Pistelli R, Muzzolon R, Valente S, Pagliari G, et al. Predicting mortality of patients hospitalized for acutely exacerbated

chronic obstructive pulmonary disease. *Am J Med.* (1995) 98:272–7. doi: 10.1016/s0002-9343(99)80374-x
26. Almagro P, Calbo E, Anna ODEE, Barreiro B, Quintana S, Heredia JL, et al. Mortality after hospitalization for COPD. *Chest.* (2002) 121:1441–8. doi: 10.1378/chest.121.5.1441
27. Tavakoli H, Chen W, Sin DD, FitzGerald JM, Sadatsafavi M. Predicting severe chronic obstructive pulmonary disease exacerbations. Developing a population surveillance approach with administrative data. *Ann Am Thorac Soc.* (2020) 17:1069–76. doi: 10.1513/AnnalsATS.202001-070OC

Serum CYR61 is Associated with Airway Inflammation and is a Potential Biomarker for Severity in Chronic Obstructive Pulmonary Disease

Zhu-Xia Tan[1,2†], *Lin Fu*[1†], *Wen-Jing Wang*[1], *Ping Zhan*[1], *Hui Zhao*[1], *Hua Wang*[2*] *and De-Xiang Xu*[2*]

[1] *Second Affiliated Hospital, Anhui Medical University, Hefei, China,* [2] *Department of Toxicology, Anhui Medical University, Hefei, China*

***Correspondence:**
De-Xiang Xu
xudex@126.com
Hua Wang
wanghuadev@126.com

† *These authors have contributed equally to this work*

Background: Cysteine-rich 61 (CYR61) and inflammation was upregulated in the lungs of patients with chronic obstructive pulmonary disease (COPD). However, the association between CYR61 and inflammation was unclear in COPD patients. This study aimed to analyze the association of serum CYR61 with pulmonary inflammation and lung function indexes in COPD patients.

Methods: One hundred and fifty COPD patients and 150 control subjects were enrolled. Serum and pulmonary CYR61 was detected. Lung function indexes were evaluated in COPD patients.

Results: Serum CYR61 level was elevated and pulmonary CYR61 expression was upregulated in COPD patients. An increased CYR61 was associated with decreased pulmonary function indexes in COPD patients. Further analyses showed that nuclear factor-kappa B (NF-κB) p65-positive nuclei was elevated in the lungs of COPD patients with high level of CYR61. Accordingly, serum monocyte chemotactic protein (MCP)-1 and tumor necrosis factor α (TNF-α), two downstream inflammatory cytokines of NF-κB pathway, were increased in parallel with CYR61, among which serum MCP-1 and TNF-α were the highest in COPD patients with high level of CYR61. Moreover, a positive correlation, determined by multivariate regression that excluded the influence of age, gender and smoking, was observed between serum CYR61 and inflammatory cytokines in COPD patients.

Conclusion: These results provide evidence that an increased CYR61 is associated with pulmonary inflammation and COPD progression. Inflammatory cytokines may be the mediators between CYR61 elevation and COPD progression.

Keywords: CYR61, COPD, NF-κB, lung function, inflammatory cytokines

BACKGROUND

Chronic obstructive pulmonary disease (COPD) is a common respiratory disease, which is characterized by lung parenchyma damage and progressive decline in lung function (1–3). Cigarette smoking is a major risk factor for the occurrence and development of COPD (4). Chronic airway inflammation, accompanied by infiltration of numerous macrophages and lymphocytes, has been implicated in the progression of COPD (5–7). Accumulating data have demonstrated that chemokines, such as monocyte chemotactic protein (MCP)-1 and interleukin (IL)-8, are involved in the recruitment of inflammatory cells (8, 9). The activation of nuclear factor-kappa B (NF-κB) may play important roles in regulating cigarette smoke-evoked inflammatory chemokines (10–13).

Cysteine-rich 61 (CYR61), also named as CCN1, is a member of CCN protein family (14). Numerous data have demonstrated that CYR61 takes part in the process of angiogenesis, embryonic development, and tissue repair (15–17). Recently, the role of CYR61 in pulmonary diseases is concerned (18). Several studies indicated that CYR61 was involved in the pathogenesis of acute lung injury and acute respiratory distress syndrome (19, 20). Moreover, CYR61 aggravated transforming growth factor (TGF)-β-induced SMAD3 activation and lung fibrosis (21). An early report showed that pulmonary CYR61 expression was upregulated in COPD patients (22). Nevertheless, the association between upregulated CYR61 and COPD progression remains unknown.

In the current study, we aimed to analyze the association among serum CYR61, pulmonary inflammation and lung function indexes in COPD patients. We showed that serum CYR61 was elevated and pulmonary CYR61 expression was upregulated in COPD patients. Moreover, an elevation of serum CYR61 was associated with lung function decline in COPD patients. Our results provide evidence that inflammatory chemokine MCP-1 is a mediator between an increased CYR61 and lung function decline in COPD patients.

METHODS

Reagents and Chemicals

Antibodies against NF-κB p65 and CYR61 were purchased from Cell Signaling Technology (MA, USA). CYR61 ELISA kits were from Cusabio (TX, USA). MCP-1 ELISA kit was from Wuhan Colorful Gene Biological Technology (Hubei, China). Chemiluminescence (ECL) detection kits were from Advansta (CA, USA). All other regents and chemicals were from Sigma Chemical Co. (MO, USA) if not specifically noted.

COPD Patients and Lung Specimen

All COPD patients who were first time diagnosed were randomly selected from Anhui COPD Cohort (AHCC) that was a hospital-based prospective cohort established by the Second Affiliated Hospital of Anhui Medical University. For the matched case-control study, 150 COPD patients were recruited from AHCC. Pulmonary function was tested in all recruited COPD patients based on standardized methods. COPD was confirmed on basis of the American Thoracic Society criteria and the Global Initiative for COPD (GOLD) criteria (23), which forced expiratory volume in 1 s (FEV1)/forced vital capacity (FVC) ratio was <70%. Total 150 sex- and age-matched control subjects were randomly collected from the physical examination center at the Second Affiliated Hospital of Anhui Medical University. To analyze the level of serum CYR61 and MCP-1, sera were collected from all COPD patients and controls. To measure pulmonary CYR61 and NF-κB, lung tissues were obtained from surgical operations between COPD patients and Controls. Lung specimens were collected from paracancerous tissue of lung cancer patients without other pulmonary disease were as controls at the Second Affiliated Hospital of Anhui Medical University. Each control subject was matched with one COPD patients in accord with age and gender (24). Finally, all 20 lung cancer patients without other pulmonary diseases and 20 COPD patients were enrolled. The current study was approved by the Ethics Committee of Anhui Medical University (2021030). All subjects have agreed and signed an informed consent.

Immunochemistry (IHC)

All lung specimens were fixed in formalin and embedded in paraffin. Lung section was dewaxed and rehydrated according to a conventional standard method (25). To punch cell membrane and suppress endogenous peroxidase, lung section was immersed in PBS containing 0.5% Triton X-100 and 3% H_2O_2 for 45 min. Antigen retrieval was performed in boiled citrate solution. After blocked, lung section was incubated with either CYR61 or NF-κB p65 antibody (1:200) at 37°C incubator for 3.5 h. After washed with PBS for three times, conjunction with streptavidin-HRP complex was incubated for 2.5 h at room temperature. Immunolabelling was evaluated using DAB solution. nucleus was stained with hematoxylin in a dark room. Pulmonary CYR61- and p65- positive cells were calculated by two independent pathologists.

Enzyme Linked Immunosorbent Assay

Serum concentrations of CYR61, monocyte chemoattractant protein 1 (MCP-1) and tumor necrosis factor α (TNF-α) were measured using enzyme linked immunosorbent assay (ELISA). CYR61 (CSB-E13884h) and MCP-1 (CSB-E04655h) ELISA kits were bought from Cusabio, Wuhan, China (https://www.cusabio.com/). TNF-α (JYM0110Hu) ELISA kits were obtained from Wuhan ColorfulGene Biological Technology Co (http://www.jymbio.com/product/286-cn.html). The detailed method referred to the reagent manual (26).

Statistical Analysis

The quantitative variables were expressed as means and standard error of mean. The categorical variables were expressed with frequencies and percentages. All statistical analysis was conducted in SPSS 21.0. Independent sample unpaired *t*-test was

---

Abbreviations: COPD, Chronic obstructive pulmonary disease; CYR61, Cysteine-rich 61; NF-κB, nuclear factor-kappa B; MCP-1, Macrophage chemoattractant protein-1; FEV1, Forced expiratory volume in 1 s; FVC, forced vital capacity.

TABLE 1 | Demographic information and clinical characteristics.

Variable	Control ($n = 150$)	COPD ($n = 150$)	P
Age (years)	67.9 ± 0.94	72.8 ± 0.61	0.132
Female, n (%)	51 (34.0)	38 (25.3)	0.100
Emphysema	N.A.	121 (80.7)	N.A.
Smoking status			<0.001
Never-smoker, n (%)	55 (36.7)	8 (5.3)	
Former-smoker, n (%)	65 (43.3)	123 (82.0)	
Current-smoker, n (%)	30 (20.0)	19 (12.7)	
WBC (10^9/L)	6.22 ± 0.121	7.45 ± 0.278	<0.01
Neutrophil (10^9/L)	3.24 ± 0.077	5.40 ± 0.270	<0.01
Lymphocyte (10^9/L)	1.83 ± 0.071	1.26 ± 0.047	<0.01
Eosinophil (10^9/L)	0.12 ± 0.010	0.18 ± 0.024	0.001
Monocyte (10^9/L)	0.41 ± 0.056	0.57 ± 0.033	<0.01
Basophil (10^9/L)	0.02 ± 0.002	0.03 ± 0.003	0.009
FEV1 (%)	N.A.	52.02 ± 2.659	N.A.
FEV1/FVC (%)	N.A.	57.79 ± 1.537	N.A.
FEV1 (L)	N.A.	1.16 ± 0.066	N.A.
FVC (L)	N.A.	1.88 ± 0.064	N.A.
PH	N.A.	7.39 ± 0.007	N.A.
PCO2 (mmHg)	N.A.	51.99 ± 2.107	N.A.
PO2 (mmHg)	N.A.	70.88 ± 2.588	N.A.
RV%TLC-SB (%)	N.A.	54.59 ± 1.564	N.A.
DLCO SB (mmol/min/kPa)	N.A.	3.82 ± 0.259	N.A.

WBC, White blood cell; FEV1, Forced expiratory volume in one second; FVC, Forced vital capacity; N.A., Not available.

used to evaluate the difference for continuous variables between two groups. The difference of continuous variables in three groups was determined through one-way ANOVA. Chi-square test was used to analyze the difference for count data. Pearson correlation analysis and linear regression analysis were used to evaluate the correlations among CYR61 and inflammatory cytokines. The association of serum CYR61 and hospital stays was accessed through logistical regression analysis. $P < 0.05$ was considered statistically significant.

RESULTS

Demographic Data and Clinical Characteristics

The demographic data and clinical characteristics were analyzed. As shown in **Table 1**, 150 COPD patients and 150 controls were recruited in this study. No significant difference on mean ages was observed between two groups (72.83 ± 0.61 in COPD patients vs. 67.94 ± 0.94 in controls, $P > 0.05$). In addition, no significant difference on sex ratio was shown between two groups (**Table 1**). There were 121 (80.7%) cases with emphysema in COPD patients (**Table 1**). Interestingly, there was obvious difference of smokers between COPD patients and control subjects. Blood routine indexes were then analyzed. As expected, the counts of white blood cell (WBC), neutrophil, eosinophil, monocyte and basophil were elevated in COPD patients (**Table 1**). By contrast, lymphocyte count was reduced in COPD patients (**Table 1**). The results of FEV1(%), FEV1/FVC, FEV1 (L), FVC (L), PH, PCO2, PO2, RV%TLC-SB (%), and DLCO SB in COPD patients was presented in **Table 1**. Not only that, the demographic data and clinical characteristics were further compared in COPD patients with different grades. As shown in **Supplementary Table 1**, no difference of emphysema and blood gas indicators was observed in COPD patients with different grades. RV%TLC-SB was lower and DLCO SB was higher in grade 1-2 (G 1-2) COPD patients than those in grade 3 and grade 4 (G 3 and G 4) COPD cases (**Supplementary Table 1**).

An Increased CYR61 Is Associated With the Severity of COPD

Serum CYR61 concentration was analyzed in COPD patients and controls. As shown in **Figure 1A**, serum CYR61 was elevated in COPD patients as compared with controls. Serum CYR61 was then compared among different grades of COPD patients. As shown in **Figure 1B**, serum CYR61 was gradually elevated in parallel with the grades of COPD patients, among which serum CYR61 level was the highest in patients with G 4. Pulmonary CYR61 was then detected in COPD patients and controls. As shown in **Figure 1C**, an obvious CYR61 staining was shown in the lungs from COPD patients. Quantitative analysis showed that pulmonary CYR61 was upregulated in COPD patients as compared with controls (**Figure 1D**). Moreover, pulmonary CYR61 was higher in G 3 and G 4 COPD patients than those in G 1-2 COPD patients (**Figures 1E,F**).

Serum CYR61 Is Negatively Correlated With Lung Function Indexes in COPD Patients

The correlation between serum CYR61 and FVC was analyzed among COPD patients. As expected, a negative correlation was observed between serum CYR61 and FVC (**Figure 2A**, $r = -0.328$, $P < 0.001$). The correlation between serum CYR61 and FEV1(L) was then analyzed among COPD patients. As shown in **Figure 2B**, there was a negative correlation between serum CYR61 and FEV1(L) ($r = -0.379$, $P < 0.001$). Next, the correlation between serum CYR61 and FEV1/FVC was evaluated among COPD patients. As shown in **Figure 2C**, there was a negative correlation between serum CYR61 and FEV1/FVC ($r = -0.144$, $P = 0.045$). The correlation between serum CYR61 and FEV1(%) is presented in **Figure 2D**. As expected, a negative correlation was observed between serum CYR61 and FEV1 (%) ($r = -0.507$, $P < 0.001$). Finally, regression analysis was used to evaluate the correlation between serum CYR61 and pulmonary function among COPD patients. Univariate regression analysis showed that there was a negative correlation between serum CYR61 and all lung function indexes in COPD patients (**Table 2**). Multivariate regression analysis was used to exclude the influence of age, gender and smoking on serum CYR61 level and pulmonary functions in COPD patients. Although no correlation between CYR61 and FEV1/FVC (%)

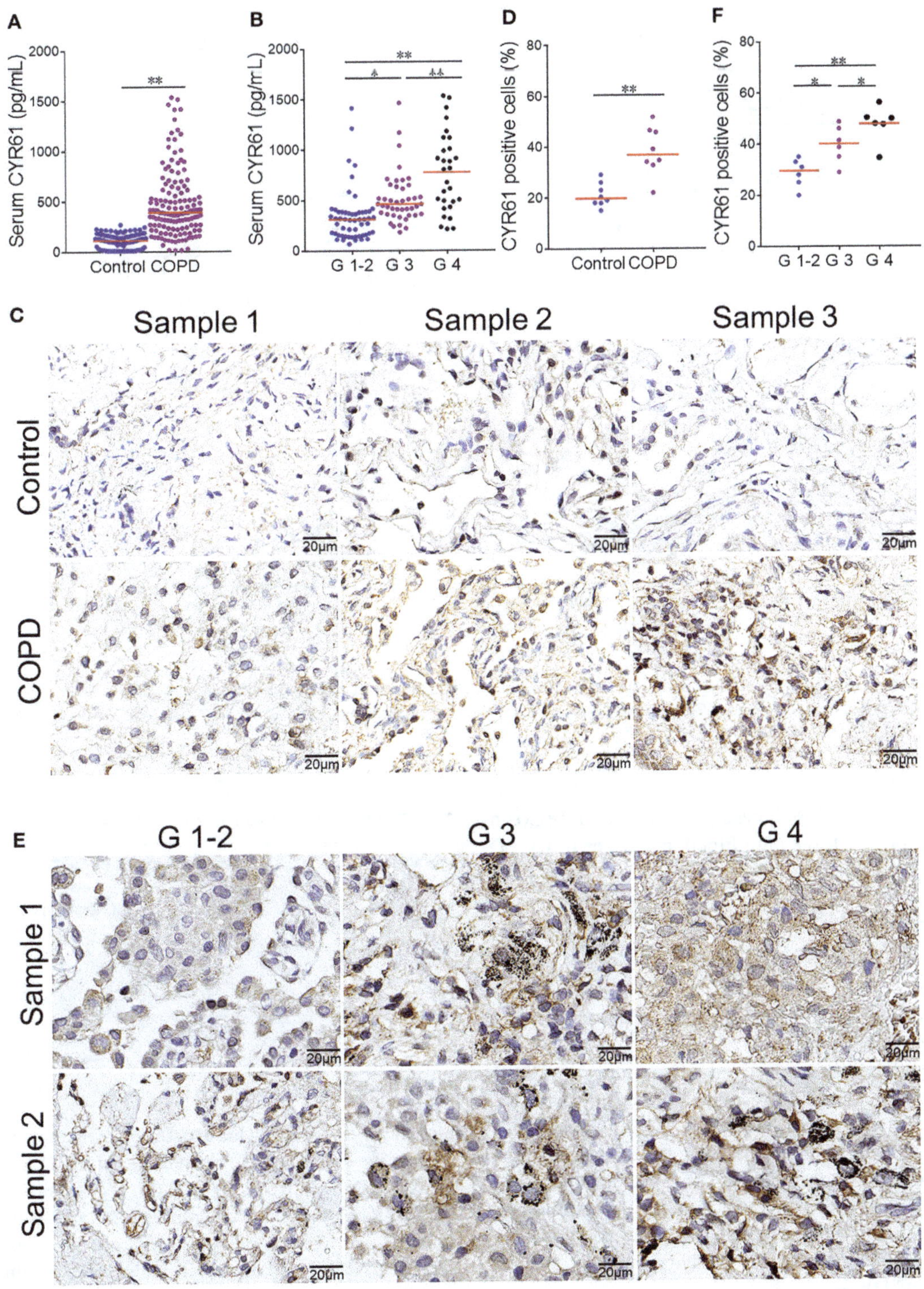

FIGURE 1 | Serum CYR61 level and its association with severity of COPD. Sera were collected from COPD patients and controls. **(A,B)** Serum CYR61 level was detected using ELISA. **(A)** Serum CYR61 level was compared between COPD patients and controls. All data were represented as means ± S.E.M. ($N = 150$). **(B)** Serum CYR61 level was compared among different grades of COPD patients. All data were represented as means ± S.E.M. ($N = 69$ for G 1-2 patients, $N = 48$ for G 3 patients, $N = 33$ for G 4 patients). **(C,D)** Pulmonary CYR61 expression was compared between COPD patients and controls. **(C)** Three representative pictures. **(D)** Quantitative analysis of CYR61-positive cells in COPD patients and controls. **(E,F)** Pulmonary CYR61 was compared among different grades of COPD patients. **(E)** Three representative pictures: arrows indicate CYR61-positive cell; **(F)** Quantitative analysis of CYR61-positive cells in COPD patients with different grades. All data were represented as means ± S.E.M. ($N = 6$). $^{*}P < 0.05$, $^{**}P < 0.01$.

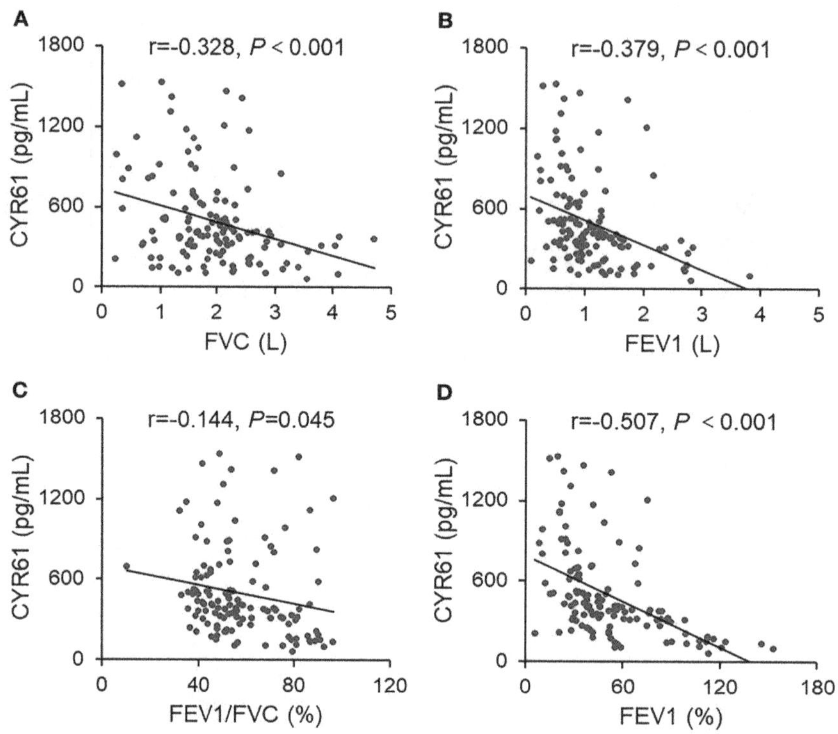

FIGURE 2 | The correlation between serum CYR61 and lung function indexes in COPD patients. Pulmonary function was measured in 150 COPD patients. Sera were collected and CYR61 was detected using ELISA. Correlation between serum CYR61 and lung function indexes was analyzed. **(A)** CYR61 vs. FVC(L); **(B)** CYR61 vs. FEV1(L); **(C)** CYR61 vs. FEV1/FVC (%); **(D)** CYR61 vs. FEV1(%).

was observed, there remains a negative correlation between serum CYR61 and other three lung function indexes in COPD patients (**Table 2**).

An Increased CYR61 Is Associated With Pulmonary NF-κB Activation in COPD Patients

Pulmonary NF-κB was evaluated among COPD patients and controls. As expected, numerous NF-κB p65-positive nuclei, as determined by IHC, were observed in the lung of COPD patients (**Figure 3A**). Quantitative analysis showed that NF-κB p65-positive nuclei were elevated in COPD patients as compared with controls (**Figure 3B**). The association between serum CYR61 and pulmonary NF-κB activation was analyzed in COPD patients. As expected, the numbers of pulmonary NF-κB p65-positive nuclei were more in COPD patients with high level of CYR61 than in COPD patients with low level of CYR61 (**Figures 3C,D**).

An Increased CYR61 Is Associated With Serum MCP-1 and TNF-α in COPD Patients

Firstly, the associations between serum CYR61 and inflammatory cytokines was analyzed among all subjects. As expected, serum MCP-1 was gradually elevated in parallel with CYR61, among which serum MCP-1 level was the highest in subjects with high level of CYR61 (**Figure 4A**). Correlation analysis showed a positive association between serum CYR61 and MCP-1 (**Figure 4D**, r = 0.518, $P < 0.001$). A positive correlation, as determined by multivariate regression analysis that excluded the influence of age, gender and smoking, was observed between serum CYR61 and MCP-1 in all subjects (**Table 3**). Next, the association between serum CYR61 and MCP-1 was analyzed among COPD patients. As expected, serum MCP-1 was gradually elevated in parallel with CYR61, among which serum MCP-1 level was the highest in subjects with high level of CYR61 (**Figure 4B**). Correlation analysis showed a positive association between serum CYR61 and MCP-1 (**Figure 4E**, r = 0.456, $P < 0.001$). Moreover, a positive correlation, as determined by multivariate regression analysis that excluded the influence

TABLE 2 | Association of serum CYR61 with lung function.

Variables	Multivariable, β (95% CI)*	*P*
FEV1 (%)	−0.466 (−0.054, −0.028)	<0.001
FEV1/FVC (%)	−0.050 (−0.011, 0.006)	0.547
FEV1 (L)	−0.408 (−0.001, 0.000)	<0.001
FVC (L)	−0.406 (−0.001, 0.000)	<0.001

**Age, gender, and smoking were adjusted.*

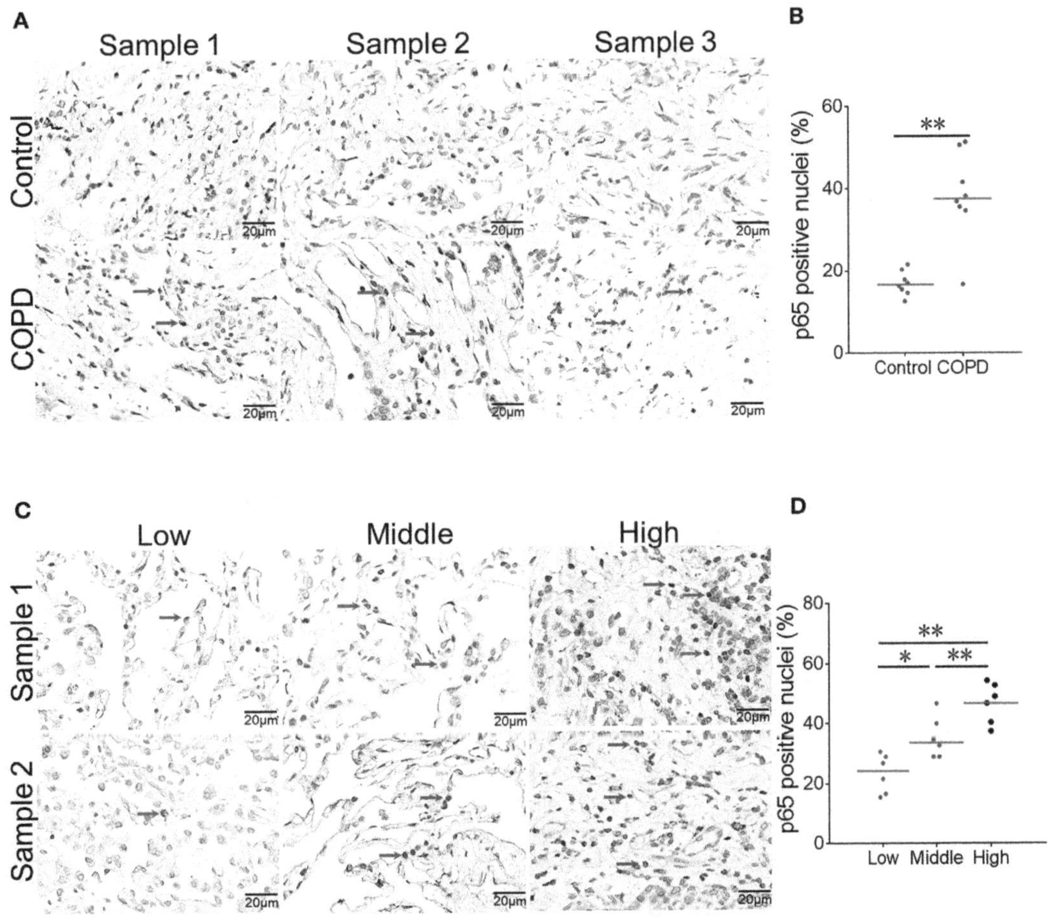

FIGURE 3 | The association between serum CYR61 and pulmonary NF-κB activation in COPD patients. Lung tissues were collected from COPD patients and controls. Pulmonary NF-κB p65 was detected using IHC. **(A,B)** Pulmonary NF-κB p65-positive nuclei were compared between COPD patients and control subjects. **(A)** Three representative pictures: arrows indicate p65-positive nuclei; **(B)** Quantitative analysis of p65-positive nuclei in COPD patients and controls. **(C,D)** Pulmonary NF-κB p65-positive nuclei were compared among COPD patients with different levels of CYR61. **(C)** Three representative pictures: arrows indicate p65-positive nuclei; **(D)** Quantitative analysis of p65-positive nuclei in COPD patients with different levels of CYR61. All data were represented as means ± S.E.M. ($N = 6$). $^*P < 0.05$, $^{**}P < 0.01$.

of age, gender and smoking, was observed between serum CYR61 and MCP-1 in COPD patients (**Table 3**). Finally, the association between serum CYR61 and MCP-1 was analyzed among control subjects. As shown in **Figure 4C**, no significant difference on serum MCP-1 was observed among different groups. Correlation and multivariate regression analyses showed that there was no association on serum CYR61 and MCP-1 (**Figure 4F**; **Table 3**, $P > 0.05$). Moreover, the association of serum CYR61 and TNF-α was evaluated in all cases. As shown in **Figure 4G**, serum TNF-α was increased in high serum CYR61 group than these in low serum CYR61 group. Besides, serum TNF-α was gradually risen in line with serum CYR61 in COPD patients (**Figure 4H**). In addition, serum TNF-α was elevated in High group than in Middle group among control cases (**Figure 4I**). Although, there was no obvious correlation of serum TNF-α with CYR61 in control cases (**Figure 4L**), serum CYR61 was positively associated with TNF-α in all cases (**Figure 4J**, $r = 0.177$, $P = 0.001$) and COPD patients (**Figure 4K**, $r = 0.329$, $P < 0.001$).

The Mediating Effect of Inflammatory Cytokines Between Increased CYR61 and Decreased Lung Function Indexes in COPD Patients

First, the direct effect of increased CYR61 on pulmonary function decline was analyzed. As shown in **Figure 5**, serum CYR61 was negatively associated with FEV1 (%) ($\beta = -0.513$, $P < 0.01$) in COPD patients. The mediating effect of inflammatory cytokines between CYR61 and lung function indexes was then evaluated in COPD patients. As shown in **Figure 5**, obvious mediating effects between increased MCP-1 ($\beta = -0.300$, $P < 0.05$) and TNF-α ($\beta = -0.111$, $P < 0.05$) with decreased lung function were observed in COPD patients. The total effect of CYR61

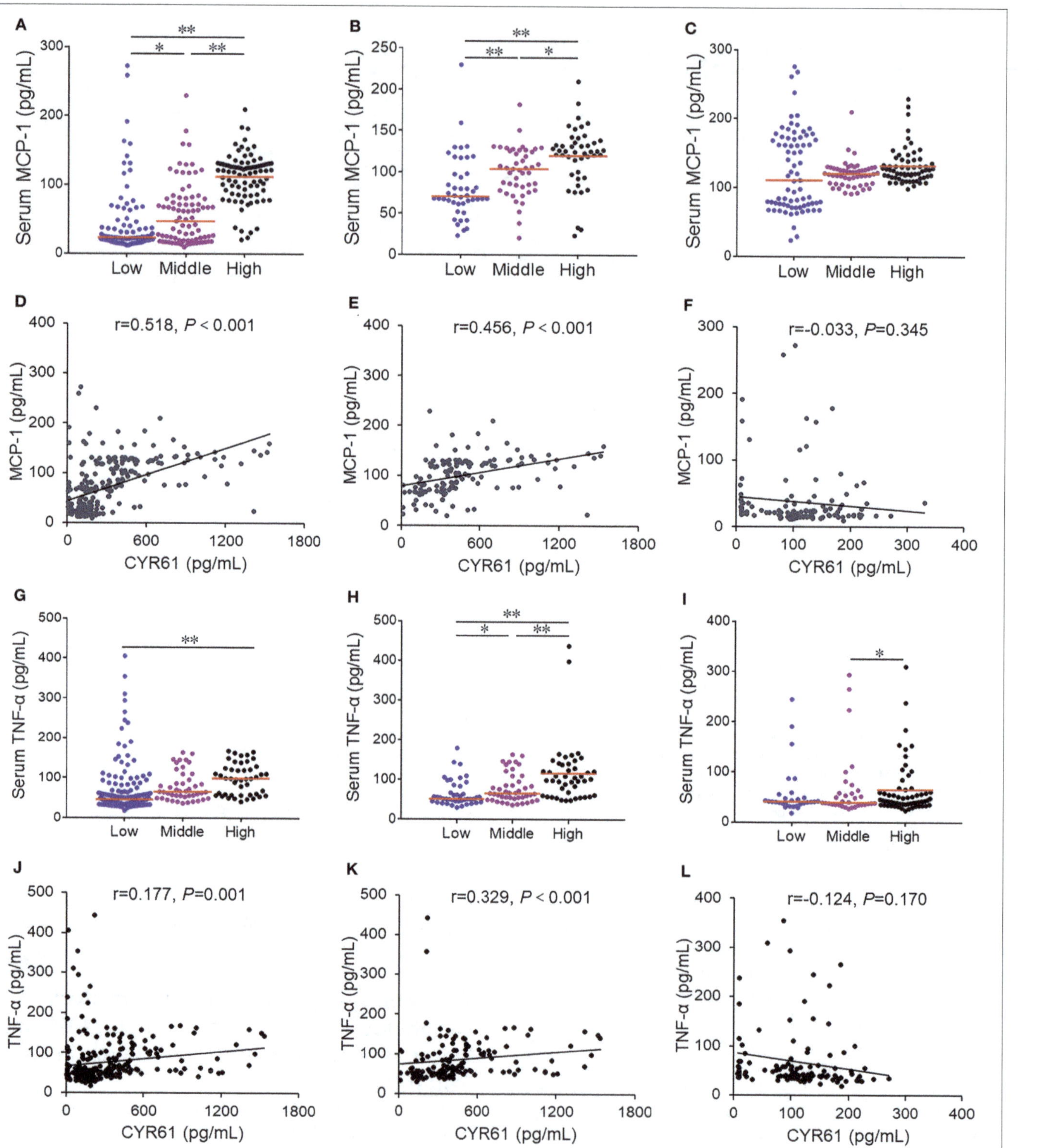

FIGURE 4 | The association of serum CYR61 level with serum inflammatory cytokines in COPD patients. Sera were collected from 150 COPD patients and 150 control subjects. Serum CYR61 and inflammatory cytokines were detected using ELISA. **(A,D)** Association between serum CYR61 and MCP-1 was analyzed among all subjects. **(A)** Serum MCP-1 was compared among subjects with different levels of CYR61. **(D)** Correlation analysis between serum CYR61 and MCP-1. **(B,E)** Association between serum CYR61 and MCP-1 was analyzed among COPD patients. **(B)** Serum MCP-1 was compared among COPD patients with different levels of CYR61. **(E)** Correlation analysis between serum CYR61 and MCP-1. **(C,F)** Association between serum CYR61 and MCP-1 was analyzed among control

(Continued)

FIGURE 4 | subjects. **(C)** Serum MCP-1 was compared among control subjects with different levels of CYR61. **(F)** Correlation analysis between serum CYR61 and MCP-1. **(G,J)** Association between serum CYR61 and TNF-α was analyzed among all subjects. **(G)** Serum TNF-α was compared among subjects with different levels of CYR61. **(J)** Correlation analysis between serum CYR61 and TNF-α. **(H,K)** Association between serum CYR61 and TNF-α was analyzed among COPD patients. **(H)** Serum TNF-α was compared among COPD patients with different levels of CYR61. **(K)** Correlation analysis between serum CYR61 and TNF-α. **(I,L)** Association between serum CYR61 and TNF-α was analyzed among control subjects. **(I)** Serum TNF-α was compared among control subjects with different levels of CYR61. **(L)** Correlation analysis between serum CYR61 and TNF-α. *$P < 0.05$, **$P < 0.01$.

TABLE 3 | Associations of serum CYR61 with MCP-1 and TNF-α.

Groups	MCP-1		TNF-α	
	Multivariable,β (95% CI)	P	Multivariable,β (95% CI)	P
All cases	0.479 (0.067, 0.102)	<0.001	0.177 (0.316, 1.685)	<0.001
Control	−0.027 (−0.145, 0.104)	0.747	−0.156 (−0.316, 0.020)	0.083
COPD	0.473 (0.041,0.077)	<0.001	0.327 (1.467, 4.365)	<0.001

Age, gender, and smoking were adjusted.

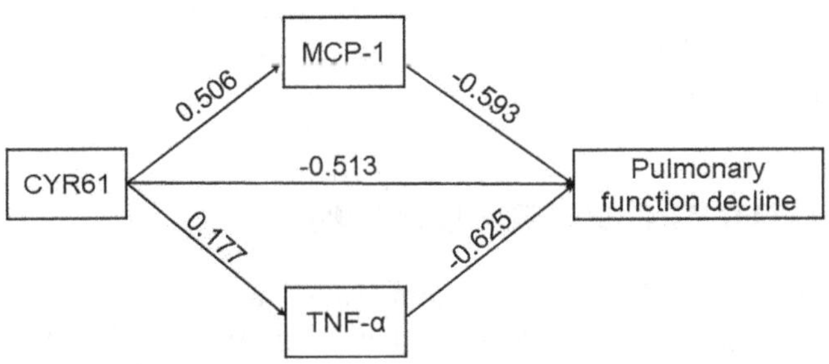

FIGURE 5 | Postulated mediational path model.

on lung function decline was −0.924 ($P < 0.01$) in COPD patients. The relative contribution of MCP-1 and TNF-α in CYR61 elevation-induced pulmonary function decline was 44.5% in COPD patients.

An Increased Serum CYR61 Is Positively Associated With Hospital Stays in COPD Patients

According to quartile, serum CYR61 was classified as Low group (<410.0 pg/ml) and High group (≥410.0 pg/ml), hospital stays were divided into Short group (<10 days) and Long group (≥10 days). Then, the effect of serum CYR61 at the early stage on hospital stay was evaluated in **Table 4**. Among 150 COPD patients, the hospital stays of 69 (46.0%) patients was longer than 10 days. The number of cases with higher hospital stays was more among COPD patients with high serum CYR61 than those with low serum CYR61 (55.1 vs. 25.9%; RR = 2.124, 95% Cl: 1.388∼3.250; $P < 0.001$).

TABLE 4 | Association of serum CYR61 and hospital stays in COPD patients.

CYR61	Cases, n	Longer hospital stays, n (%)	RR (95%)	P
Low	81	21 (25.9)	1	-
High	69	38 (55.1)	2.124 (1.388, 3.250)	<0.001

According to quartile, serum CYR61 was classified as Low group (<410.0 pg/ml) and High group (≥410.0 pg/ml), hospital stays were divided into Short group (<10 days) and Long group (≥10 days).
RR, relative risk.

DISCUSSION

The associations of serum CYR61 with pulmonary inflammation and lung function indexes were investigated in COPD patients. The major findings were as follow: Firstly, serum CYR61 level was elevated and pulmonary CYR61 expression was upregulated in COPD patients; Secondly, an increased CYR61 was associated with decreased lung function indexes in COPD patients; Thirdly, an increased CYR61 is associated with an elevation of serum MCP-1, TNF-α and activation of pulmonary inflammatory signaling in COPD patients. Fourthly, an increased CYR61 is associated with a longer hospital stays among COPD patients. Our results suggest that pro-inflammatory cytokine and chemokine are mediators between CYR61 elevation and COPD progression.

Accumulating data indicate that CYR61 is involved in the pathogenesis of COPD (18). An early study found that pulmonary CYR61 was upregulated in COPD patients as compared with controls (22). Indeed, cigarette smoking is a major risk factor for COPD (27). According to an earlier report, cigarette smoke extracts upregulated CCN1 through evoking excess reactive oxygen spices and endoplasmic reticulum stress (28). In the current study, we measured serum CYR61 level and pulmonary CYR61 expression in COPD patients. Our results showed that serum CYR61 was elevated and pulmonary CYR61 was upregulated in COPD patients. Interestingly, we found that serum CYR61 level and pulmonary CYR61 expression were positively associated with the severity of COPD. To further determine the role of CYR61 in COPD progression, the current study analyzed the association between serum CYR61 level and lung function indexes in COPD patients. We found that serum CYR61 level is negatively correlated with several lung function indexes in COPD patients. Not only that, the association of serum CYR61 and the prognosis was estimated in COPD patients. Our results indicated that serum higher CYR61 on admission prolonged the hospital stays among COPD patients. Our results provide evidence for the first time that CYR61 may be a biomarker to predict COPD progression.

The mechanism by which CYR61 associates COPD progression remains unclear. Numerous studies demonstrated that chronic airway inflammation aggravated lung function decline in COPD patients (5, 29). On the other hand, several studies found that CYR61 had proinflammatory activities (30–34). An earlier study showed that CYR61 mediated cigarette smoke extracts evoked IL-8 secretion by lung epithelial cells (28). The current study investigated the association of serum CYR61 with serum inflammatory cytokines and inflammatory signaling in the lungs of COPD patients. Our results showed that pulmonary NF-κB p65-positive nuclei were higher in COPD patients with high CYR61 than with low CYR61. Accordingly, serum MCP-1 and TNF-α, the downstream pro-inflammatory cytokine and chemokine of NF-κB signaling, were increased in parallel with CYR61, among which serum inflammatory cytokines were the highest in COPD patients with high CYR61. To determine the mediating effect of inflammatory cytokines between increased CYR61 and decreased lung function indexes, we analyzed the link between serum CYR61 and inflammatory cytokines in COPD patients. Despite no association between serum CYR61 and inflammatory cytokines among control subjects, a positive correlation of serum CYR61 with TNF-α and MCP-1, as determined by multivariate regression analysis that excluded the influence of age, gender and smoking, was observed among COPD patients. Further analysis showed an obvious mediating effect between an increased inflammatory cytokines with a decreased lung function indexes in COPD patients.

There are several flaws in the current study. First, the results of the current study were from a cross-sectional analysis, in which all COPD patients were from Anhui COPD Cohort. The causal link among CYR61, pulmonary inflammation and COPD progression was not clear. Thus, further follow-up observation and animal experiments are needed to determine the influence of CYR61 on pulmonary inflammation and lung function indexes in COPD patients. Second, the current study has not clarified the underlying mechanism through which CYR61 upregulates inflammatory cytokines in COPD patients. Indeed, an earlier study found that CYR61 upregulated MCP-1 through activating NF-κB pathway in vascular endothelial cells (33). In addition, the previous study has revealed that CYR61 elevated TNF-α via NF-κB signal in murine macrophages (30). Additional experiment is required to explore the exact mechanism by which CYR61 activates NF-κB in the lungs of COPD patients. Third, CYR61 was only detected in lung tissues and sera. But, the level of CYR61 was unclear in bronchoalveolar lavage of COPD patients. In addition, cell localization of CYR61 was not conducted in COPD patients. Further experiments are required to resolve this puzzle in the future work.

CONCLUSION

In summary, the current study investigated the association among serum CYR61, pulmonary inflammation and lung function indexes among COPD patients. Our results showed that serum CYR61 and MCP-1 were elevated in COPD patients. We found that an increased CYR61 was correlated with decreased lung function indexes in COPD patients. Moreover, an increased CYR61 was associated with pulmonary NF-κB activation and serum MCP-1 increase in COPD patients. In addition, an increased CYR61 is associated with a longer hospital stays among COPD patients. Our results provide evidence that CYR61 can be used as a biomarker to predict COPD progression. Inflammatory chemokine MCP-1 may be a mediator between CYR61 and lung function decline in COPD patients.

AUTHOR CONTRIBUTIONS

D-XX, HW, Z-XT, and LF contributed to the study design, analyzing data, and preparation manuscript. W-JW, PZ, and HZ were involved in the acquisition of data. D-XX and LF worked on the study concept, design, and final proof. All authors have read and approved the final manuscript.

ACKNOWLEDGMENTS

We greatly appreciate all doctors and nurses for recruiting participators in the Respiratory and Critical Care Medicine, the Second Affiliated Hospital of Anhui Medical University.

REFERENCES

1. Agustí A, Hogg JC. Update on the pathogenesis of chronic obstructive pulmonary disease. *N Engl J Med.* (2019) 381:1248–56. doi: 10.1056/NEJMra1900475
2. Singh D, Agusti A, Anzueto A, Barnes PJ, Bourbeau J, Celli BR, et al. Global strategy for the diagnosis, management, and prevention of chronic obstructive lung disease: the GOLD science committee report. *Eur Respir J.* (2019) 53:1900164. doi: 10.1183/13993003.00164-2019
3. Higham A, Quinn AM, Cançado JED, Singh D. The pathology of small airways disease in COPD: historical aspects and future directions. *Respir Res.* (2019) 20:49. doi: 10.1186/s12931-019-1017-y
4. Song Q, Chen P, Liu XM. The role of cigarette smoke-induced pulmonary vascular endothelial cell apoptosis in COPD. *Respir Res.* (2021) 22:39. doi: 10.1186/s12931-021-0 1630-1
5. Brightling C, Greening N. Airway inflammation in COPD: progress to precision medicine. *Eur Respir J.* (2019) 54:1900651. doi: 10.1183/13993003.00651-2019
6. OseiE T, Brandsma CA, Timens W, Heijink IH, Hackett TL. Current perspectives on the role of interleukin-1 signalling in the pathogenesis of asthma and COPD. *Eur Respir J.* (2020) 55:1900563. doi: 10.1183/13993003.00563-2019
7. Fu L, Fei J, Tan ZX, Chen YH, Hu B, Xiang HX, et al. Low vitamin D status is associated with inflammation in patients with chronic obstructive pulmonary disease. *J Immunol.* (2021) 206:515–23. doi: 10.4049/jimmunol.2000964
8. Costa C, Traves SL, Tudhope SJ, Fenwick PS, Belchamber KB, Russell RE, et al. Enhanced monocyte migration to CXCR3 and CCR5 chemokines in COPD. *Eur Respir J.* (2016) 47:1093–102. doi: 10.1183/13993003.01642-2015
9. Henrot P, Prevel R, Berger P, Dupin I. Chemokines in COPD: from implication to therapeutic use. *Int J Mol Sci.* (2019) 20:2785. doi: 10.3390/ijms20112785

10. Mortaz E, Redegeld FA, Sarir H, Karimi K, Raats D, Nijkamp FP, et al. Cigarette smoke stimulates the production of chemokines in mast cells. *J Leukoc Biol.* (2008) 83:575–80. doi: 10.1189/jlb.0907625
11. Moriyama C, Betsuyaku T, Ito Y, Hamamura T, Hata J, Takahashi H, et al. Aging enhances susceptibility to cigarette smoke-induced inflammation through bronchiolar chemokines. *Am J Respir Cell Mol Biol.* (2010) 42:304–11. doi: 10.1165/rcmb.2009-0025OC
12. Ma J, Xu H, Wu J, Qu C, Sun F, Xu S. Linalool inhibits cigarette smoke-induced lung inflammation by inhibiting NF-κB activation. *Int Immunopharmacol.* (2015) 29:708–13. doi: 10.1016/j.intimp.2015.09.005
13. Kaur G, Batra S. Regulation of DNA methylation signatures on NF-κB and STAT3 pathway genes and TET activity in cigarette smoke extract-challenged cells/COPD exacerbation model in vitro. *Cell Biol Toxicol.* (2020) 36:459–80. doi: 10.1007/s10565-020-09522-8
14. Lau LF. CCN1/CYR61: the very model of a modern matricellular protein. *Cell Mol Life Sci.* (2011) 68:3149–63. doi: 10.1007/s00018-011-0778-3
15. Chen CY, Su CM, Hsu CJ, Huang CC, Wang SW, Liu SC, et al. CCN1 Promotes VEGF production in osteoblasts and induces endothelial progenitor cell angiogenesis by inhibiting miR-126 expression in rheumatoid arthritis. *J Bone Miner Res.* (2017) 32:34–45. doi: 10.1002/jbmr.2926
16. Li XC, Jin F, Wang BY, Yin XJ, Hong W, Tian FJ. The m6A demethylase ALKBH5 controls trophoblast invasion at the maternal-fetal interface by regulating the stability of CYR61 mRNA. *Theranostics.* (2019) 9:3853–65. doi: 10.7150/thno.31868
17. Duan H, He Z, Lin M, Wang Y, Yang F, Mitteer RA, et al. Plasminogen regulates mesenchymal stem cell-mediated tissue repair after ischemia through Cyr61 activation. *JCI Insight.* (2020) 5:e131376. doi: 10.1172/jci.insight.131376
18. Zhu Y, Almuntashiri S, Han Y, Wang X, Somanath PR, Zhang D. The roles of CCN1/CYR61 in pulmonary diseases. *Int J Mol Sci.* (2020) 21:7810. doi: 10.3390/ijms21217810
19. Grazioli S, Gil S, An D, Kajikawa O, Farnand AW, Hanson JF, et al. CYR61 (CCN1) overexpression induces lung injury in mice. *Am J Physiol Lung Cell Mol Physiol.* (2015) 308:L759–65. doi: 10.1152/ajplung.00190.2014
20. Morrell ED, Grazioli S, Hung C, Kajikawa O, Kosamo S, Stapleton RD, et al. Alveolar CCN1 is associated with mechanical stretch and acute respiratory distress syndrome severity. *Am J Physiol Lung Cell Mol Physiol.* (2020) 319:L825–32. doi: 10.1152/ajplung.00073.2020
21. Kurundkar AR, Kurundkar D, Rangarajan S, Locy ML, Zhou Y, Liu RM, et al. The matricellular protein CCN1 enhances TGF-β1/SMAD3-dependent profibrotic signaling in fibroblasts and contributes to fibrogenic responses to lung injury. *FASEB J.* (2016) 30:2135–50. doi: 10.1096/fj.201500173
22. Ning E, Li CJ, Kaminski N, Feghali-Bostwick CA, Alber SM, Di YP, et al. Comprehensive gene expression profiles reveal pathways related to the pathogenesis of chronic obstructive pulmonary disease. *Proc Natl Acad Sci USA.* (2004) 101:14895–900. doi: 10.1073/pnas.0401168101
23. Vestbo J, Hurd SS, Agustí AG, Jones PW, Vogelmeier C, Anzueto A, et al. Global strategy for the diagnosis, management, and prevention of chronic obstructive pulmonary disease: GOLD executive summary. *Am J Respir Crit Care Med.* (2013) 187:347–65. doi: 10.1164/rccm.201204-0596PP
24. Fei J, Fu L, Cao W, Hu B, Zhao H, Li JB. Low vitamin D status is associated with epithelial-Mesenchymal transition in patients with chronic obstructive pulmonary disease. *J Immunol.* (2019) 203:1428–35. doi: 10.4049/jimmunol.1900229
25. Fu, L, Zhao H, Xiang Y, Xiang HX, Hu B, Tan ZX, et al. Reactive oxygen species-evoked endoplasmic reticulum stress mediates 1-nitropyrene-induced epithelial-mesenchymal transition and pulmonary fibrosis. *Environ Pollut.* (2021) 283:117134. doi: 10.1016/j.envpol.2021.117134
26. Wang JL, Chen X, Xu Y, Chen YX, Wang J, Liu YL, et al. The associations of serum IL-37 with the severity and prognosis in patients with community-acquired pneumonia: a retrospective cohort study. *Front Immunol.* (2021) 12:636896. doi: 10.3389/fimmu.2021.636896
27. Hikichi M, Mizumura K, Maruoka S, Gon Y. Pathogenesis of chronic obstructive pulmonary disease (COPD) induced by cigarette smoke. *J Thorac Dis.* (2019) 11:S2129–40. doi: 10.21037/jtd.2019.10.43
28. Moon HG, Zheng Y, An CH, Kim YK, Jin Y. CCN1 secretion induced by cigarette smoking extracts augments IL-8 release from bronchial epithelial cells. *PLoS ONE.* (2013) 8:e68199. doi: 10.1371/journal.pone.0068199
29. Guo-Parke H, Linden D, Weldon S, Kidney JC, Taggart CC. Mechanisms of virus-induced airway immunity dysfunction in the pathogenesis of COPD disease, progression, and exacerbation. *Front Immunol.* (2020) 11:1205. doi: 10.3389/fimmu.2020.01205
30. Bai T, Chen CC, Lau LF. Matricellular protein CCN1 activates a proinflammatory genetic program in murine macrophages. *J Immunol.* (2010) 184:3223–32. doi: 10.4049/jimmunol.0902792
31. Lin J, Zhou Z, Huo R, Xiao L, Ouyang G, Wang L, et al. Cyr61 induces IL-6 production by fibroblast-like synoviocytes promoting Th17 differentiation in rheumatoid arthritis. *J Immunol.* (2012) 188:5776–84. doi: 10.4049/jimmunol.1103201
32. You JJ, Yang CH, Yang CM, Chen MS. Cyr61 induces the expression of monocyte chemoattractant protein-1 via the integrin αvβ3, FAK, PI3K/Akt, and NF-κB pathways in retinal vascular endothelial cells. *Cell Signal.* (2014) 26:133–40. doi: 10.1016/j.cellsig.2013.08.026
33. Wu P, Ma G, Zhu X, Gu T, Zhang J, Sun Y, et al. Cyr61/CCN1 is involved in the pathogenesis of psoriasis vulgaris via promoting IL-8 production by keratinocytes in a JNK/NF-κB pathway. *Clin Immunol.* (2017) 174:53–62. doi: 10.1016/j.clim.2016.11.003
34. Zhou M, Ze K, Hua L, Liu L, Kuai L, Zhang M, et al. Cyr61 promotes inflammation of a gouty arthritis model in rats. *Mediators Inflamm.* (2020) 2020:1–13. doi: 10.1155/2020/8298615

10

Blood Eosinophils and Clinical Outcomes in Patients with Acute Exacerbation of Chronic Obstructive Pulmonary Disease: A Propensity Score Matching Analysis of Real-World Data in China

Yanan Cui [1], ***Zijie Zhan*** [1], ***Zihang Zeng*** [1], ***Ke Huang*** [2,3,4], ***Chen Liang*** [5], ***Xihua Mao*** [5], ***Yaowen Zhang*** [5], ***Xiaoxia Ren*** [2,3,4], ***Ting Yang*** [2,3,4*] **and** ***Yan Chen*** [1*]

[1] Department of Respiratory and Critical Care Medicine, The Second Xiangya Hospital, Central South University, Changsha, China, [2] Department of Pulmonary and Critical Care Medicine, China-Japan Friendship Hospital, Beijing, China, [3] National Clinical Research Center for Respiratory Diseases, Beijing, China, [4] Institute of Respiratory Medicine, Chinese Academy of Medical Science, Beijing, China, [5] Chinese Alliance for Respiratory Diseases in Primary Care, Beijing, China

***Correspondence:**
Yan Chen
chenyan99727@csu.edu.cn
Ting Yang
zryyyangting@163.com

Background and Objective: Elevated eosinophils in chronic obstructive pulmonary disease (COPD) are recognized as a biomarker to guide inhaled corticosteroids use, but the value of blood eosinophils in hospitalized exacerbations of COPD remains controversial. This study aimed to evaluate the accuracy of eosinophils in predicting clinical outcomes in acute exacerbation of COPD (AECOPD).

Methods: We analyzed data from the acute exacerbation of chronic obstructive pulmonary disease inpatient registry (ACURE) study, which is an ongoing nationwide multicenter, observational real-world study in patients admitted for AECOPD. Data collected between January 2018 and December 2019 in 163 centers were first reviewed. The eligible patients were divided into eosinophilic and non-eosinophilic groups, according to blood eosinophil with 2% of the total leukocyte count as the threshold. Propensity score (PS) matching was performed to adjust for confounders.

Results: A total of 1,566 patients (median age: 69 years; 80.3% male) were included and 42.7% had an eosinophilic AECOPD. Eosinophil count $<2\%$ was associated with the development of respiratory failure and pneumonia. After PS matching, 650 pairs in overall patients, 468 pairs in patients with smoking history and 177 pairs in patients without smoking were selected, respectively. Only in patients with smoking history, the non-eosinophilic AECOPD was associated with longer median hospital stays (9 vs. 8 days, $P = 0.034$), higher dosage of corticosteroid use, higher economic burden of hospitalization, and poorer response to corticosteroid therapy compared to the eosinophilic AECOPD. No significant difference was found in patients without smoking. Eosinophil levels had no relationship with the change of COPD Assessment Test scores and readmissions or death after 30 days.

Conclusion: Elevated eosinophils were associated with better short-term outcomes only in patients with a smoking history. Eosinophil levels cannot be confidently used as a predictor alone for estimating prognosis.

Keywords: AECOPD, eosinophils, smoking, prediction, corticosteroids

INTRODUCTION

Chronic obstructive pulmonary disease (COPD) is a major cause of morbidity and mortality throughout the world that incurs a considerable economic and social burden (1). Acute exacerbation of COPD (AECOPD) is an acute event characterized by a worsening of respiratory symptoms and leads to a change in therapy (2). AECOPD requiring hospitalizations are associated with an accelerated decline in lung function, a higher probability of recurrent exacerbations, an increase in healthcare costs and mortality (3). The identification of phenotypes based on biomarkers could help clinicians to establish individual treatment programs for patients with AECOPD.

Blood eosinophils are recommended by the Global Initiative for Chronic Obstructive Lung Disease (GOLD) 2020 as a biomarker to guide clinical decisions about inhaled corticosteroids (ICS) use (1). Sources of evidence include *post-hoc* analyses and pre-specified analyses, which showed a better response to ICS in stable COPD patients with higher blood eosinophil counts. However, cohort studies investigating the relationship between blood eosinophils and future exacerbation risk have produced different results (4, 5). The GOLD 2020 states that there is insufficient evidence to recommend blood eosinophils in stable COPD as a biomarker to predict exacerbation risk (1).

In patients with AECOPD, the clinical value of blood eosinophils in guiding therapy and judging prognosis is less clear. Some studies reported that higher eosinophil levels were associated with shorter hospital stays following treatment with systemic corticosteroids (6, 7), but other studies suggested a longer hospitalization (8). Scarce data exist regarding the association between blood eosinophils and 30-day readmissions or mortality. In the secondary analysis of a randomized controlled trial, there was no difference in treatment failure rates within 30 days between the eosinophilic and non-eosinophilic exacerbations treated with prednisolone (9). Recently, Hegewald et al. reported that greater eosinophil counts were associated with increased risk of 30-day COPD-related readmissions (10). Whether blood eosinophil counts at admission can predict the risk of readmissions and mortality remains controversial. In addition, most of the patients recruited had a history of smoking (6, 7, 9), which might affect the inflammatory response of eosinophils (11). Hence, there is a need for more evidence in clinically representative patient populations.

This real-world study in China aimed to evaluate the association between baseline blood eosinophil counts and the length of stay, systemic corticosteroid usage and healthcare costs, response to systemic corticosteroid therapy during hospitalization in patients with AECOPD. We also investigated whether eosinophil levels are related to the change of COPD Assessment Test (CAT) scores and readmissions or death after 30 days. In addition, clinical outcomes for different eosinophil groups were also assessed according to smoking history.

METHODS

Study Design and Study Population

We analyzed data from the acute exacerbation of chronic obstructive pulmonary disease inpatient registry (ACURE) study, which was launched to investigate the clinical features, treatments, and prognoses of AECOPD in the Chinese population. Details of the ACURE study have been previously described (12). In brief, the ACURE study is an ongoing nationwide multicenter, observational patient registry in patients admitted for AECOPD, followed up with a 3-year observing period in a real-world setting. Data collected between January 2018 and December 2019 in 163 centers were first reviewed. Only patients ≥18 years old with the discharge diagnosis of an exacerbation of COPD were included. Exacerbations were defined as an acute worsening of respiratory symptoms that result in additional therapy (1). This protocol was approved by the ethics committee of China-Japan Friendship Hospital (No. 2015-88). Informed consent was obtained from all participants in the study. This study was conducted in accordance with the Declaration of Helsinki.

In our study, the presence of a post-bronchodilator forced expiratory volume in 1 s (FEV1)/forced vital capacity (FVC) ratio <0.70 was required. Patients with a history of asthma, bronchiectasis, pulmonary embolism, pulmonary hypertension, interstitial pulmonary disease, lung cancer or other chronic lung diseases, and those with any comorbidity that could influence blood eosinophil count (allergic disorder, autoimmune disease, parasitic disease or hematologic disease) were excluded. All the included patients had documented blood eosinophil counts on admission. The subject enrollment process is shown in **Figure 1**. The eligible study population was divided into eosinophilic AECOPD group and non-eosinophilic AECOPD group. The eosinophilic AECOPD was defined as one where the blood eosinophil count at admission was ≥2% of the total white blood cell count, since this threshold had previously shown a sensitivity of 90% and specificity of 60% for predicting sputum eosinophilia in AECOPD (13). In addition, all the included patients were grouped according to their smoking history for further analyzing the effect of smoking on the effectiveness of eosinophils as a biomarker.

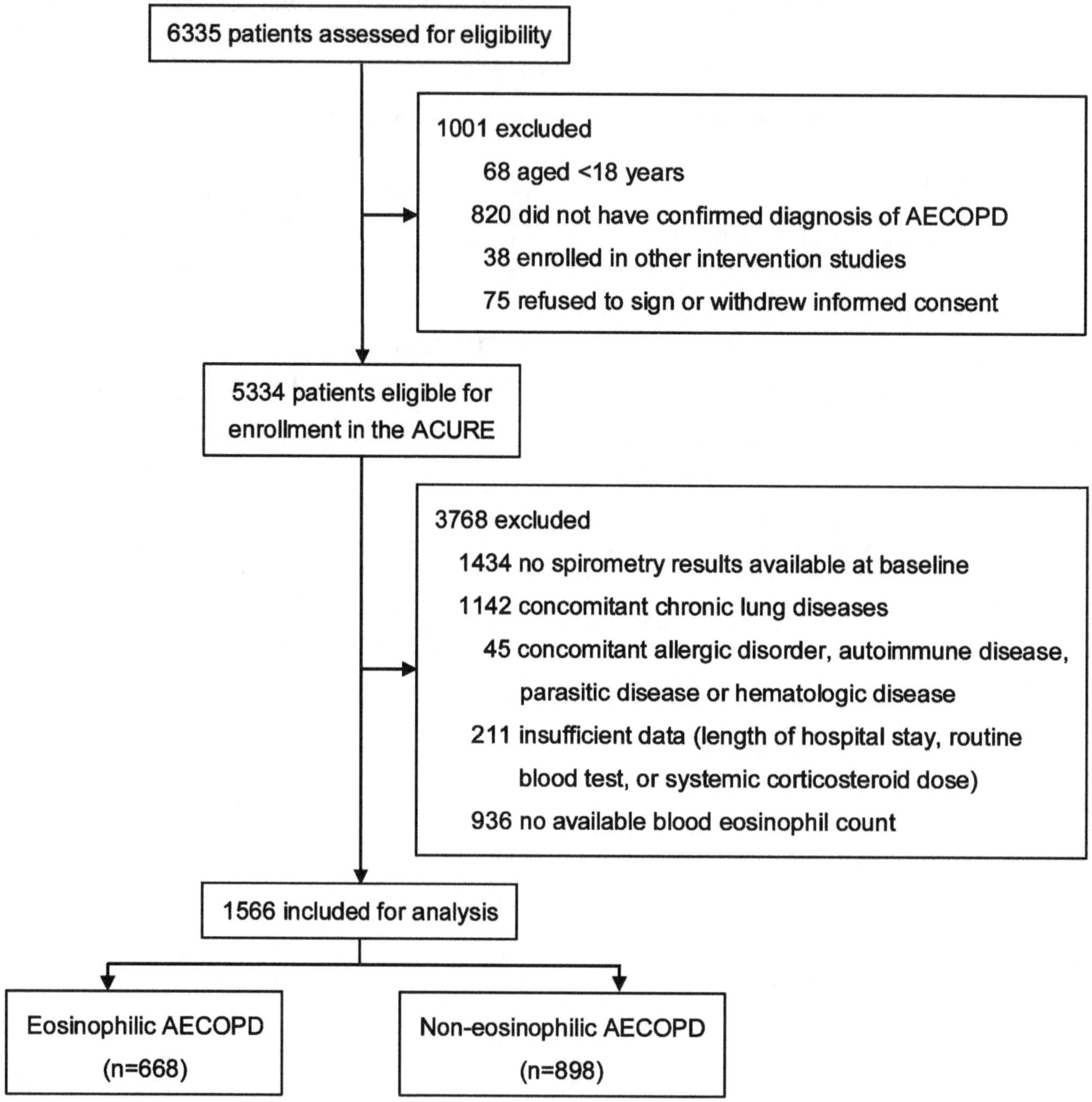

FIGURE 1 | Flowchart of patient enrollment process. AECOPD, acute exacerbations of chronic obstructive pulmonary disease; ACURE, acute exacerbation of chronic obstructive pulmonary disease inpatient registry study.

Measurements and Outcomes

Patient baseline characteristics, including age, sex, body-mass index (BMI), smoking status, pulmonary function, symptoms, modified Medical Research Council (mMRC) dyspnea grade, CAT score, the number of hospital or emergency admissions in the previous year, pre-admission medications, complications (respiratory failure and chronic cor pulmonale), comorbidities (pneumonia, hypertension, cardiac disease, diabetes, and cerebrovascular accident), blood eosinophil count, length of hospital stay, hospital corticosteroid treatment, and cost during hospitalization, were recorded. Among these variables, pulmonary function, symptoms, mMRC dyspnea grade, CAT score, respiratory failure, and pneumonia were defined upon admission. The number of hospital or emergency admissions in the previous year, pre-admission medications, chronic cor pulmonale, hypertension, cardiac disease, diabetes, and cerebrovascular accident were defined according to the historical clinical records. Specifically, respiratory failure was defined by an arterial oxygen tension (PaO2) of <8.0 kPa (60 mmHg), an arterial carbon dioxide tension (PaCO2) of >6.0 kPa (45 mmHg) or both (14). The diagnosis of pneumonia was based on the presence of certain clinical features (e.g., cough, fever, sputum production, and pleuritic chest pain) and changes on the chest radiography, which was also supported by pathogenic examination (15). In our study, cardiac disease included coronary heart disease, arrhythmia, chronic heart failure, and acute heart failure. Systemic corticosteroid use was expressed as equivalent dose of prednisolone. The primary outcome was the length of hospital stay. Secondary outcomes were cumulative systemic corticosteroid dose and cost during hospitalization, the change of CAT scores from baseline to discharge or day 30 after discharge, the early readmission with AECOPD or death, taken as those occurring in the 15 days following discharge, and readmission with AECOPD or death within 30 days. The costs were shown in US dollars using the average exchange rate in 2019 (one US dollar was equivalent to 6.90 Chinese yuan).

Subgroup Analyses

To further examine the response of eosinophils to systemic corticosteroid therapy during hospitalization, subgroup analyses of the primary outcome were performed according to if receiving hospital systemic corticosteroid therapy. In addition, all these analyses were conducted among patients who did not receive systemic corticosteroids prior to admission.

Statistical Analyses

Continuous data were expressed as median (interquartile range, IQR) and mean (standard error of mean, SEM), and categorical data were expressed as frequencies (percentage). The study variables were compared between eosinophilic and non-eosinophilic AECOPD groups using the chi-squared test for unordered categorical variables and the Mann-Whitney U-test for ordinal categorical variables. For continuous variables, the t-test and Mann-Whitney U-test were used to compare the mean and median respectively.

Given differences in the baseline characteristics between eosinophilic and non-eosinophilic AECOPD groups, propensity score (PS) matching was used to reduce potential bias. We calculated PS using a logistic regression model and used 1:1 matching with a caliper width equal to 0.02 of the standard deviation of the logit of the PS. A PS matching was performed in overall patients included in this study using the following covariates: age, sex, BMI, smoking status, mMRC dyspnea grade, respiratory failure, and pneumonia (forcing age and sex in the model but all other variables were considered only if they reached statistical significance). Further, PS matching was also carried out in patients with smoking history and patients without smoking history, respectively to balance the distributions between eosinophilic and non-eosinophilic AECOPD groups for age, sex, BMI, mMRC dyspnea grade, respiratory failure, and pneumonia.

We used Cox's proportional hazard model to evaluate the hazard ratio between eosinophil level and readmission with AECOPD or death within 15 or 30 days. The potential prognostic factors including, age, sex, BMI, post-bronchodilator FEV_1/FVC, mMRC dyspnea grade, CAT score, the number of hospital or emergency admissions in the previous year, respiratory failure, pneumonia, and hospital systemic corticosteroid therapy were adjusted in the model. All analyses were performed using the software IBM-SPSS statistics 25. A two-sided P-value <0.05 was considered statistically significant.

RESULTS

Baseline Characteristics

Of the 1,566 subjects included in the study, 668 (42.7%) had an eosinophilic AECOPD, whereas 898 subjects (57.3%) had a non-eosinophilic AECOPD. The mean age of the patients was 69 years and 80.3% were male. Most patients had a history of smoking (72.9%) and 27.1% were never smokers. Hypertension was the most common comorbidity.

Baseline characteristics of the eosinophilic and non-eosinophilic groups are shown in **Table 1**. The mMRC dyspnea grade was significantly lower in eosinophilic compared to non-eosinophilic AECOPD ($P = 0.005$). Prescription of ICS or oral corticosteroids (OCS) before admission was similar between the two groups. Patients in the non-eosinophilic group had higher frequencies of respiratory failure and pneumonia compared with those in the eosinophilic group.

During hospitalization, the cumulative systemic corticosteroid dose and total healthcare cost were lower in the eosinophilic group than in the non-eosinophilic group (P <0.001 and $P = 0.002$, respectively). There was no between-group difference for the primary outcome of length of hospital stay ($P = 0.094$; **Table 1**).

Propensity Score Matching Analyses

Of all included patients, 650 of 668 eosinophilic cases could be matched (1:1) to a non-eosinophilic control. After matching, the two groups were well-balanced regarding all baseline covariates. Notably, results from the PS matching analyses were similar to those from the unmatched analyses. The median hospitalization days of the two groups were both 9 days with no statistical difference ($P = 0.166$).

After performing PS matching for the 1,142 patients with a history of smoking in the entire 1,566 subjects, 468 matched pairs of patients were selected. In the 424 patients without smoking history, 177 matched pairs were identified. The distribution of baseline characteristics was balanced after matching between the eosinophilic and non-eosinophilic groups in patients with or without smoking history (**Supplementary Table 1**). For patients with smoking history, the median time in hospital of the eosinophilic group was significantly shorter compared with the non-eosinophilic group [median (IQR) 8 days (7–11) vs. 9 days (7–12), $P = 0.034$; **Figure 2A**], whereas no statistical difference was found between the two groups in patients who were never smokers (**Figure 2B**). The total dosage of systemic corticosteroids and total cost during hospitalization were lower in eosinophilic exacerbations than in non-eosinophilic exacerbations among patients with smoking history ($P = 0.001$ for both; **Figure 3**), but

TABLE 1 | Clinical characteristics of the study patients before and after propensity score matching.

Variables	Before propensity score matching			After propensity score matching		
	Eosinophilic AECOPD (n = 668)	Non-eosinophilic AECOPD (n = 898)	*P*-value	Eosinophilic AECOPD (n = 650)	Non-eosinophilic AECOPD (n = 650)	*P*-value
Age (years)	69 (63–76)	69 (64–76)	0.280	69 (63–76)	69 (63–76)	0.810
Male	555 (83.1%)	702 (78.2%)	0.016	537 (82.6%)	544 (83.7%)	0.604
Body-mass index (kg/m^2)	22.5 (19.8–24.6)	21.5 (19.4–24.2)	0.006	22.5 (19.7–24.5)	21.9 (19.6–24.6)	0.496
Smoking status			0.016			0.727
Ex-smoker	319 (47.8%)	370 (41.2%)		309 (47.5%)	286 (44.0%)	
Current smoker	171 (25.6%)	282 (31.4%)		164 (25.2%)	206 (31.7%)	
Non-smoker	178 (26.6%)	246 (27.4%)		177 (27.2%)	158 (24.3%)	
Post-bronchodilator FEV_1/FVC	0.5 (0.4–0.6)	0.5 (0.4–0.6)	0.893	0.5 (0.4–0.6)	0.5 (0.4–0.6)	0.924
Symptoms						
Increased cough	400 (59.9%)	569 (63.4%)	0.160	396 (60.9%)	400 (61.5%)	0.820
Increased sputum volume	262 (39.2%)	397 (44.2%)	0.054	258 (39.7%)	284 (43.7%)	0.144
Increased sputum purulence	273 (40.9%)	406 (45.2%)	0.086	267 (41.1%)	290 (44.6%)	0.197
Wheezing	561 (84.0%)	755 (84.1%)	0.960	551 (84.8%)	545 (83.8%)	0.647
mMRC dyspnea grade			0.005			0.588
0–1	119 (17.8%)	114 (12.7%)		102 (15.7%)	95 (14.6%)	
≥2	549 (82.2%)	784 (87.3%)		548 (84.3%)	555 (85.4%)	
CAT score			0.644			0.704
<10	63 (9.4%)	91 (10.1%)		59 (9.1%)	63 (9.7%)	
≥10	605 (90.6%)	807 (89.9%)		591 (90.9%)	587 (90.3%)	
Hospital admissions previous year			0.436			0.658
0	342 (51.2%)	483 (53.8%)		333 (51.2%)	344 (52.9%)	
1	169 (25.3%)	206 (22.9%)		164 (25.2%)	153 (23.5%)	
≥2	157 (23.5%)	209 (23.3%)		153 (23.5%)	153 (23.5%)	
Emergency visits previous year			0.811			0.645
0	434 (65.0%)	578 (64.4%)		424 (65.2%)	413 (63.5%)	
1	103 (15.4%)	141 (15.7%)		98 (15.1%)	111 (17.1%)	
≥2	131 (19.6%)	179 (19.9%)		128 (19.7%)	126 (19.4%)	
Pre-admission medication						
LABA	224 (33.5%)	275 (30.6%)	0.222	220 (33.8%)	220 (33.8%)	1.000
LAMA	240 (35.9%)	293 (32.6%)	0.173	236 (36.3%)	231 (35.5%)	0.773
ICS	226 (33.8%)	279 (31.1%)	0.247	223 (34.3%)	224 (34.5%)	0.953
OCS	17 (2.5%)	28 (3.1%)	0.502	17 (2.6%)	19 (2.9%)	0.735
Complications						
Respiratory failure	123 (18.4%)	211 (23.5%)	0.015	123 (18.9%)	131 (20.2%)	0.576
Chronic cor pulmonale	100 (15.0%)	144 (16.0%)	0.565	98 (15.1%)	90 (13.8%)	0.528
Comorbidities						
Pneumonia	157 (23.5%)	288 (32.1%)	<0.001	157 (24.2%)	166 (25.5%)	0.563
Hypertension	239 (35.8%)	300 (33.4%)	0.329	234 (36.0%)	217 (33.4%)	0.322
Cardiac disease	140 (21.0%)	195 (21.7%)	0.718	140 (21.5%)	116 (17.8%)	0.094
Diabetes	56 (8.4%)	90 (10.0%)	0.270	56 (8.6%)	67 (10.3%)	0.297
Cerebrovascular accident	46 (6.9%)	62 (6.9%)	0.989	46 (7.1%)	44 (6.8%)	0.827
Length of hospital stay (days)	9 (7–11)	9 (7–12)	0.094	9 (7–11)	9 (7–12)	0.166
Antibiotics during hospitalization	553 (82.8%)	770 (85.7%)	0.109	545 (83.8%)	552 (84.9%)	0.593
Systemic corticosteroids during hospitalization	457 (68.4%)	677 (75.4%)	0.002	447 (68.8%)	489 (75.2%)	0.009
Cumulative systemic corticosteroid dose (mg)	90 (0–200)	120 (0–260)	<0.001	90 (0–200)	120 (0–270)	<0.001
Total cost during hospitalization (US$)	1,333 (1,013–1,842)	1,451 (1,074–2,034)	0.002	1,333 (1,017–1,846)	1,472 (1,086–2,041)	0.002

Data are presented as n (%) or median (IQR).

AECOPD, acute exacerbations of chronic obstructive pulmonary disease; FEV_1, forced expiratory volume in 1 s; FVC, forced vital capacity; mMRC, modified Medical Research Council; CAT, COPD Assessment Test; LABA, long-acting beta-adrenoceptor agonist; LAMA, long-acting muscarinic receptor agonist; ICS, inhaled corticosteroids; OCS, oral corticosteroid.

the differences were not statistically significant in never smokers ($P = 0.053$ and 0.171, respectively; **Figure 3**). Accounting for the highest proportion of total cost, medicine fee in patients with smoking history was also numerically higher for the non-eosinophilic group, as compared with the eosinophilic group (**Figure 4A**). However, in never smokers, the eosinophilic group exhibited higher medicine fee, although the result was not statistically significant (**Figure 4B**). Antibiotics use during hospitalization showed no difference between the groups regardless of smoking history.

Subgroup Analyses

In subgroup analyses of the matched cohorts, systemic corticosteroids were prescribed in 72.0, 74.6, and 66.7% of the overall patients, the patients with smoking history and the patients with no smoking history, respectively (**Supplementary Table 2**). Length of hospital stay showed no significant difference between the eosinophilic and non-eosinophilic groups no matter whether using systemic corticosteroids or not in overall patients ($P = 0.392$ and 0.245, respectively). The hospitalization time following treatment with systemic corticosteroids was shorter in eosinophilic AECOPD compared to non-eosinophilic AECOPD in patients with smoking history [median (IQR) 8 days (7–12) vs. 9 days (7–12), $P = 0.046$] but similar between the two groups in patients with no history of smoking ($P = 0.376$). There was no statistical difference in length of hospital stay between the two groups in patients not receiving corticosteroids therapy, regardless of smoking history ($P = 0.520$ and 0.494, respectively). Limiting the analysis to patients free of OCS use prior to admission did not change these results (**Supplementary Table 3**).

Longitudinal Analyses

A total of 1,003 patients (64%) of 1,566 had follow-up data within 30 days after discharge. Clinical characteristics were largely similar among subjects with and without follow-up data (**Supplementary Table 4**). Readmission with AECOPD or death occurred in 1.6 and 3.5% of the 1,003 patients at 15 and 30 days, respectively. Cox regression analyses showed, in overall patients or patients with smoking history after matching, there was no significant difference in 15-day readmission or death between the eosinophilic and non-eosinophilic groups, nor was there a difference between the groups at 30 days (**Table 2**). Given the small number of index events in the non-smoking cohort, no further analysis was undertaken. At all timepoints evaluated, the mean change from the baseline in CAT scores did not differ between the two groups in the three matched cohorts (**Figure 5**).

DISCUSSION

To the best of our knowledge, this has been the first multicenter observational study using propensity matching analysis of real-world data to evaluate the role of eosinophils in patients with AECOPD requiring hospitalization. We found that the increased eosinophil count was associated with a better short-term prognosis only in patients with smoking history. For patients who were never smokers, the predict value of eosinophils was poor. In addition, we for the first time proposed that blood eosinophil counts might be a useful biomarker for economic burden of AECOPD during hospitalization. The nature of the exacerbation was not relevant to the change of CAT scores and readmissions for AECOPD or death after 30 days.

The prevalence of elevated blood eosinophils, defined as $\geq$2% of the total leukocyte count, was about 40% in our study, similar to recent studies in China (6, 16). According to this threshold, inpatients with eosinophilic AECOPD may have different clinical characteristics. In our study, lower eosinophil level was associated with a higher risk of respiratory failure and higher mMRC dyspnea grade. Another multicenter prospective study of 493 AECOPD patients also reported that patients with lower eosinophil counts experienced higher rates of both non-invasive mechanical ventilation and respiratory failure (17). Moreover, we found a strong relationship between low levels of eosinophils and the development of pneumonia. In a prospective observational cohort study, Kim et al. showed that eosinophils $\geq$2% at exacerbation was associated with a lower risk of bacterial infections (18). C-reactive protein as a proxy for infection correlated negatively with blood eosinophil counts (19).

In our real-world study, the difference of hospitalization time was not significant between the eosinophilic and non-eosinophilic exacerbations. The PS matching analyses did not change this result. Only in patients with a history of smoking, eosinophils $\geq$2% distinguished those with shorter median hospital stays. As we know, airway inflammation and remodeling are closely related to cigarette smoking, which is the most commonly encountered risk factor for COPD (1). However, the molecular mechanisms are not completely clear. The mechanism of inflammation in patients developing COPD without smoking is also less known. A growing number of researchers regarded eosinophils as a biomarker and proposed that eosinophilic inflammation was a common and stable phenotype in COPD (6, 16–19). It is necessary to consider the influence of smoking on eosinophilic inflammation. Chis et al. reported that the level of blood eosinophils was affected by smoking status in COPD patients (20). In another study that assessed the accuracy of inflammatory biomarkers in differentiating asthma-COPD overlap (ACO) from COPD, blood eosinophil counts had a higher sensitivity in distinguishing ACO from COPD among patients with a smoking history compared to those without smoking (21).

Many researches showed that patients presenting to hospital with an eosinophilic AECOPD had a shorter length of stay. However, a large number of these studies included patients who were former or current smokers with a minimum smoking history of 10 pack years (7, 19, 22–24). In several other studies, non-smokers were included but occupied a little proportion (<5%) (6, 25). Similar to our study, Gonzalez-Barcala et al. carried out a retrospective study including 358 patients in Spain, 26.5% of whom were never smokers. They found no significant differences in the length of stay between patients with an elevated or low blood eosinophil counts using various thresholds (26). In a study performed in three teaching hospitals in China, a longer hospital stay was observed in the non-eosinophilic group although 36.5% of the included patients had no history of

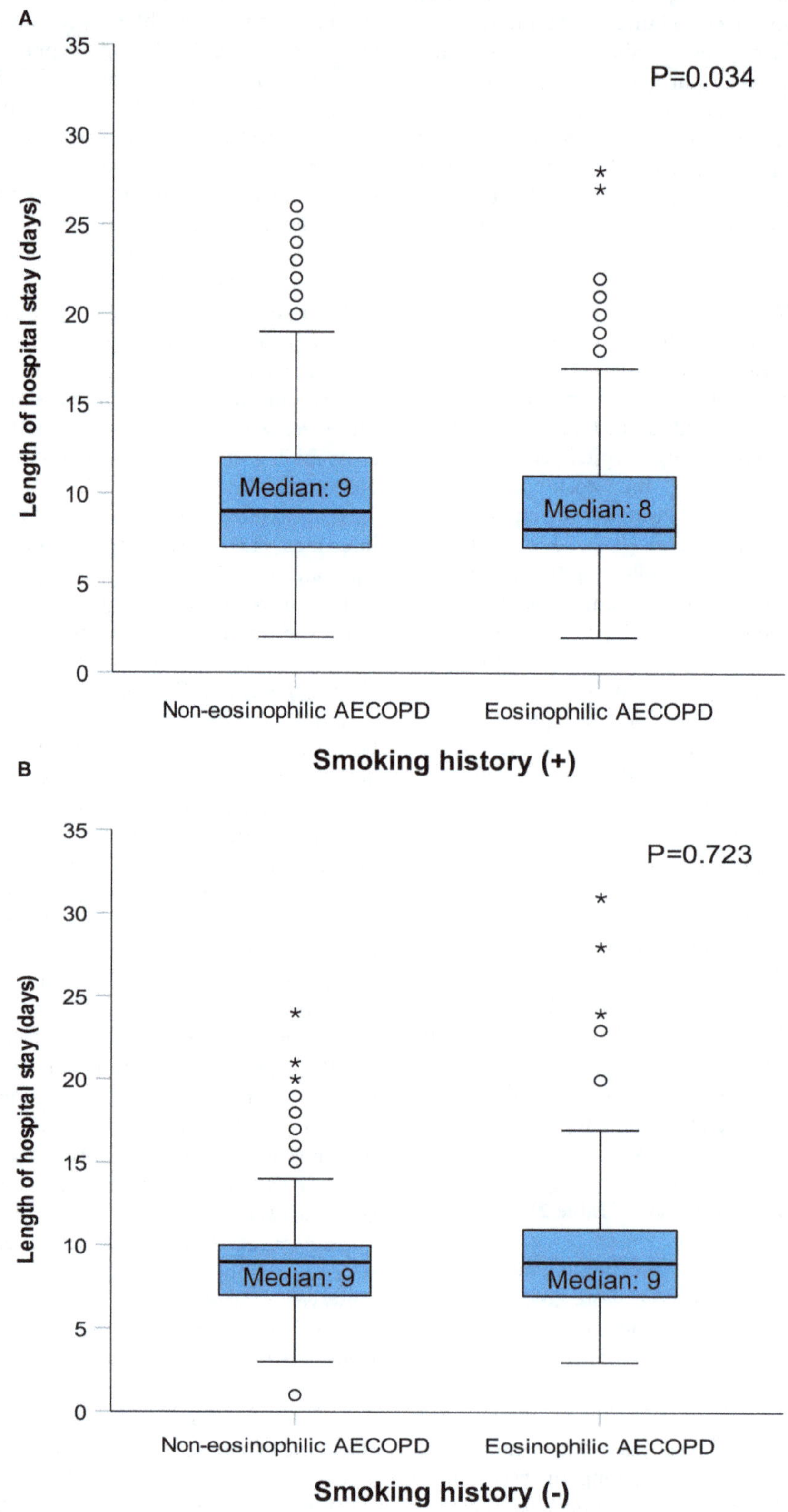

FIGURE 2 | Length of hospital stay in patients with or without smoking history after matching. AECOPD, acute exacerbations of chronic obstructive pulmonary disease. The circles and asterisks are outliers.

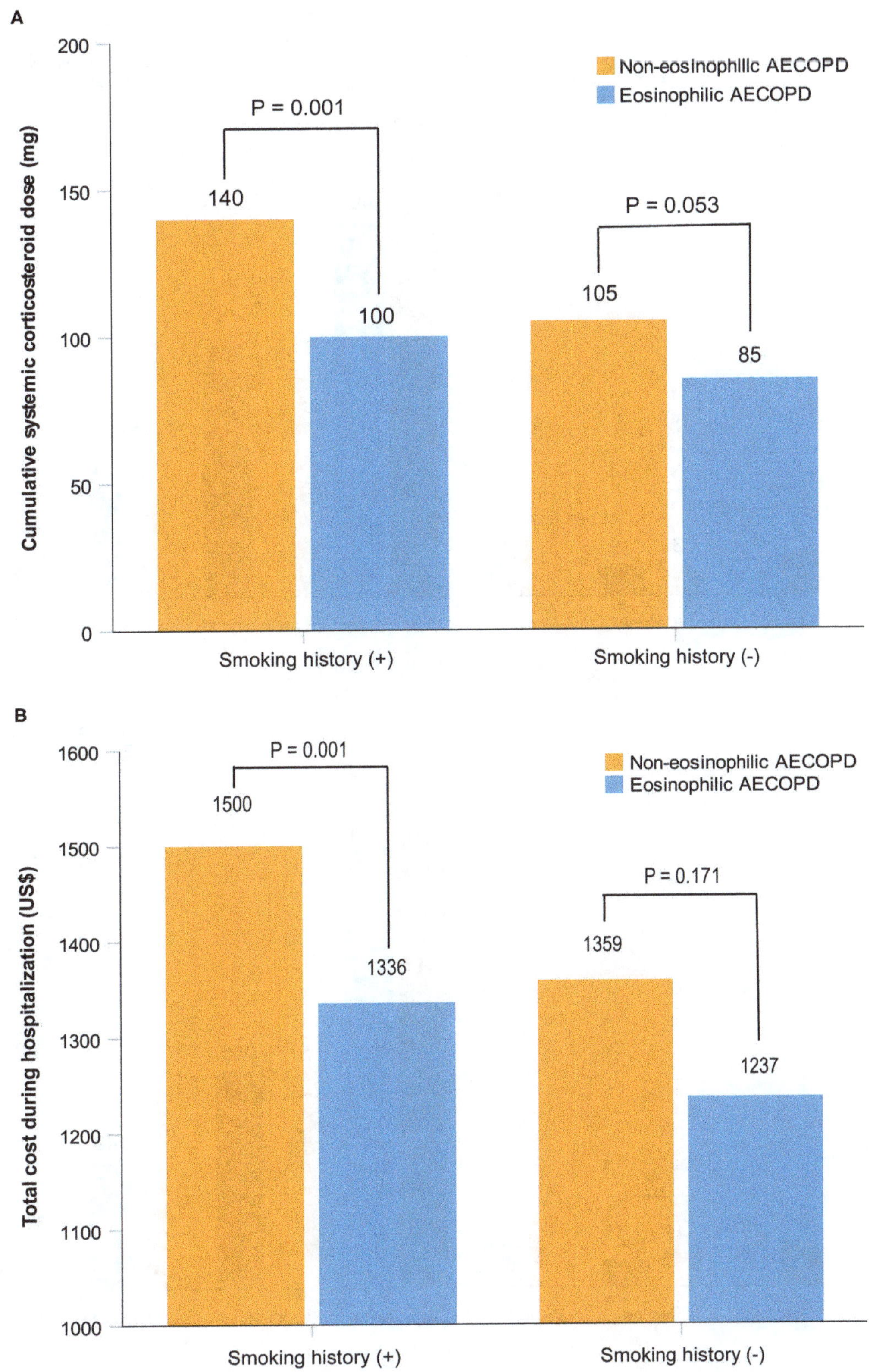

FIGURE 3 | Cumulative systemic corticosteroid dose and total cost during hospitalization in patients with or without smoking history after matching. Data are presented as median. AECOPD, acute exacerbations of chronic obstructive pulmonary disease.

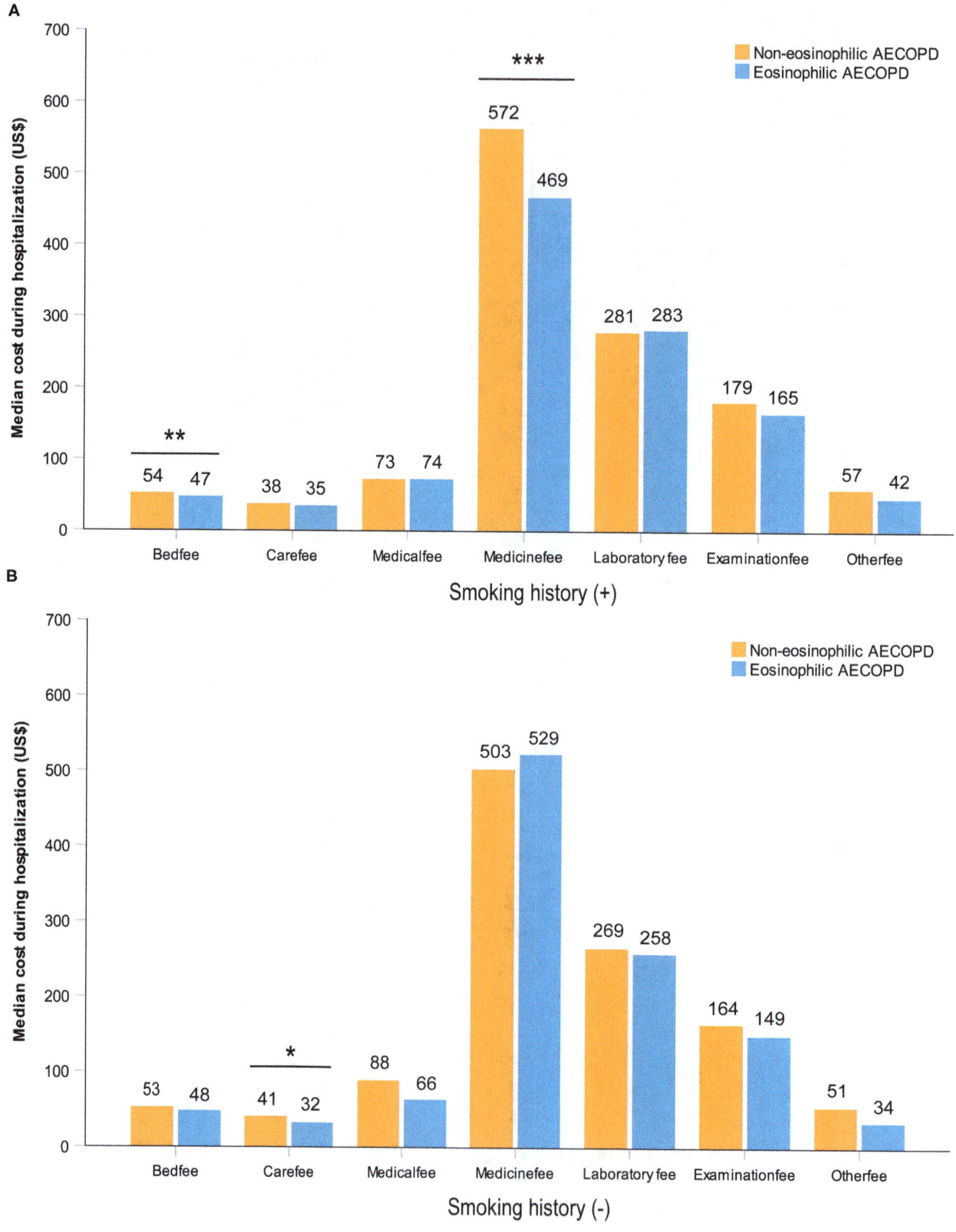

FIGURE 4 | Various cost during hospitalization in patients with or without smoking history after matching. Statistically significant differences between groups are indicated as $*P \le 0.05$, $**P \le 0.01$, and $***P \le 0.001$. Error bars show 95% confidence interval. AECOPD, acute exacerbations of chronic obstructive pulmonary disease.

TABLE 2 | Readmission with AECOPD or death within 15 and 30 days in the matched cohorts.

	Readmission with AECOPD or death within 15 days		Readmission with AECOPD or death within 30 days	
	HR (95% CI)[a]	*P*-value	HR (95% CI)[a]	*P*-value
Overall (*n* = 850)				
Non-eosinophilic AECOPD	1 (Ref)		1 (Ref)	
Eosinophilic AECOPD	1.002 (0.300–3.346)	0.998	1.264 (0.572–2.793)	0.562
Smoking history (*n* = 619)				
Non-eosinophilic AECOPD	1 (Ref)		1 (Ref)	
Eosinophilic AECOPD	1.034 (0.267–4.005)	0.962	1.064 (0.425–2.665)	0.895

[a] *Cox proportional hazards model.*
AECOPD, acute exacerbations of chronic obstructive pulmonary disease.

smoking (17). In fact, patients with lower eosinophil counts in this study experienced a higher rate of infection indicated by the higher leukocyte counts and neutrophil percentages at baseline, which also leading to longer hospital stays.

In our study, higher eosinophil levels correlated with a better response to hospital systemic corticosteroid therapy only in patients with smoking history. The association between hospital stay and blood eosinophil levels became non-statistically significant in the whole sample or in patients without smoking following treatment with corticosteroids. Previous related studies also reported that patients with non-eosinophilic exacerbations were less responsive to systemic corticosteroids, noting that almost all of the included patients had a history of smoking (6, 7, 9, 23). Few researchers have considered smoking status when studying eosinophils and the response to corticosteroids. In *The Lancet Respiratory Medicine*, Bafadhel et al. reported that smoking status was an independent predictor of response to budesonide in COPD patients in a *post-hoc* analysis of three trials and a significant interaction was observed between eosinophil count, treatment, and smoking status (27). They found in former smokers, exacerbation rate was independent of eosinophil count, but in current smokers, increased eosinophil counts were associated with increased risk of exacerbation, with a treatment effect of budesonide–formoterol as compared with formoterol alone associated with elevated eosinophil level. A *post-hoc* supervised cluster analysis showed a favorable response to fluticasone furoate/vilanterol compared with vilanterol alone in COPD patients with higher eosinophil counts or lower eosinophil counts with shorter smoking history (28). The complicated mechanisms underlying the interaction between smoking status and corticosteroid benefit remain unclear. However, in our study, never smokers had better lung function and a lower proportion of pre-admission medication usage than patients with a history of smoking. They might be more sensitive to medications like bronchodilators and antibiotics and have better compliance in the management of AECOPD, which made the differences in clinical outcomes between the eosinophilic and non-eosinophilic groups insignificant. Cigarette smoke may directly affect the response of eosinophils to corticosteroids, but the molecular mechanism and related pathway need to be further studied.

In addition, the higher dose of systemic corticosteroids as well as the number of patients treated with systemic corticosteroids in the non-eosinophilic group in our study might be due to their poorer response to corticosteroid therapy. More non-eosinophilic patients were prescribed systemic corticosteroids rather than inhaled corticosteroids and the dose of systemic corticosteroids needed in the non-eosinophilic AECOPD was also higher.

Several studies demonstrated a substantial annual burden associated with eosinophilic COPD (29, 30). In a cross-sectional study of 2,832 patients in the US, subjects with elevated eosinophil counts had numerically higher all-cause and COPD-related health care resource utilization (HCRU) and cost each year (31). However, there has been no study showing the relationship between eosinophil counts and cost during an exacerbation in hospitalized patients. Our study found that blood eosinophil counts could serve as a biomarker for the total cost during hospitalization in patients with AECOPD. The higher medicine fee in the non-eosinophilic group among patients with smoking history might be related to their higher dosage of corticosteroid use and longer hospital stay.

In our study, no relationship was found between eosinophil counts and clinical outcomes after 15 or 30 days. Gonzalez-Barcala et al. also reported that there was no relationship observed between eosinophil counts and readmissions within 15 days (26). Using data from a randomized clinical trial, Prins et al. claimed that treatment failure within 10 days was reduced in the eosinophilic group, but late treatment failure (days 11–30) did not differ significantly (22). In a randomized biomarker-directed corticosteroid vs. standard therapy study, the mean change from the baseline in CAT scores and readmissions with AECOPD or death at 30 days did not differ between the eosinophilic and non-eosinophilic groups (32). However, in another similar study, there was a greater improvement of the chronic respiratory questionnaire over 14 days in the eosinophilic exacerbations treated with prednisolone (9). Of note, the majority of the exacerbations in this study did not require hospitalization and the dosage of prednisolone in this study (30 mg once daily for 14 days) was higher than that in the real world. Recently, Hegewald et al. reported that greater eosinophil counts were associated with increased risk of COPD-related readmission at 30 days, but 26% of the included patients combined asthma and only 17.6% had spirometry results, which were likely to influence the outcome (10).

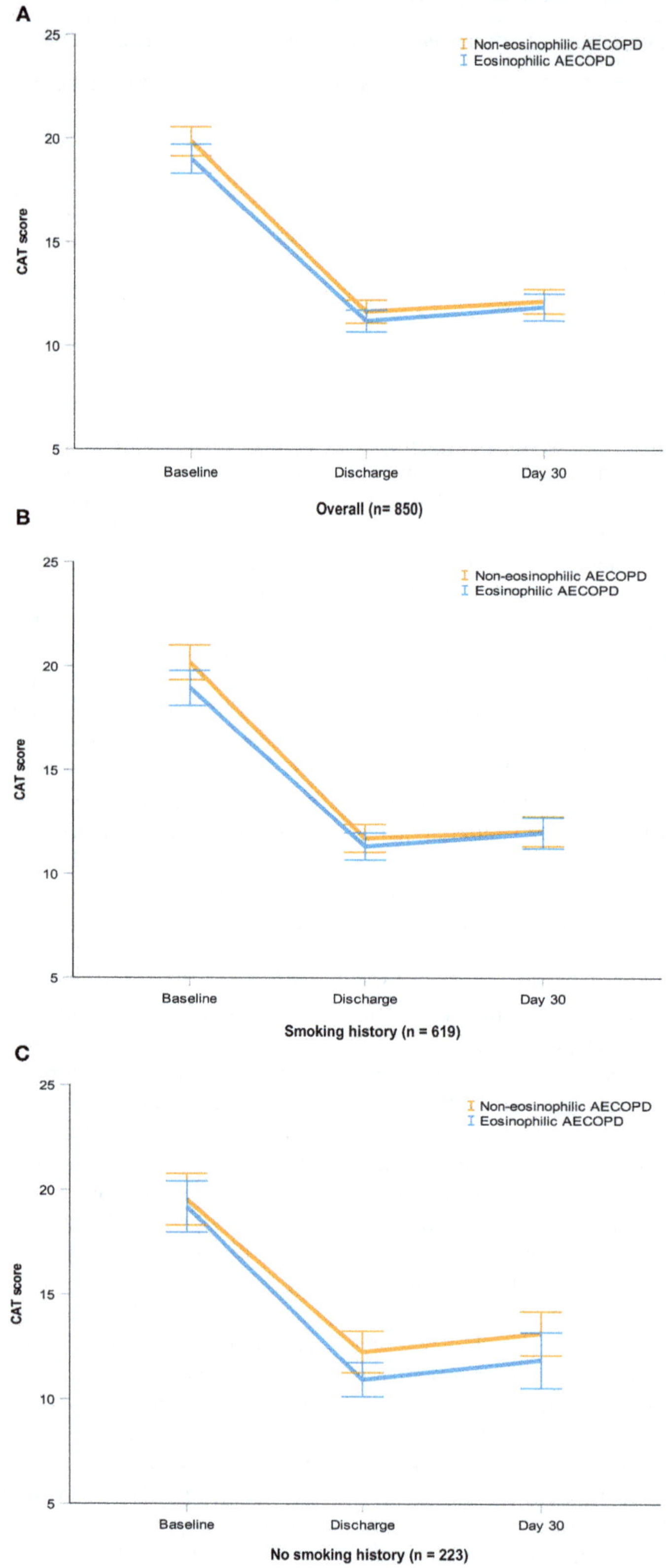

FIGURE 5 | CAT scores at baseline, discharge and day 30 in the three matched cohorts. Data are presented as mean (SEM). AECOPD, acute exacerbations of chronic obstructive pulmonary disease; CAT, COPD Assessment Test; SEM, standard error of mean.

The strength of this study was that it represented a real-world study of a large AECOPD cohort, which allowed the impact of smoking status to be discerned. Moreover, the propensity matching technique minimized bias by comparing groups with similar baseline characteristics. All patients had a diagnosis of COPD confirmed by spirometry. The present study also had several limitations. First, we used the percentage of eosinophils for analysis, which could be affected by the increased neutrophil count during exacerbations. Moreover, only the blood eosinophil count upon admission was recorded, but this value might be variable over time. Second, not all patients included in this study had follow-up data after 30 days. However, the baseline characteristics between those with or without follow-up data showed no significant differences, making selective bias less likely. Third, to date, we did not have long-term follow-up data because the ACURE study is an ongoing study with only the 30-day data available. But waiting for long-term follow-up would have delayed the reporting of these important results for several years. Fourth, only about 40% of the patients eligible for the ACURE study were recruited and we cannot be sure that our study can be implemented with the same result in patients not recruited. Finally, although PS matching was used to adjust for known baseline variables, the confounders from unmeasured variables could also influence the results.

CONCLUSION

This study found that for patients hospitalized for AECOPD with a history of smoking, eosinophil count <2% was associated with a longer length of hospital stay, a higher dosage of corticosteroid use, a higher economic burden of hospitalization, and a poor response to corticosteroid therapy. However, no significant difference was found in patients without smoking. Eosinophil levels cannot be confidently used as a predictor alone for short-term prognosis and have no relationship with 30-day clinical outcomes. Further studies are needed to assess the effect of smoking or other factors on the efficacy of eosinophils as a biomarker.

AUTHOR CONTRIBUTIONS

Concept and design of the study by YCu, YCh, TY, CL, and KH. Data collection and management by YCu, ZZh, ZZe, CL, XM, KH, YZ, XR, TY, and YCh. Statistical analysis by YCu, ZZh, CL, XM, and YZ. Drafting of the manuscript by YCu. All authors contributed to the article and approved the submitted version.

ACKNOWLEDGMENTS

We would like to thank all participants in ACURE study for collecting the data of this clinical study.

REFERENCES

1. Gold Science Committee. *Global Strategy for the Diagnosis, Management and Prevention of Chronic Obstructive Pulmonary Disease (2020 REPORT).* (2019). Available online at: http://goldcopd.com (accessed November 5, 2019).
2. Burge S, Wedzicha JA. COPD exacerbations: definitions and classifications. *Eur Respir J Suppl.* (2003) 41:46s–53. doi: 10.1183/09031936.03.00078002
3. Zhang Y, Morgan RL, Alonso-Coello P, Wiercioch W, Bała MM, Jaeschke RR, et al. A systematic review of how patients value COPD outcomes. *Eur Respir J.* (2018) 52:1800222. doi: 10.1183/13993003.00222-2018
4. Casanova C, Celli BR, de-Torres JP, Martínez-Gonzalez C, Cosio BG, Pinto-Plata V, et al. Prevalence of persistent blood eosinophilia: relation to outcomes in patients with COPD. *Eur Respir J.* (2017) 50:1701162. doi: 10.1183/13993003.01162-2017
5. Yun JH, Lamb A, Chase R, Singh D, Parker MM, Saferali A, et al. Blood eosinophil count thresholds and exacerbations in patients with chronic obstructive pulmonary disease. *J Allergy Clin Immunol.* (2018) 141:2037–47.e10. doi: 10.1016/j.jaci.2018.04.010
6. Ko FWS, Chan KP, Ngai J, Ng SS, Yip WH, Ip A, et al. Blood eosinophil count as a predictor of hospital length of stay in COPD exacerbations. *Respirology.* (2020) 25:259–66. doi: 10.1111/resp.13660
7. AE Bafadhel M, Greening NJ, Harvey-Dunstan TC, Williams JE, Morgan MD, Brightling CE, et al. Blood eosinophils and outcomes in severe hospitalized exacerbations of COPD. *Chest.* (2016) 150:320–8. doi: 10.1016/j.chest.2016.01.026
8. Holland M, Alkhalil M, Chandromouli S, Janjua A, Babores M. Eosinopenia as a marker of mortality and length of stay in patients admitted with exacerbations of chronic obstructive pulmonary disease. *Respirology.* (2010) 15:165–7. doi: 10.1111/j.1440-1843.2009.01651.x
9. Bafadhel M, McKenna S, Terry S, Mistry V, Pancholi M, Venge P, et al. Blood eosinophils to direct corticosteroid treatment of exacerbations of chronic obstructive pulmonary disease: a randomized placebo-controlled trial. *Am J Respir Crit Care Med.* (2012) 186:48–55. doi: 10.1164/rccm.201108-1553OC
10. Hegewald MJ, Horne BD, Trudo F, Kreindler JL, Chung Y, Rea S, et al. Blood eosinophil count and hospital readmission in patients with acute exacerbation of chronic obstructive pulmonary disease. *Int J Chron Obstruct Pulmon Dis.* (2020) 15:2629–41. doi: 10.2147/COPD.S251115
11. Kwon N, Pizzichini E, Bansal AT, Albers FC, Barnes N, Rile JH, et al. Factors that affect blood eosinophil counts in a non-asthmatic population: Post hoc analysis of data from Brazil. *World Allergy Organ J.* (2020) 13:100119. doi: 10.1016/j.waojou.2020.100119
12. Pei Z, Sun Y, Wang S, Chen Y, Yang T, Huang K, et al. Estimating mortality among inpatients with acute exacerbation of chronic obstructive pulmonary disease using registry data. *NPJ Prim Care Respir Med.* (2020) 30:28. doi: 10.1038/s41533-020-0186-y
13. Bafadhel M, McKenna S, Terry S, Mistry V, Reid C, Haldar P, et al. Acute exacerbations of chronic obstructive pulmonary disease: identification of biologic clusters and their biomarkers. *Am J Respir Crit Care Med.* (2011) 184:662–71. doi: 10.1164/rccm.201104-0597OC
14. Roussos C, Koutsoukou A. Respiratory failure. *Eur Respir J Suppl.* (2003) 47:3s–14. doi: 10.1183/09031936.03.00038503
15. Mandell LA, Wunderink RG, Anzueto A, Bartlett JG, Campbell GD, Dean NC, et al. Infectious Diseases Society of America/American Thoracic Society consensus guidelines on the management of community-acquired pneumonia in adults. *Clin Infect Dis.* (2007) 44(Suppl. 2):S27–72. doi: 10.1086/511159
16. Xue J, Cui YN, Chen P, Cai S, Chen L, Dai ZS, et al. Blood eosinophils: a biomarker of response to glucocorticoids and increased readmissions in severe hospitalized exacerbations of COPD. *Chin J Tuberc Respir Dis.* (2019) 42:426–31. doi: 10.3760/cma.j.issn.1001-0939.2019.06.005
17. Wu HX, Zhuo KQ, Cheng DY. Peripheral blood eosinophil as a biomarker in outcomes of acute exacerbation of chronic obstructive

pulmonary disease. *Int J Chron Obstruct Pulmon Dis.* (2019) 14:3003–15. doi: 10.2147/COPD.S226783

18. Kim VL, Coombs NA, Staples KJ, Ostridge KK, Williams NP, Wootton SA, et al. Impact and associations of eosinophilic inflammation in COPD: analysis of the AERIS cohort. *Eur Respir J.* (2017) 50:1700853. doi: 10.1183/13993003.00853-2017
19. MacDonald MI, Osadnik CR, Bulfin L, Hamza K, Leong P, Wong A, et al. Low and high blood eosinophil counts as biomarkers in hospitalized acute exacerbations of COPD. *Chest.* (2019) 156:92–100. doi: 10.1016/j.chest.2019.02.406
20. Chis AF, Pop CM. Correlations between neutrophil to lymphocyte ratio, blood eosinophils and clinical characteristics in chronic obstructive pulmonary disease. *Med Pharm Rep.* (2020) 93:169–74. doi: 10.15386/mpr-1412
21. Li M, Yang T, He R, Li A, Dang W, Liu X, et al. The value of inflammatory biomarkers in differentiating asthma-COPD Overlap from COPD. *Int J Chron Obstruct Pulmon Dis.* (2020) 15:3025–37. doi: 10.2147/COPD.S273422
22. Prins HJ, Duijkers R, Lutter R, Daniels JM, van der Valk P, Schoorl M, et al. Blood eosinophilia as a marker of early and late treatment failure in severe acute exacerbations of COPD. *Respir Med.* (2017) 131:118–24. doi: 10.1016/j.rmed.2017.07.064
23. Serafino-Agrusa L, Scichilone N, Spatafora M, Battaglia S. Blood eosinophils and treatment response in hospitalized exacerbations of chronic obstructive pulmonary disease: a case-control study. *Pulm Pharmacol Ther.* (2016) 37:89–94. doi: 10.1016/j.pupt.2016.03.004
24. Zhang Y, Liang LR, Zhang S, Lu Y, Chen YY, Shi HZ, et al. Blood eosinophilia and its stability in hospitalized COPD exacerbations are associated with lower risk of all-cause mortality. *Int J Chron Obstruct Pulmon Dis.* (2020) 15:1123–34. doi: 10.2147/COPD.S245056
25. Jabarkhil A, Moberg M, Janner J, Petersen MN, Jensen CB, Henrik Äangquist L, et al. Elevated blood eosinophils in acute COPD exacerbations: better short- and long-term prognosis. *Eur Clin Respir J.* (2020) 7:1757274. doi: 10.1080/20018525.2020.1757274
26. Gonzalez-Barcala FJ, San-Jose ME, Nieto-Fontarigo JJ, Calvo-Alvarez U, Carreira JM, Garcia-Sanz MT, et al. Blood eosinophils could be useful as a biomarker in chronic obstructive pulmonary disease exacerbations. *Int J Clin Pract.* (2019) 73:e13423. doi: 10.1111/ijcp.13423
27. Bafadhel M, Peterson S, De Blas MA, Calverley PM, Rennard SI, Richter K, et al. Predictors of exacerbation risk and response to budesonide in patients with chronic obstructive pulmonary disease: a post-hoc analysis of three randomised trials. *Lancet Respir Med.* (2018) 6:117–26. doi: 10.1016/S2213-2600(18)30006-7
28. Hinds DR, DiSantostefano RL, Le HV, Pascoe S. Identification of responders to inhaled corticosteroids in a chronic obstructive pulmonary disease population using cluster analysis. *BMJ Open.* (2016) 6:e010099. doi: 10.1136/bmjopen-2015-010099
29. Viinanen A, Lassenius MI, Toppila I, Karlsson A, Veijalainen L, Idänpään-Heikkilä JJ, et al. The burden of chronic obstructive pulmonary disease (COPD) in Finland: impact of disease severity and eosinophil count on healthcare resource utilization. *Int J Chron Obstruct Pulmon Dis.* (2019) 14:2409–21. doi: 10.2147/COPD.S222581
30. Müllerová H, Hahn B, Simard EP, Mu G, Hatipoglu U. Exacerbations and health care resource use among patients with COPD in relation to blood eosinophil counts. *Int J Chron Obstruct Pulmon Dis.* (2019) 14:683–92. doi: 10.2147/COPD.S194367
31. Ortega H, Llanos JP, Lafeuille MH, Germain G, Duh MS, Bell CF, et al. Burden of disease associated with a COPD eosinophilic phenotype. *Int J Chron Obstruct Pulmon Dis.* (2018) 13:2425–33. doi: 10.2147/COPD.S170995
32. Sivapalan P, Lapperre TS, Janner J, Laub RR, Moberg M, Bech CS, et al. Eosinophil-guided corticosteroid therapy in patients admitted to hospital with COPD exacerbation (CORTICO-COP): a multicentre, randomised, controlled, open-label, non-inferiority trial. *Lancet Respir Med.* (2019) 7:699–709. doi: 10.1016/S2213-2600(19)30176-6

11

Therapeutic Potential of Human Umbilical Cord-Derived Mesenchymal Stem Cells in Recovering from Murine Pulmonary Emphysema under Cigarette Smoke Exposure

Xiao-Yue Chen [1,2], Yi-Ying Chen [2], Willie Lin [3], Chien-Han Chen [3], Yu-Chieh Wen [3], Ta-Chih Hsiao [4], Hsiu-Chu Chou [5], Kian Fan Chung [6] and Hsiao-Chi Chuang [2,7,8]*

[1] Graduate Institute of Medical Sciences, College of Medicine, Taipei Medical University, Taipei, Taiwan, [2] School of Respiratory Therapy, College of Medicine, Taipei Medical University, Taipei, Taiwan, [3] Meridigen Biotech Co., Ltd., Taipei, Taiwan, [4] Graduate Institute of Environmental Engineering, National Taiwan University, Taipei, Taiwan, [5] Department of Anatomy and Cell Biology, School of Medicine, College of Medicine, Taipei Medical University, Taipei, Taiwan, [6] National Heart and Lung Institute, Imperial College London, London, United Kingdom, [7] Division of Pulmonary Medicine, Department of Internal Medicine, Shuang Ho Hospital, Taipei Medical University, New Taipei City, Taiwan, [8] Cell Physiology and Molecular Image Research Center, Wan Fang Hospital, Taipei Medical University, Taipei, Taiwan

***Correspondence:**
Hsiao-Chi Chuang
r92841005@ntu.edu.tw

Human umbilical cord-derived mesenchymal stem cells (hUC-MSCs) were shown to have potential for immunoregulation and tissue repair. The objective of this study was to investigate the effects of hUC-MSCs on emphysema in chronic obstructive pulmonary disease (COPD). The C57BL/6JNarl mice were exposed to cigarette smoke (CS) for 4 months followed by administration of hUC-MSCs at 3×10^6 (low dose), 1×10^7 (medium dose), and 3×10^7 cells/kg body weight (high dose). The hUC-MSCs caused significant decreases in emphysema severity by measuring the mean linear intercept (MLI) and destructive index (DI). A decrease in neutrophils (%) and an increase in lymphocytes (%) in bronchoalveolar lavage fluid (BALF) were observed in emphysematous mice after hUC-MSC treatment. Lung levels of interleukin (IL)-1β, C-X-C motif chemokine ligand 1 (CXCL1)/keratinocyte chemoattractant (KC), and matrix metalloproteinase (MMP)-12 significantly decreased after hUC-MSC administration. Significant reductions in tumor necrosis factor (TNF)-α, IL-1β, and IL-17A in serum occurred after hUC-MSC administration. Notably, the cell viability of lung fibroblasts improved with hUC-MSCs after being treated with CS extract (CSE). Furthermore, the hUC-MSCs-conditioned medium (hUC-MSCs-CM) restored the contractile force, and increased messenger RNA expressions of elastin and fibronectin by lung fibroblasts. In conclusion, hUC-MSCs reduced inflammatory responses and emphysema severity in CS-induced emphysematous mice.

Keywords: cigarette smoke, COPD, emphysema, inflammation, stem cell

INTRODUCTION

Chronic obstructive pulmonary disease (COPD) is currently one of the world's highest causes of mortality and ranks fifth worldwide in terms of disease burden (1–3). About 80–90% of COPD patients are related to cigarette smoking (4). A previous study found that exposure to cigarette smoke (CS) for 12 weeks induced emphysematous lung lesions in rats (5). This irreversible alveolar destruction and emphysematous changes due to CS exposure resulted in higher mortality and difficulties in treating COPD.

Mesenchymal stem cells (SCs; MSCs), multipotent SCs, have high self-renewal and differentiation capacities (6). Recent studies demonstrated immunoregulatory functions of MSCs in treating graft vs. host disease (7, 8). Also, tissue-repair actions of MSCs through a paracrine mechanism were explored (9, 10). Notably, most intravenously (i.v.) administered MSCs were localized in the lungs (11). Recruitment of MSCs to the lungs provides new insights that MSCs may have greater paracrine effects in the lungs. Therefore, the effects of MSCs on lung disease treatment were recently noted (12, 13).

Human umbilical cord-derived (hUC)-MSCs have a higher differential capacity, lower immunogenicity, and less age-related dysfunction compared to adult SCs (14). Other advantages of hUC-MSCs are that there are fewer ethical issues associated with them and they can be non-invasively collected (15). Anti-inflammatory effects of hUC-MSCs were found in an acute lung injury mouse model (16). Moreover, it was demonstrated that hUC-MSCs prevented bleomycin-induced lung fibrosis *in vivo* (17).

Lung fibroblasts were shown to have an important role in repairing damaged lung tissues after CS exposure (18). However, a previous study found a decrease in the proliferation of lung fibroblasts in COPD (19). Recently, the senescence-associated secretory phenotype of lung fibroblasts was found in CS-induced emphysema (20). Consequently, the loss of the ability to repair alveoli due to CS was mainly because of lung fibroblast dysfunction (21, 22). MSCs were shown to mediate the proliferation and increase the pro-collagen expression of lung fibroblasts (23).

Despite the efficacy of MSCs in ameliorating acute lung damage, few studies have investigated the effects of hUC-MSCs on chronic CS-induced emphysema. The objective of this study was to investigate the therapeutic efficacy of hUC-MSCs in emphysema.

MATERIALS AND METHODS

Animals

The animal study was approved by the Animal and Ethics Review Committee of the Laboratory Animal Center at Taipei Medical University, Taipei, Taiwan (IACUC: LAC-2017-0231). Male C57BL/6JNarl mice (8 weeks, 20–25 g, $n = 8$–10 per group) were obtained from the National Laboratory Animal Center (Taipei, Taiwan). Mice were housed in plastic cages and supplied with Lab Diet 5001 (PMI Nutrition International, St. Louis, MO, USA) and water *ad libitum*. A light/dark cycle of 12 h/12 h was maintained. The room temperature was set to 22 ± 2°C, and relative humidity to 55 ± 10%.

CS-Induced Emphysema

An emphysema mouse model was established by whole-body exposure to CS for 4 months. Details of the CS exposure system were previously reported (24). Briefly, the system consisted of a CS generator, a whole-body exposure chamber (TECNIPLAST, VA, Italy), and a particulate matter (PM) monitor. A side-stream was introduced into the whole-body exposure chamber at a flow rate of 15 L/min. There were 16 commercial cigarettes (Longlife, Taipei, Taiwan; 11 mg of tar and 0.9 mg of nicotine) combusted for 8 h/day and 5 days/week for 4 months (**Figure 1A**). The mass concentration of PM of <2.5 μm in aerodynamic diameter ($PM_{2.5}$) was monitored using a DustTrak monitor (8530, TSI, Shoreview, MN, USA). **Figure 1B** shows the distribution of the $PM_{2.5}$ mass concentration during CS exposure. The average $PM_{2.5}$ mass concentration was 90.5 ± 40.6 mg/m^3 during the first 15 min. It reached a maximum level of about 154.3 ± 58.2 mg/m^3 after 4 min of cigarette combustion, and then the mass concentration declined to the baseline level after 16 min. Simultaneously, mice exposed to CS-free high-efficiency particulate air (HEPA)-filtered room air (RA) served as the control group.

hUC-MSC Preparation and Characterization

Details of hUC-MSC preparation were previously reported (24). Briefly, umbilical cords were aseptically harvested and digested with collagenase (SERVA, Heidelberg, Germany) at 37°C. The cell pellets were expanded in α-minimal essential medium (α-MEM, Invitrogen, Carlsbad, CA, USA), and cultured in an incubator with 5% CO_2 at 37°C for 3 days. hUC-MSCs were characterized using flow cytometry (BD Stemflow™ hMSC Analysis Kit; BD Biosciences, San Jose, CA, USA) to detect expressions of cluster of differentiation (CD) markers (CD11b, CD19, CD34, CD44, CD45, CD73, CD90, and CD105) and human leukocyte antigen–antigen D related (HLA-DR). As presented in **Supplementary Table 1**, hUC-MSCs exhibited positive expressions of SC-specific surface markers (CD44, CD73, CD90, and CD105) and negative expressions of CD11b, CD19, CD34, CD45, and HLA-DR, which followed International Society for Cellular Therapy Guidelines (25). hUC-MSCs were prepared in clinical-grade normal saline supplemented with 2% clinical-grade human serum albumin and 16.7% clinical grade CS10. This study was approved by the Ethics Committee of the National Cheng Kung University Hospital Institutional Review Board (Tainan, Taiwan; IRB no.: A-BR-104-045). All subjects received written and oral informed consent before inclusion. All study processes were conducted following the approved study protocol.

hUC-MSC Administration and Sample Collection

The experimental design is shown in **Figure 1A**. After 4 months of CS exposure, emphysematous mice were randomly divided into four groups: sham control (CS), low-dose group (CS + MSC-L), medium-dose group (CS + MSC-M), and high-dose group

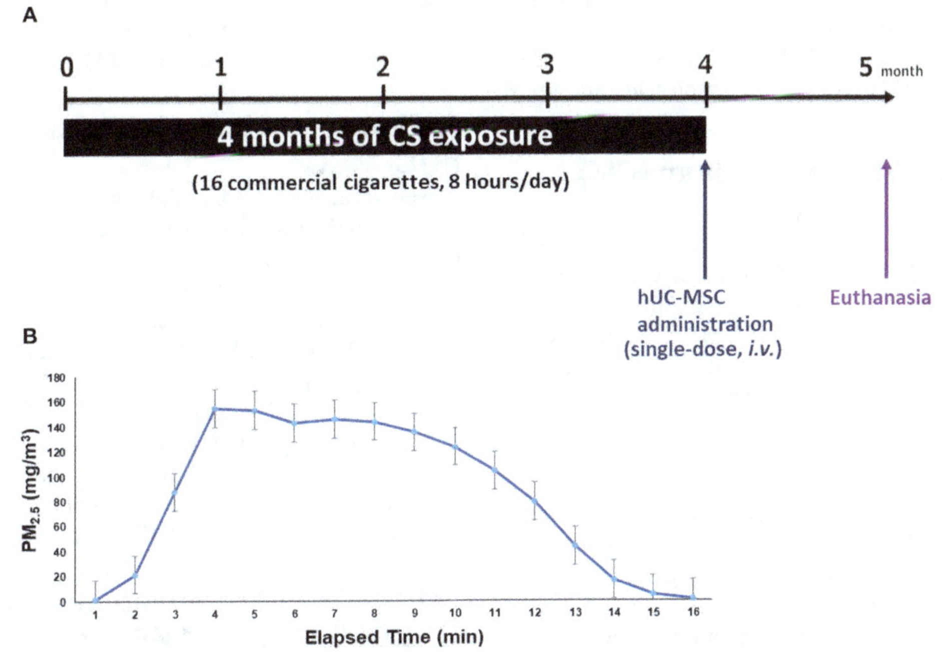

FIGURE 1 | (A) Schematic mice model of cigarette smoke (CS)-induced emphysema. **(B)** The distribution of particulate matter with an aerodynamic diameter of <2.5 μm ($PM_{2.5}$) mass concentration in the whole-body exposure system (mean ± SD). Mice (8 weeks old, 20–25 g, $n = 8$–10 per group) were exposed to CS for 4 months and received (i.v.) a single dose of human umbilical cord-derived mesenchymal stem cells (hUC-MSCs) after CS exposure (CS + MSC-L: hUC-MSCs at 3×10^6 cells/kg body weight (BW) for low-dose, CS + MSC-M: 1×10^7 cells/kg BW for medium-dose, and CS + MSC-H: 3×10^7 cells/kg BW for high-dose).

(CS + MSC-H). Mice were intravenously (i.v.) administrated a single-dose of hUC-MSCs at 3×10^6 cells/kg body weight (BW) for CS + MSC-L, 1×10^7 cells/kg BW for CS + MSC-M, and 3×10^7 cells/kg BW for CS + MSC-H. The administered dose of hUC-MSCs was referenced to our previous reports (24, 26). The control and CS sham groups were i.v. administrated the same volume of vehicle. BW was measured once a week before and after hUC-MSC administration. Mice were euthanized 4 weeks after hUC-MSC administration. Bronchoalveolar lavage fluid (BALF), lung tissues, and serum were collected. For histological analyses, lung samples were inflated with 10% (m/v) paraformaldehyde in phosphate-buffered saline (PBS) at a pressure of 21 cm H_2O.

Emphysema Evaluation

Lung tissues were embedded in paraffin and sectioned into slices for staining with hematoxylin and eosin (H&E). The mean linear intercept (MLI) and destructive index (DI) were used to evaluate the presence of emphysema. The MLI was assessed by counting the number of the alveolar walls intercepted in the grid lines, according to previously described methods (27, 28). The DI for microscopic lung lesions was previously reported (27, 28). Emphysematous defects or intramural parenchyma in at least two intersections of alveoli were considered alveolar destruction.

Hematology

BALF was centrifuged at 1,500 rpm for 10 min at 4°C. Cell pellets were resuspended in PBS. Numbers of neutrophils, lymphocytes, monocytes, and eosinophils were quantified by a hematology analyzer (ProCyte Dx, IDEXX Laboratories, Westbrook, ME, USA). Data are expressed as percentages (%) of total cell counts.

Proteins Extracted From Lung Tissues

Lysis buffer was prepared from 490 μL of lysis reagent (Sigma-Aldrich, St. Louis, MO, USA) containing 5 μL of a protease inhibitor (Geno Technology, St. Louis, MO, USA) and 5 μL of ethylenediaminetetraacetic acid. Lung tissues were homogenized in lysis buffer using a homogenizer (Minilys® personal homogenizer, Bertin, Rockville, MD, USA).

Cytometric Bead Array (CBA) and Enzyme-Linked Immunosorbent Assay (ELISA)

A CBA (BD Biosciences, San Jose, CA, USA) was used to quantify levels of tumor necrosis factor (TNF)-α, interleukin (IL)-1β, chemokine (C-X-C motif) ligand 1/keratinocyte chemoattractant (CXCL1/KC), and IL-17A in BALF, lung, and serum samples. Matrix metalloproteinase (MMP)-12 was determined in lung samples by an ELISA (Cloud-Clone, Katy, TX, USA). Quantification of these markers in lung samples was normalized to the total protein. All measurements were undertaken in accordance with the manufacturers' instructions.

Human Lung Fibroblasts

Human lung fibroblasts (MRC-5 cells) were obtained from the Food Industry Research and Development Institute (FIRDI,

Hsinchu, Taiwan) and cultured in T75 flasks with Eagle's minimum essential medium (EMEM, Lonza Group, Basel, Switzerland) supplemented with 10% fetal bovine serum (FBS), 2 mM L-glutamine, 0.1 mM non-essential amino acids, and 1 mM sodium pyruvate.

hUC-MSCs-Conditioned Medium (CM) Preparation

To collect hUC-MSCs-CM, hUC-MSCs (1.2×10^6 cells) were cultured in T75 flasks with 15 mL of hUC-MSC culture medium for 24 h. After being washed with PBS, the culture medium was replaced with 10 mL of α-MEM basal medium (Invitrogen, Carlsbad, CA, USA) and incubated for 48 h. The subsequent serum-free culture medium was collected and served as hUC-MSCs-CM.

CS Extract (CSE)

CSE was prepared from the combustion of three cigarettes (Marlboro, Philip Morris, VA, USA) by impinging onto 30 mL of α-MEM (Invitrogen) with a firm filter. The cigarette contained 10 mg of tar and 0.8 mg of nicotine. Fresh CSE was collected to serve as 100% CSE and immediately used for cell experiments.

Cell Viability of Human Lung Fibroblasts by hUC-MSCs After CSE Exposure

MRC-5 cells were treated with 8% CSE for 24 h and then indirectly cocultured with hUC-MSCs for another 48 h. Cell viability of MRC-5 cells was determined by a cell counting kit-8 (Merck, Darmstadt, Germany).

Cell Contractile Force and Elastin and Fibronectin of Human Lung Fibroblasts by hUC-MSCs-CM After CSE Exposure

MRC-5 cells (2×10^5/cells) seeded in six-well plates were treated with 8% CSE for 24 h. After CSE exposure, cells were cultured in hUC-MSCs-CM for 24 h. The cell contractile force was measured using a collagen-based cell contraction assay kit (CellBiolabs, San Diego, CA, USA). Messenger (m)RNA expressions of elastin and fibronectin were analyzed by a quantitative polymerase chain reaction (qPCR), according to the manufacturer's instructions.

Statistical Analysis

Data are presented as the mean ± standard deviation (SD). Multiple groups were compared by an analysis of variance (ANOVA) with Tukey's *post-hoc* test. An unpaired *t*-test was used for comparisons between continuous variables. All analyses were performed using GraphPad vers. 6 (San Diego, CA, USA). $p < 0.05$ was considered statistically significant.

RESULTS

hUC-MSCs Mitigated Emphysema Severity

Results of the histological analysis are shown in **Figure 2**. A significant decrease in the MLI by hUC-MSCs was observed compared to the CS group (low-dose: 87.08 ± 14.20, medium-dose: 82.34 ± 7.50, and high-dose MSCs: 79.32 ± 7.14 vs. the CS group: 103.10 ± 11.52 μm, $p < 0.001$). Furthermore, the DI (%) significantly decreased after hUC-MSC administration (medium-dose: 15.67 ± 3.30% and high-dose MSCs: 12.05 ± 2.65% vs. the CS group: 24.30 ± 2.85%, $p < 0.001$).

Reduction of Lung Infiltration by hUC-MSCs

As shown in **Figure 3A**, a significant decrease in the percentage of neutrophils was observed in the hUC-MSC group compared to the CS group (low-dose: 35.83 ± 9.50%, medium-dose: 20.64 ± 12.44%, and high-dose MSCs: 23.05 ± 12.54% vs. the CS group: 57.29 ± 27.45%, $p < 0.001$). In contrast, lymphocytes (%) significantly increased after hUC-MSC administration compared to the CS group (low-dose: 44.47 ± 13.17%, medium-dose: 65.44 ± 13.29%, and high-dose MSCs: 63.73 ± 13.08% vs. the CS group: 24.77 ± 18.41%, $p < 0.001$). There was no statistical difference in monocytes (%) or eosinophils (%) among the groups. Also, we observed no statistical difference in TNF-α, IL-1β, CXCL1/KC, or IL-17A in BALF after hUC-MSC administration (**Figure 3B**).

hUC-MSCs Decreased Levels of IL-1β, CXCL1/KC, and MMP-12 in the Lungs

Levels of IL-1β (low-dose: 0.70 ± 0.42 and medium-dose MSCs: 0.76 ± 0.42 vs. the CS group: 1.28 ± 0.47 pg/mg, $p < 0.05$) and CXCL1/KC (medium-dose: 8.20 ± 4.14 and high-dose MSCs: 9.92 ± 9.47 vs. CS group: 41.61 ± 21.56 pg/mg, $p < 0.001$) in lung lysates significantly decreased after hUC-MSC administration compared to the CS group (**Figure 4A**). Also, we found that MMP-12 in lungs of mice was significantly reduced by hUC-MSCs (low-dose: 3.83 ± 0.92, medium-dose: 3.14 ± 0.89, and high-dose MSCs: 3.13 ± 1.03 vs. the CS group: 6.40 ± 2.20 pg/mg, $p < 0.001$). There was no significant change in TNF-α or IL-17A levels among all groups.

hUC-MSCs Reduced Levels of TNF-α, IL-1β, and IL-17A in Serum

TNF-α, IL-1β, CXCL1/KC, and IL-17A levels in serum of mice were examined (**Figure 4B**). hUC-MSCs significantly reduced levels of TNF-α (low-dose MSCs: 6.49 ± 2.48 vs. the CS group: 14.71 ± 9.34 pg/mL, $p < 0.01$), IL-1β (low-dose: 14.16 ± 22.48, medium-dose: 17.69 ± 10.86, and high-dose MSCs: 21.4 ± 15.27 vs. the CS group: 56.31 ± 47.24 pg/mL, $p < 0.05$), and IL-17A (low-dose: 0.75 ± 0.59 and high-dose MSCs: 0.90 ± 0.44 vs. the CS group: 2.02 ± 1.34 pg/mL, $p < 0.05$) compared to the CS group. No significant reduction in CXCL1/KC was found when compared among all groups.

Proliferation of Lung Fibroblasts by hUC-MSCs

As shown in **Figure 5A**, the cell viability of MRC-5 cells significantly increased by hUC-MSCs after CSE treatment compared to the CSE group ($p < 0.05$). The contractile force of MRC-5 cells as determined by the collagen gel surface area was significantly reduced by hUC-MSCs-CM treatment compared to the CSE group ($p < 0.05$; **Figure 5B**). A significant increase in mRNA expressions of elastin and fibronectin were observed

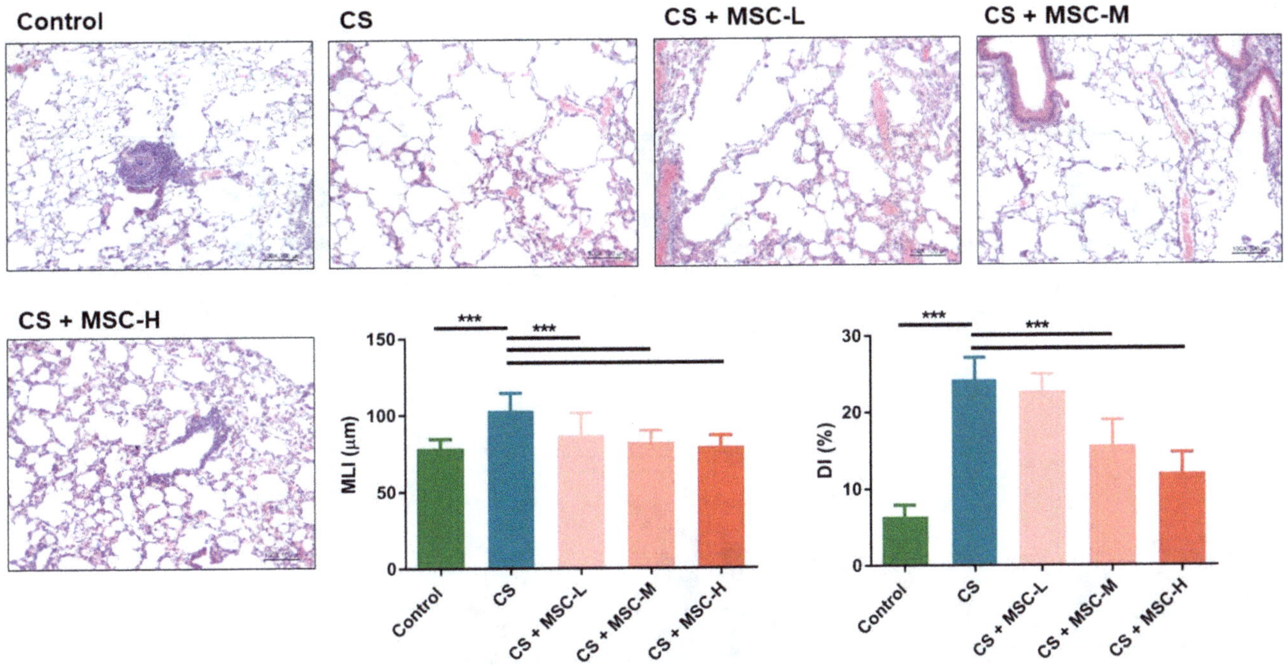

FIGURE 2 | Repair of alveolar structures by human umbilical cord-derived mesenchymal stem cells (hUC-MSCs) in a mice model of cigarette smoke (CS)-induced emphysema. Lung tissue sections were stained with hematoxylin and eosin (H&E). Lung lesions were quantified by measuring the mean linear intercept (MLI) and destructive index (DI). Significant reductions of the MLI and DI (%) were observed by hUC-MSC administration after CS exposure for 4 months. Results were determined by a one-way ANOVA with Tukey's test. $n = 8$–10 per group. $^{***}p < 0.001$.

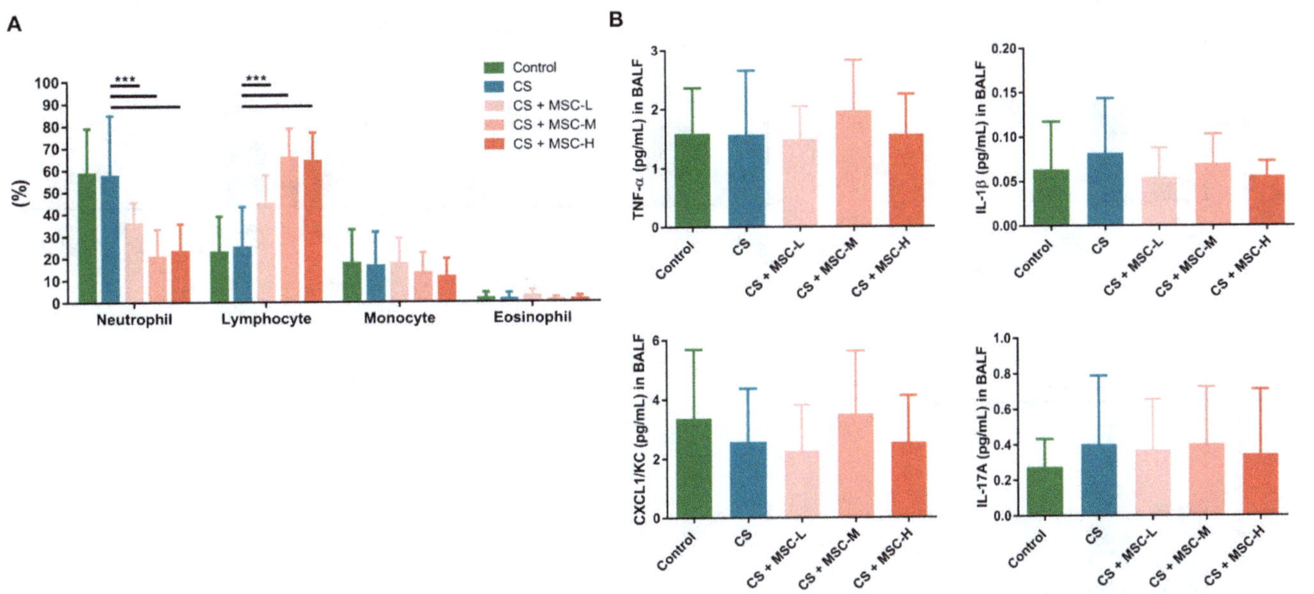

FIGURE 3 | (A) The human umbilical cord-derived mesenchymal stem cells (hUC-MSCs) reduced neutrophils and increased lymphocytes in bronchoalveolar lavage fluid (BALF) of mice. **(B)** Regulation of cytokine production (tumor necrosis factor (TNF)-α, interleukin (IL)-1β, C-X-C motif chemokine ligand 1 (CXCL1)/keratinocyte chemoattractant (KC), and IL-17A) by hUC-MSCs in BALF. A significant decrease in neutrophils (%) was observed by hUC-MSC administration, whereas lymphocytes (%) increased after hUC-MSC administration. There was no significant difference in cytokine production in BALF after hUC-MSC administration. The results were determined by a one-way ANOVA with Tukey's test. $n = 8$–10 per group. $^{***}p < 0.001$.

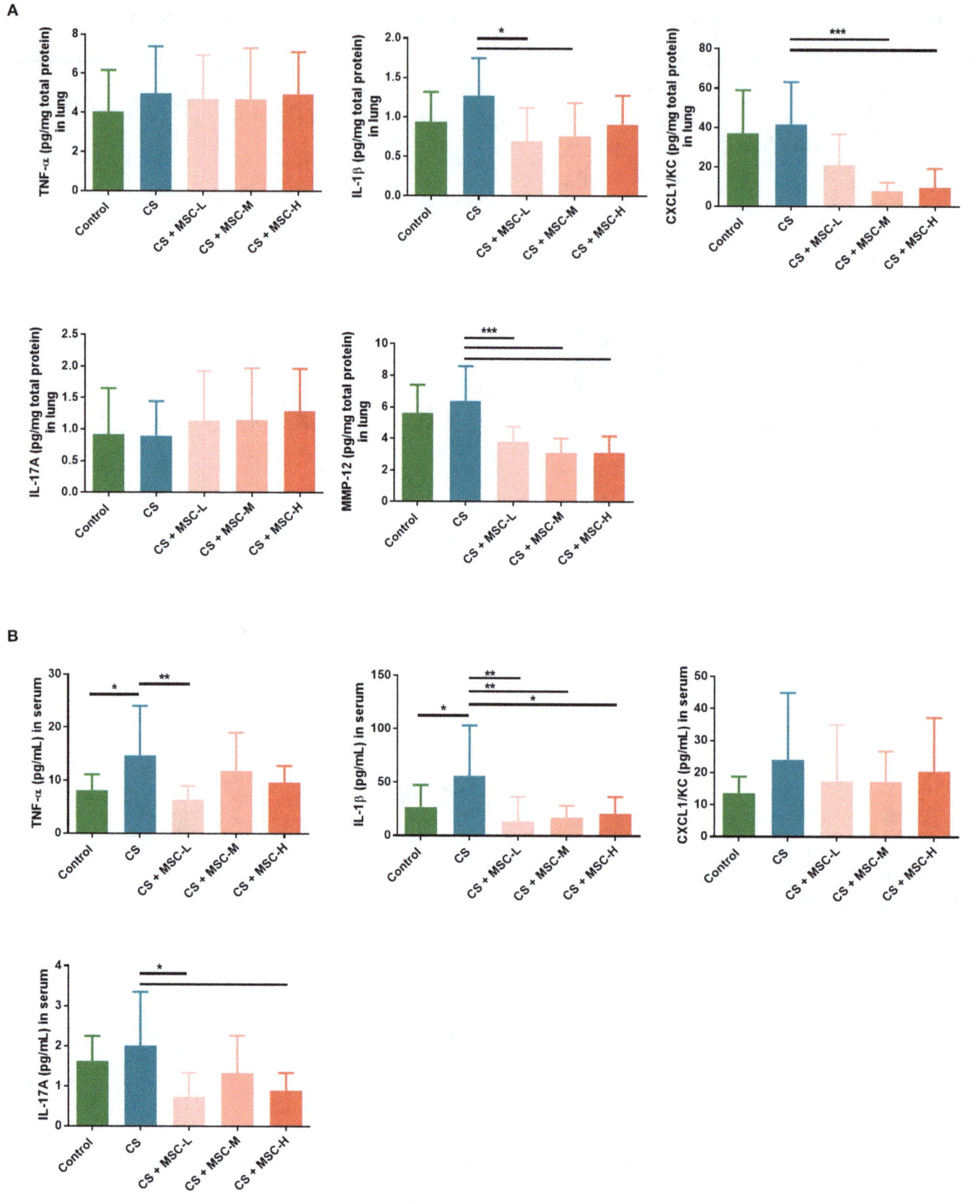

FIGURE 4 | (A) Human umbilical cord-derived mesenchymal stem cells (hUC-MSCs) downregulated interleukin (IL)-1β, C-X-C chemokine ligand 1 (CXCL1)/ keratinocyte chemoattractant (KC), and matrix metalloproteinase (MMP)-12 in lung lysates. **(B)** hUC-MSCs decreased systemic cytokine production (tumor

(Continued)

FIGURE 4 | necrosis factor (TNF)-α, IL-1β, and IL-17A) in serum. Mice lungs were homogenized, and then lung lysates and facial blood of mice were measured by a CBA or ELISA. IL-1β, CXCL1/KC, and MMP-12 in the lungs of mice were significantly reduced by hUC-MSCs. Significant decreases in TNF-α, IL-1β, and IL-17A in the serum of mice by hUC-MSCs were seen, and data were determined by a one-way ANOVA with Tukey's test. $n = 8–10$ per group. $^{*}p < 0.05$, $^{**}p < 0.01$, $^{***}p < 0.001$.

by hUC-MSCs-CM treatment compared to the CSE group ($p < 0.001$; **Figure 5C**).

DISCUSSION

MSCs were shown to have the potential for immunomodulation and tissue regeneration in different diseases (29–31). We observed that hUC-MSCs decreased the emphysema severity and reduced lung and systemic inflammatory infiltration in mice with CS-induced emphysema. Moreover, we observed that hUC-MSCs increased the proliferation of lung fibroblasts after CSE exposure. hUC-MSCs may ameliorate emphysematous lung lesions in COPD.

Mice were exposed to CS for 4 months at an average mass concentration of 90.5 ± 40.6 mg/m^3 $PM_{2.5}$ to induce development of emphysema in the present study. The CS-exposure system in this study was described previously (24). Previous reports also showed that CS exposure for 12–14 weeks was able to induce an emphysema model (32–35). During the CS exposure, the mice were significantly decreased in body weight and a significant increase in the serum level of TNF-α as compared to the control before hUC-MSC administration (**Supplementary Figures 1A,B**). After 4 months of exposure to CS, we observed significantly increased emphysema severity (MLI and DI) and elevation of pro-inflammatory factors (TNF-α and IL-1β) in serum without a significant change in BW (**Supplementary Figure 2**). The observation suggests that a mouse model of CS-induced emphysema was successfully established in the present study. However, it is worth to note that the mice were euthanized 4 weeks after the CS exposure. This may result in the decrease of inflammatory responses in the CS group.

The lungs are an important organ for accumulation of hUC-MSCs after their administration (36–38). Lung inflammatory infiltration was mitigated by hUC-MSCs in emphysematous mice. First, neutrophils were significantly reduced in BALF by hUC-MSCs. Previous studies showed that neutrophils or polymorphonuclear cells decreased in BALF by MSC administration after CS exposure for 7~16 weeks *in vivo* (35, 39). Pulmonary neutrophil activation by CS is reported to be associated with pro-inflammatory activation and alveolar destruction by releasing neutrophil elastase in COPD (40–42). Therefore, hUC-MSC administration is able to reduce increasing levels of neutrophilic inflammation. Next, we observed that lymphocytes significantly increased in BALF after hUC-MSC administration. Another study showed that intranasal delivery of MSCs slightly increased lymphocytes in BALF of mice compared to the intraperitoneal route in mice with CS-induced emphysema (43). Those results pointed out that different routes and timing of MSC administration could have distinct effects on regulating immune cell populations. MSCs transiently activate T cells to preserve the antiapoptotic function (44). For example, higher lymphocyte counts were more efficient in activating MSCs in the treatment of graft vs. host disease (45). A previous study showed that that hUC-MSCs recruited the regulatory T cells in the damaged lung (46). Together, hUC-MSCs could regulate lung neutrophil infiltration and lymphocyte activation in emphysematous mice. However, more experiments should be conducted in the future to support this.

We observed that inflammatory responses of the lungs, including IL-1β, CXCL1/KC, and MMP-12, by CS decreased after administration of hUC-MSCs. Consistent with a previous study, pro-inflammatory cytokines (TNF-α, IL-1β, and monocyte chemoattractant protein-1) and proteases (MMP-9 and−12) in the lungs of rats decreased by MSC administration after CS exposure for 11 weeks (47). In addition, we found that serum levels of TNF-α, IL-1β, and IL-17A significantly decreased by hUC-MSC administration after CS exposure. TNF-α, IL-1β, and IL-17A were shown to be key mediators in recruiting neutrophils to the lungs after CS exposure (48–53). Previous studies have found that the MMP-12 liberated the neutrophil chemoattractants (e.g., TNF-α) from the macrophage, which recruited the neutrophils and released the elastase that contributes to the lung damage (41, 54–56). It was hypothesized that MSCs may protect the pulmonary matrix structure by reducing MMP and elastase productions in alveolar macrophages and neutrophils, respectively (41, 57–59). Our results showed that decreases in serum levels of neutrophil chemotactic factors, including TNF-α, IL-1β, and IL-17A by hUC-MSCs may possibly be associated with the reduction in neutrophils in the BALF of mice after CS exposure.

The emphysema severity was significantly decreased by hUC-MSCs in emphysematous mice based on the MLI and DI results. Previous studies showed a decrease in emphysematous lesions in the lungs of mice due to bone marrow (BM)-MSCs (60, 61). Other studies found that MSCs induced neutrophil apoptosis and decreased protease secretions resulting in reduced severity of COPD (62–64). In our study, one explanation for the mitigation of the emphysema was decreased levels of pro-inflammatory factors in the lungs (IL-1β and CXCL1/KC) and circulation (TNF-α, IL-1β, and IL-17A) by hUC-MSCs which may associate with the reduction of the neutrophil infiltration in emphysematous mice. In addition, the decrease in protease secretion (MMP-12) by hUC-MSCs contributed to reducing alveolar destruction. Our results suggest that hUC-MSCs may ameliorate alveolar destruction in mice after CS-induced emphysema. However, the underlying mechanisms should be investigated in the future.

Fibroblasts play an important role in regulating COPD severity. We observed that the cell viability of lung fibroblasts increased by hUC-MSC administration after CSE exposure. In addition, hUC-MSCs-CM restored collagen's contractile force in lung fibroblasts after treatment with the CSE.

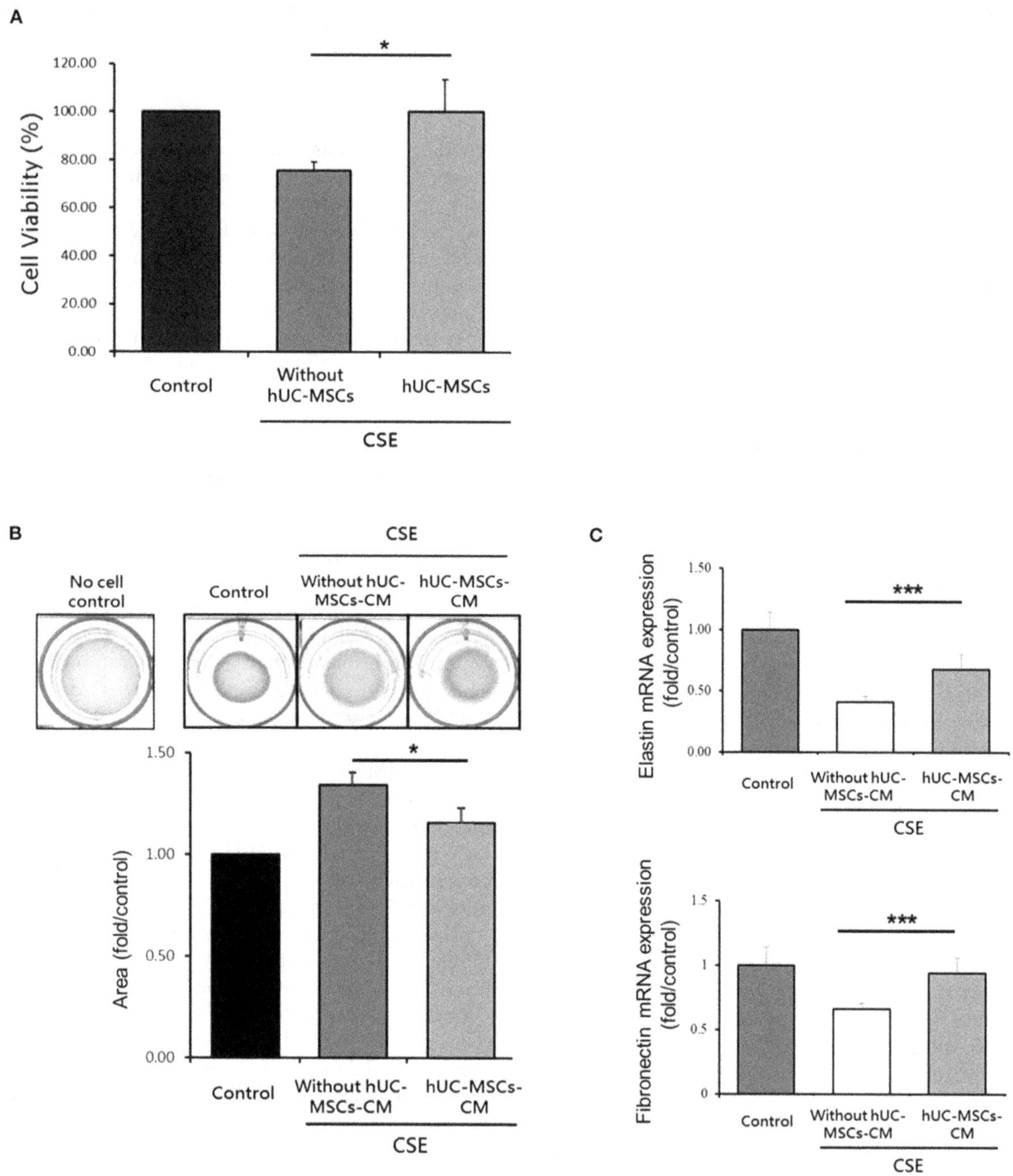

FIGURE 5 | (A) Increased cell viability of human lung fibroblasts by human umbilical cord-derived mesenchymal stem cells (hUC-MSCs) after cigarette smoke extract (CSE) exposure. **(B)** Restoration of the contractile force of lung fibroblasts by hUC-MSCs-conditioned medium (hUC-MSCs-CM). **(C)** hUC-MSCs-CM increased mRNA expressions of elastin and fibronectin in lung fibroblasts after CSE treatment. A transwell coculture system was used to determine cell viability of human lung fibroblasts (MRC5 cell line). A significant increase in cell viability (%) of MRC5 cells by hUC-MSCs was observed after CSE treatment for 24 h. MRC-5 cells were treated by CSE for 24 h and then received hUC-MSCs-CM for 24 h afterward. The contractile force was evaluated by a collagen-based cell contraction assay. The mRNA expressions of elastin and fibronectin were quantified by a qPCR. Results were examined by an unpaired *t*-test. Four independent experiments in each group. $^*p < 0.05$, $^{***}p < 0.001$.

MSCs-conditioned medium (MSCs-CM) was compatible with MSCs in attenuating inflammation in bronchopulmonary dysplasia (65). A previous study showed that MSCs-CM induced lung fibroblast proliferation and restored their repair function after CSE exposure (66). Consistent with previous findings, our results showed that mRNA expressions of elastin and fibronectin by lung fibroblasts significantly increased after treatment with hUC-MSCs-CM compared to the group treated with CSE alone. Collectively, these results suggested that paracrine factors secreted by hUC-MSCs to lung fibroblasts may be partly involved in the alveolar repair process after CS exposure.

There are a few limitations in this study. We observed an increase in lymphocytes in BALF of mice due to hUC-MSC administration. The different subgroups of lymphocytes, including regulatory T cells, were not determined in our study. In addition, interactions of hUC-MSCs with lymphocytes are not fully understood. The pulmonary function and the underlying mechanism of the hUC-MSCs in COPD will be determined in the future. Moreover, the adverse effects of fibroblasts by hUC-MSCs *in vivo* are still unclear, which should be evaluated in future work.

CONCLUSIONS

In conclusion, hUC-MSCs reduced the emphysema severity and inflammatory responses in mice with CS-induced emphysema. hUC-MSCs increased the proliferation of fibroblasts after CSE exposure. hUC-MSCs may mitigate COPD in mice after CS exposure.

AUTHOR CONTRIBUTIONS

H-CC and X-YC contributed to interpretation of the data and completion of the manuscript. H-CC, WL, and KC contributed substantially to the concept, design, interpretation of the data, and completion of the study and manuscript. Y-YC and C-HC contributed substantially to the completion of the study. T-CH contributed to the establishment of the cigarette smoke generation system and particle measurement. All authors contributed to critically revising the manuscript for important intellectual content and read and approved the final manuscript.

ACKNOWLEDGMENTS

Authors heartedly thank Ms. Yi-Syuan Lin for technical assistance during this project. KC is a Visiting Professor at Taipei Medical University.

REFERENCES

1. Garcia Castillo E, Alonso Perez T, Ancochea J, Pastor Sanz MT, Almagro P, Martinez-Camblor P, et al. Mortality prediction in chronic obstructive pulmonary disease comparing the GOLD 2015 and GOLD 2019 staging: a pooled analysis of individual patient data. *ERJ Open Res.* (2020) 6:253. doi: 10.1183/23120541.00253-2020
2. Vestbo J, Hurd SS, Agustí AG, Jones PW, Vogelmeier C, Anzueto A, et al. Global strategy for the diagnosis, management, and prevention of chronic obstructive pulmonary disease. *Am J Respir Crit Care Med.* (2013) 187:347–65. doi: 10.1164/rccm.201204-0596PP
3. May SM, Li JTC. Burden of chronic obstructive pulmonary disease: healthcare costs and beyond. *Allergy Asthma Proc.* (2015) 36:4–10. doi: 10.2500/aap.2015.36.3812
4. Kamal R, Srivastava AK, Kesavachandran CN. Meta-analysis approach to study the prevalence of chronic obstructive pulmonary disease among current, former and non-smokers. *Toxicol Rep.* (2015) 2:1064–74. doi: 10.1016/j.toxrep.2015.07.013
5. Ridzuan N, Zakaria N, Widera D, Sheard J, Morimoto M, Kiyokawa H, et al. Human umbilical cord mesenchymal stem cell-derived extracellular vesicles ameliorate airway inflammation in a rat model of chronic obstructive pulmonary disease (COPD). *Stem Cell Res Ther.* (2021) 12:54. doi: 10.1186/s13287-020-02088-6
6. Behnke J, Kremer S, Shahzad T, Chao CM, Böttcher-Friebertshäuser E, Morty RE, et al. MSC based therapies-new perspectives for the injured lung. *J Clin Med.* (2020) 9:30682. doi: 10.3390/jcm9030682
7. Cheung TS, Bertolino GM, Giacomini C, Bornhauser M, Dazzi F, Galleu A. Mesenchymal stromal cells for graft versus host disease: mechanism-based biomarkers. *Front Immunol.* (2020) 11:1338. doi: 10.3389/fimmu.2020.01338
8. Morata-Tarifa C, Macias-Sanchez MDM, Gutierrez-Pizarraya A, Sanchez-Pernaute R. Mesenchymal stromal cells for the prophylaxis and treatment of graft-versus-host disease-a meta-analysis. *Stem Cell Res Ther.* (2020) 11:64. doi: 10.1186/s13287-020-01592-z
9. Maacha S, Sidahmed H, Jacob S, Gentilcore G, Calzone R, Grivel JC, et al. Paracrine mechanisms of mesenchymal stromal cells in angiogenesis. *Stem Cells Int.* (2020) 2020:4356359. doi: 10.1155/2020/4356359
10. Pan H, Lam PK, Tong SW, Leung KK, Teoh AY, Ng EK. Mesenchymal stem cells combined with tissue fusion technology promoted wound healing in porcine bowel anastomosis. *Stem Cells Int.* (2020) 2020:5142797. doi: 10.1155/2020/5142797
11. Jasmin A, Jelicks LA, Koba W, Tanowitz HB, Mendez-Otero R, Campos de Carvalho AC, et al. Mesenchymal bone marrow cell therapy in a mouse model of chagas disease. Where do the cells go? *PLoS Negl Trop Dis.* (2012) 6:e1971. doi: 10.1371/journal.pntd.0001971
12. Liu G, Lv H, An Y, Wei X, Yi X, Yi H. Tracking of transplanted human umbilical cord-derived mesenchymal stem cells labeled with fluorescent probe in a mouse model of acute lung injury. *Int J Mol Med.* (2018) 41:2527–34. doi: 10.3892/ijmm.2018.3491
13. Hu S, Li J, Xu X, Liu A, He H, Xu J, et al. The hepatocyte growth factor-expressing character is required for mesenchymal stem cells to protect the lung injured by lipopolysaccharide *in vivo*. *Stem Cell Res Ther.* (2016) 7:66. doi: 10.1186/s13287-016-0320-5
14. Nagamura-Inoue T, He H. Umbilical cord-derived mesenchymal stem cells their advantages and potential clinical utility. *World J Stem Cells.* (2014) 6:195–202. doi: 10.4252/wjsc.v6.i2.195
15. Alatyyat SM, Alasmari HM, Aleid OA, Abdel-Maksoud MS, Elsherbiny N. Umbilical cord stem cells: background, processing and applications. *Tissue Cell.* (2020) 65:101351. doi: 10.1016/j.tice.2020.101351
16. Zhu H, Xiong Y, Xia Y, Zhang R, Tian D, Wang T, et al. Therapeutic effects of human umbilical cord-derived mesenchymal stem cells in acute lung injury mice. *Sci Rep.* (2017) 7:39889. doi: 10.1038/srep39889
17. Moroncini G, Paolini C, Orlando F, Capelli C, Grieco A, Tonnini C, et al. Mesenchymal stromal cells from human umbilical cord prevent the development of lung fibrosis in immunocompetent mice. *PLoS ONE.* (2018) 13:e0196048. doi: 10.1371/journal.pone.0196048
18. Togo S, Holz O, Liu X, Sugiura H, Kamio K, Wang X, et al. Lung fibroblast repair functions in patients with chronic obstructive pulmonary disease are altered by multiple mechanisms. *Am J Respir Crit Care Med.* (2008) 178:248–60. doi: 10.1164/rccm.200706-929OC
19. Holz O, Zuhlke I, Jaksztat E, Muller KC, Welker L, Nakashima M, et al. Lung fibroblasts from patients with emphysema show a reduced proliferation rate in culture. *Eur Respir J.* (2004) 24:575–9. doi: 10.1183/09031936.04.00143703
20. Woldhuis RR, Heijink IH, van den Berge M, Timens W, Oliver BGG, de Vries M, et al. COPD-derived fibroblasts secrete higher levels of senescence-associated secretory phenotype proteins. *Thorax.* (2020). doi: 10.1183/23120541.LSC-2020.28
21. Manevski M, Muthumalage T, Devadoss D, Sundar IK, Wang Q, Singh KP, et al. Cellular stress responses and dysfunctional Mitochondrial-cellular

senescence, and therapeutics in chronic respiratory diseases. *Redox Biol.* (2020) 33:101443. doi: 10.1016/j.redox.2020.101443
22. Miglino N, Roth M, Lardinois D, Sadowski C, Tamm M, Borger P. Cigarette smoke inhibits lung fibroblast proliferation by translational mechanisms. *Eur Respir J.* (2012) 39:705–11. doi: 10.1183/09031936.00174310
23. Salazar KD, Lankford SM, Brody AR. Mesenchymal stem cells produce Wnt isoforms and TGF-beta1 that mediate proliferation and procollagen expression by lung fibroblasts. *Am J Physiol Lung Cell Mol Physiol.* (2009) 297:L1002–11. doi: 10.1152/ajplung.90347.2008
24. Chen XY, Chen YY, Lin W, Chien CW, Chen CH, Wen YC, et al. Effects of human umbilical cord-derived mesenchymal stem cells on the acute cigarette smoke-induced pulmonary inflammation model. *Front Physiol.* (2020) 11:962. doi: 10.3389/fphys.2020.00962
25. Dominici M, Le Blanc K, Mueller I, Slaper-Cortenbach I, Marini F, Krause D, et al. Minimal criteria for defining multipotent mesenchymal stromal cells. The International Society for Cellular Therapy position statement. *Cytotherapy.* (2006) 8:315–7. doi: 10.1080/14653240600855905
26. Chen CM, Lin W, Huang LT, Chou HC. Human mesenchymal stem cells ameliorate experimental pulmonary hypertension induced by maternal inflammation and neonatal hyperoxia in rats. *Oncotarget.* (2017) 8:82366–75. doi: 10.18632/oncotarget.19388
27. Munoz-Barrutia A, Ceresa M, Artaechevarria X, Montuenga LM, Ortiz-de-Solorzano C. Quantification of lung damage in an elastase-induced mouse model of emphysema. *Int J Biomed Imaging.* (2012) 2012:734734. doi: 10.1155/2012/734734
28. Knudsen L, Weibel ER, Gundersen HJ, Weinstein FV, Ochs M. Assessment of air space size characteristics by intercept (chord) measurement: an accurate and efficient stereological approach. *J Appl Physiol.* (2010) 108:412–21. doi: 10.1152/japplphysiol.01100.2009
29. Jiang W, Xu J. Immune modulation by mesenchymal stem cells. *Cell Prolif.* (2020) 53:e12712. doi: 10.1111/cpr.12712
30. Li H, Tian Y, Xie L, Liu X, Huang Z, Su W. Mesenchymal stem cells in allergic diseases: current status. *Allergol Int.* (2020) 69:35–45. doi: 10.1016/j.alit.2019.08.001
31. Brown C, McKee C, Bakshi S, Walker K, Hakman E, Halassy S, et al. Mesenchymal stem cells: cell therapy and regeneration potential. *J Tissue Eng Regen Med.* (2019) 13:1738–55. doi: 10.1002/term.2914
32. Gotts JE, Abbott J, Fang X, Yanagisawa H, Takasaka N, Nishimura SL, et al. Cigarette smoke exposure worsens endotoxin-induced lung injury and pulmonary edema in mice. *Nicotine Tob Res.* (2017) 19:1033–9. doi: 10.1093/ntr/ntx062
33. Wittel UA, Pandey KK, Andrianifahanana M, Johansson SL, Cullen DM, Akhter MP, et al. Chronic pancreatic inflammation induced by environmental tobacco smoke inhalation in rats. *Am J Gastroenterol.* (2006) 101:148–59. doi: 10.1111/j.1572-0241.2006.00405.x
34. Serban KA, Petrache I. Mouse models of COPD. *Methods Mol Biol.* (2018) 1809:379–94. doi: 10.1007/978-1-4939-8570-8_25
35. Schweitzer KS, Johnstone BH, Garrison J, Rush NI, Cooper S, Traktuev DO, et al. Adipose stem cell treatment in mice attenuates lung and systemic injury induced by cigarette smoking. *Am J Respir Crit Care Med.* (2011) 183:215–25. doi: 10.1164/rccm.201001-0126OC
36. Zanetti A, Grata M, Etling EB, Panday R, Villanueva FS, Toma C. Suspension-expansion of bone marrow results in small mesenchymal stem cells exhibiting increased transpulmonary passage following intravenous administration. *Tissue Eng C Methods.* (2015) 21:683–92. doi: 10.1089/ten.tec.2014.0344
37. Leibacher J, Henschler R. Biodistribution, migration and homing of systemically applied mesenchymal stem/stromal cells. *Stem Cell Res Ther.* (2016) 7:7. doi: 10.1186/s13287-015-0271-2
38. Gholamrezanezhad A, Mirpour S, Bagheri M, Mohamadnejad M, Alimoghaddam K, Abdolahzadeh L, et al. *In vivo* tracking of 111In-oxine labeled mesenchymal stem cells following infusion in patients with advanced cirrhosis. *Nucl Med Biol.* (2011) 38:961–7. doi: 10.1016/j.nucmedbio.2011.03.008
39. Song L, Guan XJ, Chen X, Cui ZL, Han FF, Guo XJ, et al. Mesenchymal stem cells reduce cigarette smoke-induced inflammation and airflow obstruction in rats *via* TGF-beta1 signaling. *COPD.* (2014) 11:582–90. doi: 10.3109/15412555.2014.898032
40. Hoenderdos K, Condliffe A. The neutrophil in chronic obstructive pulmonary disease. *Am J Respir Cell Mol Biol.* (2013) 48:531–9. doi: 10.1165/rcmb.2012-0492TR
41. Voynow JA, Shinbashi M. Neutrophil elastase and chronic lung disease. *Biomolecules.* (2021) 11:1065. doi: 10.3390/biom11081065
42. Lee KH, Lee J, Jeong J, Woo J, Lee CH, Yoo CG. Cigarette smoke extract enhances neutrophil elastase-induced IL-8 production via proteinase-activated receptor-2 upregulation in human bronchial epithelial cells. *Exp Mol Med.* (2018) 50:1–9. doi: 10.1038/s12276-018-0114-1
43. Peron JP, de Brito AA, Pelatti M, Brandao WN, Vitoretti LB, Greiffo FR, et al. Human tubal-derived mesenchymal stromal cells associated with low level laser therapy significantly reduces cigarette smoke-induced COPD in C57BL/6 mice. *PLoS ONE.* (2015) 10:e0136942. doi: 10.1371/journal.pone.0136942
44. Cuerquis J, Romieu-Mourez R, Francois M, Routy JP, Young YK, Zhao J, et al. Human mesenchymal stromal cells transiently increase cytokine production by activated T cells before suppressing T-cell proliferation: effect of interferon-gamma and tumor necrosis factor-alpha stimulation. *Cytotherapy.* (2014) 16:191–202. doi: 10.1016/j.jcyt.2013.11.008
45. Hinden L, Avner M, Stepensky P, Or R, Almogi-Hazan O. Lymphocyte counts may predict a good response to mesenchymal stromal cells therapy in graft versus host disease patients. *PLoS ONE.* (2019) 14:e0217572. doi: 10.1371/journal.pone.0217572
46. Tang Z, Gao J, Wu J, Zeng G, Liao Y, Song Z, et al. Human umbilical cord mesenchymal stromal cells attenuate pulmonary fibrosis *via* regulatory T cell through interaction with macrophage. *Stem Cell Res Ther.* (2021) 12:397. doi: 10.1186/s13287-021-02469-5
47. Guan XJ, Song L, Han FF, Cui ZL, Chen X, Guo XJ, et al. Mesenchymal stem cells protect cigarette smoke-damaged lung and pulmonary function partly *via* VEGF-VEGF receptors. *J Cell Biochem.* (2013) 114:323–35. doi: 10.1002/jcb.24377
48. Chang Y, Al-Alwan L, Audusseau S, Chouiali F, Carlevaro-Fita J, Iwakura Y, et al. Genetic deletion of IL-17A reduces cigarette smoke-induced inflammation and alveolar type II cell apoptosis. *Am J Physiol Lung Cell Mol Physiol.* (2014) 306:L132–43. doi: 10.1152/ajplung.00111.2013
49. Churg A, Zhou S, Wang X, Wang R, Wright JL. The role of interleukin-1beta in murine cigarette smoke-induced emphysema and small airway remodeling. *Am J Respir Cell Mol Biol.* (2009) 40:482–90. doi: 10.1165/rcmb.2008-0038OC
50. Lappalainen U, Whitsett JA, Wert SE, Tichelaar JW, Bry K. Interleukin-1beta causes pulmonary inflammation, emphysema, and airway remodeling in the adult murine lung. *Am J Respir Cell Mol Biol.* (2005) 32:311–8. doi: 10.1165/rcmb.2004-0309OC
51. Churg A, Wang RD, Tai H, Wang X, Xie C, Wright JL. Tumor necrosis factor-alpha drives 70% of cigarette smoke-induced emphysema in the mouse. *Am J Respir Crit Care Med.* (2004) 170:492–8. doi: 10.1164/rccm.200404-511OC
52. Hong MJ, Gu BH, Madison MC, Landers C, Tung HY, Kim M, et al. Protective role of gammadelta T cells in cigarette smoke and influenza infection. *Mucosal Immunol.* (2018) 11:894–908. doi: 10.1038/mi.2017.93
53. Betsuyaku T, Hamamura I, Hata J, Takahashi H, Mitsuhashi H, Adair-Kirk TL, et al. Bronchiolar chemokine expression is different after single versus repeated cigarette smoke exposure. *Respir Res.* (2008) 9:7. doi: 10.1186/1465-9921-9-7
54. Demkow U, van Overveld FJ. Role of elastases in the pathogenesis of chronic obstructive pulmonary disease: implications for treatment. *Eur J Med Res.* (2010) 15 Suppl 2:27–35. doi: 10.1186/2047-783X-15-S2-27
55. Churg A, Wang X, Wang RD, Meixner SC, Pryzdial EL, Wright JL. Alpha1-antitrypsin suppresses TNF-alpha and MMP-12 production by cigarette smoke-stimulated macrophages. *Am J Respir Cell Mol Biol.* (2007) 37:144–51. doi: 10.1165/rcmb.2006-0345OC
56. Churg A, Zhou S, Wright JL. Series "matrix metalloproteinases in lung health and disease": Matrix metalloproteinases in COPD. *Eur Respir J.* (2012) 39:197–209. doi: 10.1183/09031936.00121611
57. Broekman W, Khedoe P, Schepers K, Roelofs H, Stolk J, Hiemstra PS. Mesenchymal stromal cells: a novel therapy for the treatment of chronic obstructive pulmonary disease? *Thorax.* (2018) 73:565–74. doi: 10.1136/thoraxjnl-2017-210672
58. Lozito TP, Tuan RS. Mesenchymal stem cells inhibit both endogenous and exogenous MMPs *via* secreted TIMPs. *J Cell Physiol.* (2011) 226:385–96. doi: 10.1002/jcp.22344
59. Jiang D, Muschhammer J, Qi Y, Kugler A, de Vries JC, Saffarzadeh M, et al. Suppression of neutrophil-mediated tissue damage-a novel skill of mesenchymal stem cells. *Stem Cells.* (2016) 34:2393–406. doi: 10.1002/stem.2417

60. Longhini-Dos-Santos N, Barbosa-de-Oliveira VA, Kozma RH, Faria CA, Stessuk T, Frei F, et al. Cell therapy with bone marrow mononuclear cells in elastase-induced pulmonary emphysema. *Stem Cell Rev Rep.* (2013) 9:210–8. doi: 10.1007/s12015-012-9419-y
61. Hoffman AM, Paxson JA, Mazan MR, Davis AM, Tyagi S, Murthy S, et al. Lung-derived mesenchymal stromal cell post-transplantation survival, persistence, paracrine expression, and repair of elastase-injured lung. *Stem Cells Dev.* (2011) 20:1779–92. doi: 10.1089/scd.2011.0105
62. Churg A, Wang R, Wang X, Onnervik PO, Thim K, Wright JL. Effect of an MMP-9/MMP-12 inhibitor on smoke-induced emphysema and airway remodelling in guinea pigs. *Thorax.* (2007) 62:706–13. doi: 10.1136/thx.2006.068353
63. Liu X, Fang Q, Kim H. Preclinical studies of mesenchymal stem cell (MSC) administration in chronic obstructive pulmonary disease (COPD): a systematic review and meta-analysis. *PLoS ONE.* (2016) 11:e0157099. doi: 10.1371/journal.pone.0157099
64. Su VY, Lin CS, Hung SC, Yang KY. Mesenchymal stem cell-conditioned medium induces neutrophil apoptosis associated with inhibition of the NF-kappaB pathway in endotoxin-induced acute lung injury. *Int J Mol Sci.* (2019) 20:92208. doi: 10.3390/ijms20092208
65. Emukah C, Dittmar E, Naqvi R, Martinez J, Corral A, Moreira A, et al. Mesenchymal stromal cell conditioned media for lung disease: a systematic review and meta-analysis of preclinical studies. *Respir Res.* (2019) 20:239. doi: 10.1186/s12931-019-1212-x
66. Kim SY, Lee JH, Kim HJ, Park MK, Huh JW, Ro JY, et al. Mesenchymal stem cell-conditioned media recovers lung fibroblasts from cigarette smoke-induced damage. *Am J Physiol Lung Cell Mol Physiol.* (2012) 302:L891–908. doi: 10.1152/ajplung.00288.2011

12

The Combination of Hemogram Indexes to Predict Exacerbation in Stable Chronic Obstructive Pulmonary Disease

Xuanqi Liu [1†], Haiyan Ge [1†], Xiumin Feng [2], Jingqing Hang [3], Fengying Zhang [3], Xiaoyan Jin [4], Hong Bao [5], Min Zhou [6], Fengfeng Han [7], Shengqing Li [8], Yechang Qian [9], Zhijun Jie [10], Wenchao Gu [11], Beilan Gao [12], Li Yu [13], Jian Wang [14], Haiying Ji [15], Jingxi Zhang [2,16] and Huili Zhu [1*]*

[1] Department of Respiratory and Critical Care Medicine, Huadong Hospital, Fudan University, Shanghai, China, [2] Department of Respiratory and Critical Care Medicine, Changji Branch of First Affiliated Hospital of Xinjiang Medical University, Xinjiang, China, [3] Department of Respiratory Medicine, Putuo People's Hospital, Shanghai, China, [4] Department of Respiratory Medicine, Tongren Hospital, Shanghai Jiaotong University School of Medicine, Shanghai, China, [5] Department of Respiratory Medicine Shanghai Pudong Hospital, Fudan University Pudong Medical Center, Shanghai, China, [6] Department of Respiratory and Critical Care Medicine, Ruijin Hospital, Shanghai Jiaotong University School of Medicine, Shanghai, China, [7] Department of Respiratory Medicine, Xinhua Hospital, Shanghai Jiaotong University School of Medicine, Shanghai, China, [8] Department of Respiratory and Critical Care Medicine, Huashan Hospital, Fudan University, Shanghai, China, [9] Baoshan District Hospital of Integrated Traditional Chinese and Western Medicine Hospital, Shanghai, China, [10] Department of Respiratory Medicine, Shanghai Fifth's Hospital, Fudan University, Shanghai, China, [11] Department of Respiratory Medicine, Pudong New District People's Hospital, Shanghai, China, [12] Department of Respiratory Medicine, Shanghai Pulmonary Hospital, Tongji University, Shanghai, China, [13] Department of Pulmonary and Critical Care Medicine, Tongji Hospital, Tongji University School of Medicine, Shanghai, China, [14] Department of Respiratory Medicine, Shanghai Ninth's Hospital, Shanghai Jiaotong University School of Medicine, Shanghai, China, [15] Department of Respiratory and Critical Care Medicine, Zhongshan Hospital, Fudan University, Shanghai, China, [16] Department of Respiratory and Critical Care Medicine, Changhai Hospital Affiliated to Navy Military Medical University, Shanghai, China

***Correspondence:**
Huili Zhu
zhuhuili001@126.com
Jingxi Zhang
jingxizhang2000@126.com

† These authors have contributed equally to this work

Background: Chronic obstructive pulmonary disease (COPD) is characterized by pulmonary and systemic inflammatory processes, and exacerbation of COPD represents a critical moment in the progression of COPD. Several biomarkers of inflammation have been proposed to have a predictive function in acute exacerbation. However, their use is still limited in routine clinical practice. The purpose of our study is to explore the prognostic efficacy of novel inflammatory hemogram indexes in the exacerbation among stable COPD patients.

Method: A total of 275 stable COPD patients from the Shanghai COPD Investigation Comorbidity Program were analyzed in our study. Blood examinations, especially ratio indexes like platelet–lymphocyte ratio (PLR), platelet × neutrophil/lymphocyte ratio [systemic immune-inflammation index (SII)], and monocyte × neutrophil/lymphocyte ratio [systemic inflammation response index (SIRI)], lung function test, CT scans, and questionnaires were performed at baseline and routine follow-ups. Clinical characteristics and information of exacerbations were collected every 6 months. The relationship between hemogram indexes and diverse degrees of exacerbation was assessed by logistic regression. The receiver operating characteristic (ROC) curve and area under the curve (AUC) were used to evaluate the ability of hemogram indexes to predict exacerbation of COPD. Furthermore, the discrimination and accuracy of combined indexes were measured by ROC and calibration curve.

Result: There was a significant positive correlation between PLR levels and total exacerbation of COPD patients in a stable stage in a year. Also, the predictive ability of PLR exceeded any other ratio indexes, with an AUC of 0.66. SII and SIRI ranked second only to PLR, with an AUC of 0.64. When combining PLR with other indexes (sex, COPD year, and St. George's Respiratory Questionnaire scores), they were considered as the most suitable panel of index to predict total exacerbation. Based on the result of the ROC curve and calibration curve, the combination shows optimal discrimination and accuracy to predict exacerbation events in COPD patients.

Conclusion: The hemogram indexes PLR, SII, and SIRI were associated with COPD exacerbation. Moreover, the prediction capacity of exacerbation was significantly elevated after combining inflammatory hemogram index PLR with other indexes, which will make it a promisingly simple and effective marker to predict exacerbation in patients with stable COPD.

Keywords: COPD, hemogram index, PLR, exacerbation, inflammation

INTRODUCTION

Chronic obstructive pulmonary disease (COPD) is characterized by persistent airflow limitation, which is usually progressive. Chronic airway and lung inflammation do exist in COPD patients (1). It is well-known that cigarette smoke inducing chronic inflammation results in the remodeling and narrowing of small airways and the destruction of lung parenchyma in COPD. According to the World Health Organization (WHO), COPD will be the third leading cause of death in the world. In the recent few years, the exacerbation of COPD has become the focus of our attention. It contributed to a series of problems (2, 3)—worsening lung function, decreasing life quality (4, 5), accelerating disease progress, and elevating the risk of hospitalization or mortality (3, 6, 7). Recently, the use of hemogram indexes indicating systemic inflammation has been determined in clinical practice for predicting hospitalization and mortality in COPD. However, there still exist obverse and reverse judgments on the usage of hemogram indexes. It is due to the exact thresholds of hemogram indexes are totally different because the target population is derived from different study designs. Meanwhile, limited data have been presented in evaluating hemogram indexes as biomarkers in patients with stable COPD. Also, the relationship between the change in these indexes and the severity of exacerbation is still uncertain.

Beyond some genetic factors, a considerable part of exacerbation cannot be explained by infection (8, 9); infection is still regarded as one of the main reasons for exacerbation in COPD (6, 10). Therefore, ratio indexes in peripheral blood, such as platelet–lymphocyte ratio (PLR), platelet × neutrophil/lymphocyte [systemic immune-inflammation index (SII)], and monocyte × neutrophil/lymphocyte [systemic inflammation response index (SIRI)], which generally served as markers of inflammation level, are studied widely, as well as hemogram indexes like platelet counts/mean platelet volume (PLT/MPV) and platelet counts/red cell distribution width (PLT/RDW) ratios on behalf of platelet and red cell activation (11, 12). What is more important is that when combining the several indexes, they are proved to be more valuable predictors in many diseases. Systemic inflammation makers SII and SIRI have been determined to play an important role in various solid tumor like lung cancer and cardiovascular diseases (13–15). It has been established that high PLR is associated with 90-day mortality in acute exacerbations of COPD (16). By contrast, conventional inflammatory indicators like C-reactive protein and procalcitonin in peripheral blood showed low specificity in predicting exacerbation of COPD (17, 18). Also, the counting of inflammatory cells in the airway is not easy and convenient to detect. Overall, the inflammatory indicators discussed earlier in the hemogram index are easier to obtain and more cost effective. It is very meaningful to analyze the inflammation-related indicators in hemogram in COPD patients.

The primary purpose of our study is to investigate the prognostic role of hemogram indexes, especially inflammation-related ones in patients with stable COPD. We also sought to explore the relationship between hemogram indexes and the severity of the exacerbation. In addition, we tried to confirm a proper combination of indexes to predict exacerbation and evaluate corresponding predictive ability, including discrimination and accuracy.

METHODS

Study Population

Patients with COPD admitted in five hospitals (Huadong Hospital, Changhai Hospital, Putuo People's Hospital, Baoshan Integrated Chinese and Western Medicine Hospital, and Pulmonary hospital) in Shanghai from June 2018 to December 2019 were enrolled. Our study has acquired the approval of the ethical committee's informed consent from Huadong Hospital. The inclusion criteria in the study were as follows: (1) Primary diagnosis of COPD in accordance with Global Initiative for Chronic Obstructive Lung Disease (GOLD) criteria (the forced expiratory volume in the first second of forced vital capacity is

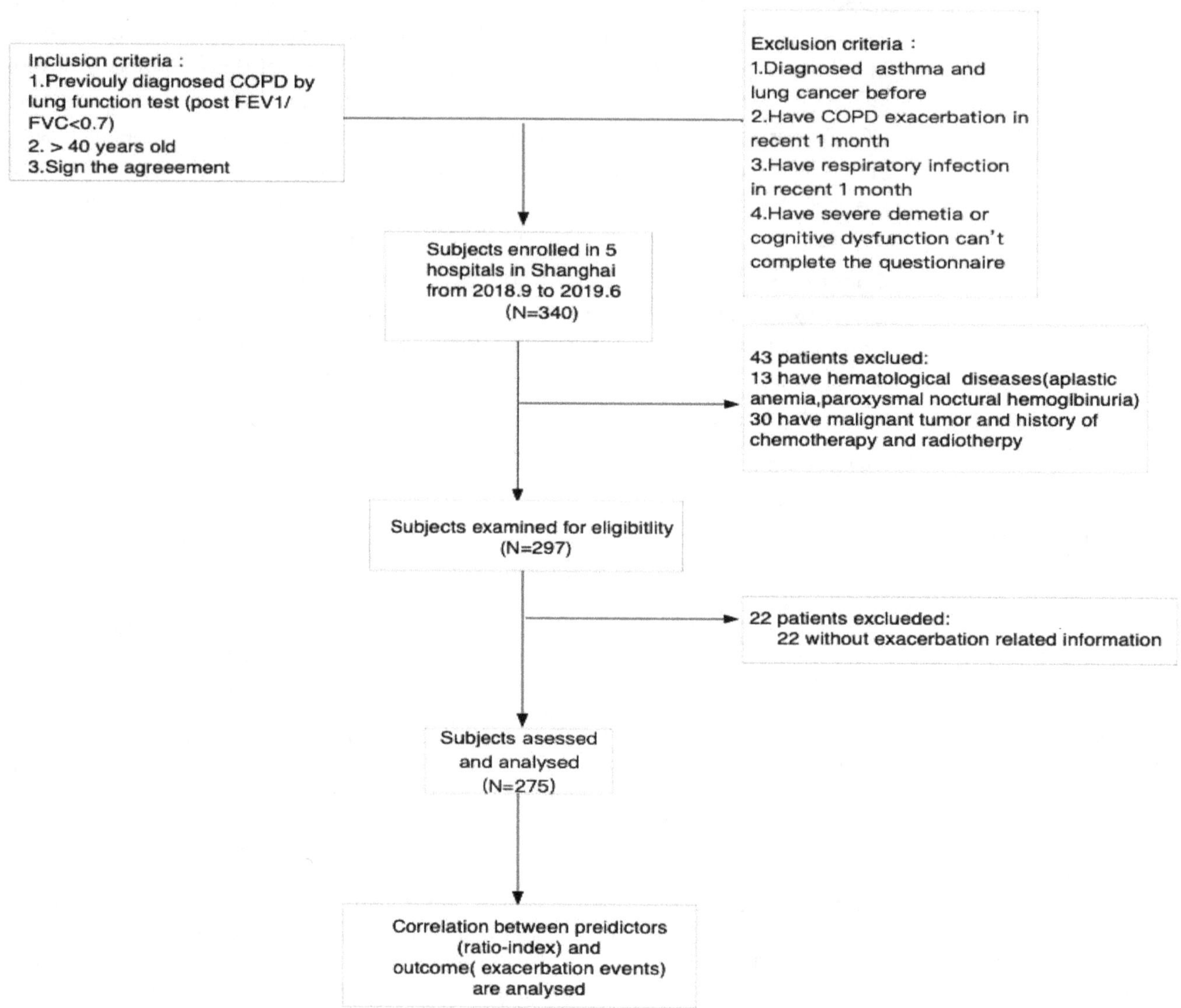

FIGURE 1 | Flowchart of the study population. Process of patient selection in this study. Finally, data from 275 patients are used to analyze and assess. COPD, chronic obstructive pulmonary disease.

<70% after inhaling bronchodilators); (2) patients whose age ≥40 years; and (3) signed the agreement of participating in the study. The exclusion criteria were as follows: (1) diagnosis of asthma or lung cancer; (2) history of COPD exacerbation in recent month, which specifically refers to a deterioration of patients' respiratory tract symptoms that were beyond the normal variation and even required steroids, antibiotics, or hospitalization; (3) history of respiratory infection in the recent month; and (4) unable to complete the questionnaire due to severe dementia and cognitive dysfunction. A total of 340 stable COPD patients were initially enrolled. Then, we exclude 43 patients; among them, 13 were suffering from hematological diseases, and 30 were receiving chemotherapy or radiotherapy, which may make an influence on hemogram. At the end of the first-year follow-up, 22 patients were lost to follow-up, and their exacerbation-related information was not available. Finally, a total of 275 subjects were used to analyze and assess. The process of patient selection is shown in **Figure 1**.

Study Design

Our study has been registered in the Chinese Clinical Trial Registry, and the registration number is ChiCTR2000030911. This is a 3 year prospective cohort study. The subjects in the study were required to complete blood examination, lung function tests, and questionnaires. The blood samples were collected at baseline during the stable stage. The exacerbation-related information was documented every 6 months. In our study, the definition of COPD exacerbation has been strictly identified according to GOLD 2018. The occurrence of exacerbation means acute worsening of respiratory symptoms that result in additional therapy. Mild exacerbation is treated with short-acting bronchodilators only. Moderate exacerbation should be treated with short-acting bronchodilators plus antibiotics and/or oral corticosteroids. Severe exacerbation always requires hospitalization, including emergency admission. Frequent exacerbation was defined as one who suffered from more than one exacerbation in a year. The platelet count, lymphocyte count, neutrophil count, mean platelet volume, and red cell distribution width were measured at each participating center. Then, we acquired the corresponding ratio index, such as PLR, PLT/MPV ratio, PLT/RDW ratio, SII, and SIRI. The baseline characteristics associated with the comorbidity of all the patients were recorded in the questionnaire, including COPD Assessment Test, Modified Medical Research Council, and St. George's Respiratory Questionnaire (SGRQ) scores evaluating patients' symptoms. Correlation between hemogram indexes and exacerbation events were then analyzed.

Statistical Analysis

Data were presented as mean ± standard deviation. Logistic regression analysis was performed to evaluate the total and diverse degrees of exacerbation in stable COPD patients. To assess the index's predictive ability of exacerbation in COPD, we constructed receiver operating characteristic (ROC) curves and tabulated the area under the curves (AUC). In the section, the results of multivariate logistic regression were regarded as predictors in a total exacerbation. Logistic regression to predict exacerbation was used to determine the weight given to each standardized index. Nomograms were operated to exhibit the model's prognostic ability of total exacerbation in detail. Then, we evaluated the model's predictive capacity from two aspects. ROC curve was utilized again to test the discrimination, whereas the accuracy of the model was certified by Hosmer–Lemeshow fitting test and calibration curve. For all tests, a two-sided $P < 0.05$ was considered significant. Data were analyzed by STATA 15.

TABLE 1 | Baseline characteristics of study patients.

Clinical characteristic	COPD
Number	275
Sex	32/243
(Female/male)	(11.6/88.4)
Age	70.8 ± 9.0
Smoking status	60/152/63
(never/ex/smoker)	(21.8/55.3/22.9)
Smoking index	33.1 ± 31.6
BMI	23.2 ± 4.1
COPD years	6.6 ± 7.7
mMRC scores	40/67/82/72/14
(1/2/3/4/5)	(14.6/24.4/29.8/26.2/5.1)
CAT score	16.6 ± 8.8
SGRQ score	35.6 ± 19.3
FEV1, %	52.2 ± 22.6
FEV1%FVC, %	56.6 ± 14.5
GOLD stage	33/76/128/78
(I/II/III/IV)	(12.0/27.6/46.6/13.8)
EOS	0.3 ± 0.9
PLR	151.1 ± 62.8
SII	745.5 ± 438.1
SIRI	1.9 ± 1.3
PLT/RDW	15.6 ± 3.9
PLT/MPV	21.5 ± 6.2

Data were shown as mean ± SD. GOLD COPD grades are defined as: grade I: post-bronchodilator FEV1 > 80% of predicted; grade II: post-bronchodilator FEV1 50–80% of predicted; grade III: post-bronchodilator FEV1 30–50% of predicted; and grade IV: post-bronchodilator FEV1 < 30% of predicted.
BMI, body mass index; smoking index, smoking packs per day; FEV1, forced expiratory volume in 1 s; FVC, first vital capacity; PLR, platelet–lymphocyte ratio; SII, platelet × neutrophil/lymphocyte; SIRI, monocyte × neutrophil/lymphocyte; PLT/RDW, platelet counts–red cell distribution width ratio; PLT/MPV, platelet counts–mean platelet volume ratio.

RESULTS

Characteristics of the Study Population

A total of 275 patients with stable COPD met our inclusion and exclusion criteria and were enrolled in this study. **Table 1** provided the summary statistics for the study population. There were 243 males and 32 females, with an average age of 71 years. Of these, 22.9% were current smokers. COPD Assessment Test scores, Modified Medical Research Council scores, and SGRQ scores were conducted to assess respiratory symptoms. The patients were classified as Global Initiative for COPD (GOLD) stages 1, 2, 3, and 4. In detail, they had 33, 76, 128, and 78 cases in each group, respectively. The clinical characteristics, pulmonary function tests, and main hemogram indexes of participants were also listed in **Table 1**.

Relationship Between Hemogram Indexes and Exacerbation in 1 Year

Univariate analysis of logistic regression revealed that all of the hemogram indexes except PLT/RDW and PLT/MPV were associated with total exacerbation. The independence of the discussed parameters as predictors for total exacerbation was determined using the entered model of multivariate logistic regression. As a result, PLR was confirmed as an independent predictor for total exacerbation in our study (**Table 2**). The other parameters were not significant in multivariate regression. Next, we repeated multivariate logistic regression in different degrees of exacerbation. Interestingly, we found that the effect of PLR in severe exacerbation still existed after adjustment for known prognostic factors. SII, SIRI, and SGRQ scores also played the prognostic role in this part. The severe exacerbation seems to be more connected with hemogram indexes compared with a moderate and mild one. In addition, SII and PLT/MPV are correlated with moderate and mild exacerbation, respectively. PLT/MPV played a prognostic role in frequent exacerbation, too (**Table 3**). Poisson regression was performed to detect the association between hemogram indices and the number of total exacerbation in a year (**Supplement 1**). All of the hemogram indexes except PLR were related to the number of total acute exacerbations whether in univariate or multivariate regression. The effect of PLR maybe minimized by other mixed factors in multivariate regression.

TABLE 2 | Univariate and multivariate logistic regression analysis for total exacerbation.

	Univariate model OR (95% CI)	*P*-value	Multivariate model OR (95% CI)	*P*-value
Sex				
Female	Reference	–	Reference	–
Male	3.0394 (1.4362–6.4321)	0.004	3.6455 (1.1323–11.7361)	0.030
Age	1.0071 (0.9785–1.0365)	0.630	NA	NA
Smoking index	1.0109 (1.0015–1.0203)	0.023	0.9999 (0.9872–1.0128)	0.993
BMI	0.9517 (0.8935–1.0138)	0.125	NA	NA
SGRQ scores	1.0653 (1.0443–1.0866)	<0.05	1.0395 (1.0140–1.0656)	<0.05
GOLD stage				
GOLD 1	Reference	–	Reference	–
GOLD 2	2.0500 (0.8845–4.7511)	0.094	1.3233 (0.4750–3.6867)	0.592
GOLD 3	8.9167 (3.8123–20.8542)	<0.05	2.6184 (0.8800–7.7903)	0.084
GOLD 4	9.3333 (3.0332–28.7195)	<0.05	1.9026 (0.4135–8.7543)	0.409
COPD years	1.1208 (1.0536–1.1924)	<0.05	1.1044 (1.0209–1.1947)	0.013
PLR	1.0093 (1.0044–1.0142)	<0.05	1.0160 (1.0051–1.0270)	0.004
SII	1.0011 (1.0004–1.0018)	0.002	1.0002 (1.0000–1.0041)	0.086
SIRI	1.5203 (1.1914–1.9399)	0.001	1.3994 (0.9070–2.1592)	0.129
PLT/MPV	0.9909 (0.9502–1.0333)	0.669	NA	NA
PLT/RDW	0.9966 (0.9335–1.0640)	0.919	NA	NA

OR, odds ratio; CI, confidence interval; PLR, platelet–lymphocyte ratio; SII, platelet × neutrophil/lymphocyte; SIRI, monocyte × neutrophil/lymphocyte; PLT/RDW, platelet counts–red cell distribution width ratio; PLT/MPV, platelet counts–mean platelet volume ratio.

TABLE 3 | Multivariate logistic regression analysis for moderate exacerbation.

	Severe O R (95% CI)	*P*-value	Moderate OR (95% CI)	*P*-value	Mild OR (95% CI)	*P*-value	Frequency OR (95% CI)	*P*-value
SGRQ score	1.0630 (1.0436–1.0827)	<0.05	–	–	–	–	1.0444 (1.0272–1.0619)	<0.05
PLR	1.0093 (1.0006–1.0180)	0.035	–	–	–	–	–	–
SII	1.0019 (1.0003–1.0036)	0.021	1.0009 (1.0002–1.0016)	0.007	–	–	–	–
SIRI	1.3785 (0.9917–1.9163)	0.056	–	–	–	–	–	–
PLT/MPV	–	–	–	–	0.9544 (0.9136–0.9971)	0.037	0.9498 (0.9089-0.9925)	0.022

OR, odds ratio; CI, confidence interval; PLR, platelet–lymphocyte ratio; SII, platelet × neutrophil/lymphocyte; SIRI, monocyte × neutrophil/lymphocyte; PLT/RDW, platelet counts–red cell distribution width ratio; PLT/MPV, platelet counts–mean platelet volume ratio.

Predictive Ability of Ratio Indexes

To compare the predictive ability of the ratio indexes, we drew the ROC of PLR, SII, SIRI, PLT/RDW, and PLT/MPV alone to predict total and severe exacerbation events. The AUC values of each index were presented in **Figure 2**. In both figures, the predictive ability of PLR exceeded that of other ratio indexes individually. It appeared that SII and SIRI also behave well in predicting exacerbation events. We further compared **Figures 2A,B** and found that the ability of all these ratio indexes (including PLR) to predict total exacerbation is universally better than severe exacerbation.

Predictive Ability of Combined Indexes

As we have mentioned in multivariate logistic regression, PLR was closely related to total exacerbation and severe exacerbation. Due to the superiority of PLR in predictive ability, we then investigated the predictive discrimination and accuracy of the logistic model: combining hemogram index PLR with other significant indexes (sex, COPD years, and SGRQ scores) to increase predictive sensitivity. Based on these four predictive indexes, we first established a predictive nomogram for total exacerbation in stable COPD patients. As shown in **Figure 3**, the result of the nomogram plot showed that PLR is one of the contributing factors. For every 88.2-unit increase in PLR value, the score in the exacerbation system will increase by one point. In addition, for every 9.58 years of increase in the course of COPD, or for every 1.11 increase in SGRQ scores, a person's exacerbation score will increase by one unit. The predictive accuracy of index combinations is exhibited in **Figure 4**.

We obtained the best AUC of 0.806 when using a combination of PLR, sex, COPD years, and SGRQ scores. As we expected, the predictive capacity of PLR was significantly augmented, combining with other indexes. These results also suggested that the model showed good discriminability. Furthermore, the

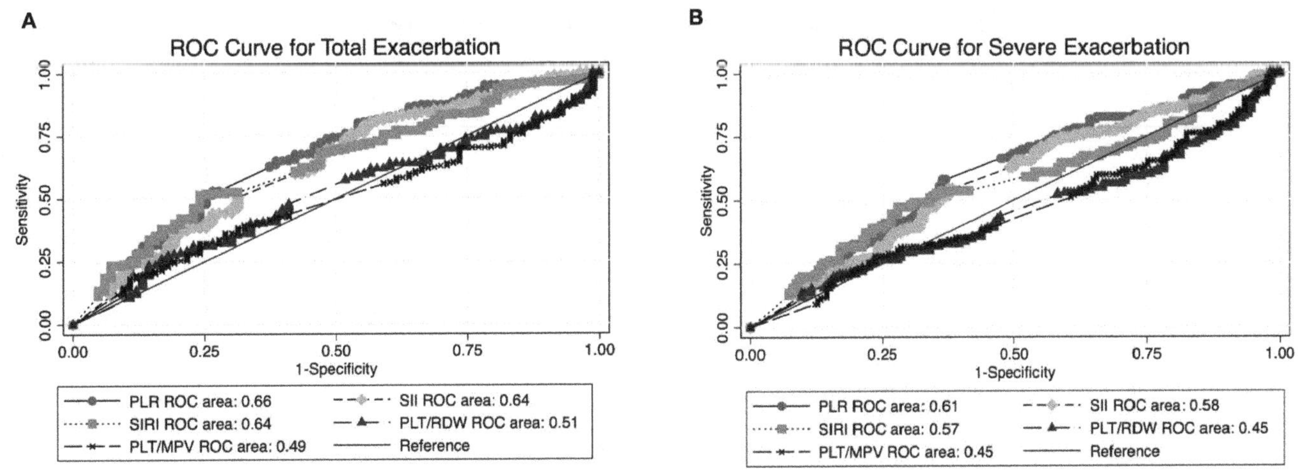

FIGURE 2 | Graph shows results of ROC analysis for predicting exacerbation among stable chronic obstructive pulmonary disease (COPD) patients by different ratio indexes (PLR, SII, SIRI, PLT/MPV, and PLT/RDW). **(A)** ROC curve analysis of ratio index to predict total exacerbation. **(B)** ROC curve analysis of ratio index to predict severe exacerbation. ROC, receiver operating characteristic, PLR, platelet–lymphocyte ratio; SII, platelet × neutrophil/lymphocyte; SIRI, monocyte × neutrophil/lymphocyte; PLT/RDW, platelet counts–red cell distribution width ratio; PLT/MPV, platelet counts–mean platelet volume ratio.

calibration curve of the model and Hosmer–Lemeshow fitness test are performed to assess the model's accuracy. The slope of the calibration curve was close to 1.0, which indicated that there was good consistency between predictive exacerbation risk and actual exacerbation risk (**Figure 5**). The result of the Hosmer–Lemeshow fitness test ($\chi^2 = 6.37$, $P = 0.606$) confirmed the accuracy. Therefore, the strong evidence in our study supported that a combination of PLR with other indexes is a qualified combination to predict total exacerbation. To conversely prove the superiority of PLR, we combine the three known indexes related to COPD (sex, COPD year, and SGRQ scores) to predict total exacerbation. The AUC is 0.7769, which is lower than the four indexes. The result suggested that PLR did play an important role, especially combined with other predictors (**Supplement 2**).

DISCUSSION

Exacerbation of COPD refers to the acute event during the clinical course of COPD (18), which is significantly associated with the clinical outcomes of patients with COPD by worsening clinical symptoms, declining lung function, and increasing mortality. Therefore, identifying a simple and reliable marker to predict exacerbation in stable COPD patients is becoming more and more urgent. By providing a comprehensive assessment of hemogram indexes, especially ratio indexes, this study confirmed that platelet related indexes such as PLR showed great predictive ability in an exacerbation. Also, we further explored the predictive discrimination and accuracy of index combinations. In the present study, we found that a combination of platelet-related index (PLR) reliably predicts total exacerbation of COPD patients in a stable stage.

Recently, the hemogram indexes, especially ratio indexes (PLR, SII, SIRI, PLT/RDW, PLT/MPV), have aroused wide public concern. Many pieces of research have proved that ratio indexes can be useful markers to predict bacterial infection in hospital mortality in patients with acute exacerbations of COPD (17). Studies related to PLT/RDW and PLT/MVP were not too much, but they have been verified in improving sepsis bacteremia diagnostics and even in predicting severe burn injury (14, 19). However, the present studies have not elucidated the clinical prognostic value of ratio indexes in stable COPD patients or compared the efficacy of different ratio indexes. Our study provided evidence supporting the relationship between hemogram indexes and exacerbation in the stable stage. Moreover, we aimed to contribute to growing area of research by exploring a combination of indexes, especially platelet-related indexes.

Platelet-related index, including PLR and MPV, are found to play important roles in total exacerbation of COPD (20). Praneel Kumar and Stephanie Law ascertained that PLR is significantly associated with 90-mortality in patients with acute exacerbation (21). Consistent with the literature, our study also observed that the levels of PLR are positively correlated with total and severe exacerbation events. When we refer to platelet in COPD, platelet activation is the kernel of the mechanism. Patients with COPD demonstrate increased platelet activation (16), with further activation occurring during acute exacerbations (13). In the status of hypoxemia, platelet behavior will change (22). The concrete performance is in several aspects: (1) The platelet survival time is shortened and can be reversed by oxygen treatment (23) (2) Activated platelet with lower platelet aggregate ratios standard for the increasing tendency to the aggregate formation in the circulation (22, 24) (3) Mean platelet volume is greater and in negative correlation with PaO_2. One hypothesis was put forward to explain it. They thought the immature platelet dropping off from megakaryocytic contributed to this (23, 25, 26). (4) Activated platelet secretes platelet factor 4 and P-selectin, and platelet–monocyte aggregate is the soluble

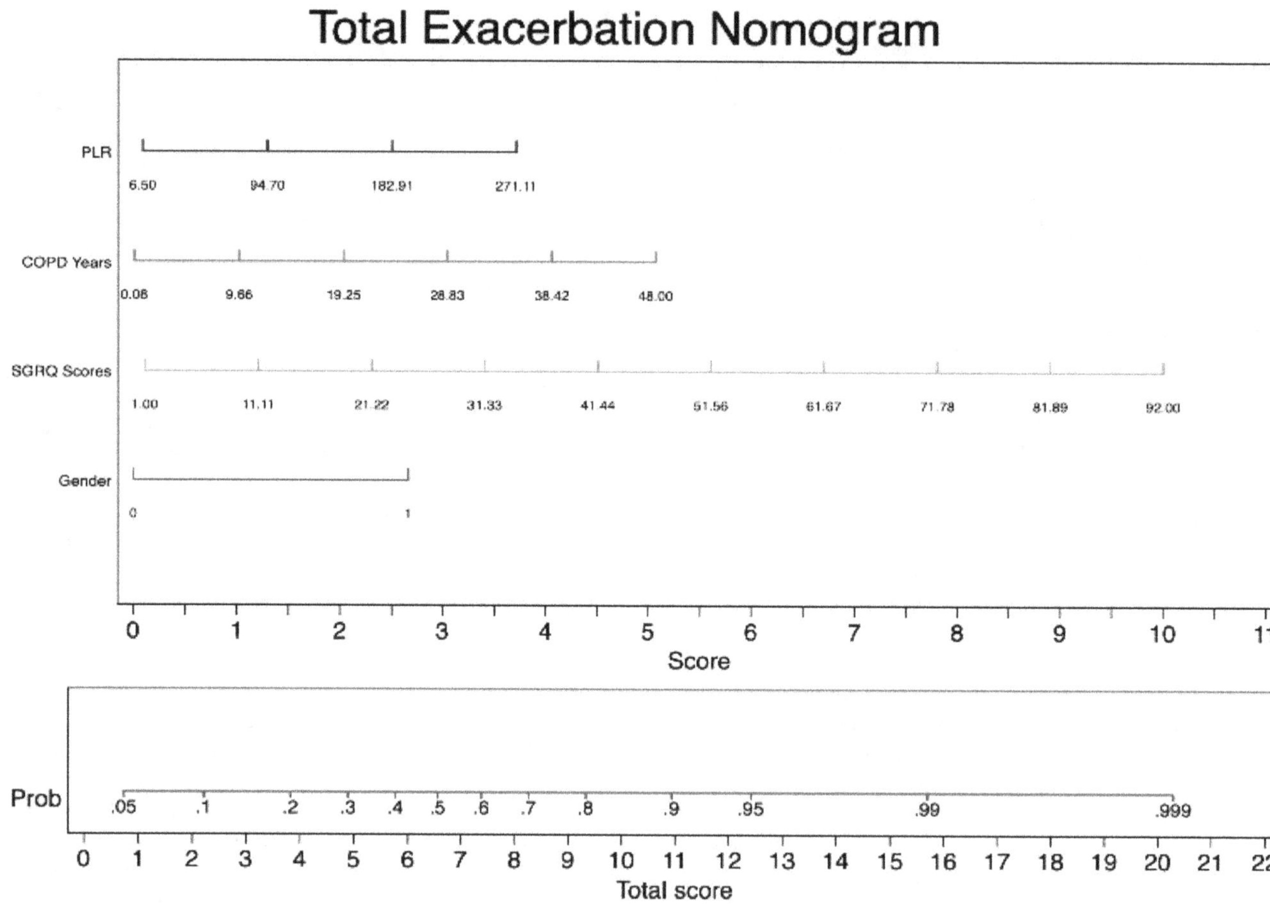

FIGURE 3 | Nomogram for predicting total exacerbation in patients with stable COPD. To use the nomogram for predicting each individual patient's exacerbation risk, first we locate the range of each variable on the horizontal scale and draw a line vertically to the bottom score line to determine the corresponding points. Then, we sum up the points of all three variables and locate the total score on the total score scale. Finally, we draw a vertical line from the dot on the total sore line to the upward risk probability line to calculate the risk of exacerbation.

marker of platelet activation (27, 28). (5) The last formation of activation is the amount. Ashraf Faway reported that those with thrombocytosis are more likely to have worse dyspnea, functional status, and quality of life compared with those with lower platelet count (27). In addition, thrombocytosis was an independent predictor of both inpatient mortality and 1 year mortality among survivors to discharge (29). All that are discussed are the external performance of platelet activation. In summary, all the evidence suggested that the relationship between platelet-related index and exacerbation exactly existed. Although PLR only reflects the change of platelet in amount, the underlying mechanism should come back to the platelet activation. When we use the combination of PLR with other indexes, we have a more comprehensive understanding of platelet activation in COPD patients. That may be the reason why index combination can predict exacerbation in COPD better than an individual one. Our results also confirmed the association between platelet activation and COPD exacerbation in a way. Also, we found that PLT/MPV is greatly correlated with mild exacerbation (**Table 3**). It is probably because the index PLT/MPV itself subsumes platelet counts and mean platelet volume, which can better reflect platelet activation. Our results offer a new thought for exploring marker in mild exacerbation of COPD patients. With the in-depth study, reactive oxidative stress (ROS) is proved to be associated with abnormal inflammation and exacerbation in patients with COPD (1, 30). Furthermore, someone holds the opinion that ROS itself is one component of inflammation by activating the oxidant-sensitive transcription factors to improve the transcription of pro-inflammatory genes in COPD (31). During the procedure of ROS, oxidized low-density lipoprotein can activate transcription factor, nuclear factor kappa B, which is related to the pathogenesis of COPD. PI3K is also activated in ROS, which can exaggerate inflammation. ROS may be the upstream in the whole regulatory networks, and platelet is one of the targets. Our result (**Table 2**) is in accordance with theirs; the higher the PLR level is, the more possible exacerbation happens.

SIRI and SII comprehensive indexes can indicate systemic inflammation and immune status. Huaping Huang reported the

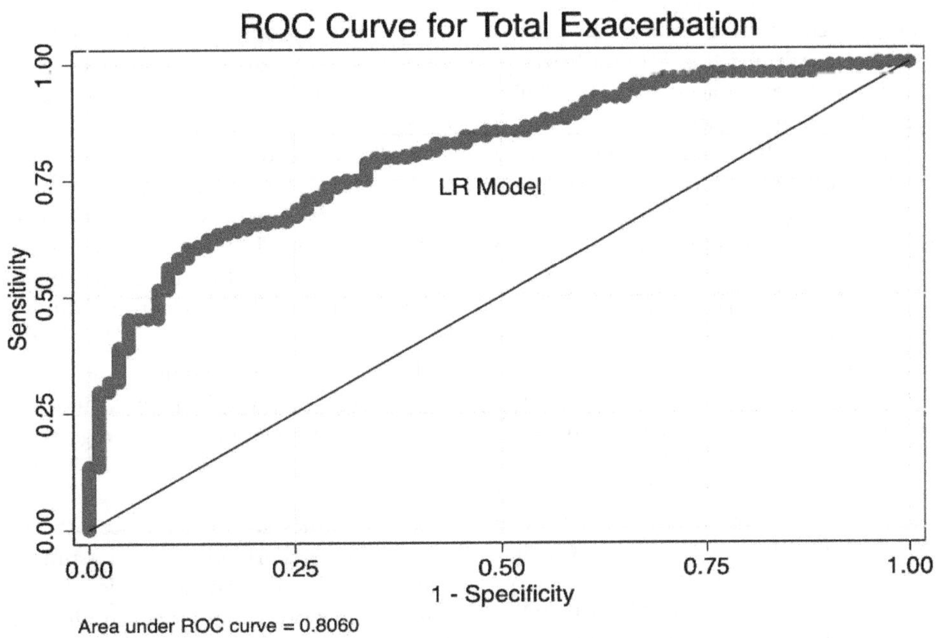

FIGURE 4 | Graph shows the results of ROC curves analysis for predictive models. Predictors were arising from multivariate logistic regression of total exacerbation among stable COPD patients [sex, COPD years, St. George's Respiratory Questionnaire (SGRQ) scores, and PLR].

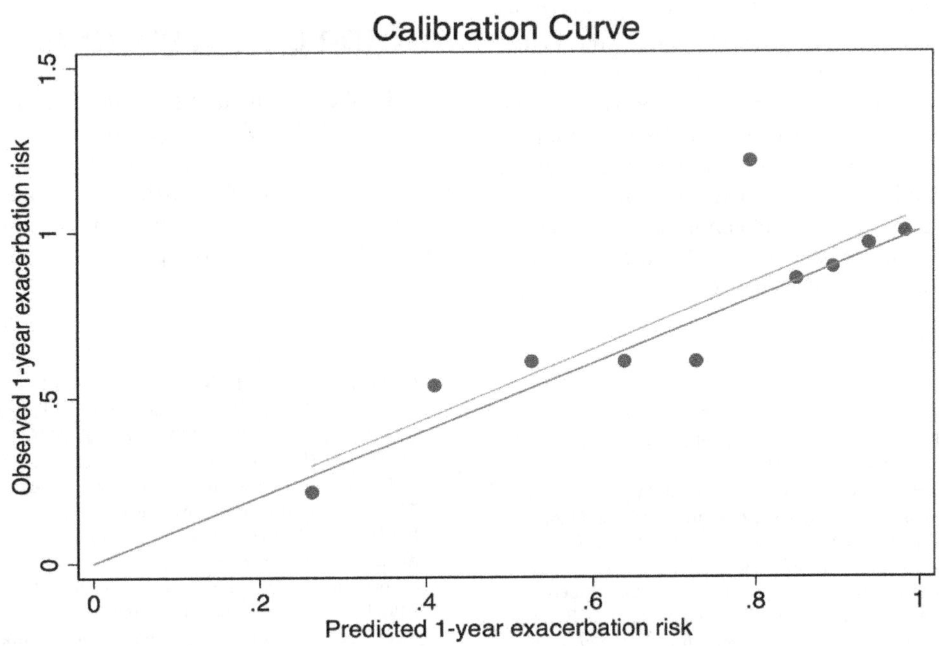

FIGURE 5 | Calibration curve of combined indexes (PLR, sex, COPD years, and SGRQ scores) to predict total exacerbation of COPD patients. Result of Hosmer–Lemeshow fitness test: $\chi^2 = 6.37$, $P = 0.606$.

prognostic value of preoperative SII in patients with cervical cancer (14). Previous research also proved the clinical utility in clear cell renal cell carcinoma and esophageal squamous cell carcinoma (32, 33). They attributed the results to the synthesis and comprehensiveness of SII and SIRI. With regard to COPD, it is widely recognized that airflow limitation is related to abnormal inflammation, which is a multicomponent inflammatory response (34). However, how SII and SIRI functioned in COPD has not been determined. SIRI is one kind of index containing platelet counts, monocytes counts, and lymphocytes counts. We confirmed that SII and SIRI are positively related to total and severe exacerbation in COPD patients in our study. What is more, the ROS may be a linking bridge between them. In ROS, oxidized low-density lipoprotein also plays a great part in other aspects. It can activate the chemotaxis of monocytes and increase the expression of monocyte chemotactic protein-1 (30). On one hand, under the influence of chemotaxis, monocyte counts will increase. On the other hand, through platelet activation, the cell surface adhesion molecules will release to recruit more monocytes (28). Someone who explored the clinical use of intercellular adhesion molecule 1 to be the biomarker of COPD found that intercellular adhesion molecule 1 is produced by bronchial epithelial cells and endothelial cell aiming to activate lung macrophages (35), maybe the discovery is also suitable in the peripheral circulation. In the present study, the predictive capacity of SIRI far exceeds PLT/MPV and PLT/RDW, whether in a total or severe exacerbation.

SII concludes platelet counts other than SIRI. It takes two aspects, inflammation and immunity, into consideration. Someone assumed that good performance of SII might owe to the integration of three indexes, which avoid being easily affected by individual differences and show greater stability (2, 21, 36). That may be exactly the same as SIRI. In our study, SII showed the same superiority as SIRI in predicting the exacerbation of COPD patients. The higher SII and SIRI generally heralds the higher systemic inflammatory level. Evidence supports that systematic inflammation is commonly seen in COPD, especially during exacerbation because of the increasing circulating cytokines, chemokines, and acute-phase proteins. However, until now, we cannot figure out whether the systematic inflammation is a "spill over" from the lung or a parallel abnormality (1). So, the extrapulmonary effects cannot be ignored (37). Further research in systemic inflammation of COPD is needed.

As a regional study, the study reflected the results of the particular population and had its limitations. First, the sample size in our study is considerably limited. Sensitivity and specificity may be improved as the samples' quantity increases. Second, compared to other western large-scale COPD clinical studies, the subjects we enrolled may be older, and we contained fewer women. So, when we extrapolated the results in population, it is not suitable for young and female COPD patients. Third, although we found that the hemogram indexes, especially PLR, are correlated with exacerbation, the mortality, and rate of descent in pulmonary function have not been evaluated.

Despite these limitations, our study still provides some new insights into the hemogram indexes and exacerbation of COPD. With the multivariate regression analysis, the result demonstrated that ratio index PLR was significantly related to the exacerbation of COPD. Also, they showed the high-powered efficacy to predict exacerbation after combining with other indexes. Furthermore, we estimated the discrimination and accuracy of combined indexes to predict exacerbation. The information will be useful in phenotyping COPD patients. Besides, it is conducive to screen high-risk patients during the stable stage. Targeted and appropriate interventions for a certain population should be performed in an early stage.

AUTHOR CONTRIBUTIONS

JZ and HZ contributed to study design. XF, JH, FZ, XJ, HB, MZ, FH, YQ, ZJ, WG, BG, LY, JW, and SL contributed to participants enrollment and contributed to study management and data collection. XL and HG contributed to manuscript writing, data analyses, and manuscript revision. All authors have read and approved the final manuscript.

REFERENCES

1. Barnes PJ. Cellular and molecular mechanisms of asthma and COPD. *Clin Sci.* (2017) 131:1541–58. doi: 10.1042/CS20160487
2. Fang H, Zhang H, Wang Z, Zhou Z, Li Y, Lu L, et al. Systemic immune-inflammation index acts as a novel diagnostic biomarker for postmenopausal osteoporosis and could predict the risk of osteoporotic fracture. *J Clin Lab Anal.* (2020) 34:e23016. doi: 10.1002/jcla.23016
3. Wedzicha JA, Miravitlles M, Hurst JR, Calverley PM, Albert RK, Anzueto A, et al. Management of COPD exacerbations: a European Respiratory Society/American Thoracic Society guideline. *Eur Respir J.* (2017) 49:1600791. doi: 10.1183/13993003.00791-2016
4. Sapey E, Bafadhel M, Bolton CE, Wilkinson T, Hurst JR, Quint JK, et al. Building toolkits for COPD exacerbations:lessons from the past and present. *Thorax.* (2019) 749:898–905. doi: 10.1136/thoraxjnl-2018-213035
5. de Miguel-Diez J, Jiménez-García R, Hernández-Barrera V, Puente-Maestu L, Girón-Matute WI, de Miguel-Yanes JM, et al. Trends in the use and outcomes of mechanical ventilation among patients hospitalized with acute exacerbations of COPD in Spain, 2001 to 2015. *J Clin Med.* (2019) 8:1621. doi: 10.3390/jcm8101621
6. Criner GJ, Bourbeau J, Diekemper RL, Quellette DR, Goodridge D, Hernandez P et al. Prevention of acute exacerbations of COPD. *Chest.* (2015) 147:894–942. doi: 10.1378/chest.14-1676
7. Labaki WW, Xia M, Murray S, Curtis JL, Barr RG, Bsatt HP, et al. NT-proBNP in stable COPD and future exacerbation risk: analysis of the SPIROMICS cohort. *Respir Med.* (2018) 140:87–93. doi: 10.1016/j.rmed.2018.06.005
8. Labaki WW, Han MK. β2 adrenergic receptor polymorphisms and COPD exacerbations: a complicated story. *Thorax.* (2019) 74:927–8. doi: 10.1136/thoraxjnl-2019-213697
9. Ingebrigtsen TS, Vestbo J, Rode L, Marott JL, Lange P, Nordestgaard PG. β2-Adrenergic genotypes and risk of severe exacerbations in COPD: a prospective cohort study. *Thorax.* (2019) 74:934–40. doi: 10.1136/thoraxjnl-2018-212340
10. Atto B, Eapen MS, Sharma P, Frey U, Ammit AJ, Markos J, et al. New therapeutic targets for the prevention of infectious acute exacerbations of COPD: role of epithelial adhesion molecules and inflammatory pathways. *Clin Sci.* (2019) 133:1663–703. doi: 10.1042/CS20181009
11. Tertemiz KC, Alpaydin AO, Sevinc C, Ellidokuz H, Acara AC, Cimrin A. Could "red cell distribution width" predict COPD severity? *Rev Port Pneumol.* (2016) 22:196–201. doi: 10.1016/j.rppnen.2015.11.006
12. Qiu L, Chen C, Li SJ, Wang C, Guo F, Peszel A, et al. Prognostic values of red blood cell distribution width, platelet count, and red cell distribution width-to-platelet ratio for severe burn injury. *Sci Rep.* (2017) 7:13720. doi: 10.1038/s41598-017-13151-3
13. Sin DD. The devastating power of platelets in COPD exacerbations: can aspirin save lives in COPD? *Thorax.* (2014) 67:603–4. doi: 10.1136/thoraxjnl-2014-205329

14. Huang H, Liu Q, Zhu L, Zhang Y, Lu XJ, Wu YW, et al. Prognostic value of preoperative systemic immune-inflammation index in patients with cervical cancer. *Sci Rep.* (2019) 9:3284. doi: 10.1038/s41598-019-39150-0
15. Valero C, Pardo L, Sansa A, Garcia Lorenzo J, López M, Quer M, et al. Prognostic capacity of Systemic Inflammation Response Index (SIRI) in patients with head and neck squamous cell carcinoma. *Head Neck.* (2019) 42:336–43. doi: 10.1002/hed.26010
16. Campo G, Pavasini R, Pollina A, Tebaldi M, Ferrari R. On-treatment platelet reactivity in patients with chronic obstructive pulmonary disease undergoing percutaneous coronary intervention: table 1. *Thorax.* (2014) 69:80–1. doi: 10.1136/thoraxjnl-2013-203608
17. Tanriverdi H, Örnek T, Erboy F, Altinsoy B, Uygur F, Atalay F, et al. Comparison of diagnostic values of procalcitonin, C-reactive protein and blood neutrophil/lymphocyte ratio levels in predicting bacterial infection in hospitalized patients with acute exacerbations of COPD. *Wien Klin Wochenschr.* (2015) 127:756–63. doi: 10.1007/s00508-014-0690-6
18. Yao C, Liu X, Tang Z. Prognostic role of neutrophil-lymphocyte ratio and platelet-lymphocyte ratio for hospital mortality in patients with AECOPD. *Int J Chron Obstruct Pulmon Dis.* (2017) 12:2285–90. doi: 10.2147/COPD.S141760
19. Tamelyte E, Vaičekauskiene G, Dagys A, Lapinskas T, Jankauskaite L. early blood biomarkers to improve sepsis/bacteremia diagnostics in pediatric emergency settings. *Medicina.* (2019) 55:99. doi: 10.3390/medicina55040099
20. Kumar P, Law S, Sriram KB. Evaluation of platelet lymphocyte ratio and 90-day mortality in patients with acute exacerbation of chronic obstructive pulmonary disease. *J Thor Dis.* (2017) 9:1509–16. doi: 10.21037/jtd.2017.05.77
21. Zhang Y, Chen B, Wang L, Wang R, Yang XJ. Systemic immune-inflammation index is a promising noninvasive marker to predict survival of lung cancer. *Medicine.* (2019) 98:e13788. doi: 10.1097/MD.0000000000013788
22. Wedzicha JA, Syndercombe-Court D, Tan KC. Increased platelet aggregate formation in patients withchronicairflowobstructionandhypoxaemia. *Thorax.* (1991) 46:504–7. doi: 10.1136/thx.46.7.504
23. Wedzicha JA, Cotter FE, Empey DW. Platelet size in patients with chronic airflow obstruction with and without hypoxaemia. *Thorax.* (1988) 43:61–4. doi: 10.1136/thx.43.1.61
24. Tariket S, Sut C, Arthaud CA, Eyraud MA, Meneveaux A, Laradi S et al. Modeling the effect of platelet concentrate supernatants on endothelial cells: focus on endocan/ESM-1. *Transfusion.* (2018) 58:439–45. doi: 10.1111/trf.14450
25. Harrison MT, Short P, Williamson PA, Singanayagam A, Chalmers JD, Schembri S. Thrombocytosis is associated with increased short and long term mortality after exacerbation of chronic obstructive pulmonary disease: a role for antiplatelet therapy? *Thorax.* (2014) 69:609–15. doi: 10.1136/thoraxjnl-2013-203996
26. Aydin I IM, Aydin M, Caliskan AM, Aren I. Neutrophil lymphocyte ratio monocyte lymphocyte ratio and mean platelet volume as systemic inflammatory markers in different states of bipolar. *Nordic J Psychiatry.* (2019) 73:372–9. doi: 10.1080/08039488.2019.1640789
27. Fawzy A, Putcha N, Paulin LM, Aaron CP, Labaki WW, Han MK, et al. Association of thrombocytosis with COPD morbidity: the SPIROMICS and COPD gene cohorts. *Respir Res.* (2018) 19:20. doi: 10.1186/s12931-018-0717-z
28. Maclay JD, Mcallister DA, Johnston S, Raftis J, Mcguinnes C, Deans A, et al. Increased platelet activation in patients with stable and acute exacerbation of COPD. *Thorax.* (2011) 66:769–74. doi: 10.1136/thx.2010.157529
29. Hodgson L. Predicting death or deterioration in patients admitted with acute exacerbation of COPD using physiological and blood parameters. *Thorax.* (2014) 69(Suppl. 2):A18. doi: 10.1136/thoraxjnl-2014-206260.37
30. Shen YC, Yang T, Guo SJ, Li XO, Chen L, Wang T. Increased serum ox-LDL levels correlated with lung function, inflammation, and oxidative stress in COPD. *Mediators Inflamm.* (2013) 2013:972347. doi: 10.1155/2013/972347
31. Drost EM, Skwarski KM, Sauleda J, Soler N, Roca J, Agustia, et al. Oxidative stress and airway inflammation in severe exacerbations of COPD. *Thorax.* (2005) 60:293–300. doi: 10.1136/thx.2004.027946
32. Murthy P, Zenati MS, Abbas AIA, Rieser CJ, Baharyn, Lotze MT, et al. Prognostic value of the systemic immune-inflammation index (sii) after neoadjuvant therapy for patients with resected pancreatic cancer. *Surg Oncol.* (2019) 27:898–906. doi: 10.1245/s10434-019-08094-0
33. Geng YT, Zhu DX, Wu C, Wu J, Wang Q, Li RQ, et al. A novel systemic inflammation response index (SIRI) for predicting postoperative survival of patients with esophageal squamous cell carcinoma. *Int Immunopharmacol.* (2018) 65:503–10. doi: 10.1016/j.intimp.2018.10.002
34. Szucs B, Szucs C, Petrekanits M, Varga JT. Molecular characteristics and treatment of endothelial dysfunction in patients with COPD: a review article. *Int J Mol Sci.* (2019) 20:4329. doi: 10.3390/ijms20184329
35. Blidberg K, Palmberg L, James A, Billing B, Henriksson E, Lantz AS, et al. Adhesion molecules in subjects with COPD and healthy non-smokers: a cross sectional parallel group study. *Respir Res.* (2013) 14:47. doi: 10.1186/1465-9921-14-47
36. Gao Y, Guo W, Cai S, Zhang F, Shao F, Zhang G, et al. Systemic immune-inflammation index (SII) is useful to predict survival outcomes in patients with surgically resected esophageal squamous cell carcinoma. *J Cancer.* (2019) 10:3188–96. doi: 10.7150/jca.30281
37. Wouters EFM, Groenewegen KH, Dentener MA, Vernooy JKJ. Systemic inflammation in chronic obstructive pulmonary disease: the role of exacerbations. *Proc Am Thor Soc.* (2007) 4:626–34. doi: 10.1513/pats.200706-071TH

13

Potential Value of Expiratory CT in Quantitative Assessment of Pulmonary Vessels in COPD

Xianxian Cao [1,2†], Xiaoyan Gao [1,3†], Nan Yu [4], Meijuan Shi [5], Xia Wei [6], Xiaoqi Huang [7], Shudi Xu [6], Jiantao Pu [8], Chenwang Jin [1] and Youmin Guo [1]*

[1] Department of Radiology, The First Affiliated Hospital of Xi'an Jiaotong University, Xi'an, China, [2] Department of Diagnostic Imaging, National Cancer Center/National Clinical Research Center for Cancer/Cancer Hospital, Chinese Academy of Medical Sciences and Peking Union Medical College, Beijing, China, [3] Medical Imaging Center, Shaanxi Provincial People's Hospital, Xi'an, China, [4] Department of Radiology, The Affiliated Hospital of Shaanxi University of Traditional Chinese Medicine, Xianyang, China, [5] Department of Radiology, The Second Affiliated Hospital of Xi'an Jiaotong University, Xi'an, China, [6] Department of Respiratory Medicine, The Ninth Hospital of Xi'an Affiliated Hospital of Xi'an Jiaotong University, Xi'an, China, [7] Department of Radiology, The Affiliated Hospital of Yan'an University, Yan'an, China, [8] Departments of Radiology and Bioengineering, University of Pittsburgh, Pittsburgh, PA, United States

***Correspondence:**
Chenwang Jin
jcw76@163.com

† These authors have contributed equally to this work

Objective: To investigate the associations between intrapulmonary vascular volume (IPVV) depicted on inspiratory and expiratory CT scans and disease severity in COPD patients, and to determine which CT parameters can be used to predict IPVV.

Methods: We retrospectively collected 89 CT examinations acquired on COPD patients from an available database. All subjects underwent both inspiratory and expiratory CT scans. We quantified the IPVV, airway wall thickness (WT), the percentage of the airway wall area (WA%), and the extent of emphysema ($LAA\%_{-950}$) using an available pulmonary image analysis tool. The underlying relationship between IPVV and COPD severity, which was defined as mild COPD (GOLD stage I and II) and severe COPD (GOLD stage III and IV), was analyzed using the Student's t-test (or Mann-Whitney U-test). The correlations of IPVV with pulmonary function tests (PFTs), $LAA\%_{-950}$, and airway parameters for the third to sixth generation bronchus were analyzed using the Pearson or Spearman's rank correlation coefficients and multiple stepwise regression.

Results: In the subgroup with only inspiratory examinations, the correlation coefficients between IPVV and PFT measures were $-0.215 \sim -0.292$ ($p < 0.05$), the correlation coefficients between IPVV and WT_{3-6} were $0.233 \sim 0.557$ ($p < 0.05$), and the correlation coefficient between IPVV and $LAA\%_{-950}$ were $0.238 \sim 0.409$ ($p < 0.05$). In the subgroup with only expiratory scan, the correlation coefficients between IPVV and PFT measures were $-0.238 \sim -0.360$ ($p < 0.05$), the correlation coefficients between IPVV and WT_{3-6} were $0.260 \sim 0.566$ ($p < 0.05$), and the correlation coefficient between IPVV and $LAA\%_{-950}$ were $0.241 \sim 0.362$ ($p < 0.05$). The multiple stepwise regression analyses demonstrated that WT were independently associated with IPVV ($P < 0.05$).

Conclusion: The expiratory CT scans can provide a more accurate assessment of COPD than the inspiratory CT scans, and the airway wall thickness maybe an independent predictor of pulmonary vascular alteration in patients with COPD.

Keywords: chronic obstructive pulmonary disease (COPD), computed tomography, intrapulmonary vessels, inspiratory, expiratory

INTRODUCTION

Chronic obstructive pulmonary disease (COPD) is very prevalent worldwide and carries high mortality and morbidity rates (1, 2). Among COPD patients, 30–70% have clinically significant pulmonary vascular disease (3–5). The major vascular alterations are vascular remodeling and vasoconstriction caused by emphysema and/or hypoxemia, and often cause pulmonary hypertension (6, 7). There are investigations showing that pulmonary vascular alterations were found in patients with mild COPD, even in non-smokers with normal lung function (8, 9). All these suggest that pulmonary vascular alterations may persist throughout the entire progress of COPD, and it is important to develop methods to quantitatively assess the pulmonary vascular alterations in COPD.

The high-resolution characteristic of computed tomography (CT) makes it possible to visualize very detailed lung structures and quantify a variety of lung abnormalities, such as emphysema, airway remodeling, and pulmonary vascular alterations in COPD (10, 11). There have been investigative efforts made to quantitatively assess pulmonary vascular alterations in COPD. Matsuoka et al. (12) proposed the total cross-sectional area (CSA) of small pulmonary vessels as an index of pulmonary vascular alterations. They reported that %CSA<5 mm^2 had a significant correlation with forced expiratory volume in 1 s (FEV_1) and FEV_1/forced vital capacity (FVC) as well as $\%LAA_{-950}$ in severe COPD. Previous studies (13–15) have demonstrated that there were quantitative pulmonary

TABLE 1 | Patient Characteristics and PFT results in the COPD subjects.

Characteristic	COPD subjects (n = 89)
Age (years)	63.6 ± 9.4
Sex, %female	19 (21.35%)
BMI (kg/m^2)	22.76 ± 3.59
GOLD stage I:II:III:IV	12:31:28:18
FEV_1/FVC%	51.45 ± 9.75
FEV_1%	47.00 (32.85)

BMI, body mass index; FEV_1/FVC, ratio of forced expiratory volume in 1 s to forced vital capacity; FEV_1, percentage predicted forced expiratory volume in 1 s.

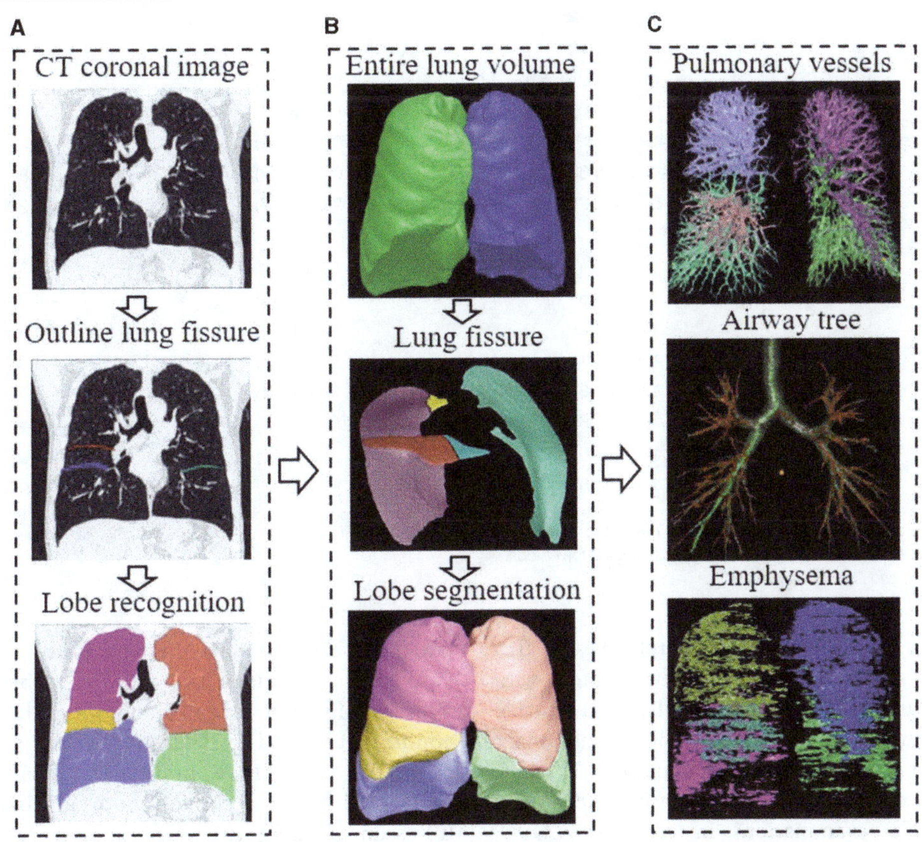

FIGURE 1 | Flow chart of CT quantitative parameter measurement. **(A)** The delineation of lung fissures and the identification of lung lobes on CT images; **(B)** The total lung volume identified by the 3D adaptive border marching algorithm, the lung fissure segmented by the computational geometry approach, and the five lung lobes segmented by implicit surface functions; **(C)** The principal curvatures and the principal directions were used to distinguish pulmonary vessels from lung tissue, and the vascular tree was automatically extracted and segmented to calculate IPVV in the whole lung and each individual lobe; The differential geometric approach to segment the airway tree, and the average values of the measurements for the 3–6th bronchial generation were automatically calculated; The extent of emphysema under the threshold of −950 HU was automatically computed, the area shown in color.

TABLE 2 | Comparisons of IPVV between mild and severe COPD.

		Mild COPD (n = 43)	Severe COPD (n = 46)	t/z-value	P-value
Inspiration IPVV					
	WL	168.94 ± 44.12	176.78 ± 48.61	−0.796	0.428
	RL	87.66 (35.42)	92.83 ± 25.05	−0.452	0.652
	LL	77.12 ± 22.36	85.15 ± 24.04	−1.628	0.107
	RUL	33.68 (15.16)	33.07 (15.26)	−0.164	0.87
	RML	12.36 (5.69)	14.13 ± 5.42	−1.355	0.176
	RLL	43.41 ± 12.46*	43.69 ± 13.11*	−0.105	0.917
	LUL	38.37 (14.95)	40.29 ± 12.98	−0.435	0.663
	LLL	37.58 ± 13.24	45.65 ± 13.84	−2.809	0.006
Expiration IPVV					
	WL	145.37 ± 49.68	171.18 ± 45.11	−2.568	0.012
	RL	79.46 ± 25.73	90.46 ± 22.90	−2.133	0.036
	LL	65.91 ± 26.06	81.93 ± 22.98	−3.081	0.003
	RUL	29.57 (16.28)	31.50 (11.32)	−1.067	0.286
	RML	10.87 (5.00)	14.32 ± 5.54	−2.451	0.014
	RLL	35.69 ± 15.26	41.58 ± 12.56*	−1.993	0.049
	LUL	34.97 ± 13.99	39.53 ± 12.33	−1.635	0.106
	LLL	30.94 ± 16.01	43.34 ± 14.83	−3.793	<0.001
Difference Value					
	WL	17.19 (32.77)	4.72 (16.95)	−3.966	<0.001
	RL	11.00 (16.12)	1.71 (10.60)	−3.834	<0.001
	LL	8.82 (13.97)	1.00 (8.16)	−3.53	<0.001
	RUL	3.15 (4.82)	0.10 (3.23)	−3.875	<0.001
	RML	0.72 (1.76)	−0.19 ± 1.24	−3.654	<0.001
	RLL	4.80 (12.39)*	0.93 (5.09)	−3.296	0.001
	LUL	4.58 ± 5.60	0.78 (3.82)	−3.851	<0.001
	LLL	5.54 (7.52)	2.07 (6.17)	−3.206	0.001
Relative Value					
	WL	1.10 (0.24)	1.03 (0.10)	−4.335	<0.001
	RL	1.14 (0.25)	1.02 (0.12)	−4.171	<0.001
	LL	1.11 (0.30)	1.02 (0.09)	−3.966	<0.001
	RUL	1.10 (0.21)	1.00 (0.10)	−3.982	<0.001
	RML	1.09 (0.13)	1.01 (0.11)	−3.752	<0.001
	RLL	1.14 (0.36)	1.02 (0.12)	−3.465	0.001
	LUL	1.11 (0.20)	1.02 (0.10)	−3.998	<0.001
	LLL	1.14 (0.55)	1.04 (0.13)	−3.563	<0.001

IPVV, intrapulmonary vascular volume; COPD, chronic obstructive pulmonary disease; WL, the whole lung; RL, the right lung; LL, the left lung; RUL, the right upper lobe; RML, the right middle lobe; RLL, the right lower lobe; LUL, the left upper lobe; LLL, the left lower lobe.
**Difference of IPVV between RUL and RLL, $P < 0.05$.*

vascular features, such as the percentage of total vessel area and the number of small vessels, closely associated with survival and PFT measures in COPD patients. It is notable that most of the available investigations about pulmonary vascular alternation were limited to the inspiratory CT scans. Although there are studies (16–18) demonstrating the unique value of expiratory CT examinations in assessing COPD, it is unclear whether the expiratory CT scans have any advantage over inspiratory CT scans in assessing pulmonary vascular alternation.

In this study, we proposed to quantify the intrapulmonary vascular volume (IPVV) depicted on CT images in COPD patients. The objective is to study whether pulmonary vascular alternations in COPD subjects are associated with emphysema extent, pulmonary functions, and airway abnormalities, and to determine which parameter can be used as predictor of IPVV in COPD patients. In particular, we performed the analyses on both inspiratory and expiratory CT scans, aiming to clarify the potential of expiratory CT examinations in assessing pulmonary vascular alternations in COPD. For this purpose, we established a dataset consisting of 89 paired inspiration-expiration CT scans. A detailed description of our dataset, methods, and experimental results follows.

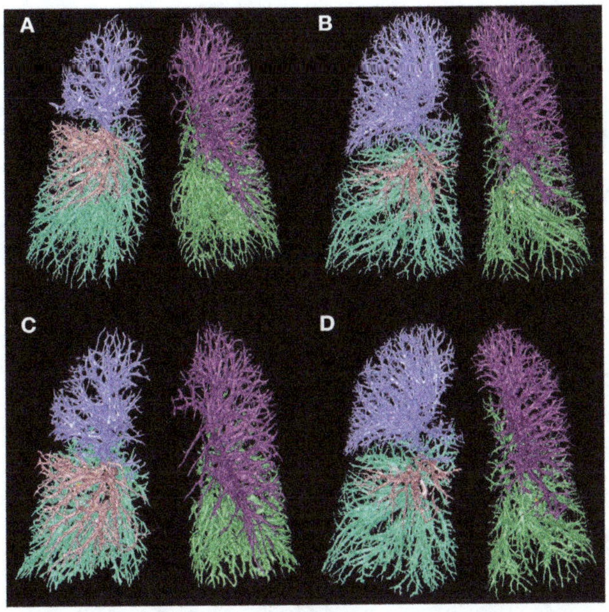

FIGURE 2 | Comparison of IPVV between mild and severe COPD in inspiratory and expiratory CT. **(A,C)** A male with mild COPD (GOLD II, 68 years): a, the IPVV of the whole lung in inspiratory CT is 209.95 ml; b, the IPVV of the whole lung in expiratory CT is 169.10 ml. **(B,D)** A male with severe COPD (GOLD III, 64 years): a, the IPVV of the whole lung in inspiratory CT is 208.31 ml; b, the IPVV of the whole lung in expiratory CT is 201.18 ml.

MATERIALS AND METHODS

Study Population

We retrospectively identified 92 patients from the "Digital Lung" Respiratory Disease Evaluation System and Diagnostic Criteria (201402013). These subjects were diagnosed with COPD and underwent both inspiratory and expiratory CT examinations. COPD was diagnosed on the basis of past history, physical examination, and spirometry data by following the Global Initiative for Chronic Obstructive Lung Disease (GOLD) (1) diagnostic criteria ($FEV_1/FVC < 70\%$ bronchodilators inhaled). Among the collected subjects, three were excluded, because of the involved issues: (1) concomitant lung diseases such as interstitial lung disease, lung cancer, infectious pneumonia, and pulmonary tuberculosis; (2) previous lung surgery; (3) insufficient CT quality of analysis; and (4) unable to complete the pulmonary function test. As a result, we have 89 subjects involved in this study and the demographics information was summarized in **Table 1**. All subjects were divided into subjects with mild COPD (GOLD I and II, $n = 43$) and subjects with severe COPD (GOLD III and IV, n=46) for comparison of IPVV. This retrospective study was approved by the Chinese Clinical Research Registry (Grant No.: ChiCTR-OCH-14004904), and written informed consent was obtained from all subjects.

Pulmonary Function Tests

All subjects underwent spirometry according to American Thoracic Society/European Thoracic Society guidelines (19). PFT measurements included forced expiratory volume during the first second of exhalation (FEV_1) percent to the predicted value (FEV_1%predicted) post inhalation of 200 μg salbutamol, FEV_1/forced vital capacity ratio (FEV_1/FVC), the ratio of residual volume to total lung capacity(RV%TLC) and the diffusing capacity for carbon monoxide (DL_{CO}). Referring to previous studies (20, 21), we only used the FEV_1% predicted and FEV_1/FVC in the subsequent analysis in this study.

CT Scan Acquisition

The CT examinations were performed at full inspiration and expiration states for the involved subjects in the supine position using 64-slice multi-detector CT scanners (SOMATOM Definition AS; Siemens, Erlangen, Germany). All subjects were given breathing training prior to examination. The scan parameters were as follows: tube voltage: 100 or 120 KV tube current, autoexposure control, exposure time: 0.5 s, and the matrix size: 512 × 512 pixels. Images were reconstructed with a 1 mm slice thickness (with 0.625 mm overlap) using a standard kernel algorithm.

Image Processing

We analyzed the CT scans using the FACT-Digital Lung Workstation (Dexin, Xi'an, China), which have both US FDA 510 K and CFDA cleared. This software system enables automated segmentation of a variety of lung structures, including right/left lungs, lung vessels, airway trees, inner/outer airway walls. On the basis of the segmentations, an automatically 3D approach was used to reconstruct the pulmonary vasculature and calculate the entire volume of the intrapulmonary vascular volume (IPVV) in the whole lung or each individual lobe. In inspiratory and expiratory CT, the measures of IPVV all includes the vascular wall and lumen of both arteries and veins, which is specified in milliliter (ml). We also measured the airway wall thickness (WT), and the percentage of the airway wall area (WA%) of the 3–6th generations and the extent of emphysema in each individual lobe of both inspiratory and expiratory CT examinations. The extent of emphysema, which is defined as the percentage of lung area with CT attenuation values <-950 HU at inspiration ($LAA\%_{-950}$), was also automatically computed at a threshold of −950 Hounsfield Unit (HU). The difference in the values between inspiratory and expiratory scans was defined as difference value, the ratio of inspiratory scans to expiratory was defined as relative value. Detailed descriptions of these computerized schemes have been reported elsewhere (22–24), and the segmentation results were shown in **Figure 1**.

Statistical Analysis

We assessed the correlations of IPVV with PFT measures, WT_{3-6}, and $LAA\%_{-950}$ using Pearson or Spearman's rank correlation analysis and multiple linear regression analysis with step-wise selection method for inspiratory and expiratory CT. Continuous data were tested for normality using the Shapiro-Wilk or Kolmogorov-Smirnov test according to the number of subjects. Data meeting the normal distribution were expressed as mean ± SD. Non-normally distributed data were expressed as median (interquartile range). The comparison of IPVV between mild COPD (GOLD stage I and II) and

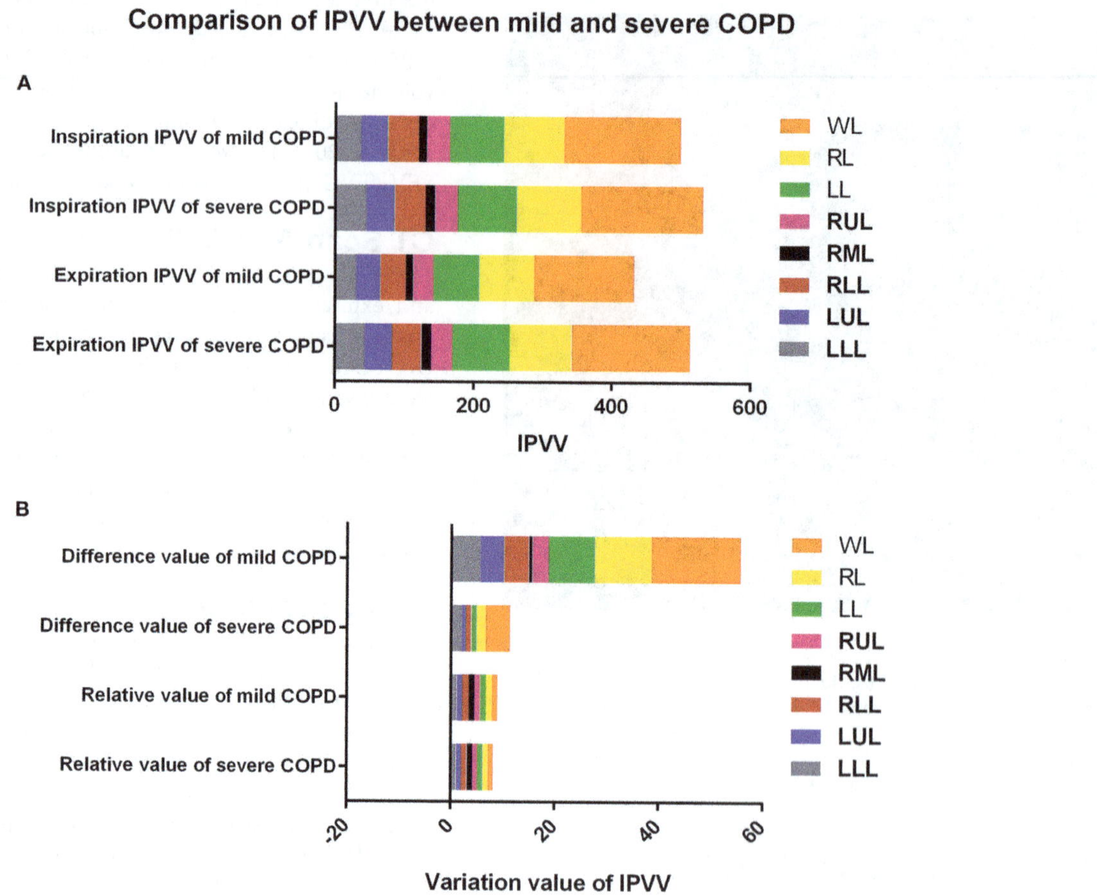

FIGURE 3 | Comparison of IPVV between mild and severe COPD in inspiratory, expiratory CT, difference value and relative value. **(A)** Comparison in inspiratory and expiratory CT; **(B)** Comparison in difference value and relative value.

severe COPD (GOLD stage III and IV) was analyzed using the Student's t-test or Mann-Whitney U-test. Statistical analysis was performed using SPSS 20.0. A p-value < 0.05 was considered statistically significant.

RESULTS

The comparison of IPVV between mild and severe COPD in inspiratory and expiratory CT were summarized in **Table 2** and **Figures 2, 3**. In the subgroup with only expiratory CT examinations, there were significant differences of IPVV between mild and severe COPD groups, except for the right upper lobe (RUL, $p = 0.286$) and left upper lobe (LUL, $p = 0.106$). In contrast, in the subgroup with only inspiratory CT examinations, only the IPVV value in the left lower lobe (LLL, $p = 0.006$) showed a difference regardless COPD severity. The IPVV values of the lower lobes were consistently higher than those of the upper lobes in both inspiratory and expiratory CT scans. For the difference values and relative values, the changes of IPVV in the severe COPD groups were significantly less than the mild.

TABLE 3 | Correlation between IPVV and PFT.

Pulmonary vascular measurement	Spirometry	
	FEV_1/FVC	FEV_1%
Inspiration		
$IPVV_{RUL}$	−0.289 (0.006)	−0.046 (0.666)
$IPVV_{RML}$	−0.280 (0.008)	−0.246 (0.020)
$IPVV_{RLL}$	−0.215 (0.043)	−0.062 (0.562)
$IPVV_{LUL}$	−0.283 (0.007)	−0.094 (0.383)
$IPVV_{LLL}$	−0.292 (0.005)	−0.230 (0.030)
Expiration		
$IPVV_{RUL}$	−0.318 (0.002)	−0.168 (0.117)
$IPVV_{RML}$	−0.346 (0.001)	−0.360 (0.001)
$IPVV_{RLL}$	−0.238 (0.024)	−0.202 (0.057)
$IPVV_{LUL}$	−0.326 (0.002)	−0.243 (0.022)
$IPVV_{LLL}$	−0.292 (0.005)	−0.297 (0.005)
Difference Value		
$IPVV_{RUL}$	0.157 (0.143)	0.393 (<0.001)

(Continued)

TABLE 3 | Continued

Pulmonary vascular measurement	Spirometry	
	FEV_1/FVC	$FEV_1\%$
$IPVV_{RML}$	0.137 (0.202)	0.353 (0.001)
$IPVV_{RLL}$	0.176 (0.099)	0.338 (0.001)
$IPVV_{LUL}$	0.162 (0.130)	0.406 (<0.001)
$IPVV_{LLL}$	0.173 (0.106)	0.311 (0.003)
Relative Value		
$IPVV_{RUL}$	0.200 (0.060)	0.412 (<0.001)
$IPVV_{RML}$	0.211 (0.047)	0.391 (<0.001)
$IPVV_{RLL}$	0.197 (0.064)	0.367 (<0.001)
$IPVV_{LUL}$	0.226 (0.033)	0.444 (<0.001)
$IPVV_{LLL}$	0.228 (0.032)	0.359 (0.001)

FEV_1/FVC, ratio of forced expiratory volume in 1 s to forced vital capacity; FEV_1, percentage predicted forced expiratory volume in 1 s; IPVV, the intrapulmonary vascular volume; All P-values were presented in parentheses.

The correlations between IPVV and PFT measures were presented in **Table 3**. For the inspiratory CT scan, there were mild negative correlations between IPVV and FEV_1/FVC in each individual lobes ($r = -0.215$ to -0.292, all $p < 0.05$), between IPVV and $FEV_1\%$ in right middle lobe (RML, $r = -0.246$, $p = 0.020$) and LLL($r = -0.230$, $p = 0.030$). $LAA\%_{-950}$ ($r = 0.221$ to 0.409, all $p < 0.05$) and WT_{3-6th} ($r = 0.233$ to 0.557, all $p < 0.05$) were significantly associated with IPVV in all lobes (see **Figures 4**, **5** and **Table 4**). In particular, the strongest correlation was consistently observed for right lower lobe (RLL) and LLL. IPVV had no association WA%, except for $WA\%_{4-5th}$ in RML ($r = -0.272, -0.236$, respectively, $p < 0.05$) and $WA\%_{6th}$ in LUL($r = -0.219$, $p = 0.045$).

For expiratory CT scans, FEV_1/FVC ($r = -0.238$ to -0.346, $p < 0.05$) and $FEV_1\%$ ($r = -0.243$ to -0.360, all $p < 0.05$) had a significant, mild-to-moderate negative correlation with IPVV, except for $FEV_1\%$ in RUL and RLL. $LAA\%_{-950}$ and WT_{3-6th} (except for WT_{5-6th} in RML) positively correlated with IPVV (see **Figures 6**, **7** and **Table 4**). Similar to the inspiratory

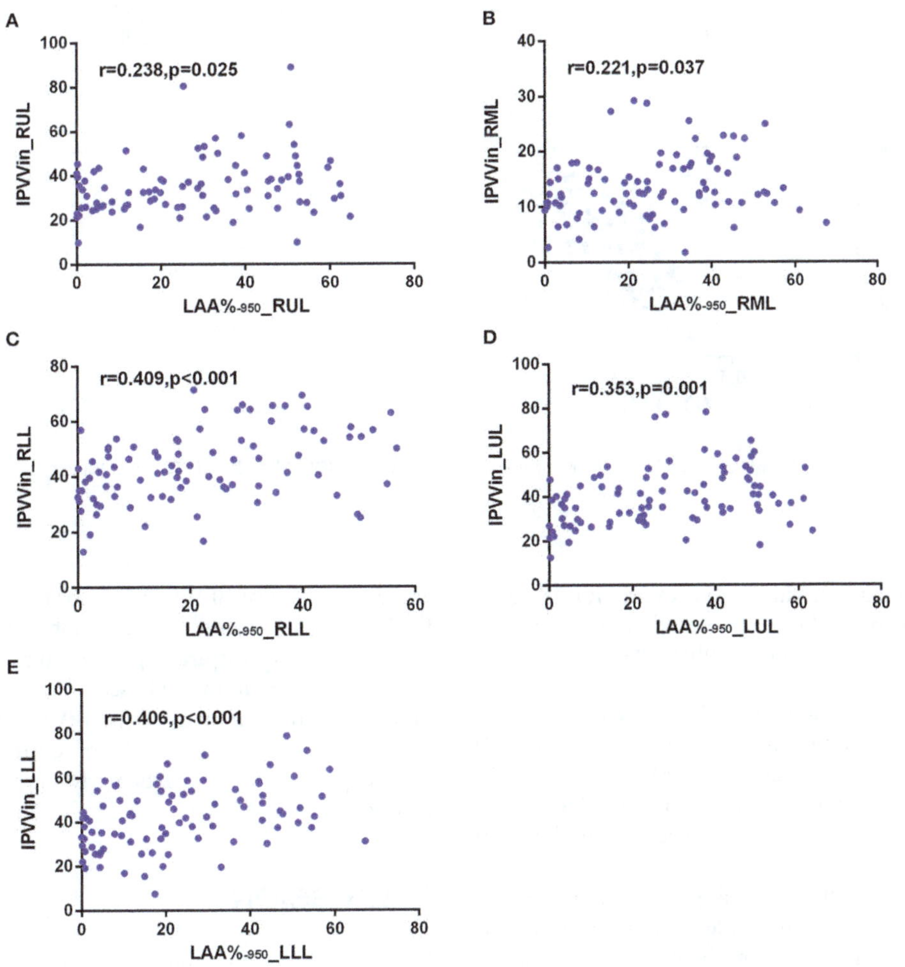

FIGURE 4 | Correlations of IPVV in individual lobes with $LAA\%_{-950}$ in the inspiratory CT scan. **(A)** RUL; **(B)** RML; **(C)** RLL; **(D)** LUL; **(E)** LLL.

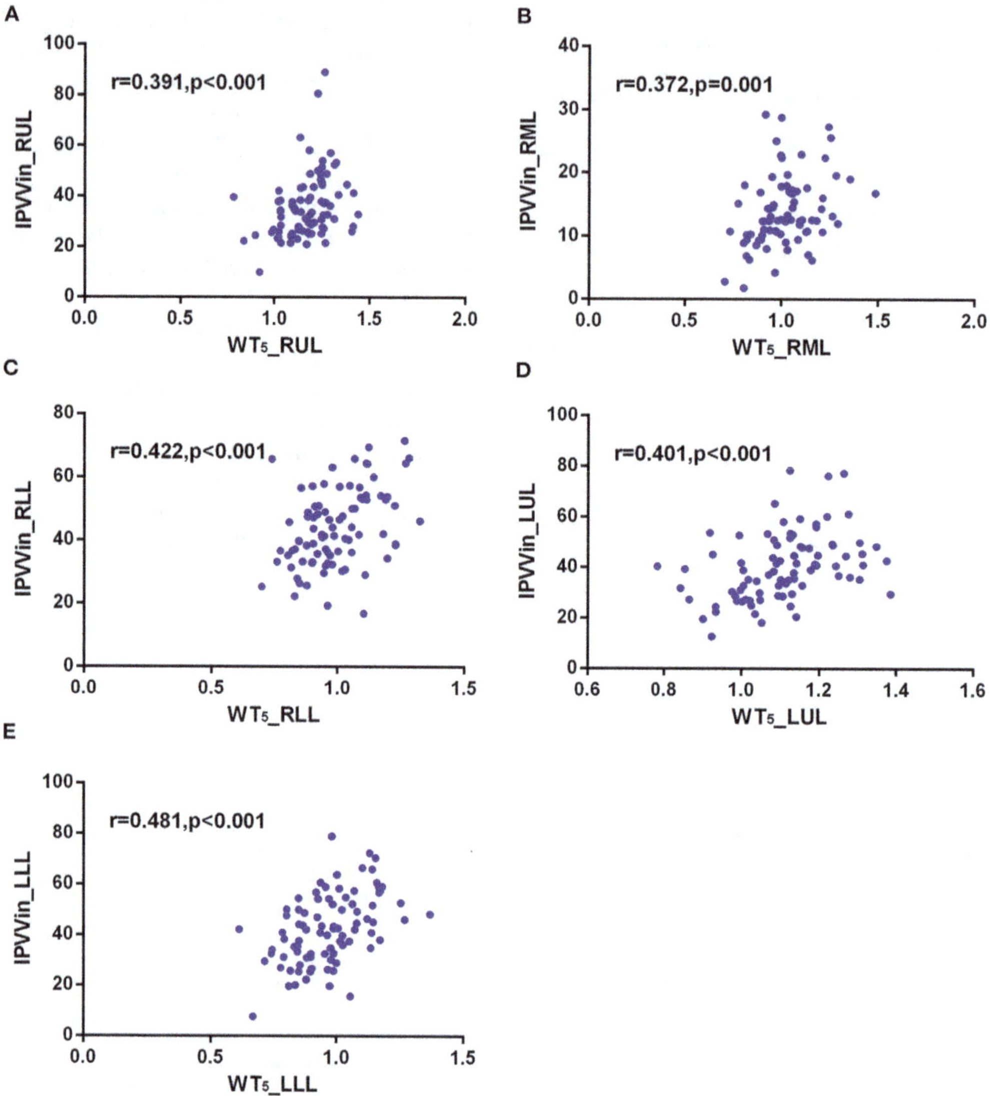

FIGURE 5 | Correlations of IPVV in individual lobes with WT_5 in the inspiratory CT scan. **(A)** RUL; **(B)** RML; **(C)** RLL; **(D)** LUL; **(E)** LLL.

CT, IPVV had no association with WA%, except for $WA\%_{3th}$ ($r = -0.266$, $p = 0.016$) in LLL. The correlation coefficients of the expiratory CT were slightly higher than that of the inspiratory CT.

For the respiratory variation, $FEV_1\%$ showed significant, moderate positive correlations with the difference value and relative value ($r = 0.350$–0.463, all $p < 0.05$), and FEV_1/FVC showed mild positive correlations with the relative value (except for RUL and RLL, $p > 0.05$). There was no correlation between FEV_1/FVC and the difference value.

Table 5 shows the results of multiple linear regression analysis, where IPVV was the dependent variable, age, BMI and other CT parameters were the independent variables. In inspiratory CT, the R^2 values of each pulmonary lobe regression equation were within the range of 0.075–0.426, while the R^2 was 0.165–0.559 in the expiratory, except for RML. The R^2 value of each lobe in the expiratory was higher than the inspiratory. The largest R^2 was observed at LLL in two respiratory phases, while the least is RML. The multiple regression analysis for IPVV revealed that WT was a significant independent predictor of IPVV at the inspiratory and expiratory CT, particularly in difference value and relative value.

DISCUSSION

In this study, we quantified IPVVs depicted on both inspiratory and expiratory CT scans and investigated their associations with pulmonary functions, airway remodeling, and disease severity in

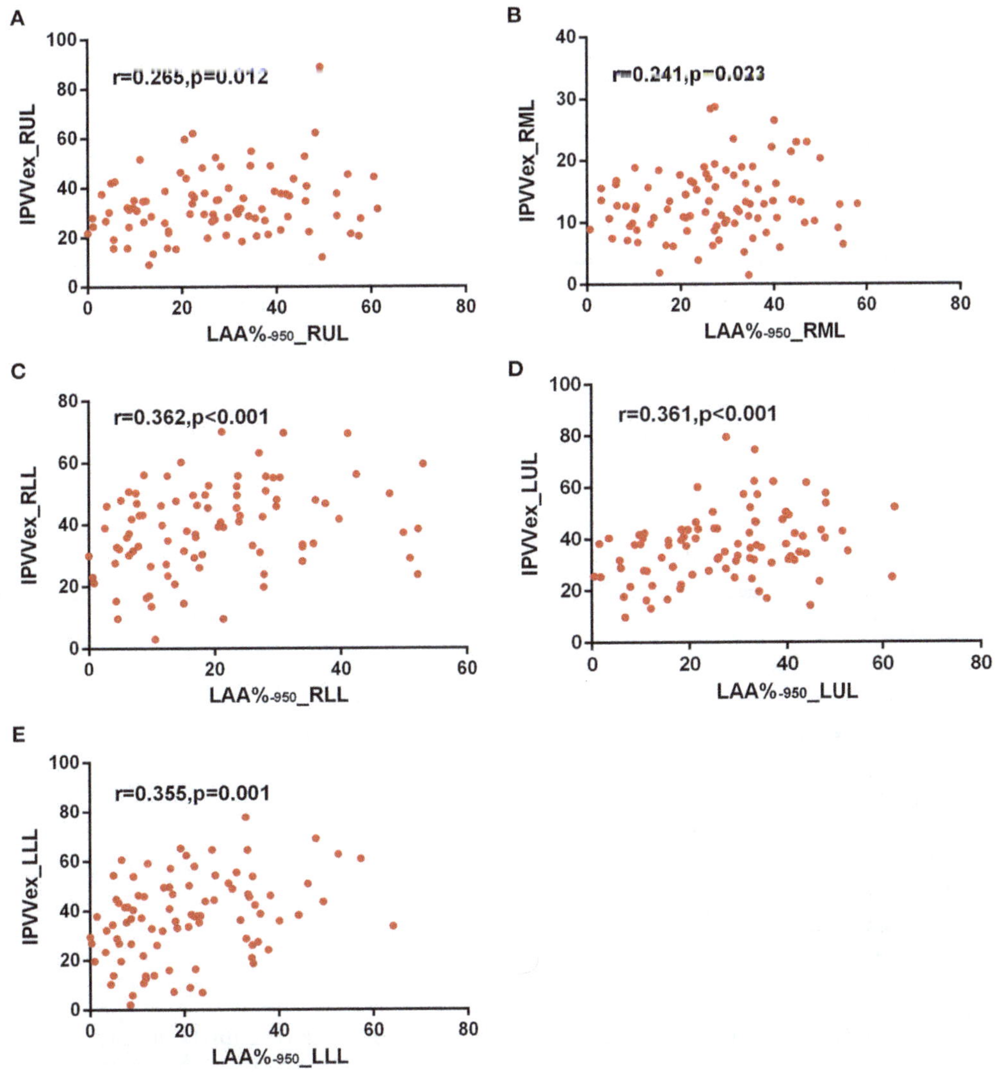

FIGURE 6 | Correlations of IPVV in individual lobes with LAA%$_{-950}$ in the expiratory CT scan. **(A)** RUL; **(B)** RML; **(C)** RLL; **(D)** LUL; **(E)** LLL.

COPD patients. The analyses were performed at the levels of the entire lungs and individual lobes. Our experimental results showed that the IPVV could serve as a quantitative index for pulmonary vascular alternations in COPD patients. In particular, the IPVVs quantified using expiratory CT examinations does not only provide a more reliable and accurate assessment of pulmonary vascular alternations and COPD as well as their progression than the inspiratory CT examinations, but also allows the calculation of the difference and relative value to show the dynamic changes of IPVV during respiration. Additionally, the multiple linear regression analyses showed that bronchial wall thickness had significant correlation with IPVV and suggested that WT might be an independent predictor of pulmonary vascular alteration in COPD.

Our findings are in consistent with Estepar et al.'s investigation (25), where there was no association between COPD severity and total blood vessel volume depicted on inspiratory CT scans. In contrast, in the expiratory CT examinations, the IPVV in severe COPD subgroup were significantly higher than those in the mild COPD subgroup at the levels of in the entire lung and individual lobes except for RUL and LUL. The difference value and relative value between inspiratory and expiratory CT revealed that the alteration of severe COPD was less than the mild. The results demonstrated that pulmonary vascular alternations between breaths decreased with the increase of COPD severity.

Stronger correlations were found between IPVV and PFT in the expiratory CT compared with the inspiratory CT. This finding reinforces the viewpoint about the value of expiratory CT in COPD patients proposed by previous studies (17, 26). Matsuoka et al. (27) reported that the correlation coefficients between airway luminal area measured at expiratory CT and PFT

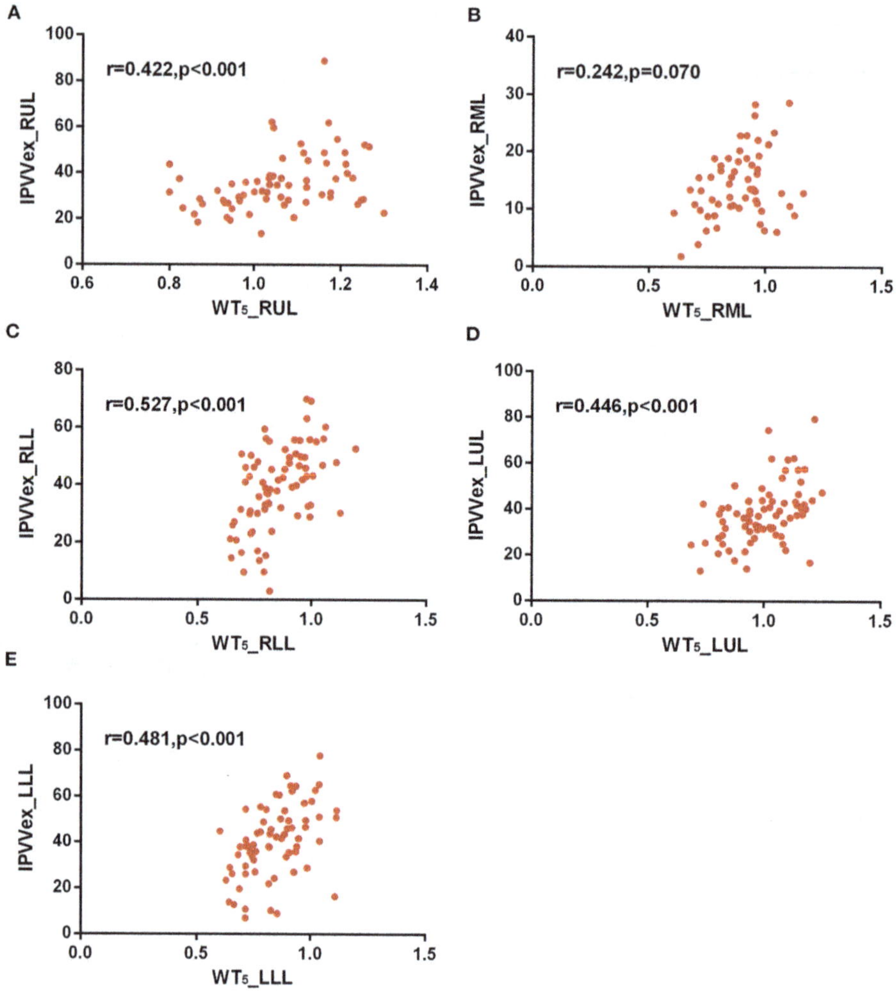

FIGURE 7 | Correlations of IPVV in individual lobes with WT_5 in the expiratory CT scan. **(A)** RUL; **(B)** RML; **(C)** RLL; **(D)** LUL; **(E)** LLL.

TABLE 4 | Correlations between IPVV and other parameters.

Pulmonary vascular measurement	Emphysema index	Airway measurements							
	$LAA\%_{-950}$	$WA\%_3$	$WA\%_4$	$WA\%_5$	$WA\%_6$	WT_3	WT_4	WT_5	WT_6
Inspiration									
$IPVV_{RUL}$	0.238 (0.025)	−0.099 (0.362)	−0.124 (0.256)	−0.062 (0.575)	−0.157 (0.176)	0.233 (0.030)	0.257 (0.017)	0.391 (<0.001)	0.415 (<0.001)
$IPVV_{RML}$	0.221 (0.037)	−0.142 (0.192)	−0.272 (0.013)	−0.236 (0.037)	−0.101 (0.437)	0.280 (0.009)	0.258 (0.019)	0.372 (0.001)	0.257 (0.043)
$IPVV_{RLL}$	0.409 (<0.001)	−0.109 (0.311)	0.045 (0.684)	0.100 (0.364)	0.219 (0.045)	0.448 (<0.001)	0.460 (<0.001)	0.422 (<0.001)	0.557 (<0.001)
$IPVV_{LUL}$	0.353 (0.001)	−0.027 (0.802)	−0.046 (0.678)	0.031 (0.776)	−0.021 (0.852)	0.383 (<0.001)	0.351 (0.001)	0.401 (<0.001)	0.425 (<0.001)
$IPVV_{LLL}$	0.406 (<0.001)	−0.036 (0.745)	0.079 (0.470)	0.181 (0.096)	0.087 (0.434)	0.440 (<0.001)	0.487 (<0.001)	0.481 (<0.001)	0.432 (<0.001)
Expiration									
$IPVV_{RUL}$	0.265 (0.012)	0.137 (0.218)	−0.030 (0.793)	−0.144 (0.248)	0.073 (0.589)	0.370 (0.001)	0.394 (<0.001)	0.422 (<0.001)	0.418 (0.001)
$IPVV_{RML}$	0.241 (0.023)	−0.160 (0.157)	−0.186 (0.124)	−0.167 (0.213)	−0.093 (0.631)	0.308 (0.005)	0.260 (0.030)	0.242 (0.070)	0.256 (0.181)
$IPVV_{RLL}$	0.362 (<0.001)	−0.027 (0.807)	−0.091 (0.425)	0.153 (0.184)	0.158 (0.182)	0.529 (<0.001)	0.383 (<0.001)	0.527 (<0.001)	0.504 (<0.001)
$IPVV_{LUL}$	0.361 (0.001)	0.040 (0.717)	0.088 (0.437)	−0.051 (0.665)	−0.048 (0.718)	0.417 (<0.001)	0.455 (<0.001)	0.446 (<0.001)	0.566 (<0.001)
$IPVV_{LLL}$	0.355 (0.001)	−0.266 (0.016)	0.139 (0.238)	−0.178 (0.140)	0.199 (0.146)	0.474 (<0.001)	0.441 (<0.001)	0.481 (<0.001)	0.535 (<0.001)

IPVV, the intrapulmonary vascular volume; $LAA\%_{-950}$, the percentage of lung area with CT attenuation values<-950HU; WT_{3-6}, airway wall thickness of the 3–6th generations; $WA\%_{3-6}$, the percentage of the airway wall area of the 3–6th generations. All P-values were presented in parentheses.

TABLE 5 | Multiple linear regression analysis of IPVV in inspiratory CT, expiratory CT, difference value and relative value.

Inspiratory IPVV		*β*	**CI**	***P*-value**
RUL (R^2 = 0.160)	BMI	−0.88	(−1.75, −0.02)	0.045
	WT_6	39.86	(14.95, 64.77)	0.002
RML (R^2 = 0.075)	WT_5	10.05	(0.40, 19.69)	0.042
RLL (R^2 = 0.373)	$LAA\%_{-950}$	0.21	(0.06, 0.35)	0.006
	WT_6	46.45	(27.91, 65.00)	<0.001
LUL (R^2 = 0.189)	WT_5	46.80	(24.17, 69.44)	<0.001
LLL (R^2 = 0.426)	Age	−0.38	(−0.66, −0.11)	0.007
	$LAA\%_{-950}$	0.18	(0.04, 0.33)	0.016
	$WA\%_4$	−46.00	(−81.93, −10.07)	0.013
	WT_4	50.17	(30.98, 69.37)	<0.001
Expiratory IPVV		*β*	**CI**	***P*-value**
RUL (R^2 = 0.165)	WT_6	41.22	(15.11, 67.33)	0.003
RLL (R^2 = 0.439)	Age	−0.32	(−0.63, −0.01)	0.045
	$LAA\%_{-950}$	0.29	(0.08, 0.50)	0.007
	$WA\%_4$	−61.44	(−108.07, −14.81)	0.011
	WT_5	67.73	(43.21, 92.24)	<0.001
LUL (R^2 = 0.330)	WT_5	61.69	(37.69, 85.68)	<0.001
LLL (R^2 = 0.559)	Age	−0.50	(−0.83, −0.16)	0.005
	$WA\%_3$	−95.39	(−144.02, −46.75)	0.001
	WT_6	67.83	(41.88, 93.79)	<0.001
	$LAA\%_{-950}$	0.24	(0.04, 0.45)	0.021
Difference Value		*β*	**CI**	***P*-value**
RUL (R^2 = 0.196)	WT_6	18.42	(7.60, 29.24)	0.001
RML (R^2 = 0.174)	WT_3	4.97	(0.30, 9.65)	0.038
RLL (R^2 = 0.247)	WT_5	27.92	(15.73, 40.10)	<0.001
LUL (R^2 = 0.191)	WT_4	14.05	(5.93, 22.17)	0.001
LLL (R^2 = 0.283)	Age	0.22	(0.04, 0.41)	0.017
	WT_4	22.50	(10.71, 34.29)	<0.001
Relative Value		*β*	**CI**	***P*-value**
RUL (R^2 = 0.359)	WT_6	0.39	(0.03, 0.76)	0.035
	$LAA\%_{-950}$	−0.11	(−0.19, −0.04)	0.004
	WT_4	0.40	(0.03, 0.76)	0.035
RML (R^2 = 0.385)	WT_3	0.79	(0.32, 1.26)	0.002
	$WA\%_3$	−0.93	(−1.70, −0.17)	0.019
RLL (R^2 = 0.119)	WT_5	1.54	(0.49, 2.59)	0.005
LUL (R^2 = 0.253)	WT_3	0.49	(0.25, 0.72)	<0.001
LLL (R^2 = 0.311)	WT_5	1.47	(0.79, 2.15)	<0.001
	$WA\%_5$	−1.11	(−1.78, −0.45)	0.002

BMI, body mass index; IPVV, the intrapulmonary vascular volume; $LAA\%_{-950}$, the percentage of lung area with CT attenuation values<-950 HU; WT_{3-6}, airway wall thickness of the 4–6th generations; $WA\%_{3-4}$, the percentage of the airway wall area of the 3–4th generations.

were higher than those for inspiratory CT. Gawlitza et al. (17) demonstrated that quantitative CT parameters of emphysema such as mean lung density and low attenuation volume in expiratory phase show stronger correlation with lung function testing than the inspiratory. Nevertheless, there are few studies on the expiratory CT involving pulmonary blood vessels. Our study not only verified higher correlations in expiratory CT but also found significant correlations between $FEV_1\%$ and the difference, relative values. Compared with the difference value, the relative value may be the better indicator of changes in pulmonary vessels during respiration. From a pathophysiological standpoint, this may be explained by promotion of pulmonary vasoconstriction and remodeling by expiratory state in patients with airflow obstruction (6).

We in particular investigated the association between pulmonary vascular disease and airway disease. Very limited investigations (28) have been conducted in this regard. We found that the airway wall thickness correlated positively with the IPVV on both inspiratory and expiratory CT. Our finding indicated that vascular alteration in COPD was influenced by both emphysema and airway remodeling, and the multiple linear regression analyses of inspiratory, expiratory CT, the difference and relative value showed that the main parameter able to explain pulmonary vascular alteration in patients with COPD was WT, which was similar in part to the result reported by Coste et al. (29). Furthermore, the higher correlations in the expiratory CT demonstrated that the expiratory CT had potential value in quantitative pulmonary vascular disease and evaluating the severity and progress of COPD, compared with the inspiratory CT.

When evaluating the distribution of pulmonary vascular alteration in different lobes, Wrobel et al. (30) quantified the percentage wall thickness to vessel diameter and showed that there was increased pulmonary arterial remodeling in the upper lobes compared with the lower lobes in subjects with COPD. Our results were in consistent with Estepar et al.'s (25) but contradict with Wrobel et al.'s (30) in that the IPVV of the lower lobes was higher than that of the upper lobes. However, this study failed to observe significant difference in IPVV between LUL and LLL. This may be due to the influence of cardiac motion in the left lung, resulting in some errors in IPVV measurement (31) and the limitation of the small datasets. Additional efforts are needed to verify this.

We are aware that the primary limitations with this study is the relatively small dataset for the analyses. There is significant imbalance with the study population in many aspects, such as gender, disease severity, and lung functions. All these along with other potential confounding factors (e.g., image quality and acquisition protocols) could unavoidably lead to some biases in both conclusion and analyses, and this may also be the reason why the correlation coefficient of this study is small. Nevertheless, the findings in this study suggest the unique potential of expiratory CT scans in analyzing pulmonary vascular alternations and the potential association of pulmonary vascular alternations with COPD and other airway diseases.

In conclusion, the quantitative parameter IPVV demonstrated significant associations with PFT, emphysema and airway disease in patients with COPD, the expiratory CT and the relative values showed potential values in quantifying pulmonary vascular alterations and evaluating the severity of COPD. Additionally, the airway wall thickness may be the independent predictor of pulmonary vascular alteration in COPD. Further work is required to clarify and validate the exact value of expiratory CT in quantitative pulmonary vessels in COPD with advanced quantitative technique.

AUTHOR CONTRIBUTIONS

XC, CJ, and YG conceived of the idea. XC conducted statistical analyses. XG, NY, XW, and XH collected the data. XC and XG wrote the manuscript with inputs from all authors. All authors contributed to the article and approved the submitted version.

REFERENCES

1. Vogelmeier CF, Criner GJ, Martinez FJ, Anzueto A, Barnes PJ, Bourbeau J, et al. Global strategy for the diagnosis, management, and prevention of chronic obstructive lung disease 2017 report: GOLD executive summary. *Eur Respir J.* (2017) 49:1700214. doi: 10.1183/13993003.00214-2017
2. Wang C, Xu J, Yang L, Xu Y, Zhang X, Bai C, et al. Prevalence and risk factors of chronic obstructive pulmonary disease in China (the China Pulmonary Health [CPH] study): a national cross-sectional study. *Lancet.* (2018) 391:1706–17. doi: 10.1016/S0140-6736(18)30841-9
3. Chatila WM, Thomashow BM, Minai OA, Criner GJ, Make BJ. Comorbidities in chronic obstructive pulmonary disease. *Proc Am Thorac Soc.* (2008) 5:549–55. doi: 10.1513/pats.200709-148ET
4. Chaouat A, Naeije R, Weitzenblum E. Pulmonary hypertension in COPD. *Eur Respir J.* (2008) 32:1371–85. doi: 10.1183/09031936.00015608
5. Rahaghi FN, Wells JM, Come CE, De La Bruere IA, Bhatt SP, Ross JC, et al. Arterial and venous pulmonary vascular morphology and their relationship to findings in cardiac magnetic resonance imaging in smokers. *J Comput Assist Tomogr.* (2016) 40:948–52. doi: 10.1097/RCT.0000000000000465
6. Rahaghi FN, van Beek EJ, Washko GR. Cardiopulmonary coupling in chronic obstructive pulmonary disease: the role of imaging. *J Thorac Imaging.* (2014) 29:80–91. doi: 10.1097/RTI.0000000000000076
7. Minai OA, Chaouat A, Adnot S. Pulmonary hypertension in COPD: epidemiology, significance, and management: pulmonary vascular disease: the global perspective. *Chest.* (2010) 137:39S–51S. doi: 10.1378/chest.10-0087
8. Matsuura Y, Kawata N, Yanagawa N, Sugiura T, Sakurai Y, Sato M, et al. Quantitative assessment of cross-sectional area of small pulmonary vessels in patients with COPD using inspiratory and expiratory MDCT. *Eur J Radiol.* (2013) 82:1804–10. doi: 10.1016/j.ejrad.2013.05.022
9. Uejima I, Matsuoka S, Yamashiro T, Yagihashi K, Kurihara Y, Nakajima Y. Quantitative computed tomographic measurement of a cross-sectional area of a small pulmonary vessel in nonsmokers without airflow limitation. *Jpn J Radiol.* (2011) 29:251–5. doi: 10.1007/s11604-010-0551-9
10. Washko GR, Coxson HO, O'Donnell DE, Aaron SD. CT imaging of chronic obstructive pulmonary disease: insights, disappointments, and promise. *Lancet Respir Med.* (2017) 5:903–8. doi: 10.1016/S2213-2600(17)30345-4
11. Schroeder JD, McKenzie AS, Zach JA, Wilson CG, Curran-Everett D, Stinson DS, et al. Relationships between airflow obstruction and quantitative CT measurements of emphysema, air trapping, and airways in subjects with and without chronic obstructive pulmonary disease. *Am J Roentgenol.* (2013) 201:W460–70. doi: 10.2214/AJR.12.10102
12. Matsuoka S, Washko GR, Dransfield MT, Yamashiro T, San Jose Estepar R, Diaz A, et al. Quantitative CT measurement of cross-sectional area of small pulmonary vessel in COPD: correlations with emphysema and airflow limitation. *Acad Radiol.* (2010) 17:93–9. doi: 10.1016/j.acra.2009.07.022
13. Cho YH, Lee SM, Seo JB, Kim N, Bae JP, Lee JS, et al. Quantitative assessment of pulmonary vascular alterations in chronic obstructive lung disease: associations with pulmonary function test and survival in the KOLD cohort. *Eur J Radiol.* (2018) 108:276–82. doi: 10.1016/j.ejrad.2018.09.013
14. Wang Z, Chen X, Liu K, Xie W, Wang H, Wei Y, et al. Small pulmonary vascular alteration and acute exacerbations of COPD: quantitative computed tomography analysis. *Int J Chron Obstruct Pulmon Dis.* (2016) 11:1965–71. doi: 10.2147/COPD.S112651
15. Yu N, Wei X, Li Y, Deng L, Jin CW, Guo Y. Computed tomography quantification of pulmonary vessels in chronic obstructive pulmonary disease as identified by 3D automated approach. *Medicine.* (2016) 95:e5095. doi: 10.1097/MD.0000000000005095
16. Akira M, Toyokawa K, Inoue Y, Arai T. Quantitative CT in chronic obstructive pulmonary disease: inspiratory and expiratory assessment. *Am J Roentgenol.* (2009) 192:267–72. doi: 10.2214/AJR.07.3953
17. Gawlitza J, Trinkmann F, Scheffel H, Fischer A, Nance JW, Henzler C. et al. Time to exhale: additional value of expiratory chest CT in chronic obstructive pulmonary disease. *Can Respir J.* (2018) 2018:9493504. doi: 10.1155/2018/9493504
18. Gawlitza J, Haubenreisser H, Henzler T, Akin I, Schonberg S, Borggrefe M, et al. Finding the right spot: where to measure airway parameters in patients with COPD. *Eur J Radiol.* (2018) 104:87–93. doi: 10.1016/j.ejrad.2018.05.003

19. Miller MR, Hankinson J, Brusasco V, Burgos F, Casaburi R, Coates A, et al. Standardisation of spirometry. *Eur Respir J.* (2005) 26:319–38. doi: 10.1183/09031936.05.00034805
20. Yahaba M, Kawata N, Iesato K, Matsuura Y, Sugiura T, Kasai H, et al. The effects of emphysema on airway disease: correlations between multi-detector CT and pulmonary function tests in smokers. *Eur J Radiol.* (2014) 83:1022–8. doi: 10.1016/j.ejrad.2014.03.003
21. Onoe R, Yamashiro T, Handa H, Azagami S, Matsuoka S, Inoue T, et al. 3D-measurement of tracheobronchial angles on inspiratory and expiratory chest CT in COPD: respiratory changes and correlation with airflow limitation. *Int J Chron Obstruct Pulmon Dis.* (2018) 13:2399–407. doi: 10.2147/COPD.S165824
22. Pu J, Roos J, Yi CA, Napel S, Rubin GD, Paik DS. Adaptive border marching algorithm: automatic lung segmentation on chest CT images. *Comput Med Imaging Graph.* (2008) 32:452–62. doi: 10.1016/j.compmedimag.2008.04.005
23. Pu J, Leader JK, Zheng B, Knollmann F, Fuhrman C, Sciurba FC, et al. A computational geometry approach to automated pulmonary fissure segmentation in CT examinations. *IEEE Trans Med Imaging.* (2009) 28:710–9. doi: 10.1109/TMI.2008.2010441
24. Pu J, Zheng B, Leader JK, Fuhrman C, Knollmann F, Klym A, et al. Pulmonary lobe segmentation in CT examinations using implicit surface fitting. *IEEE Trans Med Imaging.* (2009) 28:1986–96. doi: 10.1109/TMI.2009.2027117
25. Estepar RS, Kinney GL, Black-Shinn JL, Bowler RP, Kindlmann GL, Ross JC, et al. Computed tomographic measures of pulmonary vascular morphology in smokers and their clinical implications. *Am J Respir Crit Care Med.* (2013) 188:231–9. doi: 10.1164/rccm.201301-0162OC
26. Lynch DA, Austin JH, Hogg JC, Grenier PA, Kauczor HU, Bankier AA, et al. CT-definable subtypes of chronic obstructive pulmonary disease: a statement of the Fleischner Society. *Radiology.* (2015) 277:192–205. doi: 10.1148/radiol.2015141579
27. Matsuoka S, Kurihara Y, Yagihashi K, Hoshino M, Nakajima Y. Airway dimensions at inspiratory and expiratory multisection CT in chronic obstructive pulmonary disease: correlation with airflow limitation. *Radiology.* (2008) 248:1042–9. doi: 10.1148/radiol.2491071650
28. Dournes G, Laurent F, Coste F, Dromer C, Blanchard E, Picard F, et al. Computed tomographic measurement of airway remodeling and emphysema in advanced chronic obstructive pulmonary disease. Correlation with pulmonary hypertension. *Am J Respir Crit Care Med.* (2015) 191:63–70. doi: 10.1164/rccm.201408-1423OC
29. Coste F, Dournes G, Dromer C, Blanchard E, Freund-Michel V, Girodet PO, et al. CT evaluation of small pulmonary vessels area in patients with COPD with severe pulmonary hypertension. *Thorax.* (2016) 71:830–7. doi: 10.1136/thoraxjnl-2015-207696
30. Wrobel JP, McLean CA, Thompson BR, Stuart-Andrews CR, Paul E, Snell GI, et al. Pulmonary arterial remodeling in chronic obstructive pulmonary disease is lobe dependent. *Pulm Circ.* (2013) 3:665–74. doi: 10.1086/674339
31. Karayama M, Lnui N, Mori K, Kono M, Hozumi H, Suzuki Y, et al. Respiratory impedance is correlated with morphological changes in the lungs on three-dimensional CT in patients with COPD. *Sci Rep.* (2017) 7:41709. doi: 10.1038/srep41709

14

Association Between Air Pollution and Lung Lobar Emphysema in COPD

Nguyen Thanh Tung[1,2†], Shu-Chuan Ho[3†], Yueh-Hsun Lu[4,5], Tzu-Tao Chen[6], Kang-Yun Lee[6,7], Kuan-Yuan Chen[6], Chih-Da Wu[8,9], Kian Fan Chung[10], Han-Pin Kuo[7], Huynh Nguyen Xuan Thao[11], Hoang Ba Dung[2], Tran Phan Chung Thuy[12], Sheng-Ming Wu[6,7], Hsiao-Yun Kou[3], Yueh-Lun Lee[13] and Hsiao-Chi Chuang[3,6,14]*

[1] International Ph.D. Program in Medicine, College of Medicine, Taipei Medical University, Taipei, Taiwan, [2] Otorhinolaryngology Department, Cho Ray Hospital, Ho Chi Minh City, Vietnam, [3] School of Respiratory Therapy, College of Medicine, Taipei Medical University, Taipei, Taiwan, [4] Department of Radiology, Shuang Ho Hospital, Taipei Medical University, New Taipei City, Taiwan, [5] Department of Radiology, School of Medicine, College of Medicine, Taipei Medical University, Taipei, Taiwan, [6] Division of Pulmonary Medicine, Department of Internal Medicine, Shuang Ho Hospital, Taipei Medical University, New Taipei City, Taiwan, [7] Division of Pulmonary Medicine, Department of Internal Medicine, School of Medicine, College of Medicine, Taipei Medical University, Taipei, Taiwan, [8] Department of Geomatics, National Cheng Kung University, Tainan City, Taiwan, [9] National Institute of Environmental Health Sciences, National Health Research Institutes, Miaoli, Taiwan, [10] National Heart and Lung Institute, Imperial College London, London, United Kingdom, [11] Otorhinolaryngology Department, Ho Chi Minh City University of Medicine and Pharmacy, Ho Chi Minh City, Vietnam, [12] Otorhinolaryngology Department, Faculty of Medicine, Vietnam National University Ho Chi Minh City, Ho Chi Minh City, Vietnam, [13] Department of Microbiology and Immunology, School of Medicine, College of Medicine, Taipei Medical University, Taipei, Taiwan, [14] Cell Physiology and Molecular Image Research Center, Wan Fang Hospital, Taipei Medical University, Taipei, Taiwan

***Correspondence:**
Hsiao-Chi Chuang
r92841005@ntu.edu.tw

† These authors have contributed equally to this work and share first authorship

The development of emphysema has been linked to air pollution; however, the association of air pollution with the extent of lobar emphysema remains unclear. This study examined the association of particulate matter <2.5 μm in aerodynamic diameters ($PM_{2.5}$) ($\leq 2.5\,\mu m$), nitrogen dioxide (NO_2), and ozone (O_3) level of exposure with the presence of emphysema in 86 patients with chronic obstructive pulmonary disease (COPD). Exposure to the air pollution estimated using the land-use regression model was associated with lung function, BODE (a body mass index, degree of obstruction, dyspnea severity, and exercise capacity index) quartiles, and emphysema measured as low-attenuation areas on high-resolution CT (HR-CT) lung scans. Using paraseptal emphysema as the reference group, we observed that a 1 ppb increase in O_3 was associated with a 1.798-fold increased crude odds ratio of panlobular emphysema ($p < 0.05$). We observed that $PM_{2.5}$ was associated with BODE quartiles, modified Medical Research Council (mMRC) dyspnea score, and exercise capacity (all $p < 0.05$). We found that $PM_{2.5}$, NO_2, and O_3 were associated with an increased degree of upper lobe emphysema and lower lobe emphysema (all $p < 0.05$). Furthermore, we observed that an increase in $PM_{2.5}$, NO_2, and O_3 was associated with greater increases in upper lobe emphysema than in lower lobe emphysema. In conclusion, exposure to O_3 can be associated with a higher risk of panlobular emphysema than paraseptal emphysema in patients with COPD. Emphysema severity in lung lobes, especially the upper lobes, may be linked to air pollution exposure in COPD.

Keywords: air pollution, BODE, computed tomography, COPD, LAA

DEFINITION

Lobar percent emphysema, the voxel numbers <-950 Hounsfield units (HUs) in a lung lobe field divided by the total voxel numbers in that lung lobe field; centrilobular emphysema, low attenuated areas (LAAs) located within the central portion of the pulmonary lobe; paraseptal emphysema, LAA in the more distal alveoli adjacent to the visceral pleura or interlobular septa; and panlobular emphysema, diffuse LAA that distributes throughout the pulmonary lobe.

INTRODUCTION

Chronic obstructive pulmonary disease (COPD) is an irreversible and progressive respiratory condition. COPD is currently the chronic disease associated with one of the highest mortality in the world, and also ranks fifth worldwide in terms of disease burden (1, 2). In previous studies, air pollution has been associated with increased risk of COPD and reduced lung function (3–6). Specifically, a 5 $\mu g/m^3$ increase in 1-year particulate matter <2.5 μm in aerodynamic diameters ($PM_{2.5}$ concentrations has been associated with 1.52-fold increased odds ratio (OR) of COPD prevalence (95% CI: 1.42–1.62), while a 10 $\mu g/m^3$ increase in 1-year nitrogen dioxide (NO_2) concentrations was associated with 1.12-fold increased OR of COPD prevalence (95% CI: 1.10–1.14) (7). Therefore, air pollution can be considered as a risk factor for the development of COPD by the Chronic Obstructive Lung Disease (GOLD) guideline (8).

The hybrid kriging/land-use regression (LUR) combined two methods (i.e., kriging interpolation and LUR) to detect small-scale variation in air pollution. This model also takes into consideration the local emission sources (i.e., temples and restaurants) to achieve a more accurate prediction of annual NO_2 variability ($R^2 = 0.90$) (9). Another study in Taiwan captured 85% of annual $PM_{2.5}$ variation by using this method (10). Utilizing estimates from the hybrid kriging/LUR, our previous study showed that 0.99 $\mu g/m^3$ increase in $PM_{2.5}$ resulted in 0.011 kg increase in right arm fat mass, whereas 2.45 ppb increase in NO_2 resulted in 0.181 kg decrease in muscle mass ($p < 0.05$) (11).

Lung emphysema is characterized by the destruction of alveolar septal structures and the loss of lung parenchyma (12). Emphysema is categorized into three major subtypes based on its distribution in secondary lung lobules: centrilobular, paraseptal, and panlobular emphysema (13–15). Centrilobular emphysema has been characterized as low attenuated areas (LAAs) in the central portion of the pulmonary lobe, paraseptal emphysema as LAA in the more distal alveoli adjacent to the visceral pleura or interlobular septa, and panlobular as diffuse LAA that distributes throughout the pulmonary lobe (14, 16, 17). Previous studies have reported an association between smoking and increased risk of centrilobular emphysema (14, 18).

Emphysema can be examined quantitatively on high-resolution CT (HRCT) imaging by measuring the LAA of the lung. The percentage of LAA (or percent emphysema) on HRCT scans has been associated with the decrease in lung function in patients with COPD (19). It was reported that cigarette smoke affected emphysema preferentially in the upper lobes (14, 20). Previous studies have demonstrated the association of air pollution with emphysema severity of the total lung (21, 22). However, the link between exposure to air pollution and the degree of emphysema at the lobular level has not been reported. We hypothesized that exposure to air pollution was associated with the emphysema severity at the lung lobular level. Meanwhile, lung function and BODE index [a composite measure of body-mass index (BMI), degree of obstruction, dyspnea severity, and exercise capacity (23)] were considered clinical outcomes related to the severity of COPD and emphysema. Therefore, we examined the association of 1-year exposure to $PM_{2.5}$, NO_2, and ozone (O_3) with the extent of emphysema in different lung lobes of COPD subjects, while also assessing the associations between 1-year exposure to air pollutants with lung function and the degree of incapacity as measured by the BODE index.

MATERIALS AND METHODS

Study Subjects

We conducted a retrospective cross-sectional study in 86 patients with COPD recruited from the COPD clinic of a respiratory department of a hospital in New Taipei, Taiwan. The patients underwent HRCT of the thorax between April 2010 and October 2019. The inclusion criteria in this study were: (1) having been diagnosed with COPD by a post-bronchodilator forced expiratory volume in the first second (FEV_1)/forced vital capacity (FVC) ratio of <70% (1) and (2) being between 40 years old and 90 years old. The smoking statuses of the patients were collected by oral questionnaire. Patients with a known malignancy, progressive inflammatory condition (i.e., bronchiectasis, asthma, or other non-COPD-related diseases), or exacerbation during the 3 months before the study were excluded. The Ethics Committee of the Taipei Medical University-Joint Institutional Review Board approved this study (Approval No. N202003075).

Ambient Air Pollution Exposure

Individual-level exposure to air pollutants ($PM_{2.5}$, NO_2, and O_3) was predicted by a hybrid kriging/LUR approach, which was previously demonstrated (9, 10). Briefly, mean air pollutant data were obtained from Taiwan Environmental Protection Administration (EPA) air quality monitoring stations (https://airtw.epa.gov.tw/). The Environment Resource Database, Point of Interest, Land-use Investigation of Taiwan, Traffic Network Digital Map, Digital Terrain Model, Industrial Development Bureau Database, and Normalized Difference Vegetation Index were included to build the model. The regression model takes into consideration the traffic intensity, weather, population density, industry emissions, elevation, vegetation distribution, the number of temples, and the number of restaurants to calculate residential air pollution levels. Daily $PM_{2.5}$, NO_2, and O_3 levels were then accumulated into 1-year average concentrations. Land-use predictors with a Spearman's correlation coefficient larger than 0.4 with an effect on air pollutants were entered into a stepwise linear regression. Furthermore, to improve the robustness of the LUR model, a set of pollutant levels was created through a leave-one-out kriging interpolation and added to the model. Average individual exposure to air pollution was estimated for 1 year before the HRCT assessment.

Lung Function

Lung function data were collected from each subject retrospectively from the hospital records of the subject. Spirometry was conducted according to the American Thoracic Society/European Respiratory Society guidelines (24). Lung function tests were performed once right before conducting the HRCT.

BODE Index

BODE index, namely, BMI, degree of obstruction, dyspnea severity, and exercise capacity, has proven to be a predictor of COPD mortality and severity (23, 25). Previous studies reported that exposure to air pollution could cause adverse effects on dyspnea and exercise capacity (26, 27). A subgroup of four variables (i.e., the BMI scale, airflow obstruction index, modified Medical Research Council (mMRC) dyspnea scale (28), and the exercise capacity index) is included in the BODE index, which is shown in **Supplementary Table 1**. Airflow obstruction index was defined as the FEV_1 (% predicted). Exercise capacity index was defined as the distance walked in 6 min (meters). The BODE index was categorized into four quartiles: quartile 1 by a score of 0–2; quartile 2 by a score of 3–4; quartile 3 by a score of 5–6; and quartile 4 by a score of 7–10 as previously described (29). Quartile 1 represents the least severity, while quartile 4 represents the most severity.

Emphysema Severity

HRCT scans were acquired at suspended full inspiration. APOLLO version 1.2 software (VIDA Diagnostics, Coralville, IA, USA) was employed to assess the image attenuation on full-lung scans at a single reading center by trained readers without the knowledge of the characteristics of participants. The lung volume was calculated, and all voxels in the lung were identified. The percent emphysema (%LAA) on CT scans was determined as the voxel numbers <-950 Hounsfield units in a lung field divided by the total voxel numbers in that lung field based upon pathological comparisons (30, 31). Emphysema severity was categorized into three levels: level 1 if $1\% \leq \%LAA < 5\%$, level 2 if $5\% \leq \%LAA < 25\%$, and level 3 if $25\% \leq \%LAA < 50\%$.

Statistical Analysis

Tests of normality were used to determine if the data were normally distributed. The extremely low and high values outside percentiles 1 and 99 were replaced by using a winsorization approach to minimize the influence of severe outliers (32). Upper lobe LAA was defined as right upper lobe LAA plus left upper lobe LAA. Lower lobe LAA was defined as right lower lobe LAA plus left lower lobe LAA. We performed a generalized linear model, adjusted for age, sex, BMI, and smoking pack-years, to identify the associations of 1-year air pollution exposure in the five lung lobes with lung function, BODE quartiles, and the percent emphysema in the left upper lobe, left lower lobe, left lung, right upper lobe, right middle lobe, right lower lobe, right lung, upper lobes, lower lobes, and total lung. The beta coefficients (β) were calculated to estimate the contribution of each of the individual variables. Also, the crude OR of outcome variables of predominant centrilobular and panlobular emphysema with the reference group (paraseptal emphysema group) was investigated by a multinomial logistic regression model. To calculate the adjusted OR, we performed the multinomial logistic regression adjusting for age, sex, BMI, and smoking pack-years. SPSS version 22.0.0.0 for Windows statistical software (SPSS Inc., Chicago, IL, USA) was used for data analysis. The value of $p < 0.05$ was set as statistically significant.

RESULTS

Characteristics of the Study Subjects

The baseline characteristics of 86 patients enrolled in our study are summarized in **Table 1**. Overall, the patients had a mean age of 70.4 ± 7.9 years, and 91.9% were men. Their BMI was 23.3 ± 4.4 kg/m^2. About 40.7% of the subjects were current smokers, 51.2% were ex-smokers, and 8.1% were non-smokers. The average smoking pack-years was 50.4 ± 37.9 years. In terms of lung function, the patients had a mean FEV_1 (% predicted) of 56.6 ± 19.8%, an average FEV_1 of 1.3 ± 0.5 L, and FEV_1/FVC ratio of 52.3 ± 10.0%. Mean outcomes were as follows: BODE quartiles (1.8 ± 1.1 points), mean BMI scale (0.3 ± 0.5 points), mean airflow obstruction index (1.3 ± 1.1 points), mean mMRC dyspnea scale (0.7 ± 0.8 points), and mean exercise capacity index (0.7 ± 1.0 points).

Based on HRCT scans, pulmonary emphysema was further classified into different subtypes (i.e., centrilobular, paraseptal, and panlobular emphysema). The percentage of predominant centrilobular, paraseptal, and panlobular emphysema were 66.3, 22.1, and 11.6%, respectively. The mean degree of emphysema in the total lung was 15.6 ± 9.4%. The mean emphysema severity was 2.1 ± 0.5 points.

Air Pollution

One-year mean air pollution levels are depicted in **Table 1**. Levels of 1-year concentrations of $PM_{2.5}$, NO_2, and O_3 to which study subjects were exposed were 28.02 ± 3.38 μg/m^3, 18.20 ± 2.23 ppb, and 24.44 ± 3.31 ppb, respectively.

Association of O_3 With Predominant Panlobular Emphysema

The association of air pollution with emphysema subtypes is shown in **Table 2**. We observed that a 1 ppb increase in O_3 was associated with 1.798-fold increased crude OR of panlobular subtype (95% CI: 1.073, 3.013; $p < 0.05$). After adjusting for age, sex, BMI, and smoking pack-years, 1 ppb increase in O_3 was associated with 1.854-fold increased adjusted OR of panlobular subtype (95% CI: 1.069, 3.216; $p < 0.05$).

Associations of $PM_{2.5}$, NO_2, and O_3 With BODE and Degree of Emphysema

One-year mean air pollution levels and the association of $PM_{2.5}$, NO_2, and O_3 on BODE quartiles and percent emphysema are depicted in **Table 3**. Levels of 1-year concentrations of

TABLE 1 | Demographic characteristics of study subjects.

Characteristics	Mean ± SD
Total	*N* = 86
Age, years	70.4 ± 7.9
Male, % (*n*)	91.9 (79)
Body mass index, kg/m^2	23.3 ± 4.4
Smoking, % (*n*)	
Current	40.7 (35)
Ex-smoker	51.2 (44)
Non-smoker	8.1 (7)
Lung function	
FEV_1, %	56.6 ± 19.8
FEV_1, L	1.3 ± 0.5
FEV_1/FVC, %	52.3 ± 10.0
BODE quartiles, point	1.8 ± 1.1
BMI scale, point	0.3 ± 0.5
Airflow obstruction index, point	1.3 ± 1.1
mMRC dyspnea scale, point	0.7 ± 0.8
Exercise capacity index, point	0.7 ± 1.0
Emphysema subtypes	
Centrilobular, % (*n*)	66.3 (57)
Paraseptal, % (*n*)	22.1 (19)
Panlobular, % (*n*)	11.6 (10)
Percent emphysema	
Left upper lobe LAA, %	17.0 ± 11.7
Left lower lobe LAA, %	14.0 ± 11.1
Left lung LAA, %	15.8 ± 10.8
Right upper lobe LAA, %	16.5 ± 11.2
Right middle lobe LAA, %	17.3 ± 10.4
Right lower lobe LAA, %	13.1 ± 9.1
Right lung LAA, %	15.4 ± 9.0
Upper lung LAA, %	33.5 ± 22.1
Lower lung LAA, %	27.2 ± 18.8
Total lung LAA, %	15.6 ± 9.4
Emphysema severity, point	2.1 ± 0.5
Air pollution	
$PM_{2.5}$, μg/m^3	28.02 ± 3.38
NO_2, ppb	18.20 ± 2.23
O_3, ppb	24.44 ± 3.31

BMI, body mass index; FEV_1, forced expiratory volume in the first second; FVC, forced vital capacity; LAA, low attenuation area; mMRC, modified Medical Research Council.

$PM_{2.5}$, NO_2, and O_3 to which study subjects were exposed were 28.02 ± 3.38 μg/m^3, 18.20 ± 2.23 ppb, and 24.44 ± 3.31 ppb, respectively. After adjusting for age, sex, BMI, and smoking pack-years, we observed significant associations between $PM_{2.5}$ and left upper lobe LAA (β = 1.476), right upper lobe LAA (β = 1.296), left lower lobe LAA (β = 1.293), right middle lobe LAA (β = 1.202), right lower lobe LAA (β = 0.978), and emphysema severity (β = 0.059). Furthermore, we observed significant associations between $PM_{2.5}$ and BODE quartiles, mMRC dyspnea scale, and exercise capacity scale.

Similarly, significant associations were observed between NO_2 and right upper lobe LAA (β = 1.946), left upper lobe LAA (β = 1.434), right lower lobe LAA (β = 0.883), and emphysema severity (β = 0.055).

Meanwhile, we observed significant associations between O_3 and right upper lobe LAA (β = 1.560), left upper lobe LAA (β = 1.492), right middle lobe LAA (β = 1.126), left lower lobe LAA (β = 0.866), right lower lobe LAA (β = 0.860), and emphysema severity (β = 0.044).

Furthermore, we observed that an increase in $PM_{2.5}$, NO_2, and O_3 was associated with greater increases in upper lobe LAA than in lower lobe LAA.

DISCUSSION

We showed an association between O_3 exposure and panlobular emphysema subtype. Importantly, air pollution ($PM_{2.5}$, NO_2, and O_3) was associated with an increased degree of lobar emphysema, especially in the upper lobes. Our results suggest that particulate and gaseous pollution could have distinct impacts on lung lobes emphysema.

The annual $PM_{2.5}$, NO_2, and O_3 levels in our study were following previous studies conducted in Taipei (33, 34). However, the mean $PM_{2.5}$ levels in our study were nearly 3-fold higher than the WHO acceptable upper limit (annual $PM_{2.5}$ of 10 μg/m^3) (35). Meanwhile, the mean O_3 levels in our study were lower than the acceptable upper limit of the United States EPA (annual O_3 of 70 ppb) (36). Using paraseptal emphysema as the reference group, we found that exposure to O_3 was associated with a higher OR of panlobular emphysema. O_3 is formed by the photochemical dissociation of molecular oxygen into two oxygen atoms, followed by a combination between the oxygen atom and the molecular oxygen. Previous studies reported the role of apoptosis of alveolar epithelial cells and endothelial cells in the pathogenesis of emphysema (37–39). O_3-induced oxidative stress could induce the activation of proteases (caspase-3) (40–42). Moreover, a previous *in vivo* study reported that exposure to 2.5 ppm O_3 for 6 weeks resulted in alveolar enlargement and airway wall destruction associated with an increase in matrix metalloproteinase-12 (MMP-12) and caspase-3 (42). It was also reported that interleukin (IL)-13 may modulate O_3-induced neutrophilic inflammation (43). Furthermore, IL-13 could promote alveolar macrophage elastase (MMP-12) upregulation, thus leading to emphysema (44–46). Moreover, previous studies reported that O_3 was diffused in the alveolar periphery (47–49). It is also suggested that panlobular emphysema represents a more advanced phase of emphysema and COPD (14, 50). Together, this suggests that exposure to O_3 can be associated with a higher risk of panlobular emphysema than paraseptal emphysema in patients with COPD. However, the association of O_3 with panlobular emphysema warrants further investigations.

Next, we examined the association between air pollution and BODE quartiles and demonstrated that exposure to $PM_{2.5}$ was associated with the increased BODE quartiles, the mMRC dyspnea scale, and the exercise capacity index. Our findings are

TABLE 2 | Associations [odds ratio (OR)] of centrilobular and panlobular emphysema subtypes with paraseptal emphysema (reference) by 1-year average air pollution concentrations of $PM_{2.5}$, NO_2, and O_3.

Air pollution	Crude OR (95% CI)			Adjusted OR (95% CI)		
	Paraseptal	Centrilobular	Panlobular	Paraseptal	Centrilobular	Panlobular
$PM_{2.5}$, μg/m^3	1	0.937 (0.799, 1.098)	1.151 (0.922, 1.436)	1	0.923 (0.784, 1.087)	1.110 (0.883, 1.395)
NO_2, ppb	1	0.868 (0.683, 1.103)	0.870 (0.613, 1.236)	1	0.865 (0.680, 1.101)	0.850 (0.587, 1.232)
O_3, ppb	1	0.933 (0.788, 1.106)	**1.798 (1.073, 3.013)***	1	0.923 (0.774, 1.100)	**1.854 (1.069, 3.216)***

NO_2, nitrogen dioxide; O_3, ozone; $PM_{2.5}$, particulate matter <2.5 μm in aerodynamic diameters.
Adjusted for age, sex, body mass index, and smoking pack-years.
*Values in bold characters are deemed statistically significant. *$p < 0.05$.*

consistent with previous studies showing that mMRC scores of patients with COPD when the air quality index (AQI) > 100 were higher than when AQI ≤ 100 (27). Moreover, exposure to diesel engine exhaust significantly decreased the exercise capacity compared to exposure to clean air in heart failure patients (26). The results indicate that exposure to air pollution increased the risk of COPD severity. Together, our data further suggested the adverse effects of exposure to $PM_{2.5}$ to the BODE quartiles (i.e., BMI, airflow obstruction, dyspnea, and physical activities) in patients with COPD.

We identified air pollution (i.e., $PM_{2.5}$, NO_2, and O_3) associated with increased percent emphysema of the total lung and emphysema severity. Previous studies showed that air pollutants may penetrate deeply into the lung and destroy the alveolar septa through the excessive reactive oxygen species (ROS) generation (51). It was reported that the ROS played an important role in the apoptosis of alveolar epithelial cells (52–55). ROS was necessary to activate the BCL2-associated X (Bax) protein, leading to cell death (53, 56, 57). Furthermore, the ROS can cause endothelial cell apoptosis (58, 59). Our results are consistent with previous studies (21, 22). Using 1-year average air pollution exposure, a previous study found that 5 μg/m^3 increase in $PM_{2.5}$ and 25 ppb increase in oxides of nitrogen (NO_x) were associated with 0.6 (95% CI: 0.1, 1.2%) and 0.5 (95% CI: 0.1, 0.9%) increase in percent emphysema (21). A cohort study involving 19-year exposure to air pollutants demonstrated that 2 μg/m^3 increase in $PM_{2.5}$, 10 ppb increase in NO_x, and 3 ppb increase in O_3 resulted in 0.11 (95% CI: 0.03, 0.19), 0.06 (95% CI: 0.01, 0.12), and 0.13 (95% CI: 0.03, 0.24) increase in percent emphysema, respectively (22). In a study including 10-year exposure to O_3, 5 ppb increase in O_3 concentration was associated with increased emphysema severity ($\beta = 0.94$; 95% CI: 0.25, 1.64; $p < 0.05$) (60). However, the associations between air pollution and lobar emphysema are still unclear.

Due to the lung anatomy and aerodynamic motion of inhaled particles, we suspect that air pollution (especially particulate pollution) may have different impacts on the lung lobes. Our results further showed that air pollution was associated with lobar emphysema, especially in the upper lobes, by $PM_{2.5}$, NO_2, and O_3. Our previous study found that a 1 μg/m^3 increase in $PM_{2.5}$ deposition in each lung lobe was associated with increases in %LAA (beta coefficient) of the same lung lobe ($p < 0.05$) (61). Because of particle physicochemical characteristics, lung geometric difference, and breathing pattern, the associations between air pollutants with lung lobe percent emphysema could be associated with our findings. In this study, we observed that an increase in $PM_{2.5}$, NO_2, and O_3 was associated with greater increases in upper lobe LAA than in lower lobe LAA. This was consistent with a previous study showing that $PM_{2.5}$ deposition was associated with higher emphysema severity in upper lobes than in lower lobes (61). This suggested that upper lobes might be preferentially impacted by air pollution than lower lobes. Furthermore, smoking-induced emphysema was also commonly observed in the upper lung lobes (13, 18). Smoking was also reported to be associated with centrilobular emphysema, which is mostly observed in upper lobe emphysema (14, 18, 20). The reasons for this upper lobe predominant distribution may include regional differences in lung physiology (i.e., ventilation/perfusion ratio, lymphatic flow, particle clearance, and intrapleural pressure) (13, 62). Although the ventilation predominated in the lower lung lobes, the ratio of ventilation to perfusion was higher in the upper lobes than in the lower lobes, which could favor the pathogenesis of upper lobe emphysema (63, 64). Meanwhile, the decrease in the lymphatic drainage in the upper lobes due to gravity could result in a decline in particle clearance, thus facilitating the development of emphysema (18, 63). Furthermore, the higher mechanical stress and more intrapleural pressures in the upper lung lobes may also result in the high distribution of emphysema in the upper lung lobes (65–67). However, this needs further investigations in future studies. Together, our data suggest that upper lung lobes could be more susceptible to impairment by air pollution.

The limitation of this study included its small sample size because the subjects recruited for this study depended on the number of admissions diagnosed with COPD during the study period. Furthermore, the lack of female representation in our study could be a limitation. The chemical components of $PM_{2.5}$ (i.e., water-soluble ions, heavy metals, and polycyclic aromatic hydrocarbon) were not examined in our study. The effects of indoor pollution should also be clarified in future studies. We observed the associations between air pollution and the extent of emphysema, but the

TABLE 3 | Associations between lung function, BODE quartiles, and percent emphysema (95% CI) with 1-year average air pollution concentrations of $PM_{2.5}$, NO_2, and O_3.

Air pollution	$PM_{2.5}$ β coefficient (95% CI)	NO_2 β coefficient (95% CI)	O_3 β coefficient (95% CI)
Lung function			
FEV_1, %	−0.724 (−1.976, 0.529)	−0.135 (−2.013, 1.742)	0.468 (−0.817, 1.753)
FEV_1, L	−0.022 (−0.053, 0.010)	−0.003 (−0.050, 0.044)	−0.006 (−0.038, 0.027)
FEV_1/FVC, %	−0.358 (−0.995, 0.278)	0.038 (−0.915, 0.992)	0.148 (−0.506, 0.801)
BODE quartiles, point	**0.099 (0.024, 0.175)***	−0.066 (−0.182, 0.050)	0.054 (−0.027, 0.135)
BMI scale, point	0.003 (−0.021, 0.027)	−0.015 (−0.060, 0.031)	0.003 (−0.029, 0.034)
Airflow obstruction, point	0.024 (−0.052, 0.100)	−0.085 (−0.197, 0.026)	0.007 (−0.069, 0.083)
mMRC dyspnea, point	**0.076 (0.023, 0.130)***	0.019 (−0.065, 0.102)	0.017 (−0.043, 0.077)
Exercise capacity, point	**0.083 (0.017, 0.150)***	0.046 (−0.056, 0.148)	0.031 (−0.040, 0.103)
Percent emphysema			
Left upper lobe LAA, %	**1.476 (0.813, 2.139)***	**1.434 (0.387, 2.481)***	**1.492 (0.813, 2.171)***
Left lower lobe LAA, %	**1.293 (0.660, 1.927)***	0.922 (−0.086, 1.929)	**0.866 (0.185, 1.546)***
Left lung LAA, %	**1.414 (0.811, 2.018)***	**1.236 (0.269, 2.203)***	**1.206 (0.568, 1.845)***
Right upper lobe LAA, %	**1.296 (0.665, 1.927)***	**1.946 (1.008, 2.883)***	**1.560 (0.939, 2.180)***
Right middle lobe LAA, %	**1.202 (0.604, 1.800)***	0.687 (−0.269, 1.642)	**1.126 (0.507, 1.746)***
Right lower lobe LAA, %	**0.978 (0.481, 1.474)***	**0.883 (0.106, 1.661)***	**0.860 (0.342, 1.378)***
Right lung LAA, %	**1.138 (0.640, 1.635)***	**1.242 (0.462, 2.021)***	**1.209 (0.705, 1.712)***
Upper lobe LAA, %	**2.772 (1.535, 4.009)***	**3.380 (1.473, 5.286)***	**3.052 (1.812, 4.291)***
Lower lobe LAA, %	**2.271 (1.238, 3.303)***	**1.805 (0.154, 3.455)***	**1.726 (0.621, 2.830)***
Total lung LAA, %	**1.283 (0.769, 1.797)***	**1.282 (0.461, 2.102)***	**1.198 (0.662, 1.735)***
Emphysema severity, point	**0.059 (0.029, 0.089)***	**0.055 (0.008, 0.103)***	**0.044 (0.012, 0.076)***

BMI, body mass index; FEV_1, forced expiratory volume in the first second; FVC, forced vital capacity; LAA, low attenuation area; mMRC, modified Medical Research Council; NO_2, nitrogen dioxide; O_3, ozone; $PM_{2.5}$, particulate matter <2.5 μm in aerodynamic diameters.
Adjusted for age, sex, body mass index, and smoking pack-years.
*Values in bold characters are deemed statistically significant. *$p < 0.05$.*

inflammatory responses and underlying mechanisms need to be investigated in the future. Because the sample size in our study was small, we did not adjust for previous pulmonary infections, alpha-1 antitrypsin levels, and socioeconomic status. These confounding factors should be included in future works. The subjects in our study were exposed to 1-year air pollution concentrations, which could be a limitation. Longitudinal analyses with long-term exposure to air pollution may better clarify these associations with percent emphysema.

CONCLUSIONS

In conclusion, exposure to air pollution was associated with the degree and type of lobar emphysema in COPD. Our findings suggested that exposure to O_3 was preferentially associated with panlobular emphysema than paraseptal emphysema in patients with COPD. Particulate and gaseous pollution may have distinct impact on the lung lobes. Moreover, this study showed an association between air pollution and the degree of emphysema, especially in the upper lobes. Air pollution could be associated with the severity of lobar emphysema in COPD.

AUTHOR CONTRIBUTIONS

H-CC planned the study and designed the experiments. NT and S-CH completed the manuscript. Y-HL, T-TC, K-YL, K-YC, S-MW, and H-YK completed the COPD data collection. C-DW completed the personal exposure assessment. HT, HD, and TT conducted the Multiple-Path Particle Dosimetry (MPPD) model. KC, H-PK, and Y-LL critically revised the manuscript. All authors analyzed and discussed the results, commented on the manuscript, and read and approved the final version of the manuscript for publication.

ACKNOWLEDGMENTS

The authors wish to thank the Department of Radiology in Shuang Ho Hospital for the technical assistance of this research. KC is a Visiting Professor at Taipei Medical University.

REFERENCES

1. Vestbo J, Hurd SS, Agust,í AG, Jones PW, Vogelmeier C, Anzueto A, et al. Global strategy for the diagnosis, management, and prevention of chronic obstructive pulmonary disease. *Am J Respir Crit Care Med.* (2013) 187:347–65. doi: 10.1164/rccm.201204-0596PP
2. May SM, Li JTC. Burden of chronic obstructive pulmonary disease: healthcare costs and beyond. *Allergy Asthma Proc.* (2015) 36:4–10. doi: 10.2500/aap.2015.36.3812
3. Adam M, Schikowski T, Carsin AE, Cai Y, Jacquemin B, Sanchez M, et al. Adult lung function and long-term air pollution exposure. ESCAPE: a multicentre cohort study and meta-analysis. *Euro Res J.* (2015) 45:38–50. doi: 10.1183/09031936.00130014
4. Rice MB, Ljungman PL, Wilker EH, Dorans KS, Gold DR, Schwartz J, et al. Long-term exposure to traffic emissions and fine particulate matter and lung function decline in the framingham heart study. *Am J Respir Crit Care Med.* (2015) 191:656–64. doi: 10.1164/rccm.201410-1875OC
5. De Jong K, Vonk JM, Zijlema WL, Stolk RP, Van Der Plaat DA, Hoek G, et al. Air pollution exposure is associated with restrictive ventilatory patterns. *Euro Res J.* (2016) 48:1221–4. doi: 10.1183/13993003.00556-2016
6. Guo C, Zhang Z, Lau AKH, Lin CQ, Chuang YC, Chan J, et al. Effect of long-term exposure to fine particulate matter on lung function decline and risk of chronic obstructive pulmonary disease in Taiwan: a longitudinal, cohort study. *Lancet Planet Health.* (2018) 2:e114–25. doi: 10.1016/S2542-5196(18)30028-7
7. Doiron D, De Hoogh K, Probst-Hensch N, Fortier I, Cai Y, De Matteis S, et al. Air pollution, lung function and COPD: results from the population-based UK Biobank study. *Euro Res J.* (2019) 54:1802140. doi: 10.1183/13993003.02140-2018
8. Global Initiative for Chronic Obstructive Lung Disease. *Global Strategy for Prevention, Diagnosis and Management of COPD (2020 Report).* Global Initiative for Chronic Obstructive Lung Disease (2020).
9. Chen TH, Hsu YC, Zeng YTC, Su HJ, Chao HJ, Wu C-D, et al. A hybrid kriging/land-use regression model with Asian culture-specific sources to assess NO2 spatial-temporal variations. *Environ Pollut.* (2020) 259:113875. doi: 10.1016/j.envpol.2019.113875
10. Wu CD, Zeng YT, Lung SCC. A hybrid kriging/land-use regression model to assess PM2.5 spatial-temporal variability. *Sci Total Environ.* (2018) 645:1456–64. doi: 10.1016/j.scitotenv.2018.07.073
11. Tung NT, Lee YL, Lin SY, Wu D, Dung HB, Thuy TPC, et al. Associations of ambient air pollution with overnight changes in body composition and sleep-related parameters. *Sci Total Environ.* (2021) 791:148265. doi: 10.1016/j.scitotenv.2021.148265
12. Taraseviciene-Stewart L, Voelkel NF. Molecular pathogenesis of emphysema. *J Clin Invest.* (2008) 118:394–402. doi: 10.1172/JCI31811
13. Takahashi M, Fukuoka J, Nitta N, Takazakura R, Nagatani Y, Murakami Y, et al. Imaging of pulmonary emphysema: a pictorial review. *Int J Chron Obstruct Pulmon Dis.* (2008) 3:193–204. doi: 10.2147/COPD.S2639
14. Smith BM, Austin JHM, Newell, J. D. Jr., D'souza BM, Rozenshtein A, Hoffman EA, et al. Pulmonary emphysema subtypes on computed tomography: the MESA COPD study. *Am J Med.* (2014) 127:94.e97–23. doi: 10.1016/j.amjmed.2013.09.020
15. Lynch DA, Austin JHM, Hogg JC, Grenier PA, Kauczor, H.-U., Bankier AA, et al. CT-definable subtypes of chronic obstructive pulmonary disease: a statement of the fleischner society. *Radiology.* (2015) 277:192–205. doi: 10.1148/radiol.2015141579
16. Hansell DM, Bankier AA, Macmahon H, Mcloud TC, Müller NL, Remy J. Fleischner society: glossary of terms for thoracic imaging. *Radiology.* (2008) 246:697–722. doi: 10.1148/radiol.2462070712
17. Hochhegger B, Dixon S, Screaton N, Silva VCD, Marchiori E, Binukrishnan S, et al. Emphysema and smoking-related lung diseases. *Imaging.* (2008) 20:219–35. doi: 10.1259/imaging/18176184
18. Nemec SF, Bankier AA, Eisenberg RL. Upper lobe-predominant diseases of the lung. *Am J Roentgenol.* (2013) 200:W222–37. doi: 10.2214/AJR.12.9253
19. Mohamed Hoesein FA, Van Rikxoort E, Van Ginneken B, De Jong PA, Prokop M, Lammers JW, et al. Computed tomography-quantified emphysema distribution is associated with lung function decline. *Eur Respir J.* (2012) 40:844–50. doi: 10.1183/09031936.00186311
20. Sousa C, Rodrigues M, Carvalho A, Viamonte B, Cunha R, Guimarães S, et al. Diffuse smoking-related lung diseases: insights from a radiologic-pathologic correlation. *Insights Imaging.* (2019) 10:73. doi: 10.1186/s13244-019-0765-z
21. Adar SD, Kaufman JD, Diez-Roux AV, Hoffman EA, D'souza J, Stukovsky KH, et al. Air pollution and percent emphysema identified by computed tomography in the multi-ethnic study of atherosclerosis. *Environ Health Perspect.* (2015) 123:144–51. doi: 10.1289/ehp.1307951
22. Wang M, Aaron CP, Madrigano J, Hoffman EA, Angelini E, Yang J, et al. Association between long-term exposure to ambient air pollution and change in quantitatively assessed emphysema and lung function. *JAMA.* (2019) 322:546–56. doi: 10.1001/jama.2019.10255
23. Celli BR, Cote CG, Marin JM, Casanova C, Montes De Oca M, Mendez RA, et al. The body-mass index, airflow obstruction, dyspnea, and exercise capacity index in chronic obstructive pulmonary disease. *N Engl J Med.* (2004) 350:1005–12. doi: 10.1056/NEJMoa021322
24. Miller MR, Hankinson J, Brusasco V, Burgos F, Casaburi R, Coates A, et al. Standardisation of spirometry. *Euro Res J.* (2005) 26:319–38. doi: 10.1183/09031936.05.00034805
25. Ong KC, Earnest A, Lu SJ. A multidimensional grading system (BODE index) as predictor of hospitalization for COPD. *Chest.* (2005) 128:3810–6. doi: 10.1378/chest.128.6.3810
26. Vieira JL, Guimaraes GV, De Andre PA, Saldiva PH, Bocchi EA. Effects of reducing exposure to air pollution on submaximal cardiopulmonary test in patients with heart failure: analysis of the randomized, double-blind and controlled FILTER-HF trial. *Int J Cardiol.* (2016) 215:92–7. doi: 10.1016/j.ijcard.2016.04.071
27. Liu PF, Yan P, Zhao DH, Shi WF, Meng S, Liu Y, et al. The effect of environmental factors on the differential expression of miRNAs in patients with chronic obstructive pulmonary disease: a pilot clinical study. *Int J Chron Obstruct Pulmon Dis.* (2018) 13:741–51. doi: 10.2147/COPD.S156865
28. Mahler DA, Wells CK. Evaluation of clinical methods for rating dyspnea. *Chest.* (1988) 93:580–6. doi: 10.1378/chest.93.3.580
29. Li CL, Lin MH, Chen PS, Tsai YC, Shen LS, Kuo HC, et al. Using the BODE index and comorbidities to predict health utilization resources in chronic obstructive pulmonary disease. *Int J Chron Obstruct Pulmon Dis.* (2020) 15:389–95. doi: 10.2147/COPD.S234363
30. Gevenois PA, De Maertelaer V, De Vuyst P, Zanen J, Yernault JC. Comparison of computed density and macroscopic morphometry in pulmonary emphysema. *Am J Respir Crit Care Med.* (1995) 152:653–7. doi: 10.1164/ajrccm.152.2.7633722
31. Hoffman EA, Ahmed FS, Baumhauer H, Budoff M, Carr JJ, Kronmal R, et al. Variation in the percent of emphysema-like lung in a healthy, nonsmoking multiethnic sample. The MESA lung study. *Ann Am Thorac Soc.* (2014) 11:898–907. doi: 10.1513/AnnalsATS.201310-364OC
32. Tsai DH, Riediker M, Wuerzner G, Maillard M, Marques-Vidal P, Paccaud F, et al. Short-term increase in particulate matter blunts nocturnal blood pressure dipping and daytime urinary sodium excretion. *Hypertension.* (2012) 60:1061–9. doi: 10.1161/HYPERTENSIONAHA.112.195370
33. Chen CC, Chiu HF, Yang CY. Air pollution exposure and daily clinical visits for allergic rhinitis in a subtropical city: Taipei, Taiwan. *J Toxicol Environ Health A.* (2016) 79:494–501. doi: 10.1080/15287394.2016.1182002
34. Liu JY, Hsiao TC, Lee KY, Chuang HC, Cheng TJ, Chuang KJ. Association of ultrafine particles with cardiopulmonary health among adult subjects in the urban areas of northern Taiwan. *Sci Total Environ.* (2018) 627:211–5. doi: 10.1016/j.scitotenv.2018.01.218
35. World Health Organization O, Environmental Health T. *WHO Air Quality Guidelines for Particulate Matter, Ozone, Nitrogen Dioxide and Sulfur Dioxide: Global Update 2005: Summary of Risk Assessment.* Geneva: World Health Organization (2006).
36. Epa U. *Overview of EPA's Updates to the Air Quality Standards for Ground-Level Ozone.* (2015). Available online at: https://www.epa.gov/sites/production/files/2015-10/documents/overview_of_2015_rule.pdf
37. Kasahara Y, Tuder RM, Cool CD, Lynch DA, Flores SC, Voelkel NF. Endothelial cell death and decreased expression of vascular endothelial growth factor and vascular endothelial growth factor receptor 2 in emphysema. *Am J Respir Crit Care Med.* (2001) 163:737–44. doi: 10.1164/ajrccm.163.3.2002117
38. Yokohori N, Aoshiba K, Nagai A. Increased levels of cell death and proliferation in alveolar wall cells in patients with pulmonary emphysema. *Chest.* (2004) 125:626–32. doi: 10.1378/chest.125.2.626
39. Imai K, Mercer BA, Schulman LL, Sonett JR, D'armiento JM. Correlation of lung surface area to apoptosis and proliferation in human emphysema. *Eur Respir J.* (2005) 25:250–8. doi: 10.1183/09031936.05.00023704

40. Voynow JA, Fischer BM, Zheng S, Potts EN, Grover AR, Jaiswal AK, et al. NAD(P)H quinone oxidoreductase 1 is essential for ozone-induced oxidative stress in mice and humans. *Am J Respir Cell Mol Biol.* (2009) 41:107–13. doi: 10.1165/rcmb.2008-0381OC
41. Pallepati P, Averill-Bates DA. Mild thermotolerance induced at 40°C protects HeLa cells against activation of death receptor-mediated apoptosis by hydrogen peroxide. *Free Rad Biol Med.* (2011) 50:667–79. doi: 10.1016/j.freeradbiomed.2010.11.022
42. Triantaphyllopoulos K, Hussain F, Pinart M, Zhang M, Li F, Adcock I, et al. A model of chronic inflammation and pulmonary emphysema after multiple ozone exposures in mice. *Am J Physiol Lung Cell Mol Physiol.* (2011) 300:L691–700. doi: 10.1152/ajplung.00252.2010
43. Williams AS, Nath P, Leung, S.-Y., Khorasani N, Mckenzie ANJ. Modulation of ozone-induced airway hyperresponsiveness and inflammation by interleukin-13. *Euro Res J.* (2008) 32:571–8. doi: 10.1183/09031936.00121607
44. Hautamaki RD, Kobayashi DK, Senior RM, Shapiro SD. Requirement for macrophage elastase for cigarette smoke-induced emphysema in mice. *Science.* (1997) 277:2002–4. doi: 10.1126/science.277.5334.2002
45. Zheng T, Zhu Z, Wang Z, Homer RJ, Ma B, Riese J Jr, et al. Inducible targeting of IL-13 to the adult lung causes matrix metalloproteinase- and cathepsin-dependent emphysema. *J Clin Invest.* (2000) 106:1081–93. doi: 10.1172/JCI10458
46. Doyle AD, Mukherjee M, Lesuer WE, Bittner TB, Pasha SM, Frere JJ, et al. Eosinophil-Derived IL-13 promotes emphysema. *Eur Respir J.* (2019) 53:1801291. doi: 10.1183/13993003.01291-2018
47. Gertner A, Bromberger-Barnea B, Traystman R, Berzon D, Menkes H. Responses of the lung periphery to ozone and histamine. *J Appl Physiol Respir Environ Exerc Physiol.* (1983) 54:640–6. doi: 10.1152/jappl.1983.54.3.640
48. Gertner A, Bromberger-Barnea B, Traystman R, Menkes H. Effects of ozone on peripheral lung reactivity. *J Appl Physiol.* (1983) 55:777–84. doi: 10.1152/jappl.1983.55.3.777
49. Möller W, Felten K, Sommerer K, Scheuch G, Meyer G, Meyer P, et al. Deposition, retention, and translocation of ultrafine particles from the central airways and lung periphery. *Am J Respir Crit Care Med.* (2008) 177:426–32. doi: 10.1164/rccm.200602-301OC
50. Sverzellati N, Lynch DA, Pistolesi M, Kauczor HU, Grenier PA, Wilson C, et al. Physiologic and quantitative computed tomography differences between centrilobular and panlobular emphysema in COPD. *Chronic Obstr Pulm Dis.* (2014) 1:125–32. doi: 10.15326/jcopdf.1.1.2014.0114
51. Xing YF, Xu YH, Shi MH, Lian YX. The impact of PM2.5 on the human respiratory system. *J Thorac Dis.* (2016) 8:E69–74. doi: 10.3978/j.issn.2072-1439.2016.01.19
52. Upadhyay D, Panduri V, Ghio A, Kamp DW. Particulate matter induces alveolar epithelial cell DNA damage and apoptosis. *Am J Respir Cell Mol Biol.* (2003) 29:180–7. doi: 10.1165/rcmb.2002-0269OC
53. Buccellato LJ, Tso M, Akinci OI, Chandel NS, Budinger GRS. Reactive oxygen species are required for hyperoxia-induced bax activation and cell death in alveolar epithelial cells*. *J Biol Chem.* (2004) 279:6753–60. doi: 10.1074/jbc.M310145200
54. Kosmider B, Loader JE, Murphy RC, Mason RJ. Apoptosis induced by ozone and oxysterols in human alveolar epithelial cells. *Free Radic Biol Med.* (2010) 48:1513–24. doi: 10.1016/j.freeradbiomed.2010.02.032
55. Chen YW, Yang YT, Hung DZ, Su CC, Chen KL. Paraquat induces lung alveolar epithelial cell apoptosis via Nrf-2-regulated mitochondrial dysfunction and ER stress. *Arch Toxicol.* (2012) 86:1547–58. doi: 10.1007/s00204-012-0873-8
56. Byun JY, Kim MJ, Eum DY, Yoon CH, Seo WD, Park KH, et al. Reactive oxygen species-dependent activation of Bax and poly(ADP-ribose) polymerase-1 is required for mitochondrial cell death induced by triterpenoid pristimerin in human cervical cancer cells. *Mol Pharmacol.* (2009) 76:734–44. doi: 10.1124/mol.109.056259
57. Sobhan PK, Seervi M, Deb L, Varghese S, Soman A, Joseph J, et al. Calpain and reactive oxygen species targets bax for mitochondrial permeabilisation and caspase activation in zerumbone induced apoptosis. *PLoS ONE.* (2013) 8:e59350. doi: 10.1371/journal.pone.0059350
58. Thomashow MA, Shimbo D, Parikh MA, Hoffman EA, Vogel-Claussen J, Hueper K, et al. Endothelial microparticles in mild chronic obstructive pulmonary disease and emphysema. The multi-ethnic study of atherosclerosis chronic obstructive pulmonary disease study. *Am J Res Crit Care Med.* (2013) 188:60–8. doi: 10.1164/rccm.201209-1697OC
59. Redza-Dutordoir M, Averill-Bates DA. Activation of apoptosis signalling pathways by reactive oxygen species. *Biochim Biophys Acta.* (2016) 1863:2977–92. doi: 10.1016/j.bbamcr.2016.09.012
60. Paulin LM, Gassett AJ, Alexis NE, Kirwa K, Kanner RE, Peters S, et al. Association of long-term ambient ozone exposure with respiratory morbidity in smokers. *JAMA Intern Med.* (2020) 180:106–15. doi: 10.1001/jamainternmed.2019.5498
61. Tung NT, Ho SC, Lu YH, Chen T, Lee KY, Chen KY, et al. Higher alveolar deposition of particulate matter in emphysematous lobes of COPD. *ERJ Open Res.* (2021) 7:00324-2021. doi: 10.1183/23120541.00324-2021
62. Gurney JW. Cross-sectional physiology of the lung. *Radiology.* (1991) 178:1–10. doi: 10.1148/radiology.178.1.1984285
63. Gurney JW, Schroeder BA. Upper lobe lung disease: physiologic correlates. Review. *Radiology.* (1988) 167:359–66. doi: 10.1148/radiology.167.2.3282257
64. Petersson J, Glenny RW. Gas exchange and ventilation–perfusion relationships in the lung. *Euro Res J.* (2014) 44:1023–41. doi: 10.1183/09031936.00037014
65. West JB. Distribution of mechanical stress in the lung, a possible factor in localisation of pulmonary disease. *Lancet.* (1971) 1:839–41. doi: 10.1016/S0140-6736(71)91501-7
66. Kononov S, Brewer K, Sakai H, Cavalcante FS, Sabayanagam CR, Ingenito EP, et al. Roles of mechanical forces and collagen failure in the development of elastase-induced emphysema. *Am J Respir Crit Care Med.* (2001) 164:1920–6. doi: 10.1164/ajrccm.164.10.2101083
67. Pellegrino R, Antonelli A. Unfolding the mechanisms of progression of pulmonary emphysema in COPD. *Euro Res J.* (2012) 40:801–3. doi: 10.1183/09031936.00030112

15

Yifei Sanjie Formula Treats Chronic Obstructive Pulmonary Disease by Remodeling Pulmonary Microbiota

Yueying Wu [1,2†], Hui Meng [1†], Bo Qiao [1†], Ning Li [1,2], Qiang Zhang [3], Wenqing Jia [1], Haijing Xing [1], Yuqing Li [1], Jiali Yuan [1] and Zhongshan Yang [1*]*

[1] Yunnan Provincial Key Laboratory of Molecular Biology for Sinomedicine, Kunming, China, [2] First Clinical School of Medicine, Yunnan University of Chinese Medicine, Kunming, China, [3] Basic Medical School, Shanghai University of Chinese Medicine, Shanghai, China

***Correspondence:**
Zhongshan Yang
yangzhongshan@ynutcm.edu.cn
Jiali Yuan
2748132800@qq.com

† These authors have contributed equally to this work and share first authorship

Chronic obstructive pulmonary disease (COPD) is one of the most common pulmonary diseases. Evidence suggests that dysbiosis of pulmonary microbiota leads to the COPD pathological process. Yifei Sanjie Formula (YS) is widely used to treat diseases in respiratory systems, yet little is known about its mechanisms. In the present study, we first established the fingerprint of YS as the background for UHPLC-QTOF-MS. Components were detected, including alkaloids, amino acid derivatives, phenylpropanoids, flavonoids, terpenoids, organic acids, phenols, and the like. The therapeutic effect of YS on COPD was evaluated, and the pulmonary function and ventilatory dysfunction (EF50, TV, and MV) were improved after the administration of YS. Further, the influx of lymphocytes was inhibited in pulmonary parenchyma, accompanied by down-regulation of inflammation cytokines *via* the NLRP3/caspase-1/IL-1β signaling pathway. The severity of pulmonary pathological damage was reversed. Disturbed pulmonary microbiota was discovered to involve an increased relative abundance of *Ralstonia* and *Mycoplasma* and a decreased relative abundance of *Lactobacillus* and *Bacteroides* in COPD animals. However, the subversive effect was shown. The abundance and diversity of pulmonary microflora were remodeled, especially increasing beneficial genua *Lactobacillus* and *Bacteroides*, as well as downregulating pathogenic genua *Ralstonia* and *Mycoplasma* in the YS group. Environmental factor correlation analysis showed that growing pulmonary microbiota was positively correlated with the inflammatory factor, referring to *Ralstonia* and *Mycoplasma*, as well as negatively correlated with the inflammatory factor, referring to *Lactobacillus* and *Bacteroides*. These results suggest that the effects of YS involved remodeling lung microbes and anti-inflammatory signal pathways, revealing that intervention microbiota and an anti-inflammatory may be a potential therapeutic strategy for COPD.

Keywords: chronic obstructive pulmonary disease, pulmonary microbiota, inflammation, Yifei Sanjie Formula, NLRP3/caspase-1/IL-1β signaling pathway

INTRODUCTION

Chronic obstructive pulmonary disease (COPD) is a complex respiratory system disease characterizing continuous respiratory symptoms and airflow limitation followed by a progressive and irreversible decline in lung function. This disease has become the third-most-common life-threatening disease worldwide, leading to substantial social and economic burdens (1, 2). The complex pathogenesis of COPD includes inflammation, oxidative stress, and protease/antiprotease imbalance (3, 4). The inflammatory immune response runs throughout the whole disease process of COPD to reduce inflammation. It is beneficial in delaying the development and improving symptoms of COPD (5). Chronic inflammation in COPD is attributed to the infiltration of various immune cells, macrophages, lymphocytes, neutrophils, and the like, leading to epithelial cell injury and fibrocyte activation to remodel the airway structure (6). The nod-like receptor protein 3 (NLRP3) is known as a potent inducer of inflammation to process Interleukin-1β (IL-1β) and IL-18 (7, 8). NLRP3 inflammasome is essential for the development of COPD in animal or clinical research of human respiratory system samples (9, 10). Activating NLRP3 may be initiate the inflammatory response by binding to cytoplasmic pathogen-associated molecular patterns or damage-associated molecular patterns to aggravate COPD (11). Targeted anti-inflammatory therapy is likely to benefit COPD (12).

In the lungs and airways, there are enormous and complicated microbes that have a profound effect on the host's health, nutrition, and disease progression (13). Microbial community structure and distribution are crucial in maintaining a homeostasis environment (14). Research suggests that bacteria in the respiratory tract resist colonization by foreign pathogens, and cigarette smoking alters the composition of the pulmonary microbiota (15). Pulmonary microbiota dysbiosis is related to inflammation, pathological airway alterations, immune responses, and the aggravation of clinical symptoms in patients with COPD (16). Pathogens stimulate inflammatory cells to produce inflammatory media that often destroy the immune function of the airway and mucosa, leading to chronic inflammation and pulmonary microbiota dysbiosis, further aggravating COPD (17). Undeniably, remodeling pulmonary microbiota structure and proportion is a novel strategy for treating COPD.

Much attention has been paid to the development of Chinese herbal medicines to treat COPD (18). Yifei Sanjie Formula (YS), a traditional Chinese medicine, comprises eight medicinal herbs [*Hedysarum Multijugum Maxim*, *Atractylodes Macrocephala Koidz*, *Saposhnikoviae Radix*, *Sinapis Semen*, *Fritillariae Thunbrgii Bulbus*, *Mori Cortex*, *Curcumae Rhizoma*, and *Panax Notoginseng (Burk.) F. H. Chen Ex C. Chow*] and has been shown to possess extensive pharmacological effects against pulmonary disease, including the reduction of lung injury and inflammatory responses (19, 20). Nevertheless, the pharmacological mechanisms of YS on COPD remain poorly understood. Therefore, we explored the efficacy mechanism of YS on COPD in alleviating lung injury and the ventilatory function and the relationship between the efficacy of YS and pulmonary microflora. We aimed to support YS's efficacy in correcting pulmonary microbiota dysbiosis (**Figure 1**).

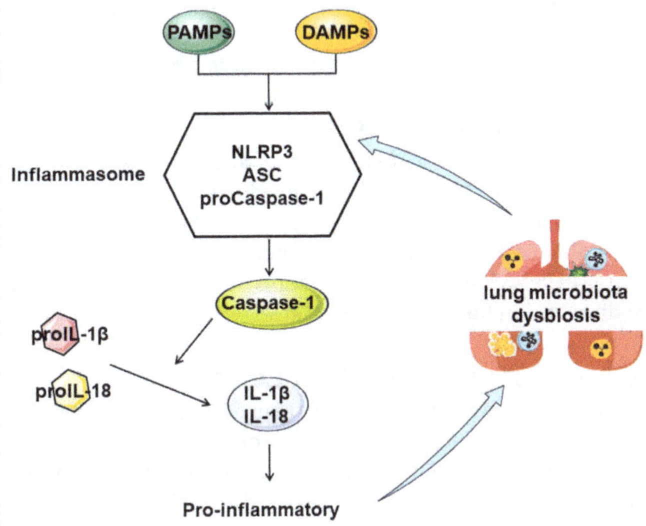

FIGURE 1 | The proposed mechanism by which YS treats COPD.

TABLE 1 | Prescription of YS.

NO.	Chinese Pinyin name	Latin name
1	Huangqi	*Hedysarum Multijugum Maxim*
2	Baizhu	*Atractylodes Macrocephala Koidz*
3	Fangfeng	*Saposhnikoviae Radix*
4	Jiezi	*Sinapis Semen*
5	Zhe Beimu	*Fritillariae Thunbrgii Bulbus*
6	Sang Baipi	*Mori Cortex*
7	Ezhu	*Curcumae Rhizoma*
8	Sanqi	*Panax Notoginseng (Burk.) F. H. Chen Ex C. Chow*

MATERIALS AND METHODS

Groups and Treatments

According to the "Guidelines for the Care and Use of Laboratory Animals" published by the National Institutes of Health, all rat experiments were approved by the Animal Ethics Experiment Committee of Yunnan University of Traditional Chinese Medicine and were conducted following the guidelines of the committee. SPF Wistar rats ($n = 18$; 200 ± 20 g; male) were provided by Chengdu Dossy Experimental Animals Co., Ltd. [Chengdu, China; license No. SCXK (Chuan)−2020-030]. The rats were randomly divided into the control (CT), COPD, and COPD + YS groups. Besides the CT group, the rat COPD model was replicated by using cigarette smoke exposure (Hongyun cigarette, tar 11 mg, nicotine 1.1 mg, CO12 mg) combined with airway instillation of lipopolysaccharide (LPS, Sigma) (21). 11.6 g/kg once per day of YS was administered daily by intragastric administration from days 57 to 84 (the same dosage is used clinically) (**Figure 2A**). Animal weight and behaviorism were monitored regularly and recorded. The composition of YS is shown in **Table 1**.

Pulmonary Function Testing

Pulmonary function testing was performed with a whole-body plethysmograph (EMMS, Alton, Hants, UK) after the experiment was over (12 weeks). According to the whole-body plethysmograph, data for EF50 (Expiratory Flow at 50%), tidal volume (TV), and minute volume (MV) were collected. All of the raw data were obtained from **Supplementary Material S17**.

Histological Evaluation

The upper lobe of the right lung of the rat was fixed with 4% formalin for 48 h and then embedded in paraffin, stained with hematoxylin and eosin (H&E) and Masson. Finally, it was evaluated histopathologically under an optical microscope (OLYMPUS VS200). All of the full scans of the entire original gels are displayed in **Supplementary Materials S1–12**.

Serum Cytokine/Protein Levels

Protein was extracted from lung tissue. Protein quantification was performed using the BCA protein quantification kit (P0012, Beyotime, Jiangsu, China) to calculate loading capacity. Samples were added to a precast SDS polyacrylamide gel for electrophoretic separation, and proteins in the gel were electrotransferred to a PVDF membrane using water bath electroblotting. The primary antibodies were added, anti-TGF-β1 (rabbit polyclonal antibody, Abcam, ab179695) and anti-NLRP3 (rabbit polyclonal antibody, Bioss, bs-10021R), overnight at 4°C. After washing the membrane, a secondary antibody was added, shook at 4°C, and incubated for 1 h. PVDF was dropped, and ECL luminescence liquid was developed and photographed (GeneGnome). The grayscale values of individual bands were analyzed using gene tools software. All of the full scans of the entire original gels are displayed in S13 to S16. ELISA kit (Jiangsu Enzyme-Linked Biotechnology Co., Ltd.) was used to detect the concentration of TNF-α and IL-6 in serum and the concentration of IL-1β, IL-18, and SIgA in the lung. The method and procedure were completed according to the kit operating instructions. Finally, read the absorbance at 450 nm after adding the stop solution within 15 min. All of the raw data were obtained from **Supplementary Material S17**.

16S rRNA Gene High-Throughput Sequencing to Detect the Pulmonary Microbiota

The total genome DNA from samples of the pulmonary microbiota was extracted using the CTAB/SDS method. DNA concentration and purity were monitored on 1% agarose gels. According to the concentration, DNA was diluted to 1 ng/μL using sterile water. 16S rRNA genes of distinct regions (16S V4/16S V3/16S V3-V4) were amplified using a specific primer (16S V4:515F-806R) with the barcode. PCR products were mixed in equidensity ratios. Then, the mixture of PCR products was purified with Qiagen Gel Extraction Kit (Qiagen, Germany). Sequencing libraries were generated using TruSeq® DNA PCR-Free Sample Preparation Kit (Illumina, USA) following the manufacturer's recommendations, and index codes were added. The library quality was assessed on the Qubit@ 2.0 Fluorometer (Thermo Scientific) and AgilentBioanalyzer 2100 system. Finally, the library was sequenced on an Illumina NovaSeq platform, and 250 bp paired-end reads were generated. The data on pulmonary microbiota were obtained from the online tool-NovoMagic at https://magic.novogene.com *via* a personal account. All of the raw data were obtained from **Supplementary Material S17**.

UHPLC-QE-MS to Screen the Components of YS

We used UHPLC-QE-MS to detect and analyze the potential active components of YS to exert its medicinal effect and further clarify the components of YS. LC-MS/MS analysis was performed on a UHPLC system (Vanquish, Thermo Fisher Scientific) with a Waters UPLC BEH C18 column (1.7 μm 2.1 *100 mm). The flow rate was set at 0.4 mL/min, and the sample injection volume was set at 5 μL. The mobile phase consisted of 0.1% formic acid in water (A) and 0.1% formic acid in acetonitrile (B). The multi-step linear elution gradient program was as follows: 0–3.5 min, 95–85% A; 3.5–6 min, 85–70% A; 6–6.5 min, 70–70% A; 6.5–12 min, 70–30% A; 12–12.5 min, 30–30% A; 12.5–18 min, 30–0% A; 18–25 min, 0–0% A; 25–26 min, 0–95% A; 26–30 min, 95–95% A.

An Orbitrap Exploris 120 mass spectrometer coupled with an Xcalibur software was employed to obtain the MS and MS/MS data based on the IDA acquisition mode. During each acquisition cycle, the mass range was from 100 to 1,500, and the top four of every cycle were screened. The corresponding MS/MS data were further acquired. Sheath gas flow rate: 30 Arb, Aux gas flow rate: 10 Arb, Ion Transfer Tube Temp: 350°C, Vaporizer Temp: 350°C, Full ms resolution: 60,000, MS/MS resolution: 15,000, Collision energy: 16/38/42 in NCE mode, Spray Voltage: 5.5 kV (positive) or−4 kV (negative).

Statistical Analysis

Data were expressed as means ± standard deviation ($\bar{x}$ ±s). The normal distribution of the data was assessed with the Shapiro-Wilk test. Depending on the data normality distribution, significant differences in the variance of parameters were evaluated either with ANOVA or the Kruskal-Wallis test in SPSS 22.0. All statistical tests were two-sided, and a P-value of < 0.05, or FDR adjusted $Padj$ value < 0.05 was considered statistically significant. The analysis of pulmonary microbiota was performed using the online tool-NovoMagic at https://magic.novogene.com *via* a personal account. All raw data were obtained from S17 and the file of statistical programs (original).

RESULTS

YS Improved Pulmonary Function in COPD Rats

The pulmonary function is an important index in evaluating COPD, including TV, MV, and EF50, reflecting a small airway obstruction. Studies found that COPD patients had decreased TV and MV. Our data showed that EF50, TV, and MV were significantly lower in COPD rats ($P < 0.05$), while EF50, TV, and MV were higher after YS intervention ($P < 0.05$) (**Figures 2C–E**). COPD rats exhibited hair withering, slow action, and shortness of breath. There were significant improvements in animal behaviors after treatment with YS. The body weights of COPD rats significantly decreased ($P < 0.05$). And, the body weights in the YS+ COPD group significantly increased ($P < 0.05$) (**Figure 2B**).

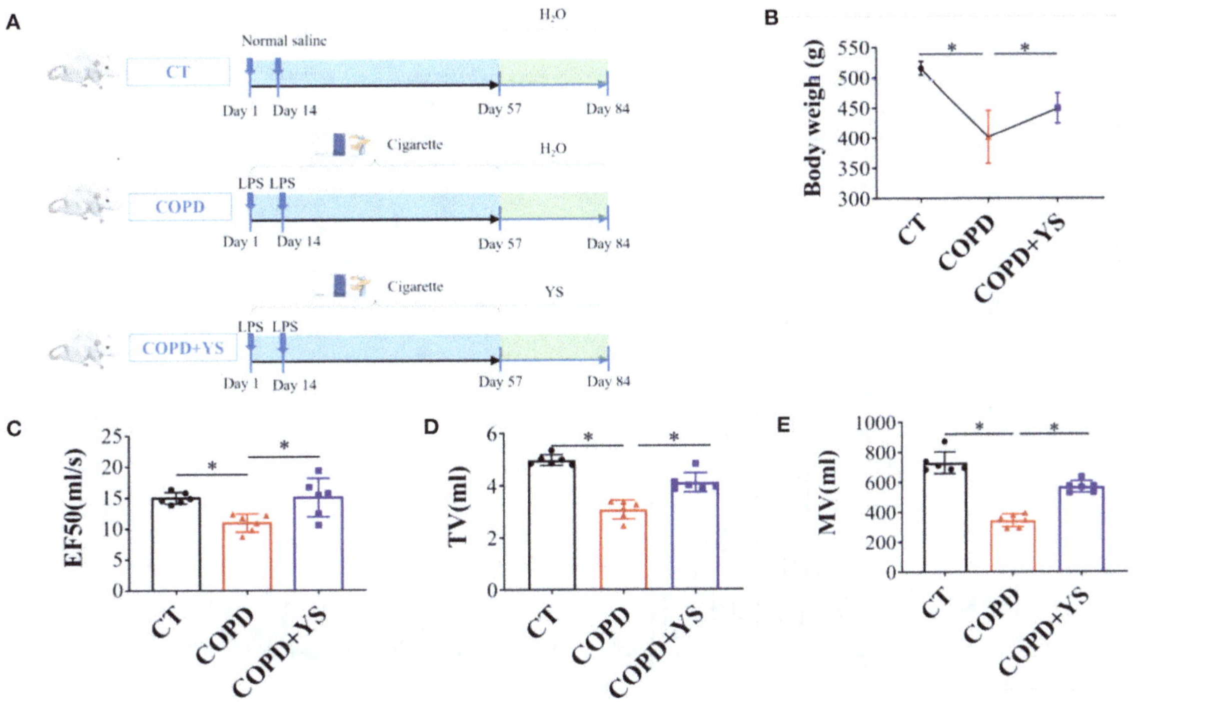

FIGURE 2 | (A) Timeline diagrams of the experimental design ($n = 6$). **(B)** Body weight of the three groups including CT, COPD, and COPD + YS ($n = 6$). **(C)** EF50 of CT, COPD, and COPD + YS ($n = 6$). **(D)** TV of CT, COPD and COPD + YS ($n = 6$). **(E)** MV of CT, COPD and COPD+ YS ($n = 6$). The data are presented as the means ± SEM of three experiments (*$P < 0.05$).

These findings suggest that YS improves animal behaviors and pulmonary ventilatory functions in COPD rats.

Screening Components of YS With UHPLC-QTOF-MS

YS is a Chinese herbal medicine formula. It is composed of *Hedysarum Multijugum Maxim, Atractylodes macrocephala Koidz, Saposhnikoviae Radix, Sinapis Semen, Fritillaria Thunbrgii Bulbus, Mori Cortex, Curcumae Rhizoma* and *Panax Notoginseng (Burk.) F. H. Chen Ex C. Chow.* We performed UHPLC-QTOF-MS to screen for the components of YS. We established the fingerprint of YS as the background for UHPLC-QTOF-MS, including the positive ion mode and negative ion mode. We analyzed the top 20 components by peak areas with the main peaks separated (**Figures 3A,B**). Among these, eight kinds of components were detected, including alkaloids, amino acid derivatives, carbohydrates and their derivatives, carboxylic acids and their derivatives, phenylpropanoids, flavonoids, terpenoids, organic acids and their derivatives, phenols, and aliphatic acyl based on a comparison with standard materials (**Table 2**). The main active products may be one or more of these components.

YS Improved Immune Function in COPD Rats

The spleen and thymus are critical immune organs, and their organ indexes reflect the strength of immune function to a certain extent (22). Our results showed that the thymus index and spleen index were decreased significantly in COPD rats ($P < 0.05$); after being treated with YS, the thymus and spleen indexes significantly increased ($P < 0.05$) (**Figures 4A,B**). SIgA is a major effector molecule of the mucosal immune defense system against the colonization and adhesion of pathogenic microorganisms on mucosal surfaces (23). Local SIgA deficiency on small airway surfaces is associated with COPD progression (24). In this present study, the SIgA was decreased in COPD rats ($P < 0.05$), whereas the SIgA in the COPD + YS group was significantly increased ($P < 0.05$) (**Figure 4C**). These data suggest that YS could enhance the local mucosal immunity and improve immune function in COPD rats.

YS Ameliorated Inflammation in COPD Rats

The inflammatory response of COPD primarily involves neutrophil infiltration. TNF-α activates neutrophils, and IL-6 inhibits apoptosis (25). HE staining showed that substantial amounts of neutrophil infiltration plugged the bronchi. The lumens were significantly narrowed, and the alveolar walls became thinner and fused in COPD rats. There were fewer pathological changes in the YS intervention group (**Figure 5A**). Masson staining exhibited that much collagen fiber deposition occurred around the trachea and pulmonary interstitium in COPD rats. Collagen deposition was less severe in COPD+YS rats than in COPD rats (**Figure 5B**). The levels of TNF-α and

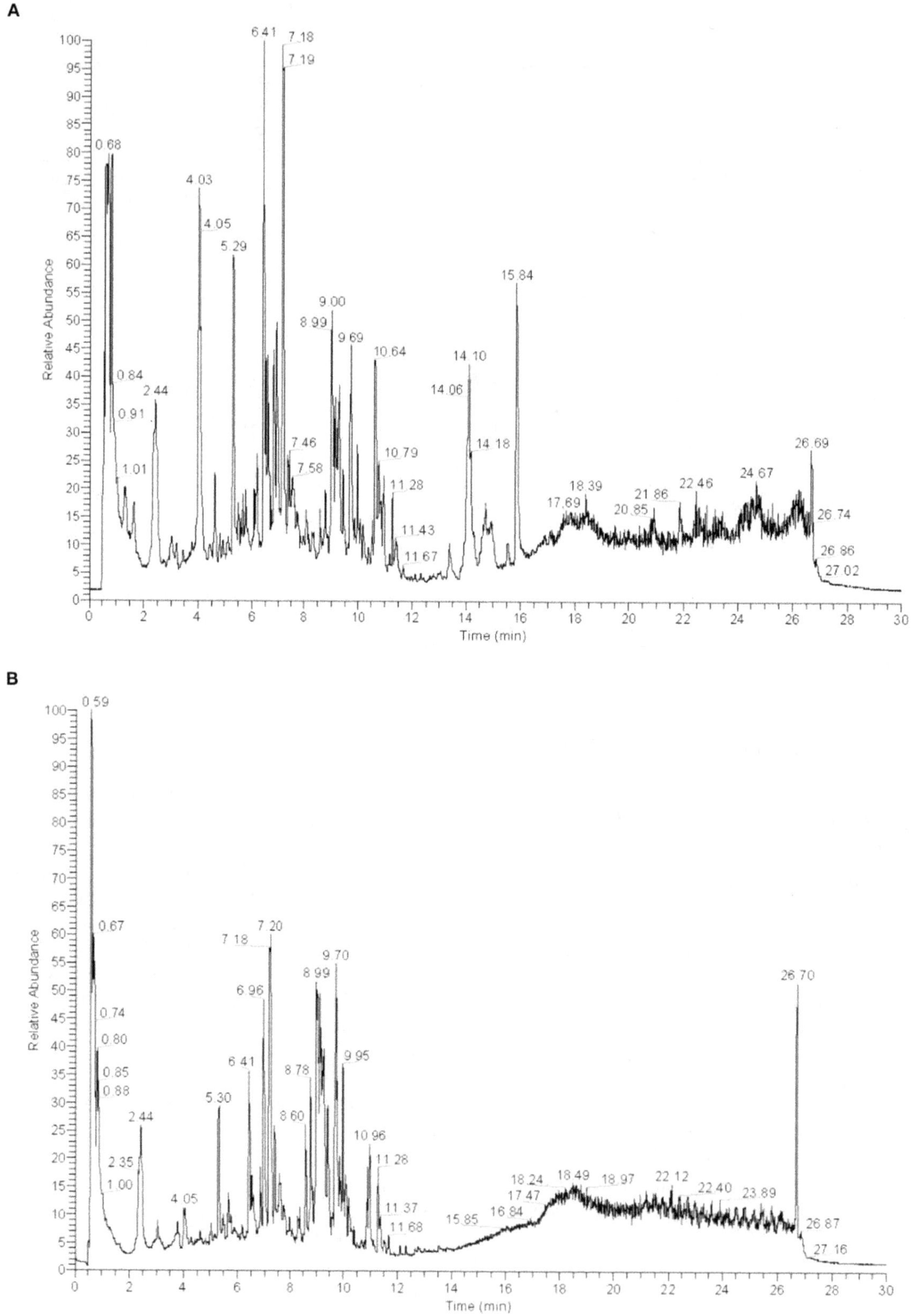

FIGURE 3 | (A) UHPLC-QTOF-MS analysis base peak intensity chromatograms of YS in positive mode. **(B)** UHPLC-QTOF-MS analysis base peak intensity chromatograms of YS in negative mode.

TABLE 2 | Screening the top 20 components of YS with UHPLC-QTOF-MS.

No.	Components	CompositeScore	Class	Electric	Rtmed(s)	Peak area
1	4-Hydroxybenzoylcholine	0.831	Alkaloid	+H	98.380	4E+09
2	Arginine	0.984	Amino acid derivatives	+H	36.876	2.8E+09
3	4-Amino-2-methylenebutanoic acid	0.998	Others	+H	41.834	2.7E+09
4	SUCROSE	0.688	Carbohydrates and derivatives	-H	38.728	2E+09
5	Citric acid	0.990	Carboxylic acids and derivatives	-H	44.239	1.8E+09
6	Adenosine	1.000	Alkaloid	+H	48.666	1.6E+09
7	p-Coumaric acid	1.000	Phenylpropanoids	+H	98.380	1.5E+09
8	Phenylalanine	0.976	Amino acid derivatives	+H	80.181	1.5E+09
9	Prunetin	0.987	Flavonoids	+H	454.896	1.3E+09
10	Biochanin-7-O-glucoside	0.911	Flavonoids	+H	339.706	1.2E+09
11	Isoleucine	0.967	Amino acid derivatives	+H	55.474	1.2E+09
12	Ginsenoside F1	0.860	Terpenoids	-H	556.663	1.E+09
13	N2-Fructopyranosylarginine	1.000	Others	+H	36.630	8.1E+08
14	2-Chloro-DL-Phenylalanine	1.000	Internal standards	+H	150.892	8E+08
15	Tectochrysin	0.972	Flavonoids	+H	559.658	6.1E+08
16	Acacetin	0.990	Flavonoids	-H	390.813	5.5E+08
17	O-Methylcorypalline	0.969	Alkaloid	+H	207.566	5.4E+08
18	Ginsenoside Re	0.958	Terpenoids	-H	429.754	5.3E+08
19	Formononetin-7-O-glucoside	0.610	Flavonoids	+H	429.358	4.9E+08
20	D-Gluconic acid	0.958	Organic acids and derivatives	-H	38.028	4.5E+08
21	Curdione	0.986	Terpenoids	+H	671.712	4.1E+08
22	3-Hydroxy-5-isopropylidene-3,8-dimethyl-2,3,3a,4,5,8a-hexahydro-6(1H)-azulenone	0.987	Terpenoids	+H	403.394	4.1E+08
23	8-(2-hydroxy-1-methoxy-3-methylbut-3-enyl)-7-methoxychromen-2-one	0.922	Phenylpropanoids	+H	446.978	4E+08
24	Formononetine	0.999	Flavonoids	-H	560.193	3.5E+08
25	Ginsenoside Rf	0.991	Terpenoids	-H	528.602	3.2E+08
26	ADENOSINE 3′,5′-CYCLIC MONOPHOSPHATE	0.900	Alkaloid	+H	44.421	3.1E+08
27	Adenine	1.000	Alkaloid	+H	48.666	3E+08
28	p-Hydroxybenzyl glucosinolate	0.638	Others	-H	43.373	2.9E+08
29	3,4,5-trimethoxycinnamic acid	0.952	Phenylpropanoids	+H	146.417	2.7E+08
30	2-AMINO-2-METHYLPROPANOATE	0.633	Organic acids and derivatives	-H	146.038	2E+08
31	5-OXO-D-PROLINE	0.978	Amino acid derivatives	-H	48.733	1.8E+08
32	Salicylic acid	0.978	Phenols	-H	384.737	1.8E+08
33	MANNITOL	0.991	Others	-H	38.283	1.7E+08
34	Formononetin-7-O-glucoside	0.645	Flavonoids	-H	428.785	1.3E+08
35	Glutaric acid	0.967	Organic acids and derivatives	-H	89.709	1.2E+08
36	L-ASPARAGINE	0.963	Amino acid derivatives	-H	34.140	1.2E+08
37	Inositol	0.789	Others	-H	38.473	1.1E+08
38	2-METHYLMALEATE	0.968	Aliphatic acyl	-H	61.769	9.1E+07
39	Sativanone	0.684	Others	-H	485.593	8.5E+07
40	Azuleno(5,6-c)furan-1(3H)-one, 4,4a,5,6,7,7a,8,9-octahydro-3,4,8-trihydroxy-6,6,8-trimethyl	0.720	Terpenoids	-H	217.031	7.8E+07

IL-6 were significantly higher in the serum of COPD rats ($P < 0.05$) with YS intervention (**Figures 5C,D**). TGF-β1 is a powerful profibrotic cytokine that participates in inflammatory repair (26). The expression of TGF-β1 was significantly elevated in lung tissue of COPD rats ($P < 0.05$). TGF-β1 in the COPD + YS groupwas significantly lower ($P < 0.05$) (**Figure 5E**). These findings suggest that YS ameliorates lung tissue damage *via* attenuating inflammatory responses and reducing collagen deposition in COPD rats.

YS Reduced NLRP3/Caspase-1/IL-1β Signaling Expression in COPD Rats

NLRP3 promotes the release of downstream inflammatory cytokines, inducing acute and chronic inflammatory responses. When NLRP3 is overactivated, ASC acts as an adaptor protein to recruit the precursor caspase-1, promotes IL-1β and IL-18 secreted outside the cell, and exerts proinflammatory effects (27). Compared with control, the protein levels of NLRP3 were significantly greater in lung tissues of COPD rats ($P < 0.05$).

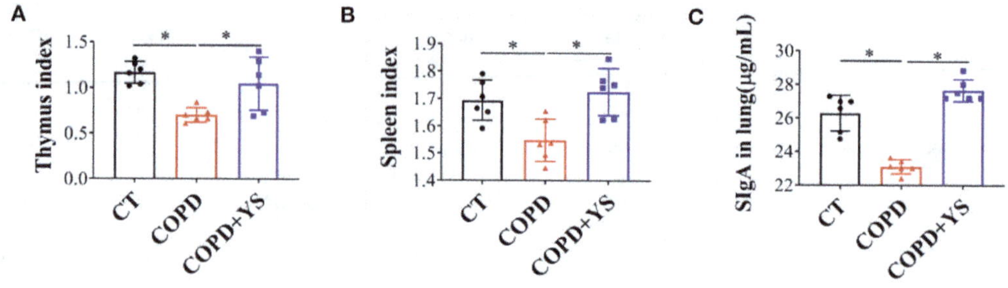

FIGURE 4 | (A) Thymus index of CT, COPD, and COPD + YS ($n = 6$). **(B)** Spleen index of CT, COPD, and COPD + YS($n = 6$). **(C)** The SIgA in the lung of CT, COPD, and COPD + YS ($n = 6$). The data are presented as the means ± SEM of three experiments (*$P < 0.05$).

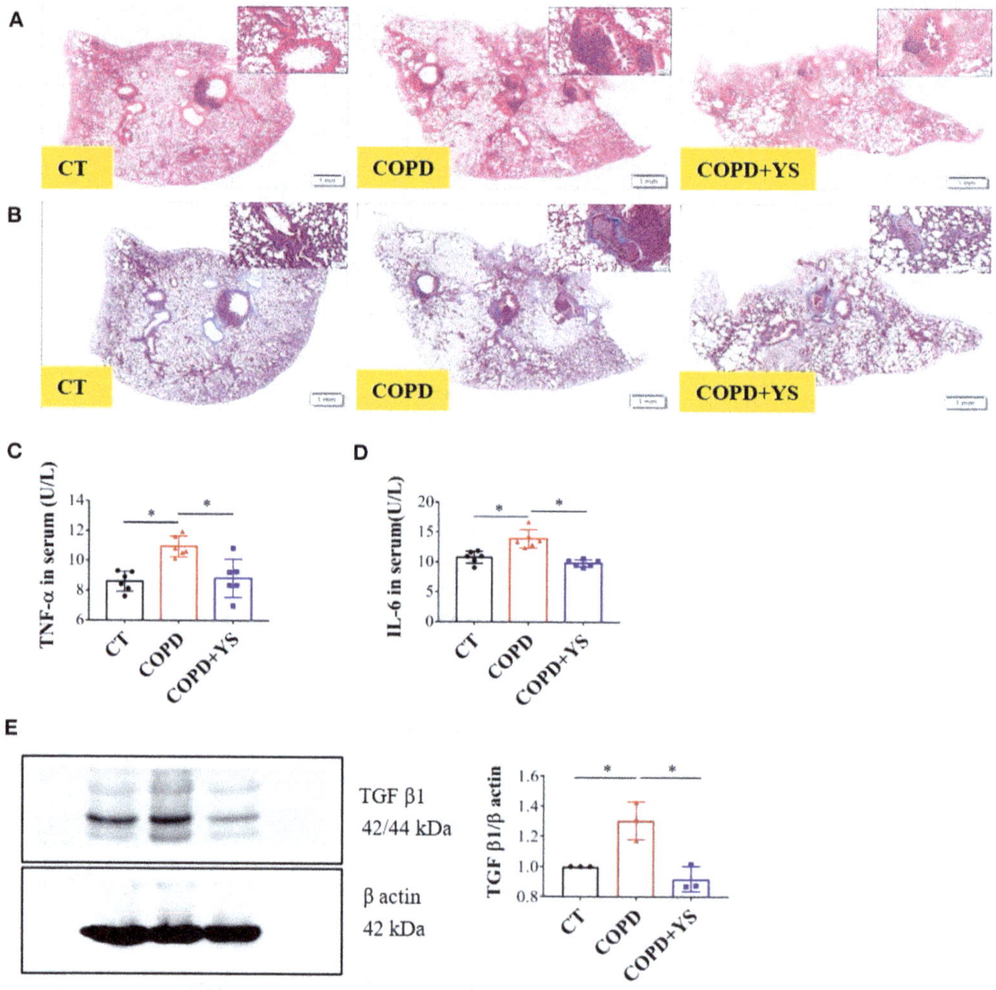

FIGURE 5 | (A) H&E staining of lung tissues of CT, COPD, and COPD + YS. **(B)** Masson staining of lung tissues of CT, COPD, and COPD + YS. **(C)** TNF-α in serum of CT, COPD, and COPD + YS ($n = 6$). **(D)** IL-6 in serum of CT, COPD, and COPD + YS ($n = 6$). **(E)** The relative expression of TGF-β1 in the lung of CT, COPD, and COPD + YS ($n = 3$). The data are presented as the means ± SEM of three experiments (*$P < 0.05$).

Caspase-1 and ASC were significantly increased in lung tissues ($P < 0.05$), and IL-1β and IL-18 were significantly higher in serum ($P < 0.05$). In the COPD + YS group, NLRP3 protein expression was lower in the lung ($P > 0.05$), caspase-1 and ASC were lower in lung tissue ($P > 0.05$), and IL-18 levels of serum were significantly lower ($P < 0.05$). These results suggest

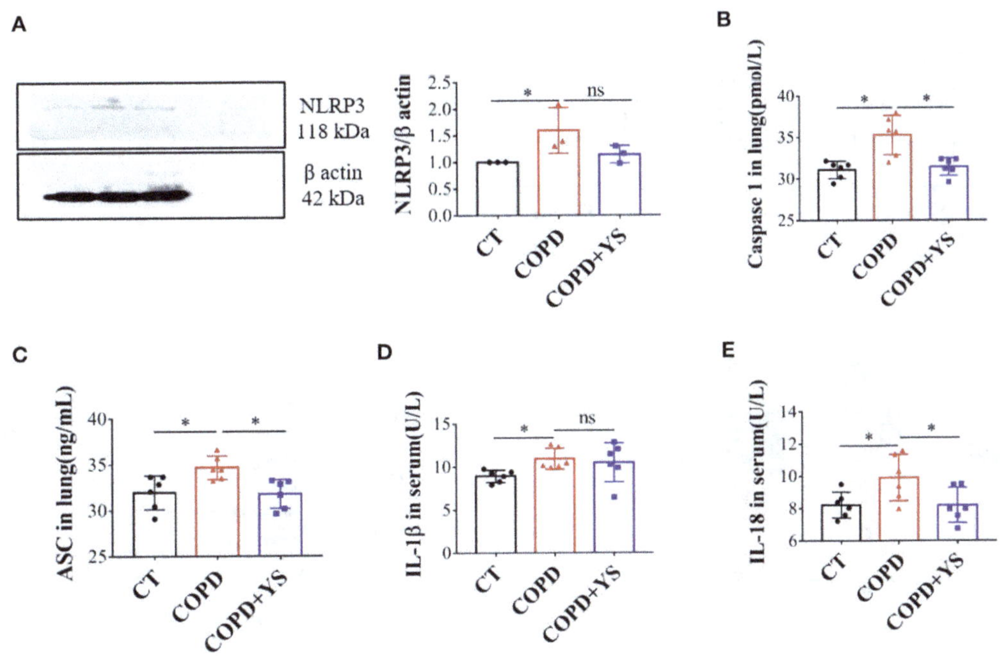

FIGURE 6 | (A) NLRP3 in the lung of CT, COPD, and COPD + YS ($n = 3$). **(B)** Caspase1 in the lung of CT, COPD, and COPD + YS ($n = 6$). **(C)** ASC in the lung of CT, COPD, and COPD + YS ($n = 6$). **(D)** IL-1β in the serum of CT, COPD, and COPD+YS ($n = 6$). **(E)** IL-18 in the serum of CT, COPD, and COPD + YS ($n=6$). The data are presented as the means ± SEM of three experiments (ns, non-significant, $^*P < 0.05$).

that YS inhibits the NLRP3/caspase-1/IL-1β signaling pathway (**Figures 6A–E**) to alleviate the inflammatory response.

Effect of YS on Pulmonary Microbiota in COPD Rats

The pulmonary microbiota is strongly associated with COPD. 16s rDNA gene high-throughput sequencing was employed to analyze the pulmonary microbiota to explore the mechanisms. The Chao1 index reflects the relative abundance of pulmonary microbiota, and the Shannon index reflects the diversity of pulmonary microbiota. The relative abundance of pulmonary microbiota was decreased in COPD rats. After YS treatment, the relative abundance of pulmonary microbiota showed no significant change. Meanwhile, the diversity of the pulmonary microbiota was reduced in COPD rats. ($P > 0.05$), which was significantly greater after the YS intervention ($P < 0.05$) (**Figure 7A**).

Next, we observed the bacteria in phylum and genera levels among the CT, COPD, and COPD + YS groups. At the phylum level, the pulmonary microbiota was dominated by Proteobacteria, Firmicutes, and Bacteroidota. It's shown that Proteobacteria and Firmicutes increased in COPD rats, while Bacteroidota decreased in COPD rats. After YS intervention, Proteobacteria and Firmicutes decreased while Bacteroidota increased (**Figures 7B,C**). At the genera level, the pulmonary microbiota was dominated by *Ralstonia, Mycoplasma, Halomonas, Lactobacillus, Dizetzia,* and *Bacteroides*. The COPD group showed an increased relative abundance of *Ralstonia, Mycoplasma, Halomonas,* and *Dizetzia* over the CT group. Meanwhile, there was a decreased relative abundance of *Lactobacillus* and *Bacteroides*. The relative abundance of *Halomonas, Lactobacillus, Dizetzia,* and *Bacteroides* were increased, and there was a lower relative abundance of *Ralstonia* and *Mycoplasma* after being treated with YS (**Figures 7D,E**).

Linear discriminant analysis of effect size showed that the iconic microorganisms in each group contributed significantly to differences in microbial structures. *Mycoplasma* was more abundant in the pulmonary microbiota of the COPD group. *Mycoplasma* was significantly increased in COPD patients. Meanwhile, *Halomonas, Dietzia,* and *Nesterenkonia* were enriched after the YS intervention. These results suggest that YS changes the relative abundance of specific bacteria and modulates the pulmonary microbiota in COPD rats (**Figures 7F,G**).

Environmental Factor Correlation Analysis

Correlation heatmap plots were used to assess the top 35 genera and correlations with 12 environmental factors (EF50, TV, MV, SIgA, TGF-β1, IL-6, TNF-α, Caspasel, IL-18, IL-1β, ASC, and NLRP3). As shown in the **Figure 8**, EF50 was positively correlated with *Clostridium_sensu_stricto_1* and *Klebsiella* ($P < 0.05$). TV was positively correlated with *Pseudolabrys* ($P < 0.05$). MV was negatively related with *Mycoplasma* ($P < 0.05$) and positively related with *Clostridium_sensu_stricto_1* ($P < 0.05$). SIgA had a positive correlation with *Methylobacterium, Methylorubrum, Halomonas, Dietzia, Parabacteroides, Bacteroides, Roseburia, Clostridium_sensu_stricto_1, Blautia, Pseudolabrys* and *Klebsiella* ($P < 0.05$). TGF-β1 was negatively correlated with *Bacteroides, Clostridium_sensu_stricto_1*

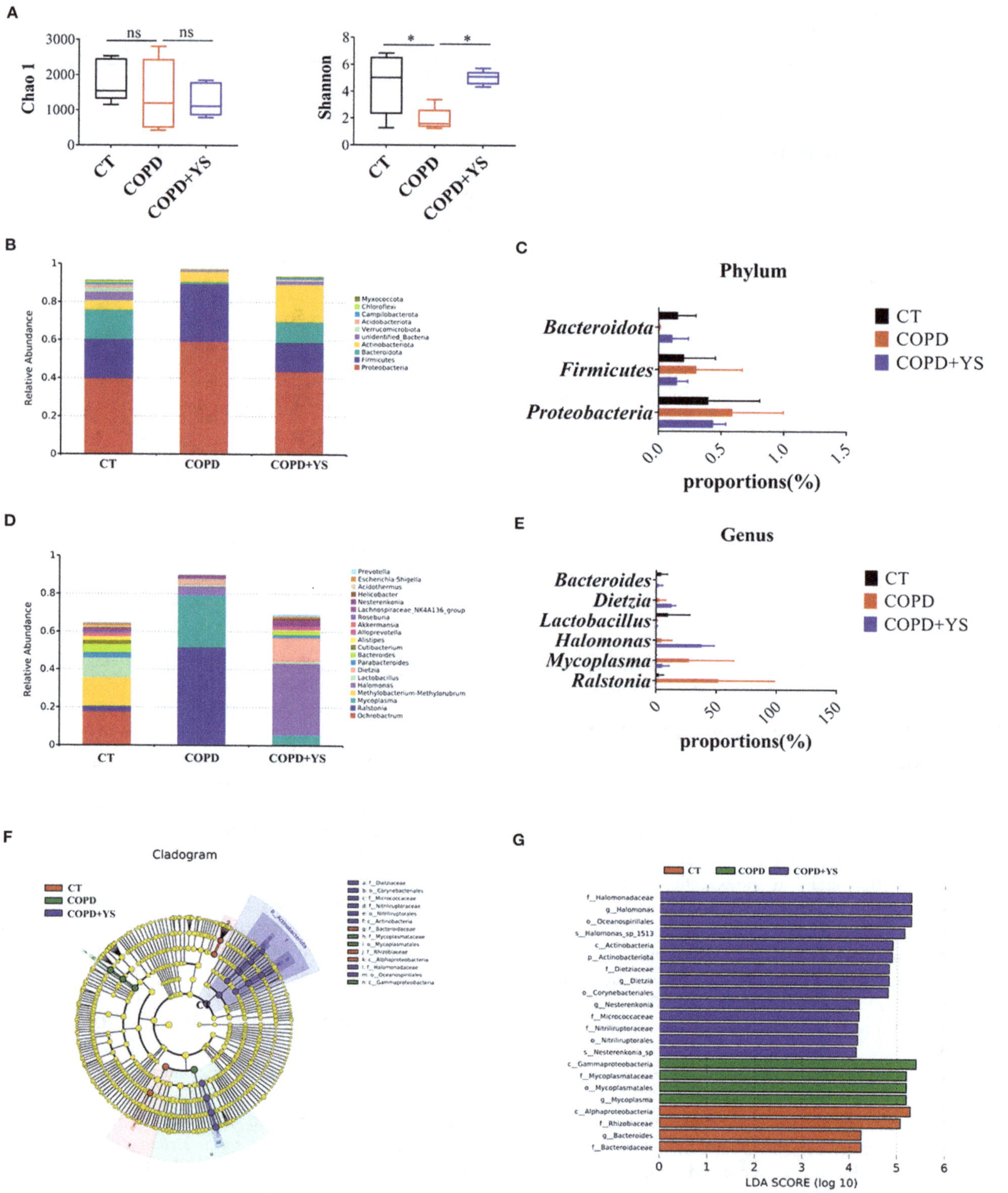

FIGURE 7 | (A) Analysis of alpha diversity: Chao1 and Shannon index ($n = 5$). **(B)** The relative abundance of top ten pulmonary microbiota in the phylum ($n = 5$). **(C)** The advantage of pulmonary microbiota in the phylum ($n = 5$). **(D)** The relative abundance of the top twenty pulmonary microbiota in the genera ($n = 5$). **(E)** The advantage of pulmonary microbiota in the genera ($n = 5$). **(F)** Taxonomic differences of pulmonary microbiota among different groups. The taxonomic cladogram was obtained by LEfSe. Differences are represented by the color of the most abundant class. The diameter of each circle is proportional to the taxon's abundance ($n = 5$). **(G)** Linear discriminant analysis score of each group of gut microbiota ($n = 5$). The data are presented as the means ± SEM of three experiments (ns, non-significant, $^{*}P < 0.05$).

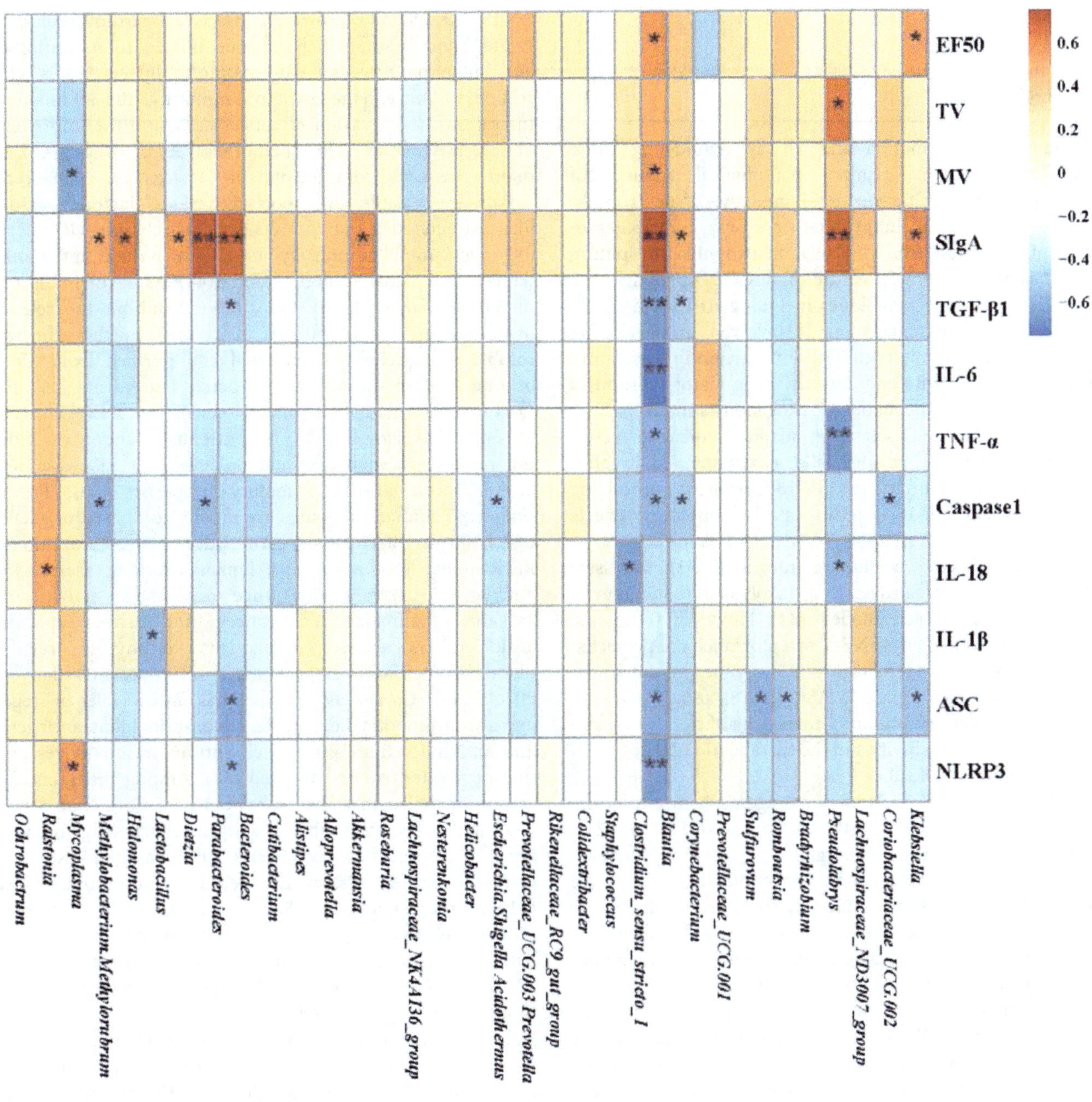

FIGURE 8 | Heatmap of the correlation among the pulmonary microbiota related to environmental factors (*$P < 0.05$, **$P < 0.01$; blue represents a negative correlation; red represents a positive correlation).

and *Blautia* ($P < 0.05$). IL-6 was negatively associated with *Clostridium_sensu_stricto_1* ($P < 0.01$). TNF-α had a negative correlation with *Clostridium_sensu_stricto_1* and *Pseudolabrys* ($P < 0.05$). Caspase1 negatively correlated with *Methylobacterium, Methylorubrum, Parabacteroides, Escherichia, Shigella, Clostridium_sensu_stricto_1, Blautia* and *Coriobacteriaceae_UCG.002* ($P < 0.05$). IL-18 had a positive correlation with *Ralstonia* ($P < 0.05$) and a negative correlation with *Staphylococcus, Pseudolabrys* ($P < 0.05$). IL-1β was negatively correlated with *Lactobacillus* ($P < 0.05$). NLRP3 was positively correlated with *Mycoplasma* ($P < 0.05$) and negatively correlated with *Bacteroides, Clostridium_sensu_stricto_1* ($P < 0.05$) (**Figure 8**). Among them, *Clostridium_sensu_stricto_1* was associated with more than half of the environmental factors, which may be the potential target bacteria of pulmonary microbiota for COPD progression and YS therapy. At the same time, SIgA in the lung was more correlated with pulmonary microbiota.

DISCUSSION

A well-known inflammation and airway remodeling cause airflow limitation, the primary pathological features of COPD (28). The infiltration of lymphocytes, neutrophils, and monocytes into the lung tissue or airway contributes to chronic inflammation (6). Clinically, neutrophilia of sputum and blood is a characteristic feature of all COPD patients (29), which is derived from chemokines including IL-1β and CXCL (30). The NLRP3 inflammasome is involved in developing diseases by promoting the release of downstream inflammatory cytokines, inducing acute and chronic inflammatory responses (31). In response to endogenous or exogenous stimuli, NLRP3 is activated. Further, ASC acts as an adaptor protein to recruit the precursor caspase-1, which has an enzymatic activity after cleaving pro-interleukin-1β and IL-18 precursor, producing mature IL-1β and IL-18, exerting proinflammatory effects (32). Superfluous inflammasome activation is a feature of numerous lung diseases, including infections (33). Excessive inflammatory factors are proven to be involved in tissue injuries and remodeling in mouse models (34). However, transgenic animal knockout IL-1β and TNF-α receptor mice are protected from developing airway remodeling (35). In the present study, the levels of NLRP3, caspase-1, ASC, IL-18, and IL-1β were decreased in YS administration animals. Insufficiently, we did not evaluate COPD sensitivity and the therapeutic effect of YS in transgenic animals of NLRP3.

Bronchodilators, anti-inflammatory agents, and hormones may improve symptoms in patients with COPD (36). The four main types (Anticholinergics, β2-Agonists, inhaled corticosteroids, and combination bronchodilator therapy) are found in GOLD reports to reduce dynamic hyperinflation at rest and during exercise and improve exercise performance (37). Antioxidant and anti-inflammatory agents were applied to treat COPD *in vitro* and *in vivo* (38). Anti-inflammatory and entire modeling effects of muscarinic receptors and antagonists were confirmed in COPD (39). All of them are important for improving symptoms. The contribution is limited in halting the progressive deterioration of pulmonary function and the progression of the disease. YS, as traditional Chinese medicine, is a clinically effective empirical formula for the treatment of lung disease, which is composed of *Hedysarum Multijugum Maxim*, *Atractylodes Macrocephala Koidz*, *Saposhnikoviae Radix*, *Sinapis Semen*, *Fritillariae Thunbrgii Bulbus*, *Mori Cortex*, *Curcumae Rhizoma*, and *Panax Notoginseng (Burk.) F. H. Chen Ex C. Chow* (19, 40). Pharmacological studies indicate that the main components of "*Hedysarum Multijugum Maxim*," include astragalus polysaccharides (APS), flavonoids, saponins, alkaloids, and the like. Astragalus polysaccharide is the most important natural active ingredient in *Hedysarum Multijugum Maxim*, with immunomodulatory, antiviral, antifibrotic, and other pharmacological effects (41). Astragaloside IV (AS-IV) is one of the main compounds in the water extract of *Hedysarum Multijugum Maxim*. Studies have shown that AS-IV has effective protective effects on cardiovascular, lung, kidney, and brain, which may be related to its antioxidant, anti-inflammatory, and anti-apoptotic effects. It is closely related to the enhancement of immunity, the attenuation of migrations, the invasion of cancer cells, and the improvement of chemosensitivity to chemotherapeutic drugs (42). The main chemical components of *Atractylodes Macrocephala Koidz* are volatile oils, polysaccharides, lactones, and the like. Atractylodes macrocephala polysaccharide (PAMK) can improve animal immunity (43) and reduce inflammatory damage and oxidative stress in mice (44). As the main ingredient of *Saposhnikoviae Radix* (SR), SR can inhibit the release of histamine for an anti-allergic effect (45). Further, the water-soluble polysaccharides extracted and purified from SR may be one of its main anti-allergic active ingredients (46). Prim-O-glucosylcimifugin Attenuates, one of the active ingredients of *Saposhnikoviae Radix*, can attenuate endotoxin-induced inflammatory response in macrophages (47). Likewise, *Sinapis Semen* shows anti-inflammatory properties (48). *Fritillaria thunbergii Miq* and its bulbs are mainly composed of alkaloids, essential oils, diterpenoids, carbohydrates, sterols, amino acids, nucleotides, fatty acids, and lignans. Among them, Nepeta and its bulbs have a wide range of biological activities, such as anti-inflammatory, anticancer, antitussive, expectorant, antiulcer, antibacterial, antioxidant, antithyroid, regulating blood rheology, antidiarrheal, neuroprotective, and sedative pain effects (49). *Curcumae Rhizoma* has anti-platelet aggregation and antithrombotic, hepatoprotective, antioxidant, antibacterial, and antiviral activities, in which antitumor activity research is the most extensive and focused (50). Among them, curcumin, as one of the main active components of *Curcumae Rhizoma*, is a highly effective antibacterial agent effective against various types of cancer, diabetes, obesity, cardiovascular disease, lung disease, nervous system disease, and autoimmune disease (51). *Panax Notoginseng (Burk.) F. H. Chen Ex C. Chow* can reduce reactive oxygen species, lysozyme, prostaglandins, leukotrienes, and inflammatory cytokines, such as IL-1, IL-12, and TNF-α, to reduce potential damage to surrounding tissues, exerting anti-inflammatory effects (52). The main active ingredient of *Panax Notoginseng (Burk.) F. H. Chen Ex C. Chow* has been widely studied for its applications such as anti-inflammatory effects (53, 54). Pharmacologically, the function of YS has been confirmed to improve pulmonary function and ventilatory dysfunction and played an important role in repairing inflammatory damage in COPD animals.

The study of the airway microbiota is in its infancy. Still, it has been gradually recognized that the microbiota of the respiratory tract is associated with pulmonary disease (55). Abundant microbial diversity is regarded as beneficial in development and immune system domestication, affecting the susceptibility to allergic asthma, cystic fibrosis, respiratory infection, and lung cancer (56–58). Current reports suggest that the development of COPD is primarily achieved through microbiota. However, risk factors for COPD, including cigarette smoke and inhaling contaminated air, can affect the composition of the pulmonary microbiota (59). In contrast to healthy individuals, the influence of the lung microenvironment on the microbiome in COPD could be obvious (60). The diversity of the sputum microbiome is decreased in COPD patients (61), such as *Haemophilis influenzae* increasing at the exacerbation of COPD (62). We observed lower microbial alpha diversity in the COPD group than in the control group. The lung microbial alpha diversity of mice in the COPD+YS groups differed from that of the COPD group. Analysis of flora diversity showed that YS prevented pulmonary microbiota dysbiosis in COPD rats. Consistent with this finding, linear discriminant analysis of effect size showed different lung microbial compositions in these groups. *Mycoplasma* belongs to *Firmicutes*, which accelerates disease processes by promoting chronic inflammation (63). *Halomonas* are gram-positive bacteria. Various oligotypes of *Christensenella* and *Clostridium* were detected in lung tissue and a few oligotypes of *Halomonas* in both airway fluid and lung tissue from pulmonary fibrosis and lung cancer patients, suggesting the involvement of these microbial communities in fibrotic diseases (64). *Nesterenkonia* belongs to *Actinobacteria* and *Lactobacillaceae*. The microbiome might play a significant role in maintaining normal lung function, including structural and immune barriers (65). These findings suggest that in COPD treatment, the relative abundance of *Halomonas* and *Nesterenkonia* are increased by decreasing the relative abundance of *Mycoplasma*, potentially inhibiting the inflammatory factors IL-1β, TNF-α, IL-6, IL-1β, and TGF-β1. This further increases SIgA expression, which enhances immunity, alleviates collagen deposition and improves lung function. We used the correlation heatmap plots to assess the top 35 genera and correlations with 12 environmental factors (EF50, TV, MV, SIgA, TGF-β1, IL-6, TNF-α, Caspasel, IL-18, IL-1β, ASC, and NLRP3) to further explore the relationship between pulmonary microbiota and pulmonary ventilation function, inflammatory factors, and immunity. Clostridium_sensu_stricto_1 may be the potential target bacteria of pulmonary microbiota for COPD progression and YS therapy. Besides, SIgA in the lung may be an important factor affecting the pulmonary microbiota.

SUMMARY AND PROSPECTS

In this work, we confirmed the function of YS in improving the pulmonary ventilatory function in COPD rats referring to EF50, TV, and MV. Histopathological findings showed that inflammatory injury associated with COPD was weakened. The inflammatory mediators of NLRP3/caspase-1/IL-1βsignaling were involved in pulmonary pathological damage. Furthermore, disturbed pulmonary microbiota was discovered in COPD animals. However, after administration with YS, the abundance and diversity of pulmonary microflora were remodeled, especially increasing the beneficial genua. The replacement of flora is associated with inflammation by environmental factor correlation analysis. In general, we provided some evidence that dysbiosis of pulmonary microbiota leads to the COPD pathological process. The function of the Yifei Sanjie Formula was involved in remodeling lung microbes and anti-inflammatory signal pathways. To evaluate the sensitivity of COPD or pharmacodynamic tests is positive in animals with germ-free lungs, which is verified for further study in the future. It is certain targeting intervention microbiota to anti-inflammatory may be a potential therapeutic strategy for COPD.

AUTHOR CONTRIBUTIONS

ZY and JY: study design. YW: data collection. YW, HM, and BQ: statistical analysis and data interpretation. NL, QZ, WJ, HX, and YL: manuscript preparation. ZY, JY, and YW: funds collection. All authors contributed to the article and approved the submitted version.

FUNDING

This work was funded in part by a grant from the National Natural Science Foundation of China (81860646, 81760819), Yunnan Provincial Science and Technology Department (202201AS070084, 202005AC160058, 202101AZ070001-012, 202005AF150063, 202102AE090031), the Science Research Foundation of Yunnan Provincial Department of Education (2020Y0204), Yunnan Science and Technology Planning Project-Joint Major Project of Traditional Chinese Medicine (2019FF002[-002]), and the Provincial Innovation Team of the Yunnan University of Chinese Medicine for Traditional Chinese Medicine to Regulate Human Microecology (No. 2018HC011).

ACKNOWLEDGMENTS

We are very grateful to Prof. Xu Ou of Fuwai Cardiovascular Hospital Yunnan Province in the guidance for the pulmonary function experiment.

REFERENCES

1. Agustí A, Vogelmeier C, Faner R, COPD. 2020: changes and challenges. Lung cellular and molecular physiology. *Am J Physiol.* (2020) 319:L879–83. doi: 10.1152/ajplung.00429.2020
2. Adeloye D, Chua S, Lee C, Basquill C, Papana A, Theodoratou E, et al. Global and regional estimates of COPD prevalence: Systematic review and meta-analysis. *J Glob Health.* (2015) 5:020415. doi: 10.7189/jogh.05.020415
3. Barnes PJ. Inflammatory mechanisms in patients with chronic obstructive pulmonary disease. *J Aller Clin Immunol.* (2016) 138:6–27. doi: 10.1016/j.jaci.2016.05.011
4. McGuinness AJ, Sapey E. Oxidative stress in COPD: sources, markers, and potential mechanisms. *J Clin Med.* (2017) 6:2. doi: 10.3390/jcm6020021
5. Wang C, Xu J, Yang L, Xu Y, Zhang X, Bai C, et al. Prevalence and risk factors of chronic obstructive pulmonary disease in China (the China Pulmonary Health [CPH] study): a national cross-sectional study. *Lancet.* (2018) 391:1706–17. doi: 10.1016/S0140-6736(18)30841-9
6. Wang Y, Xu J, Meng Y, Adcock IM, Yao X. Role of inflammatory cells in airway remodeling in COPD. *Int J Chronic Obstr.* (2018) 13:3341–8. doi: 10.2147/COPD.S176122
7. Rotta Detto Loria J, Rohmann K, Droemann D, Kujath P, Rupp J, Goldmann T, et al. Nontypeable haemophilus influenzae infection upregulates the nlrp3 inflammasome and leads to caspase-1-dependent secretion of Interleukin-1β - a possible pathway of exacerbations in COPD. *PLoS ONE.* (2013) 8:e66818. doi: 10.1371/journal.pone.0066818

8. Wang H, Lv C, Wang S, Ying H, Weng Y, Yu W. NLRP3 inflammasome involves in the acute exacerbation of patients with chronic obstructive pulmonary disease. *Inflammation.* (2018) 41:1321–33. doi: 10.1007/s10753-018-0780-0
9. Pauwels NS, Bracke KR, Dupont LL, Van Pottelberge GR, Provoost S, Vanden Berghe T, et al. Role of IL-1α and the Nlrp3/caspase-1/IL-1β axis in cigarette smoke-induced pulmonary inflammation and COPD. *Eur Respir J.* (2011) 38:1019–28. doi: 10.1183/09031936.00158110
10. Di Stefano A, Caramori G, Barczyk A, Vicari C, Brun P, Zanini A, et al. Innate immunity but not NLRP3 inflammasome activation correlates with severity of stable COPD. *Thorax.* (2014) 69:516–24. doi: 10.1136/thoraxjnl-2012-203062
11. Nachmias N, Langier S, Brzezinski RY, Siterman M, Bar-Shai A. NLRP3 inflammasome activity is upregulated in an in-vitro model of COPD exacerbation. *PLoS ONE.* (2019) 14:e0214622. doi: 10.1371/journal.pone.0214622
12. Markelić I, Hlapčić I, Ceri A, Radić Antolic M, SamarŽija M, Popović-Grle S, et al. Activation of NLRP3 inflammasome in stable chronic obstructive pulmonary disease. *Sci Rep.* (2022) 12:7544. doi: 10.1038/s41598-022-11164-1
13. Invernizzi R, Lloyd CM, Molyneaux PL. Respiratory microbiome and epithelial interactions shape immunity in the lungs. *Immunology.* (2020) 160:171–82. doi: 10.1111/imm.13195
14. Dang AT, Marsland BJ. Microbes, metabolites, and the gut-lung axis. *Mucosal Immunol.* (2019) 12:843–50. doi: 10.1038/s41385-019-0160-6
15. Wypych TP, Wickramasinghe LC, Marsland BJ. The influence of the microbiome on respiratory health. *Nat Immunol.* (2019) 20:1279–90. doi: 10.1038/s41590-019-0451-9
16. Belkaid Y, Hand TW. Role of the microbiota in immunity and inflammation. *Cell.* (2014) 157:121–41. doi: 10.1016/j.cell.2014.03.011
17. Erb-Downward JR, Thompson DL, Han MK, Freeman CM, McCloskey L, Schmidt LA, et al. Analysis of the lung microbiome in the "healthy" smoker and in COPD. *PLoS ONE.* (2019) 6:e16384. doi: 10.1371/journal.pone.0016384
18. Li J, Zhao P, Li Y, Tian Y, Wang Y. Systems pharmacology-based dissection of mechanisms of Chinese medicinal formula Bufei Yishen as an effective treatment for chronic obstructive pulmonary disease. *Sci Rep.* (2015) 5:15290. doi: 10.1038/srep15290
19. Yu JZ, Ying Y, Liu Y, Sun CB Dai C, Zhao S, et al. Antifibrotic action of Yifei Sanjie formula enhanced autophagy via PI3K-AKT-mTOR signaling pathway in mouse model of pulmonary fibrosis. *Biomed Pharmacother.* (2019) 118:109293. doi: 10.1016/j.biopha.2019.109293
20. Sun CB, Ying Y, Wu QY, Liu Y, Yu JZ, Xing HJ, et al. The main active components of Curcuma zedoaria reduces collagen deposition in human lung fibroblast via autophagy. *Mol Immunol.* (2020) 124:109–16. doi: 10.1016/j.molimm.2020.05.017
21. Song YP, Cui DJ, Mao PY, A. new way of establishing a rat chronic obstructive pulmonary disease model and the effects of drugs on them. *Acad J Pla Postgrad Med Sch.* (2001). 39:51–52+73–74.
22. Li Y, Chen J, Zhang L, Wei W. Research advance of tumor necrosis factor receptor-associated factors in inflammatory immune regulation. *Chin Pharmacol Bull.* (2015) 31:1206–11. doi: 10.3969/j.issn.1001-1978.2015.09.006
23. Li Y, Jin L, Chen T. The effects of secretory IgA in the mucosal immune system. *Biomed Res Int.* (2020) 2020:2032057. doi: 10.1155/2020/2032057
24. Du RH, Richmond BW, Blackwell TS, Cates JM, Massion PP, Ware LB, et al. Secretory IgA from submucosal glands does not compensate for its airway surface deficiency in chronic obstructive pulmonary disease. *Virch Arch.* (2015) 467:657–65. doi: 10.1007/s00428-015-1854-0
25. Cheng Q, Fang L, Feng D, Tang S, Yue S, Huang Y, et al. Memantine ameliorates pulmonary inflammation in a mice model of COPD induced by cigarette smoke combined with LPS. *Biomed Pharmacother.* (2019) 109:2005–13. doi: 10.1016/j.biopha.2018.11.002
26. Wang L, Meng J, Wang C, Yang C, Li Y. Hydrogen sulfide alleviates cigarette smoke-induced COPD through inhibition of the TGF- β 1/smad pathway. *Exp Biol Med.* (2020) 245:153537022090434. doi: 10.1177/1535370220904342
27. Peng Z, Zhang W, Qiao J, He B. Melatonin attenuates airway inflammation via SIRT1 dependent inhibition of NLRP3 inflammasome and IL-1β in rats with COPD. *Int Immunopharmacol.* (2018) 62:23–8. doi: 10.1016/j.intimp.2018.06.033
28. Berg K, Wright JL. The pathology of chronic obstructive pulmonary disease: progress in the 20th and 21st centuries. *Arch Pathol Lab Med.* (2016) 140:1423–8. doi: 10.5858/arpa.2015-0455-RS
29. Dima E, Rovina N, Gerassimou C, Roussos C, Gratziou C. Pulmonary function tests, sputum induction, and bronchial provocation tests: diagnostic tools in the challenge of distinguishing asthma and COPD phenotypes in clinical practice. *Int J Chronic Obstr.* (2010) 5:287–96. doi: 10.2147/COPD.S9055
30. Baek KJ, Cho JY, Rosenthal P, Alexander L, Nizet V, Broide DH. Hypoxia potentiates allergen induction of HIF-1α, chemokines, airway inflammation, TGF-β1, and airway remodeling in a mouse model. *Clin Immunol.* (2013) 147:27–37. doi: 10.1016/j.clim.2013.02.004
31. Mangan M, Olhava EJ, Roush WR, Seidel HM, Glick GD, Latz E. Targeting the NLRP3 inflammasome in inflammatory diseases. *Nat Rev Drug Discov.* (2018) 17:588–606. doi: 10.1038/nrd.2018.97
32. Wang L, Hauenstein AV. The NLRP3 inflammasome: mechanism of action, role in disease and therapies. *Mol Aspects Med.* (2020) 76:100889. doi: 10.1016/j.mam.2020.100889
33. Kim RY, Pinkerton JW, Gibson PG, Cooper MA, Horvat JC, Hansbro PM. Inflammasomes in COPD and neutrophilic asthma. *Thorax.* (2015) 70:1199–201. doi: 10.1136/thoraxjnl-2014-206736
34. Yang Y, Di TT, Zhang ZX, Liu JX, Fu CL, Wu Y, et al. Dynamic evolution of emphysema and airway remodeling in two mouse models of COPD. *BMC Pulm Med.* (2021) 21:134. doi: 10.1186/s12890-021-01456-z
35. Churg A, Zhou S, Wang X, Wang R, Wright JL. The role of interleukin-1beta in murine cigarette smoke-induced emphysema and small airway remodeling. *Am J Resp Cell Mol.* (2009) 40:482–90. doi: 10.1165/rcmb.2008-0038OC
36. Tashkin DP. Smoking cessation in chronic obstructive pulmonary disease. *Semin Resp Crit Care.* (2015) 36:491–507. doi: 10.1055/s-0035-1555610
37. Terry PD, Dhand R. Inhalation therapy for stable COPD: 20 years of GOLD reports. *Adv Ther.* (2020) 37:1812–28. doi: 10.1007/s12325-020-01289-y
38. Sadowska AM. Manuel-Y-Keenoy B, De Backer WA. Antioxidant and anti-inflammatory efficacy of NAC in the treatment of COPD: discordant *in vitro* and *in vivo* dose-effects: a review. *Pulm Pharmacol Ther.* (2007) 20:9–22. doi: 10.1016/j.pupt.2005.12.007
39. Karakiulakis G, Roth M. Muscarinic receptors and their antagonists in COPD: anti-inflammatory and antiremodeling effects. *Mediat Inflamm.* (2012) 2012:409580. doi: 10.1155/2012/409580
40. Wei N, Wang XX, Wang YQ Li N, Cheng Y, Tian SZ, et al. Effect of Yupingfengsan improved decoction on airway inflammatory microenvironment in rats with COPD. *Mod J Integr Trad Chin West Med.* (2018) 27:457–61. doi: 10.3969/j.issn.1008-8849.2018.05.001
41. Zheng YJ, Ren WY, Zhang LN, Zhang YM, Liu DL, Liu YQ, et al. Review of the pharmacological action of astragalus polysaccharide. *Front Pharmacol.* (2020) 11:349. doi: 10.3389/fphar.2020.00349
42. Zhang JQ, Wu CX, Gao L, Du GH, Qin XM. Astragaloside IV derived from Astragalus membranaceus: A research review on the pharmacological effects. *Adv Pharmacol.* (2020) 87:89–112. doi: 10.1016/bs.apha.2019.08.002
43. Lin Z, Liu YF, Qu Y, Shi LY, Dou DQ, Kuang HX. Characterisation of oligosaccharides from Baizhu by HILIC-MS. *Nat Prod Res.* (2015) 29:1194–200. doi: 10.1080/14786419.2014.995652
44. Guo SX Li WY, Chen FY, Yang SZ, Huang YM, Tian YB, et al. Polysaccharide of Atractylodes macrocephala Koidz regulates LPS-mediated mouse hepatitis through the TLR4-MyD88-NFκB signaling pathway. *Int Immunopharmacol.* (2021) 98:107692. doi: 10.1016/j.intimp.2021.107692
45. Jia QQ, Sun W, Zhang LY, Fu J, Lv YN, Lin YY, et al. Screening the anti-allergic components in Saposhnikoviae Radix using high-expression Mas-related G protein-coupled receptor X2 cell membrane chromatography online coupled with liquid chromatography and mass spectrometry. *J Sep Sci.* (2019) 42:2351–9. doi: 10.1002/jssc.201900114
46. Gao YY, Jiang Y, Chen GC Li SS, Yang F, Ma Q. Saposhnikoviae RadixA sensitive and rapid UPLC-MS/MS method for determination of monosaccharides and anti-allergic effect of the polysaccharides extracted from. *Molecules.* (2018) 23:1924. doi: 10.3390/molecules23081924
47. Zhou J, Sun YY, Sun MY, Mao WA, Wang L, Zhang J. et al. Prim-O-glucosylcimifugin attenuates lipopolysaccharideinduced inflammatory response in RAW 2647 macrophages. *Pharmacogn Mag.* (2017) 13:378–84. doi: 10.4103/pm.pm_323_16
48. Xian YF, Hu Z, Ip SP, Chen JN, Su ZR, Lai XP, et al. Comparison of the anti-inflammatory effects of Sinapis alba and Brassica juncea in mouse models of inflammation. *Phytomedicine.* (2018) 50:196–204. doi: 10.1016/j.phymed.2018.05.010

49. Nile SH, Su J, Wu D, Wang L, Hu J, Sieniawska E, et al. Fritillaria thunbergii Miq (Zhe Beimu): a review on its traditional uses, phytochemical profile and pharmacological properties. *Food Chem Toxicol.* (2021) 153:112289. doi: 10.1016/j.fct.2021.112289
50. Zhou Y, Xie M, Song Y, Wang WP, Zhao HR, Tian YX, et al. Two Traditional Chinese Medicines Curcumae Radix and Curcumae Rhizoma: an ethnopharmacology, phytochemistry, and pharmacology review. *Evid Based Comp Altern Med.* (2016) 2016:4973128. doi: 10.1155/2016/4973128
51. Kunnumakkara AB, Bordoloi D, Padmavathi G, Monisha J, Roy NK, Prasad S, et al. Curcumin, the golden nutraceutical: multitargeting for multiple chronic diseases. *Br J Pharmacol.* (2017) 174:1325–48. doi: 10.1111/bph.13621
52. Xu Y, Tan HY Li S, Wang N, Feng Y. Panax notoginseng for inflammation-related chronic diseases: a review on the modulations of multiple pathways. *Am J Chin Med.* (2018) 46:971–96. doi: 10.1142/S0192415X18500519
53. Ruan JY, Zhang Y, Zhao W, Sun F, Han LF Yu HY, et al. Panax notoginsengNew 12,23-epoxydammarane type saponins obtained from leaves and their anti-inflammatory activity. *Molecules.* (2020) 25:3784. doi: 10.3390/molecules25173784
54. Zheng YR, Fan CL, Chen Y, Quan JY, Shi LZ, Tian CY, et al. Anti-inflammatory, anti-angiogenetic and antiviral activities of dammarane-type triterpenoid saponins from the roots of Panax notoginseng. *Food Funct.* (2022) 13:3590–602. doi: 10.1039/D1FO04089H
55. O'Dwyer DN, Ashley SL, Gurczynski SJ, Xia M, Wilke C, Falkowski NR, et al. Lung microbiota contribute to pulmonary inflammation and disease progression in pulmonary fibrosis. *Am J Resp Crit Care.* (2019) 199:1127–38. doi: 10.1164/rccm.201809-1650OC
56. Daley D. The evolution of the hygiene hypothesis: the role of early-life exposures to viruses and microbes and their relationship to asthma and allergic diseases. *Curr Opin Allergy Clin.* (2014) 14:390–6. doi: 10.1097/ACI.0000000000000101
57. Gray J, Oehrle K, Worthen G, Alenghat T, Whitsett J, Deshmukh H. Intestinal commensal bacteria mediate lung mucosal immunity and promote resistance of newborn mice to infection. *Sci Transl Med.* (2017) 9:eaaf9412. doi: 10.1126/scitranslmed.aaf9412
58. Dayama G, Priya S, Niccum DE, Khoruts A, Blekhman R. Interactions between the gut microbiome and host gene regulation in cystic fibrosis. *Genome Med.* (2020) 12:12. doi: 10.1186/s13073-020-0710-2
59. Bassis CM, Erb-Downward JR, Dickson RP, Freeman CM, Schmidt TM, Young VB, et al. Analysis of the upper respiratory tract microbiotas as the source of the lung and gastric microbiotas in healthy individuals. *MBio.* (2015) 6:e00037. doi: 10.1128/mBio.00037-15
60. Mammen MJ, Sethi S. COPD and the microbiome. *Respirology.* (2016) 21:590–9. doi: 10.1111/resp.12732
61. Galiana A, Aguirre E, Rodriguez JC, Mira A, Santibañez M, Candela I, et al. Sputum microbiota in moderate versus severe patients with COPD. *Eur Respir J.* (2014) 43:1787–90. doi: 10.1183/09031936.00191513
62. Short B, Carson S, Devlin AC, Reihill JA, Crilly A, MacKay W, et al. Haemophilus influenzaeNon-typeable chronic colonization in chronic obstructive pulmonary disease (COPD). *Crit Rev Microbiol.* (2021) 47:192–205. doi: 10.1080/1040841X.2020.1863330
63. Chaudhry R, Ghosh A, Chandolia A. Pathogenesis of mycoplasma pneumoniae: an update. *Indian J Med Microbiol.* (2016) 34:7–16. doi: 10.4103/0255-0857.174112
64. D'Alessandro-Gabazza CN, Méndez-García C, Hataji O, Westergaard S, Watanabe F, Yasuma T, et al. Identification of halophilic microbes in lung fibrotic tissue by oligotyping. *Front Microbiol.* (2018) 9:1892. doi: 10.3389/fmicb.2018.01892
65. Harrison OJ, Maloy KJ. Innate immune activation in intestinal homeostasis. *J Innate Immun.* (2011) 3:585–93. doi: 10.1159/000330913

16

Triple Therapy in COPD: Can we Welcome the Reduction in Cardiovascular Risk and Mortality?

Paolo Solidoro [1,2], *Carlo Albera* [1,2], *Fulvia Ribolla* [1], *Michela Bellocchia* [1], *Luisa Brussino* [2,3†] *and Filippo Patrucco* [4,5*†]

[1] Division of University Respiratory Medicine, Cardiovascular and Thoracic Department, AOU Città della Salute e della Scienza di Torino, Turin, Italy, [2] Department of Medical Sciences, University of Turin, Turin, Italy, [3] Allergy and Clinical Immunology Unit, AO Ordine Mauriziano Hospital, Turin, Italy, [4] Division of Respiratory Diseases, Medical and Specialistic Department, AOU Maggiore della Carità, Novara, Italy, [5] Translational Medicine Department, University of Piemonte Orientale, Novara, Italy

Correspondence:
Filippo Patrucco
filippo.patrucco@gmail.com

† These authors have contributed equally to this work

Chronic obstructive pulmonary disease (COPD) is a complex disease which consists in the reduction of the airflow and leads to the disruption of the pulmonary tissue due to a chronic inflammation. The progression of the disease is characterized by an exacerbation of the symptoms and the presence of life-threatening systemic complications, such as stroke and ischemic heart disease, with a progressive decline in lung function which can deeply impact the quality of life. Mortality represents the most important COPD outcome, with an increased risk in patients with cardiovascular comorbidities. The efficacy and safety of triple inhaled therapy were demonstrated by numerous controlled trials. Above all, many robust data are now available on the effectiveness of the triple therapy to reduce mortality in COPD patients.

Keywords: chronic obstructive pulmonary disease (COPD), triple inhaled therapy, ICS, LAMA, LABA, CV mortality

INTRODUCTION

Chronic obstructive pulmonary disease (COPD) is a slowly progressive (1) complex disease, which consists in the reduction of the airflow and leads to the disruption of the pulmonary tissue due to a chronic inflammation (2, 3). According to the Global Initiative for Chronic Obstructive Lung Disease (GOLD) initiative, the airflow limitation “is usually both progressive and associated with an abnormal inflammatory response of the lungs to noxious particles or gases” (4). Over the lifetime, COPD might predispose to exacerbations and serious illness (5). According to the World Health Organization (WHO), 251 million cases of COPD were globally reported in 2016 and it is estimated that 3.17 million deaths were caused by the disease in 2015 (5). Moreover, COPD prevalence is likely to increase in the coming years due to higher smoking habits and aging populations (5).

Although the development of COPD might be considered multifactorial (6), smoking can be considered the most important environmental risk factor in the development of COPD (7), leading to a rapid decline in lung function and an increase in mortality in smokers compared to non-smokers (8). However, multiple risk factors might be involved in the development of the disease which can be classified into environment-related risk factors and patient-related risk factors, such as respiratory infections, occupational exposures, ambient air pollution, passive smoke exposure, and diet. Moreover, some other genetic factors can be involved in the establishment of COPD, such as the Alpha1-antitrypsin deficiency (9).

Another important risk factor is reduced Daily Physical Activity (DPA), which might be considered an important cause of cardiovascular (CV) morbidity (10).

COPD pathophysiology is also influenced by toxic particles inhalation (11), which indeed may lead to chronic inflammation that might exacerbate the COPD prognosis (12). These substances act by activating both epithelial cells and alveolar macrophages, which are involved in the release of proinflammatory cytokines and proteases, such as matrix metalloproteinases (MMPs) and neutrophil elastase. The release of neutrophil elastase leads to elastin degradation and the alveolar wall destruction (11).

COPD clinical course is characterized by persistent and productive cough, dyspnea, and chest tightness (1). The progression of the disease is characterized by an exacerbation of the symptoms and the presence of life-threatening systemic complications (1), such as stroke and ischemic heart disease (13), which are associated with a progressive decline in lung function, and can deeply impact the quality of life (14).

Acute Exacerbations of COPD are mainly triggered by respiratory infections, environmental factors (15), or both (14). Moreover, disorders of the immune system may increase the frequency of AECOPDs, which are associated with an increase of airway inflammation, mucus hypersecretion and gas trapping, and are characterized by both minor (wheeze, sore throat, cough, fever, chest tightness, fatigue, sleep disturbance) and major symptoms (dyspnea, increased sputum volume and purulence) (14). Often, after recurrent exacerbations, respiratory failure might occur, due to hypoxia which is usually characterized by the dropping of the blood oxygen levels during rest, sleep, or activity (16).

MORTALITY AND CARDIOVASCULAR RISK IN COPD

Mortality represents the most important COPD outcome (17), even though this event is often underestimated (18), or underreported (19). With 3.23 million deaths in 2019, COPD represents the third cause of death worldwide (20). In the last years, mortality for COPD rapidly increased, particularly among old women, with an increase of three-fold higher among women ≥75 years old (21). This could be due to the high susceptibility to secondary COPD complications, but also to the high smoking prevalence among the global population (22). To date, in Italy 3.5 million people suffer for COPD, with approximately 55% of death due to the respiratory disease. However, the prevalence of the disease is high and often variable between Italian regions, and is related to a late diagnosis after hospitalization for exacerbations, while mild-to-moderate disease are often underdiagnosed. The national PNE (Programma Nazionale Esiti) estimated a high number of hospitalizations for COPD (>100.000/year), with a rate of mortality of 9.8% and 13.45% hospital readmissions at 30 days (https://pne.agenas.it/).

Multiple risk factors may contribute to increase the mortality risk in patients with COPD.

In particular, the reduction in the forced expiratory volume in one second (FEV_1) is a strong risk factor of all-cause mortality in moderate COPD (23, 24).

Fletcher and Peto for the first time demonstrated that the initial value of measured FEV_1 correlated with the increased risk of death in patients with COPD (25).

Since COPD patients are frequently affected by other comorbidities, cardiovascular disease and malignancy are still the predominant causes of death. Moreover, AECOPDs represent another important risk factor which may influence the mortality rate (26).

Nowadays, multidimensional indexes including BODE, ADO (age, dyspnea, airflow obstruction) and DOSE (dyspnea, obstruction, smoking, exacerbation) indexes, have been used in order to predict the risk of mortality in COPD patients. Several papers, underline this increased risk as also associated with low exercise capacity and increased number of exacerbations (27, 28).

The decrease of morbidity and mortality in COPD is one of the main objectives of GOLD initiative, which represents the most important guide for the management and staging of COPD (29). Last updates, matched spirometry staging, symptoms and exacerbations in the ABCD Classifications in order to choose the best treatment approach (30).

Indeed, from 2015 to 2019, mortality was taken into account was reconsidered because of similar variability between ABCD groups (30).

Cardiovascular diseases (CVD) represent the most frequent cause of death worldwide (29) and it is an important comorbidity in the prediction of all-cause mortality in COPD patients (31). This could be due to the risk shared among two diseases, such as old age, smoking history and increased systemic inflammation (32, 33).

Ischemic heart disease, heart failure and cardiac arrhythmias are the most commonly observed CVDs in COPD patients (34). Numerous mechanisms might be involved in the development of COPD-related CVD, including lung hyperinflation, hypoxemia, pulmonary hypertension (PH), systemic inflammation, oxidative stress, and exacerbations.

Hyperinflation is the major cause of COPD mortality (35) and it deeply impacts the respiratory system. As a matter of the fact, hyperinflation results from the destruction of the lung parenchyma and subsequent loss of lung elasticity, or it occurs when the air becomes trapped during the subsequent respiratory cycle (36), being the trigger of dyspnea (37). The direct consequence is an airflow limitation which causes increased pressure in the cardiopulmonary system, right-ventricular dysfunction, impaired left-ventricular filling and reduced cardiac output (38). Moreover, the airflow limitation results in a mismatch between ventilation and perfusion, which contributes to the development of hypoxemia (39). Finally, the increase of intrapulmonary pressure can lead to the dilation and hypertrophy of the right ventricle (RV), causing the septum displacement to the left ventricle, with compromission of ventricular filling, stroke volume (SV) and cardiac output (40, 41). Moreover, hypoxemia is responsible for pulmonary vasoconstriction, which results in a diastolic disfunction in the right ventricle (42).

Ventricular arrhythmias are common in COPD patients, especially during exacerbations (43) and include supraventricular or ventricular premature beats, atrial fibrillation, atrial flutter, multifocal atrial tachycardia, supraventricular tachycardia, and non-sustained ventricular tachycardia (44).

The mechanism responsible for the increased risk of cardiovascular disease in patients with COPD is not known; however, several processes have been proposed as alternatives, which are involved in the pathogenesis of cardiovascular disease, playing an important role in driving the increased cardiovascular risk associated with enhanced mortality in COPD (45). Indeed, several biomarkers demonstrated a prognostic value for COPD such as C-reactive protein, fibrinogen, brain type natriuretic peptide (BNB), N- terminal pro-BNP (NT Pro BNP), troponin, VEGF, surfactant protein D and the neutrophil/lymphocyte ratio (NLR) (46, 47). **Figure 1** summarizes the link and the possible mechanism between COPD and CV risk.

The role of medications for cardiovascular diseases needs to be fully understood. A concomitant COPD treatment with angiotensin-converting enzyme inhibitors (ACEIs), angiotensin receptor blockers (ARBs), β-blockers and statins have been correlated with a better management of the disease (48). On the other hand, some COPD treatments might increase CV risk (49–52), such as methylxanthines (53) (which have been now withdrawn), β-agonist drugs (54), inhaled short-acting β-agonists (31), inhaled long-acting β-agonists and anticholinergic drugs (short and long acting) (54). Single dose of indacaterol (55) reduces lung hyperinflation in acute conditions, with a clinically relevant improvement of dyspnea in patients with COPD and CV pathology.

These modifications are associated with a significant increase of the right ventricular compliance indexes and may have a role in improving left ventricular preload leading to a reduction in cardiac frequency (55). In 2018, Hohfòeld et al. (56) conducted a s double-blind, randomized, two-period crossover, placebo-controlled, single-center study aimed to evaluate whether dual bronchodilation with indacaterol/glycopirronium improved cardiac function. This dual bronchodilation significantly improved cardiac function as measured by left-ventricular end-diastolic volume (56).

Systemic corticosteroids are often administered in COPD patients during exacerbations. Schols et al. (57) conducted a study aimed to evaluate the role of systemic corticosteroids, administered orally, in the CV risk for COPD patients. In this study, an oral glucocorticoid use (10 mg/day) was associated with an increased risk, which was even higher when the administered dose has been increased. In conclusion, maintenance treatment with oral glucocorticoids was associated with increased mortality in a dose-dependent manner (57).

TRIPLE INHALED THERAPY

Nowadays, COPD treatment follows a stepwise approach, where a different treatment regimen is indicated for each class (15). Patients belonging to group A present one or fewer exacerbations, without hospitalizations, and not severe symptoms. In this case, patients should receive a short- or long-acting bronchodilator. Group B patients present one or fewer exacerbations, without hospitalization, but are characterized by severe symptoms. A long-acting bronchodilator, either a long-acting muscarinic antagonist (LAMA) or long-acting β 2-agonist (LABA) are indicated for these patients. Group C includes patients with two or more exacerbations which can lead to hospitalization; they do not present severe symptoms and they should be treated with LAMA as first-line therapy. Finally, group D includes symptomatic patients with an history of two or more exacerbations with the need of hospitalization. For these patients, the first-line therapy is a LAMA and for patients with very severe symptoms (COPD Assessment Test Score [CAT] greater than or equal to 20) a LAMA/LABA combination is recommended (58). Moreover, when the eosinophil count is above the threshold of ≥300 eosinophils/μl, a combination on LABA/ICS is strongly recommended as first approach (15).

GOLD recommends triple inhaled therapy for patients who experience recurrent exacerbations despite treatment with either a dual bronchodilator or LABA/ICS combination (59). Triple inhaled therapy includes an inhaled corticosteroid (ICS), a long-acting β 2-agonist (LABA) and a long-acting muscarinic antagonist (LAMA) (58). Indeed, it can improve FEV1 and health status (60).

Nowadays, there are three available inhaled ICS/LABA/LAMA fixed-dose combinations (FDCs): Budesonide/Formoterol/Glycopyrronium (61), Beclometasone/Formoterol/Glycopyrronium (62) and Fluticasone Furoate/Vilanterol/Umeclidinium (63). The three available triple combinations are delivered by three different devices: the aerosphere MDI (61), the Ellipta DPI (63) and a MDI (64). Inhaled ICS/LABA/LAMA FDCs are characterized by different mechanisms of action which provide benefits on exacerbations' reduction, lung function and health status improvement as well by reducing the risk of death (compared with increasing the dose of the single bronchodilator) (64).

Corticosteroids bind the C-terminal of glucocorticoid receptor which is localized in the cytoplasm of target cells. Corticosteroids directly regulate 10–100 genes per cell, but the interaction with other transcription factors indirectly regulates many other genes. The most anti-inflammatory effect of ICS is the inhibition of inflammatory proteins' synthesis, such as cytokines 18. Moreover, ICS increase their effectiveness by inducing the expression of β2-adrenoreceptors, and human genes for β2 receptors have three potential glucocorticoid response elements (65). For this reason ICS can positively impact the cardiovascular outcomes through the reduction of serum CRP levels (66).

LAMAs act by blocking the endogenous cholinergic tone. In particular, vascular innervation of the airways results in the contraction of the smooth bronchial musculature. Acetylcholine can play different roles in this function, being responsible both as a neurotransmitter at the ganglia level, a function mediated through M1 muscarine receptors, and as a neurotransmitter in the neuromuscular junction, resulting in the contraction of smooth musculature through the muscarinic receptor M3 (67). The M2 receptors, located in the post-gangliary neuron, inhibits

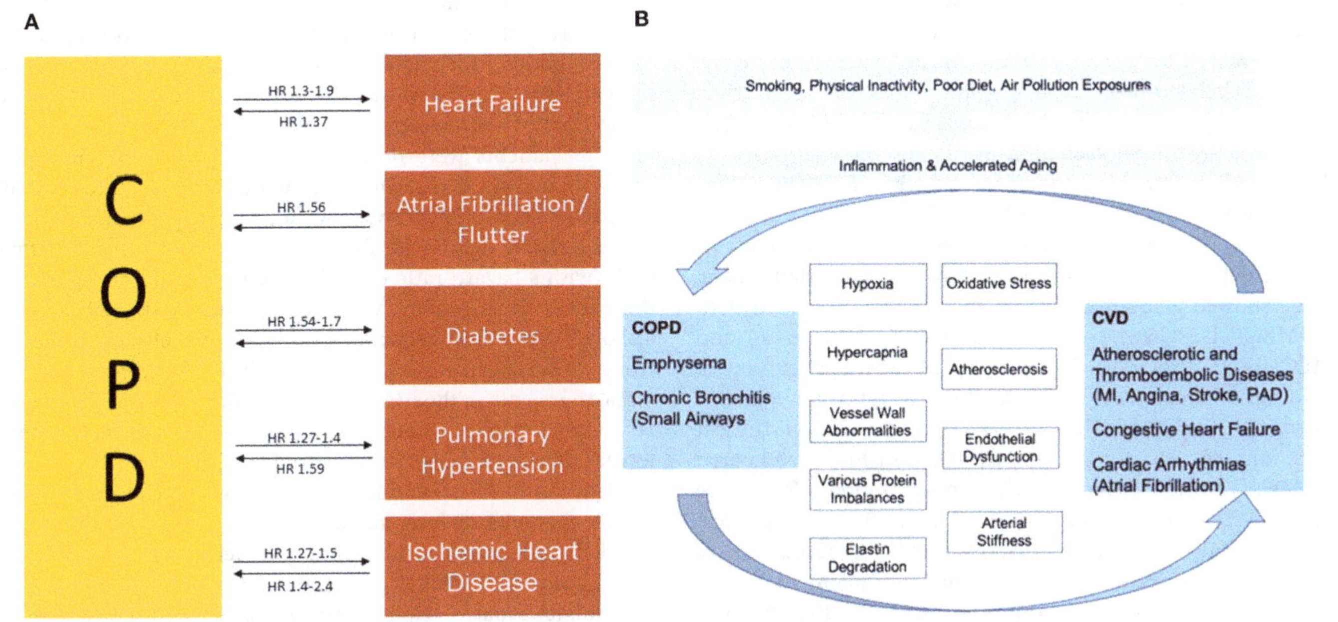

FIGURE 1 | (A) Association between COPD, cardiovascular disease and risk factors and their interrelationship. **(B)** Both diseases are closely linked for several features. COPD, Chronic Obstructive Pulmonary Disease; CVD, Cardiovascular Disease, HR, Hazard Ratio; MI, Myocardial Infraction; and PAD, Peripheral Arterial Disease. Figure adapted from Rabe et al., (38) and adapted from Morgan et al., (34).

the release of acetylcholine. Anticholinergic bronchodilators have been designed to prevent contraction of smooth muscles primarily by blocking the M3 receptor in the neuromuscular junction (67).

Beta2-agonist induce smooth bronchial muscles relaxation through their action on beta2-adrenergic receptors. These receptors, located in the bronchial smooth musculature surface, consist of G-proteins which are able to increase the adenosine monophosphate levels, resulting in the activation of the protein kinase A and in the subsequent relaxation of the smooth bronchial musculature (68).

Combining each family molecule in a single inhaler is the easiest way to deliver triple therapy (69). This therapeutic approach demonstrated a significant reduction in AECOPDs and hospitalizations, as well as a reduction of all-cause mortality (70).

The efficacy and safety of inhaled ICS/LABA/LAMA FDCs in patients with COPD have been evaluated in several clinical trials.

TRIBUTE was a randomized, parallel-group, double-blind study that aimed to compare a single-inhaler triple combination of beclometasone dipropionate, formoterol fumarate, and glycopyrronium (BDP/FF/G) vs. a single-inhaler dual bronchodilator combination of indacaterol plus glycopyrronium (IND/GLY), evaluating the rate of moderate-to-severe AECOPDs over 52 weeks of treatment. Eligible patients were 40 years or older, current or ex-smokers, with a diagnosis of COPD, a FEV_1/FVC post-bronchodilator (salbutamol 400 μg) ratio of less than 0·7, and severe or very severe airflow limitation (FEV_1 <50%). Patients had at least one moderate or severe COPD exacerbation in the previous 12 months, a COPD Assessment Test total score of at least 10 and, for at least 2 months before screening had used an inhaled corticosteroid plus a long-acting β2-agonist, an inhaled corticosteroid plus a long-acting muscarinic antagonist, a long-acting β2-agonist plus a long-acting muscarinic antagonist, or long-acting muscarinic antagonist monotherapy, but not triple therapy. 1532 patients were enrolled among 17 countries and randomized 1:1 to receive 52 weeks of treatment with two inhalations of extrafine BDP/FF/G (87 μg/5 μg/9 μg) twice per day (764 patients) or one inhalation of IND/GLY (85 μg/43 μg) per day (768 patients). The primary endpoint was the rate of moderate-to-severe COPD exacerbations across 52 weeks of treatment. Results showed a rate of moderate-to-severe exacerbation of 0.50 per patient per year (95% CI 0.45–0.57) for BDP/FF/G group and 0.59 per patient per year (0.53–0.67) for IND/GLY group. Adverse events were reported by 490 of 764 patients (64%) receiving BDP/FF/G and 516 of 768 (67%) patients receiving IND/GLY (71). Additional analyses on mortality were assessed by Vestbo et al. in a pooled analysis for all extrafine ICS-containing treatments. The rate of fatal events was 2.1% in the BDP/FF/G and 2.7% in the IND/GLY group. However, no statistical significance in the reduction in the risk of death was observed within 1 year of observation (72).

The IMPACT trial was a randomized study involving 10,355 patients with symptomatic COPD (CAT>10; FeV_1 <80%) and a history of moderate/severe exacerbations. Patients were randomized to receive fluticasone furoate/umeclidium/vilanterol (FF/UMEC/VI) (100 μg/62.5 ug/25 ug) OR fluticasone furoate/vilanterol (FF/VI) (100 ug/25 ug) OR umeclidinium/vilanterol (UMEC/VI) (62.5 ug/25 ug). Results showed that the reduction of moderate to severe COPD exacerbations rate was significantly greater for triple therapy with FF/UMEC/VI group than fluticasone furoate-vilanterol or umeclidinium-vilanterol groups, with rates of 0.91 per year, 1.07 per year and 1.21 per year, respectively. The COPD-related hospitalization rate was lower in the triple therapy group than umeclidinium-vilanterol (0.13 vs. 0.19). Moreover, a significant reduction in all-cause mortality (ACM) risk was demonstrated in patients treated with FF/UMEC/VI vs. UMEC/VI, with a hazard ratio of 0.58 (73). In 2020, a *post-hoc* analysis was performed to report any ACM and the impact of stepping down therapy using the additional vital status data. Results showed a lower rate of death in patients treated with FF/UMEC/VI (2.36%) compared to both FF/VI (2.64%) and UMEC/VI (3.19%) (74). Time to ACM was also evaluated, including off-treatment data: the hazard ratio for patients treated with FF/UMEC/VI was 0.72 compared with UMEC/VI group, and was 0.82 for patients treated with FF/VI compared to UMEC/VI ones. Because of the randomization, 40% of the patients were stepped down to FF/VI and 20% were stepped down to UMEC/VI. Results demonstrated a reduced risk of on/off-treatment death for patients who were maintained on a triple therapy compared to those who underwent step down to one of the dual therapies (FF/VI or UMEC/VI) (hazard ratio of 0.71 compared with patients stepped down to FF/VI; hazard ratio of 0.62 compared to patients who stepped down to UMEC/VI). It is worth to note that 76.9% of the patients were treated with a therapeutic regimen including an ICS at the time of enrollment: in these patients, mortality was lower if they were maintained on an ICS-containing regimen compared with UMEC/VI (74).

The ETHOS (75)study was a phase 3 randomized trial that evaluated efficacy and safety of triple therapy at two dose levels of inhaled glucocorticoid over 52 weeks. The study included 40–80 years old patients with symptomatic COPD (defined as a score of ≥10 on the COPD Assessment Test, on which scores range from 0 to 40, with higher scores indicating more symptoms; the minimum clinically important difference is 2 points). Patients were receiving at least two inhaled maintenance therapies at the time of screening, with a post-bronchodilator FEV_1/FVC ratio of <0.7, and a postbronchodilator FEV_1 of 25 to 65% of the predicted normal value. Patients were smokers or ex smokers and had a documented history of at least one moderate or severe COPD exacerbation (if their FEV_1 was <50% of the predicted normal value) or at least two moderate or at least one severe COPD exacerbation (if their FEV_1 was ≥50% of the predicted normal value) in the year before screening. 8,509 patients were included in the study and randomly assigned to the groups receiving: inhaled budesonide/glycopyrronium/formoterol, 320 μg/18 ug/ 9.6 ug (320-BGF; 2,137 patients); inhaled budesonide/glycopyrronium/formoterol, 160 ug/18 ug/ 9.6 ug (160-BGF; 2,121 patients); glycopyrronium/formoterol-18 ug/9.6 ug- (GFF; 2,120 patients); budesonide/formoterol-320 ug/9.6 ug (BFF; 2,131 patients). The primary endpoint was to assess the annual rate of moderate or severe COPD exacerbations. BGF triple therapy resulted in a lower rate of moderate or severe COPD exacerbations (1.08 and 1.07 for the 320 ug and 160 ug, respectively) than GFF (1.42) or BFF (1.24) (75). Moreover, the rate was significantly lower with 320- μg–budesonide triple therapy group than with GFF (24% lower) or BFF ones (13% lower). Mortality was evaluated as key secondary endpoint, and a lower risk of death from any cause was observed only in the 320-μg–budesonide triple-therapy group (75). Overall, the risk of death from any cause was 46% lower for 320-μg–budesonide triple therapy vs. glycopyrronium- formoterol (75). Since 384 of 8,509 patients were missing vital status at Week 52 in the original analyses, a *post-hoc* analysis was performed to evaluate the robustness of the ETHOS mortality findings. Results showed that the risk of death with BGF 320 was significantly lower than GFF (with a hazard ratio of 0.51), and there were no significant differences in mortality when comparing BGF 320 to BFF, although numerical reductions of 28% were observed. Deaths from cardiovascular causes occurred in 0.5%, 0.8%, 1.4%, and 0.5% of patients in the BGF 320, BGF 160, GFF, and BFF groups, respectively (76). Overall, the risk of death was significantly lower (49%) with BGF 320 compared to GFF (76).

Other studies were conducted to evaluate the effect of triple vs. double therapies on lung function.

TRILOGY was a randomized, parallel-group, double-blind, active-controlled study aimed to compare the efficacy of the single inhaler triple therapy vs. inhaled corticosteroid plus long-acting β2-agonist therapy [beclometasone dipropionate, formoterol fumarate, and glycopyrronium bromide (BDP/FF/GB) with beclometasone dipropionate and formoterol fumarate (BDP/FF)] over 52 weeks of treatment. Patients were 40 years or older, with a diagnosis of COPD, a $FEV_1 < 50\%$, a $FEV_1/FVC < 0{\cdot}7$, and at least one moderate or severe COPD exacerbation in the previous 12 months. Previous treatment included an inhaled corticosteroid plus a long-acting β2 agonist, or an inhaled corticosteroid plus a long-acting muscarinic antagonist, or a long-acting β2 agonist plus a long-acting muscarinic antagonist, or long-acting muscarinic antagonist monotherapy for at least 2 months before screening. Patients receiving triple therapy of an inhaled corticosteroid plus a long-acting β2 agonist plus a long-acting muscarinic antagonist were not eligible. Additionally, all patients needed to be symptomatic for inclusion, classified as a COPD Assessment Test (CAT) total score of 10 or more and a Baseline Dyspnea Index (BDI) focal score of 10 or less at screening, with the BDI criterion also confirmed at the randomization visit. 1,367 patients with symptomatic COPD have been enrolled. Three primary endpoints were assessed: change from baseline in pre-dose (morning) FEV_1, change from baseline in 2-h post-dose FEV_1, and Transition Dyspnea Index (TDI) focal score assessed at week 26. Results showed that BDP/FF/GB improved the morning pre-dose trough FEV_1, and 2-h post dose FEV_1 vs. ICS/LABA, and reduced exacerbations by 23% when compared with BDP/FF (77).

KRONOS study aimed to compare the efficacy of triple therapy with other dual therapies in patients with moderate to very severe COPD, with or without a history of exacerbations, over 24 weeks. This double-blind, parallel-group, multicenter phase 3 randomized controlled trial involved 1,902 patients. Participants were randomly assigned to receive triple therapy (budesonide/glycopyrronium /Formoterol Fumarate Metered Dose Inhaler -BGF MDI-) or dual therapies (glycopyrronium/formoterol fumarate [GFF] MDI and budesonide/formoterol fumarate [BFF] MDI, BUD/FORM DPI). BGF significantly improved morning pre-dose trough FEV_1 when compared to GFF and BFF. This improvement was also observed for FEV_1 AUC_{0-4}. A significant reduction in the rate of moderate/severe exacerbations was observed in the triple therapy arm when compared to GFF (52% of reduction for moderate-to-severe exacerbation and 64% of reduction for severe exacerbations). Results showed that BGF MDI was more effective to improve FEV_1 and to reduce exacerbation. Also, it was well-tolerated compared to the corresponding dual therapies among symptomatic patients with moderate to very severe COPD, with or without exacerbation history (78).

A *post-hoc* analysis (76) evaluated whether the benefits observed were driven by patients with ≥ 1 exacerbation in the 12 months prior to the study, considering that 74.4% were symptomatic patients without a prior history of exacerbations. Independently of eosinophil count, triple therapy results in exacerbations control in those symptomatic patients without exacerbations history. Respectively 52% and 58% of moderate/severe and severe exacerbations were reduced in this group, supporting the hypothesis that the exacerbations reduction in KRONOS was not driven by the subset of patients with a prior history of exacerbations (76).

DISCUSSION

Mortality represents the most important COPD outcome (17). In particular, cardiovascular diseases are important comorbidities in the prediction of all-cause mortality in COPD patients (31, 79).

So far, oxygen therapy, smoking discontinuation and surgical reduction of lung volume (in selected cases) were the only treatments able of reducing mortality.

Recently, the effectiveness of the triple inhaled therapy in the reduction of mortality was largely demonstrated, even though mortality was not the primary endpoint in the trials (80). The IMPACT study was the first large trial reporting significant mortality reduction data in patients who received triple inhaled therapy, with a hazard ratio for triple therapy vs. the dual bronchodilator umeclidinium/vilanterol of 0.58 (95% CI 0.38–0.88) and 0.61 (95% CI 0.40–0.93), although this finding derived from another endpoint (73, 74). Later on, the ETHOS study showed that the risk of death from any cause in the 320-μg budesonide triple therapy group was 49% lower than the glycopyrronium/formoterol group, including this analysis among key secondary endpoints (75, 76). For the reasons mentioned above, triple inhaled therapy was recommended in the latest GOLD guidelines as a potential option to reduce mortality in COPD patients with concomitant chronic diseases (57). Additionally, the choice of a device must be taken into account also evaluating the patient's clinical condition, as well as their ability to coordinate the inhalation maneuver and to generate sufficient inspiratory flow and their adherence to the treatment (81).

It is worth to note that previous large, controlled trials, comparing inhaled therapy with placebo, failed to demonstrate a significant effect on mortality. The TORCH trial aimed to evaluate the mortality reduction among patients with COPD treated with the combination of the long-acting b-agonist salmeterol and the inhaled corticosteroid fluticasone propionate compared with usual care (with each of the components alone) and with placebo over a 3-year period. 6,112 patients were enrolled in the study. The hazard ratio for death was 0.825 in the combination-therapy group (comparison to placebo) even if the reduction of death from all causes among patients with COPD in the combination-therapy group did not reach the predetermined level of statistical significance (82).

The SUMMIT trial was the largest randomized controlled COPD trial, where more than 16,000 patients with moderate airflow limitation (⩾50% and ⩽70% predicted forced expiratory volume in 1 s) and a history or an increased risk for cardiovascular disease were enrolled. The study aimed to compare the effectiveness of a combined treatment of fluticasone furoate and vilanterol compared with placebo. Results showed a non-significant reduction of all-cause mortality (12%) with ICS/LABA compared to placebo (83).

The UPLIFT trial evaluated the long-term effects of tiotropium therapy compared to placebo. The study included 5,993 COPD patients with a FEV1 of 70% or less after bronchodilation. Patients were evaluated in a 4-years follow up. Results showed a non-significant decrease in mortality (hazard ratio 0.89, 95% CI 0.79–1.02; $p = 0.09$) compared to placebo (84).

The OUTPUL study enrolled 18,615 patients and assessed whether in COPD patients adding an ICS to a long-acting bronchodilators (LB) would lead to a mortality reduction in patients discharged from hospital. Mortality rates were 110 and 143 cases per 1,000 person-years in the "LB plus ICS" and "LB alone" groups, respectively. The mortality reduction was much more pronounced in patients with frequent exacerbations, with a hazard ratio of 0.63 (95% CI: 0.44–0.90; p value: 0.012) (85).

Beneficial effects of triple inhaled therapy on the mortality reduction might be due to several mechanisms, such as reduction of hyperinflation, reduction of exacerbations risk, stabilization of atherosclerotic plaques and the improvement of cardiac perfusion.

COPD is characterized by a low-grade systemic inflammation (with the release of numerous proinflammatory cytokines and CRP) which can contribute to the pathogenesis of atherosclerosis and cardiovascular disease (86). In particular, high CRP levels are correlated with poor CV outcomes, such as atherosclerotic plaque genesis, rupture, and subsequent thrombofibrosis of vulnerable vessels. The efficacy of corticosteroids in the reduction of CRP and cytokines blood concentrations, which regulate CRP (such as interleukin 6), is well known. Especially, fluticasone demonstrated to be effective in the reduction of the serum CRP levels (66). ICSs are able to reduce the local inflammation and subsequent cardiovascular morbidity: Lofdahl et al. (87) demonstrated that budesonide was involved in the reduction of ischemic cardiac events, as well as angina pectoris, myocardial infarction and coronary artery disease. Moreover, ICS demonstrated to be involved in a reduction of the risk from myocardial infarction. This may be due to the reduction of COPD exacerbations, the reduction in systemic inflammation or the reduction in the adaptive immune response (88).

It is known that lung hyperinflation is associated with an increase in all-cause mortality in COPD patients. In particular, increased levels of static lung hyperinflation and emphysema are associated with a reduction in the cardiac chamber size and function, responsible of death for CV reasons. Triple inhaled therapies demonstrated to improve the right ventricular end-diastolic volume index and to reduce residual volume (89).

In conclusion, cardiovascular diseases represent an important comorbidity in the prediction of all-cause mortality in COPD patients. Numerous mechanisms may be involved in the development of COPD-related CVD: among these, a major role could be played by lung hyperinflation, hypoxemia, pulmonary hypertension (PH), systemic inflammation, oxidative stress, and exacerbations. The efficacy and safety of triple inhaled therapy were demonstrated by numerous controlled trials: above all, many robust data are now available on the effectiveness of the triple therapy to reduce mortality in COPD patients. Mechanisms involved need to be fully understood and they most likely include the reduction of hyperinflation, the improvement in the risk of exacerbations, the stabilization in the atherosclerotic plaques and the improvement of the cardiac perfusion. Thus, triple therapy may represent a valid option to reduce mortality in COPD patients, although it is still necessary to optimize the ideal patient profile.

AUTHOR CONTRIBUTIONS

PS and FP designed the project, selected the literature, and wrote and reviewed the manuscript. CA reviewed the manuscript. FR selected the literature and reviewed the manuscript. MB selected the literature and wrote the manuscript. LB designed the project and wrote the manuscript. All authors have reviewed and approved the manuscript.

ACKNOWLEDGMENTS

Editorial and writing assistance was provided by Edra S.p.A., Milan, Italy and funded by AstraZeneca.

REFERENCES

1. Devine JF. Chronic obstructive pulmonary disease: an overview. *Am Health Drug Benefits.* (2008) 1:34–42.
2. Singh D, Agusti A, Anzueto A, Barnes PJ, Bourbeau J, Celli BR, et al. Global strategy for the diagnosis, management, and prevention of chronic obstructive lung disease: the GOLD science committee report 2019. *Eur Respir J.* (2019) 53:1900164. doi: 10.1183/13993003.00164-2019
3. Barnes PJ. Chronic obstructive pulmonary disease. *N Engl J Med.* (2000) 343:269–80. doi: 10.1056/NEJM200007273430407
4. Pauwels RA, Buist AS, Calverley PM, Jenkins CR, Hurd SS, GOLD Scientific Committee. Global strategy for the diagnosis, management, and prevention of chronic obstructive pulmonary disease NHLBI/WHO Global Initiative for Chronic Obstructive Lung Disease (GOLD) Workshop summary. *Am J Respir Crit Care Med.* (2001) 163:1256–76. doi: 10.1164/ajrccm.163.5.2101039
5. Organization WH. *Chronic obstructive pulmonary disease (COPD) 2020.* Available online at: https://www.who.int/news-room/fact-sheets/detail/chronic-obstructive-pulmonary-disease-(copd)
6. Vijayan VK. Chronic obstructive pulmonary disease. *Indian J Med Res.* (2013) 137:251–69.
7. Rennard SI. Overview of causes of COPD. New understanding of pathogenesis and mechanisms can guide future therapy. *Postgrad Med.* (2002) 111:28–38. doi: 10.3810/pgm.2002.06.1223
8. Hogea SP, Tudorache E, Fildan AP, Fira-Mladinescu O, Marc M, Oancea C. Risk factors of chronic obstructive pulmonary disease exacerbations. *Clin Respir J.* (2020) 14:183–97. doi: 10.1111/crj.13129
9. Silverman EK. Genetics of COPD. *Annu Rev Physiol.* (2020) 82:413–31. doi: 10.1146/annurev-physiol-021317-121224
10. Albarrati AM, Gale NS, Munnery MM, Cockcroft JR, Shale DJ. Daily physical activity and related risk factors in COPD. *BMC Pulm Med.* (2020) 20:60. doi: 10.1186/s12890-020-1097-y
11. Hikichi M, Mizumura K, Maruoka S, Gon Y. Pathogenesis of chronic obstructive pulmonary disease (COPD) induced by cigarette smoke. *J Thorac Dis.* (2019) 11:S2129–40. doi: 10.21037/jtd.2019.10.43
12. Wang Y, Xu J, Meng Y, Adcock IM, Yao X. Role of inflammatory cells in airway remodeling in COPD. *Int J Chron Obstruct Pulmon Dis.* (2018) 13:3341–8. doi: 10.2147/COPD.S176122
13. Tkác J, Man SF, Sin DD. Systemic consequences of COPD. *Ther Adv Respir Dis.* (2007) 1:47–59. doi: 10.1177/1753465807082374
14. Ritchie AI, Wedzicha JA. Definition, causes, pathogenesis, and consequences of chronic obstructive pulmonary disease exacerbations. *Clin Chest Med.* (2020) 41:421–38. doi: 10.1016/j.ccm.2020.06.007
15. Global Initiative for Chronic Obstructive Lung Disease (GOLD). *Global Strategy for the Diagnosis, Management, and Prevention of Chronic Obstructive Pulmonary Disease* (2021 report).
16. Negewo NA, Gibson PG, McDonald VM. COPD and its comorbidities: impact, measurement and mechanisms. *Respirology.* (2015) 20:1160–71. doi: 10.1111/resp.12642
17. Cazzola M, MacNee W, Martinez FJ, Rabe KF, Franciosi LG, Barnes PJ, et al. Outcomes for COPD pharmacological trials: from lung function to biomarkers. *Eur Respir J.* (2008) 31:416–69. doi: 10.1183/09031936.00099306
18. Sin DD, Anthonisen NR, Soriano JB, Agusti AG. Mortality in COPD: role of co-morbidities. *Eur Respir J.* (2006) 28:1245–57. doi: 10.1183/09031936.00133805
19. Drummond MB, Wise RA, John M, Zvarich MT, McGarvey LP. Accuracy of death certificates in COPD: analysis from the TORCH trial. *COPD.* (2010) 7:179–85. doi: 10.3109/15412555.2010.481695
20. World Health Organization. *Chronic Obstructive Pulmonary Disease (COPD).* (2019). Available online at: https://www.who.int/news-room/fact-sheets/detail/chronic-obstructive-pulmonary-disease-(copd) (accessed November 17, 2021).
21. National Institutes of Health and National Heart, Lung, and Blood Institute (NHLBI). *Morbidity and Mortality: 2009 Chartbook on Cardiovascular, Lung, and Blood Diseases.* NIH (2009).
22. Berry CE, Wise RA. Mortality in COPD: causes, risk factors, and prevention. *COPD.* (2010) 7:375–82. doi: 10.3109/15412555.2010.510160
23. Bikov A, Lange P, Anderson JA, Brook RD, Calverley PMA, Celli BR, et al. FEV_1 is a stronger mortality predictor than FVC in patients with moderate COPD and with an increased risk for cardiovascular disease. *Int J Chron Obstruct Pulmon Dis.* (2020) 15:1135–42. doi: 10.2147/COPD.S242809
24. David S, Edwards CW. *Forced Expiratory Volume.* Treasure Island, FL: StatPearls Publishing (2021). Available online at: https://www.ncbi.nlm.nih.gov/books/NBK540970/ (accessed September 14, 2020).
25. Fletcher C, Peto R. The natural history of chronic airflow obstruction. *Br Med J.* (1977) 1:1645–8.
26. Hoogendoorn M, Hoogenveen RT. Rutten-van Mölken MP, Vestbo J, Feenstra TL. Case fatality of COPD exacerbations: a meta-analysis and statistical modelling approach. *Eur Respir J.* (2011) 37:508–15. doi: 10.1183/09031936.00043710

27. Vieira EB, Degani-Costa LH, Amorim BC, Oliveira LB, Miranda-Silva T, Sperandio PC, et al. Modified BODE index to predict mortality in individuals with COPD: the role of 4-min step test. *Respir Care.* (2020) 65:977–83. doi: 10.4187/respcare.06991
28. Prudente R, Frano E, Mesquita C, Ferrari R, de Godoy I, Tanni S. Predictors of mortality in patients with COPD after 9 years. *Int J Chron Obstruct Pulmon Dis.* (2018) 13:3389–98. doi: 10.2147/COPD.S174665
29. Wood-Baker R, Cochrane B, Naughton MT. Cardiovascular mortality and morbidity in chronic obstructive pulmonary disease: the impact of bronchodilator treatment. *Intern Med J.* (2010) 40:94–101. doi: 10.1111/j.1445-5994.2009.02109.x
30. García Castillo E, Alonso Pérez T, Ancochea J, Pastor Sanz MT, Almagro P, Martínez-Camblor P, et al. Mortality prediction in chronic obstructive pulmonary disease comparing the GOLD 2015 and GOLD 2019 staging: a pooled analysis of individual patient data. *ERJ Open Res.* (2020) 6:00253-2020. doi: 10.1183/23120541.00253-2020
31. Huiart L, Ernst P, Suissa S. Cardiovascular morbidity and mortality in COPD. *Chest.* (2005) 128:2640–6. doi: 10.1378/chest.128.4.2640
32. Magnussen H, Watz H. Systemic inflammation in chronic obstructive pulmonary disease and asthma: relation with comorbidities. *Proc Am Thorac Soc.* (2009) 6:648–51. doi: 10.1513/pats.200906-053DP
33. Roversi S, Fabbri LM, Sin DD, Hawkins NM, Agustí A. Chronic obstructive pulmonary disease and cardiac diseases. An urgent need for integrated care. *Am J Respir Crit Care Med.* (2016) 194:1319–36. doi: 10.1164/rccm.201604-0690SO
34. Morgan AD, Zakeri R, Quint JK. Defining the relationship between COPD and CVD: what are the implications for clinical practice? *Ther Adv Respir Dis.* (2018) 12:1753465817750524. doi: 10.1177/1753465817750524
35. Global Initiative for Chronic Obstructive Lung Disease (GOLD). *Global Strategy for the Diagnosis, Management, and Prevention of Chronic Obstructive Pulmonary Disease (2018 Report).* Available online at: https://goldcopd.org/wp-content/uploads/2017/11/GOLD-2018-v6.0-FINAL-revised-20-Nov_WMS.pdf (accessed November 28, 2017).
36. Rossi A, Aisanov Z, Avdeev S, Di Maria G, Donner CF, Izquierdo JL, et al. Mechanisms, assessment and therapeutic implications of lung hyperinflation in COPD. *Respir Med.* (2015) 109:785–802. doi: 10.1016/j.rmed.2015.03.010
37. Parshall MB, Schwartzstein RM, Adams L, Banzett RB, Manning HL, Bourbeau J, et al. An official American Thoracic Society statement: update on the mechanisms, assessment, and management of dyspnea. *Am J Respir Crit Care Med.* (2012) 185:435–52. doi: 10.1164/rccm.201111-2042ST
38. Rabe KF, Hurst JR, Suissa S. Cardiovascular disease and COPD: dangerous liaisons? [published correction appears in Eur Respir Rev. 2018 Nov 21;27(150)]. *Eur Respir Rev.* (2018) 27(149):180057. doi: 10.1183/16000617.0057-2018
39. Kent BD, Mitchell PD, McNicholas WT. Hypoxemia in patients with COPD: cause, effects, and disease progression. *Int J Chron Obstruct Pulmon Dis.* (2011) 6:199–208. doi: 10.2147/COPD.S10611
40. MacNee W. Pathophysiology of cor pulmonale in chronic obstructive pulmonary disease. *Part One Am J Respir Crit Care Med.* (1994) 150:833–52. doi: 10.1164/ajrccm.150.3.8087359
41. Vonk-Noordegraaf A. The shrinking heart in chronic obstructive pulmonary disease. *N Engl J Med.* (2010) 362:267–8. doi: 10.1056/NEJMe0906251
42. Zangiabadi A, De Pasquale CG, Sajkov D. Pulmonary hypertension and right heart dysfunction in chronic lung disease. *Biomed Res Int.* (2014) 2014:739674
43. Rusinowicz T, Zielonka TM, Zycinska K. Cardiac arrhythmias in patients with exacerbation of COPD. *Adv Exp Med Biol.* (2017) 1022:53–62. doi: 10.1007/5584_2017_41
44. Bhatt SP, Dransfield MT. Chronic obstructive pulmonary disease and cardiovascular disease. *Transl Res.* (2013) 162:237–51. doi: 10.1016/j.trsl.2013.05.001
45. Maclay JD, MacNee W. Cardiovascular disease in COPD: mechanisms. *Chest.* (2013) 143:798–807. doi: 10.1378/chest.12-0938
46. André S, Conde B, Fragoso E, Boléo-Tomé JP, Areias V, Cardoso J. GI DPOC-Grupo de Interesse na Doença Pulmonar Obstrutiva Crónica. COPD and Cardiovascular Disease. *Pulmonology.* (2019) 25:168–76. doi: 10.1016/j.pulmoe.2018.09.006
47. Song M, Graubard BI, Rabkin CS, Engels EA. Neutrophil-to-lymphocyte ratio and mortality in the United States general population. *Sci Rep.* (2021) 11:464. doi: 10.1038/s41598-020-79431-7
48. Almagro P, Salvadó M, Garcia-Vidal C, Rodriguez-Carballeira M, Delgado M, Barreiro B, et al. Recent improvement in long-term survival after a COPD hospitalisation. *Thorax.* (2010) 65:298–302. doi: 10.1136/thx.2009.124818
49. Suissa S. Dell'Aniello S, Ernst P. Long-term natural history of chronic obstructive pulmonary disease: severe exacerbations and mortality. *Thorax.* (2012) 67:957–63. doi: 10.1136/thoraxjnl-2011-201518
50. Suissa S, Hemmelgarn B, Blais L, Ernst P. Bronchodilators and acute cardiac death. *Am J Respir Crit Care Med.* (1996) 154:1598–602. doi: 10.1164/ajrccm.154.6.8970341
51. Maxwell SR, Moots RJ, Kendall MJ. Corticosteroids: do they damage the cardiovascular system? *Postgrad Med J.* (1994) 70:863–70.
52. Sholter DE, Armstrong PW. Adverse effects of corticosteroids on the cardiovascular system. *Can J Cardiol.* (2000) 16:505–11.
53. McKenzie DK, Frith PA, Burdon JG, Town GI. The COPDX plan: Australian and New Zealand guidelines for the management of chronic obstructive pulmonary disease 2003. *Med J Aust.* (2003) 178(Suppl):S7–39. doi: 10.5694/j.1326-5377.2003.tb05213.x
54. Sestini P, Renzoni E, Robinson S, Poole P, Ram FS. Short-acting beta 2 agonists for stable chronic obstructive pulmonary disease. *Cochrane Database Syst Rev.* (2002) 2002:CD001495. doi: 10.1002/14651858.CD001495
55. Santus P, Radovanovic D, Di Marco S, Valenti V, Raccanelli R, Blasi F, et al. Effect of indacaterol on lung deflation improves cardiac performance in hyperinflated COPD patients: an interventional, randomized, double-blind clinical trial. *Int J Chron Obstruct Pulmon Dis.* (2015) 10:1917–23. doi: 10.2147/COPD.S91684
56. Hohlfeld JM, Vogel-Claussen J, Biller H, Berliner D, Berschneider K, Tillmann HC, et al. Effect of lung deflation with indacaterol plus glycopyrronium on ventricular filling in patients with hyperinflation and COPD (CLAIM): a double-blind, randomised, crossover, placebo-controlled, single-centre trial. *Lancet Respir Med.* (2018) 6:368–78. doi: 10.1016/S2213-2600(18)30054-7
57. Schols AM, Wesseling G, Kester AD, de Vries G, Mostert R, Slangen J, et al. Dose dependent increased mortality risk in COPD patients treated with oral glucocorticoids. *Eur Respir J.* (2001) 17:337–42. doi: 10.1183/09031936.01.17303370
58. Petite SE. What is the role of triple inhaled therapy in COPD? *JAAPA.* (2019) 32:44–5. doi: 10.1097/01.JAA.0000580568.79593.55
59. Global Initiative for Chronic Obstructive Lung Disease (GOLD). *Global Strategy for the Diagnosis, Management, and Prevention of Chronic Obstructive Pulmonary Disease* (2021 report). Available online at: https://goldcopd.org/wp-content/uploads/2020/11/GOLD-REPORT-2021-v1.1-25Nov20_WMV.pdf
60. Zheng Y, Zhu J, Liu Y, Lai W, Lin C, Qiu K, et al. Triple therapy in the management of chronic obstructive pulmonary disease: systematic review and meta-analysis. *BMJ.* (2018) 363:k4388. doi: 10.1136/bmj.k4388
61. Trixeo. *Summary of Product Characteristics.* Available online at: https://www.ema.europa.eu/en/medicines/human/EPAR/trixeo-aerosphere
62. Trimbow. *Summary of Product Characteristics.* Available online at: https://www.ema.europa.eu/en/medicines/human/EPAR/trimbow
63. Trelegy. *Summary of Product Characteristics.* Available online at: https://www.ema.europa.eu/en/medicines/human/EPAR/trelegy-ellipta
64. Vanfleteren L, Fabbri LM, Papi A, Petruzzelli S, Celli B. Triple therapy (ICS/LABA/LAMA) in COPD: time for a reappraisal. *Int J Chron Obstruct Pulmon Dis.* (2018) 13:3971–81. doi: 10.2147/COPD.S185975
65. Aksoy MO, Mardini IA, Yang Y. Glucocorticoid effects on the beta-adrenergic receptor-adenylyl cyclase system of human airway epithelium. *J Allergy Clin Immunol.* (2002) 109:491–7. doi: 10.1067/mai.2002.122154
66. Sin DD, Lacy P, York E, Man SF. Effects of fluticasone on systemic markers of inflammation in chronic obstructive pulmonary disease. *Am J Respir Crit Care Med.* (2004) 170:760–5. doi: 10.1164/rccm.200404-543OC
67. Barnes PJ. Muscarinic receptor subtypes in airways. *Life Sci.* (1993) 52:521–7.
68. Barnes PJ. *Chronic Obstructive Pulmonary Disease.* London: Chapman and Hall (1995).

69. Montuschi P, Malerba M, Macis G, Mores N, Santini G. Triple inhaled therapy for chronic obstructive pulmonary disease. *Drug Discov Today.* (2016) 21:1820–7. doi: 10.1016/j.drudis.2016.07.009
70. Bourbeau J, Bafadhel M, Barnes NC, Compton C, Di Boscio V, Lipson DA, et al. Benefit/risk profile of single-inhaler triple therapy in COPD. *Int J Chron Obstruct Pulmon Dis.* (2021) 16:499–517. doi: 10.2147/COPD.S291967
71. Papi A, Vestbo J, Fabbri L, Corradi M, Prunier H, Cohuet G, et al. Extrafine inhaled triple therapy versus dual bronchodilator therapy in chronic obstructive pulmonary disease (TRIBUTE): a double-blind, parallel group, randomised controlled trial [published correction appears in Lancet. 2018 Feb 26]. *Lancet.* (2018) 391:1076–84. doi: 10.1016/S0140-6736(18)30206-X
72. Vestbo J, Fabbri L, Papi A, Petruzzelli S, Scuri M, Guasconi A, et al. Inhaled corticosteroid containing combinations and mortality in COPD. *Eur Respir J.* (2018) 52:1801230. doi: 10.1183/13993003.01230-2018
73. Lipson DA, Barnhart F, Brealey N, Brooks J, Criner GJ, Day NC, et al. Once-daily single-inhaler triple versus dual therapy in patients with COPD. *N Engl J Med.* (2018) 378:1671–80. doi: 10.1056/NEJMoa1713901
74. Lipson DA, Crim C, Criner GJ, Day NC, Dransfield MT, Halpin DMG, et al. Reduction in all-cause mortality with fluticasone furoate/umeclidinium/vilanterol in patients with chronic obstructive pulmonary disease. *Am J Respir Crit Care Med.* (2020) 201:1508–16. doi: 10.1164/rccm.201911-2207OC
75. Rabe KF, Martinez FJ, Ferguson GT, Wang C, Singh D, Wedzicha JA, et al. Triple inhaled therapy at two glucocorticoid doses in moderate-to-very-severe COPD. *N Engl J Med.* (2020) 383:35–48. doi: 10.1056/NEJMoa1916046
76. Martinez FJ, Ferguson GT, Bourne E, Ballal S, Darken P, Aurivillius M, et al. Budesonide/glycopyrrolate/formoterol fumarate metered dose inhaler improves exacerbation outcomes in patients with COPD without a recent exacerbation history: a subgroup analysis of KRONOS. *Int J Chron Obstruct Pulmon Dis.* (2021) 16:179–89. doi: 10.2147/COPD.S286087
77. Singh D, Papi A, Corradi M, Pavlišová I, Montagna I, Francisco C, et al. Single inhaler triple therapy versus inhaled corticosteroid plus long-acting β2-agonist therapy for chronic obstructive pulmonary disease (TRILOGY): a double-blind, parallel group, randomised controlled trial. *Lancet.* (2016) 388:963–73. doi: 10.1016/S0140-6736(16)31354-X
78. Ferguson GT, Rabe KF, Martinez FJ, Fabbri LM, Wang C, Ichinose M, et al. Triple therapy with budesonide/glycopyrronium/formoterol fumarate with co-suspension delivery technology versus dual therapies in chronic obstructive pulmonary disease (KRONOS): a double-blind, parallel-group, multicentre, phase 3 randomised controlled trial [published correction appears in *Lancet Respir Med.* 2018 Oct 4] [published correction appears in *Lancet Respir Med.* 2019;7(2):e9]. *Lancet Respir Med.* (2018) 6:747–58. doi: 10.1016/S2213-2600(18)30327-8
79. Divo M, Cote C, de Torres JP, Casanova C, Marin JM, Pinto-Plata V, et al. Comorbidities and risk of mortality in patients with chronic obstructive pulmonary disease. *Am J Respir Crit Care Med.* (2012) 186:155–61. doi: 10.1164/rccm.201201-0034OC
80. Andreas S, Taube C. Inhaled therapy reduces COPD mortality. *ERJ Open Res.* (2020) 6:00634-2020. doi: 10.1183/23120541.00634-2020
81. Scichilone N, Benfante A, Bocchino M, Braido F, Paggiaro P, Papi A, et al. Which factors affect the choice of the inhaler in chronic obstructive respiratory diseases? *Pulm Pharmacol Ther.* (2015) 31:63–7. doi: 10.1016/j.pupt.2015.02.006
82. Calverley PM, Anderson JA, Celli B, Ferguson GT, Jenkins C, Jones PW, et al. Salmeterol and fluticasone propionate and survival in chronic obstructive pulmonary disease. *N Engl J Med.* (2007) 356:775–89. doi: 10.1056/nejmoa063070
83. Vestbo J, Anderson JA, Brook RD, Calverley PM, Celli BR, Crim C, et al. Fluticasone furoate and vilanterol and survival in chronic obstructive pulmonary disease with heightened cardiovascular risk (SUMMIT): a double-blind randomised controlled trial. *Lancet.* (2016) 387:1817–26. doi: 10.1016/S0140-6736(16)30069-1
84. Tashkin DP, Celli B, Senn S, Burkhart D, Kesten S, Menjoge S, et al. A 4-year trial of tiotropium in chronic obstructive pulmonary disease. *N Engl J Med.* (2008) 359:1543–54. doi: 10.1056/nejmoa0805800
85. Di Martino M, Agabiti N, Cascini S, Kirchmayer U, Bauleo L, Fusco D, et al. The effect on total mortality of adding inhaled corticosteroids to long-acting bronchodilators for COPD: a real practice analysis in Italy. *COPD.* (2016) 13:293–302. doi: 10.3109/15412555.2015.1044861
86. Sin DD, Man SF. Why are patients with chronic obstructive pulmonary disease at increased risk of cardiovascular diseases? The potential role of systemic inflammation in chronic obstructive pulmonary disease. *Circulation.* (2003) 107:1514–9. doi: 10.1161/01.CIR.0000056767.69054.B3
87. Löfdahl CG, Postma DS, Pride NB, Boe J, Thorén A. Possible protection by inhaled budesonide against ischaemic cardiac events in mild COPD. *Eur Respir J.* (2007) 29:1115–9. doi: 10.1183/09031936.00128806
88. Macie C, Wooldrage K, Manfreda J, Anthonisen NR. Inhaled corticosteroids and mortality in COPD. *Chest.* (2006) 130:640–6. doi: 10.1378/chest.130.3.640
89. Stone IS, Barnes NC, James WY, Midwinter D, Boubertakh R, Follows R, et al. Lung deflation and cardiovascular structure and function in chronic obstructive pulmonary disease. A Randomized Controlled Trial. *Am J Respir Crit Care Med.* (2016) 193:717–26. doi: 10.1164/rccm.201508-1647OC

17

Prevalence and Risk Factors for COPD at High Altitude: A Large Cross-Sectional Survey of Subjects Living Between 2,100–4,700 m Above Sea Level

Yanfei Guo [1,2,3†], Zhenzhen Xing [2,3†], Guangliang Shan [4†], Jean-Paul Janssens [5†], Tieying Sun [1,2,3†], Di Chai [2], Weiming Liu [6,7], Yuxia Wang [2,3], Yali Ma [2,3], Yaqi Tong [2,3], Yilin Huang [2,3], Yang Cao [2,3] and Chen Wang [1,8,9,10,11*]*

[1] National Clinical Research Center for Respiratory Diseases, Beijing, China, [2] Department of Respiratory and Critical Care Medicine, Beijing Hospital, Beijing, China, [3] National Center of Gerontology, Beijing, China, [4] School of Basic Medicine, Institute of Basic Medical Sciences, Peking Union Medical College, Chinese Academy of Medical Sciences, Beijing, China, [5] Division of Pulmonary Diseases, Department of Medicine, Geneva University Hospitals, Geneva, Switzerland, [6] Department of Intensive Care Medicine, Beijing Boai Hospital, Beijing, China, [7] Rehabilitation Research Center, Beijing, China, [8] Department of Pulmonary and Critical Care Medicine, Center of Respiratory Medicine, China-Japan Friendship Hospital, Beijing, China, [9] Chinese Academy of Medical Sciences and Peking Union Medical College, Beijing, China, [10] Department of Respiratory Medicine, Capital Medical University, Beijing, China, [11] WHO Collaboration Center for Tobacco Cessation and Respiratory Diseases Prevention, Beijing, China

***Correspondence:**
Yanfei Guo
yanfeiguo2003@126.com
Chen Wang
wangchen@pumc.edu.cn;
cyh-birm@263.net*

† These authors have contributed equally to this work

Aim of Study: Four hundred million people live at high altitude worldwide. Prevalence and risk factors for COPD in these populations are poorly documented. We examined the prevalence and risk factors for COPD in residents living at an altitude of 2,100–4,700 m.

Methods: We performed a cross-sectional survey in Xinjiang and Tibet autonomous region. A multistage stratified sampling procedure was used to select a representative population aged 15 years or older from eight high altitude regions. All participants underwent pre- and post-bronchodilator measurement of forced expiratory volumes. COPD was diagnosed according to 2019 Global Initiative for Chronic Obstructive Lung Disease (GOLD) criteria.

Results: Between June, 2015 and August 2016, 4,967 subjects were included. Median age was 38.0 years (range: 15–91 years; inter-quartile range: 28–49 years); 51.4% participants were female. Overall prevalence of spirometry-defined COPD was 8.2% (95% CI 7.4–8.9%): 9.3% in male (95% CI 8.2–10.4%), and 7.1% in female (95% CI 6.1–8.2%). By multivariable logistic regression analysis, COPD was significantly associated with being aged ≥40 years (odds ratio: 2.25 [95% CI 1.72–2.95], $P < 0.0001$), exposure to household air pollution (OR: 1.34 [95% CI 1.01–1.79], $P = 0.043$), and a history of tuberculosis (OR: 1.79 [95% CI 1.23–2.61], $P = 0.030$), while living at a higher altitude (OR: 0.45 [95% CI 0.33–0.61], $P < 0.0001$) and having a higher educational level (OR: 0.64 [95% CI 0.43–0.95], $P = 0.025$) were associated with a lower prevalence of COPD.

Conclusions: Our results show that the spirometry-defined COPD is a considerable health problem for residents living at high altitudes and COPD prevalence was inversely correlated with altitude. Preventing exposure to household air pollution and reducing the incidence of tuberculosis should be public health priorities for high altitude residents.

Keywords: risk factors, prevalence, tuberculosis, high altitude, household air pollution, Chronic Obstructive Pulmonary Disease (COPD)

INTRODUCTION

Chronic obstructive pulmonary disease (COPD) is one of the leading causes of death from non-communicable diseases in the world, accounting for 5.4% of all deaths globally in 2016 (1–3). In China, COPD has been one of the top four causes of death over the past 30 years (4). The Global Burden of Disease study estimated that there were 299 million adults with prevalent COPD worldwide in 2017 (5), and 99.9 million individuals aged ≥20 years with COPD in China in 2015 (6), causing a substantial clinical, economic, and societal burden. Globally, around 400 million people live at high altitude (defined as >1,500 m above sea-level) (7). However, to date, few studies have focused on the prevalence of COPD in high altitude regions, especially for areas with altitudes above 4,000 m.

Living at high altitude results in exposure to colder temperatures, a lower humidity, and hypobaric hypoxic conditions. These conditions could induce physiological adaptations such as changes in lung volumes or diffusing capacity in residents at high altitude (8). At 4,000 m, ambient arterial partial pressure of oxygen (PaO_2) is ~63% that of PaO_2 measured at sea level (9, 10). These variables may impact on respiratory health in general and prevalence of COPD in particular. Approximately 90% of deaths from COPD occur in low- and middle-income countries (11). Thus the high altitude setting combines social-economic factors and environmental conditions which may affect respiratory health.

In the present study, we aimed to determine the prevalence of COPD and to explore potential risk factors for COPD in residents living at high altitude.

METHODS

Study Design and Participants

Between June, 2015 and August 2016, a multistage stratified sampling procedure was used to select a representative sample of subjects living at an altitude of 2,100–4,700 m. Firstly, eight districts or counties were selected in both urban (2 districts) and rural (6 counties) areas using the probability proportional to size method. Lhasa Chengguan District (altitude 3,650 m above sea level) and Shigatse City (altitude 3,900 m) were selected as urban sites. Six counties were also selected: Linzhi County (altitude 3,000 m), Anduo County (4,700 m), Xietongmen County (4,100 m), Duilongdeqing County (4,500 m), Aheqi County (2,100 m) and Tashkurgan County (3,200 m). Subsequently, using a simple random sampling method, two streets or townships were selected from each district or county, and three communities or village communities were selected from each street or township. Finally, using the same method, we chose participants from each of the sex/age strata from communities or villages. The proportion of samples from each gender and age group was based on the 2010 census of Chinese population. We selected only one participant from each household. We included permanent residents (i.e., living in their current residence for more than 1 year) aged ≥15 years for this analysis.

Exclusion criteria were: treatment for tuberculosis during study period; myocardial infarction or cerebrovascular accident during the previous 3 months; pregnancy; heart rate >120 beats/min or blood pressure >180/120 mmHg, and any condition that would impede the use of spirometry (such as recent thoracic, abdominal, or eye surgery, or retinal detachment).

The study protocol was approved by the Institutional Review Board and ethics committee of Beijing Hospital (2013BJYYEC-042C-01). Each participant received detailed information about the study and study methods, and provided written informed consent before data collection.

Procedures

A standardized questionnaire covering demographic data, living conditions, respiratory symptoms, history of respiratory diseases and comorbidities, and potential risk factors for COPD was administered by experienced interviewers. Forced expiratory volumes were measured in all qualified study participants (spirometry) with a MasterScreen™ Pneumo PC spirometer (CareFusion, Yorba Linda, CA) according to ATS/ERS recommendations (12). The spirometer was calibrated daily using a 3 L syringe to ensure measured volumes within 3% of syringe volume, before data collection; ambient temperature, humidity, and altitude were also recorded daily. Each participant underwent the same procedure twice, before and after receiving a bronchodilator (400 ug of salbutamol through a 500 ml spacer). The forced expiratory maneuvers were performed 3–8 times until the forced vital capacity (FVC) and forced expiratory volume in 1 s (FEV_1) were reproducible within 150 ml. Acceptability of FVC and FEV_1 was scored using the grading system (A-F) of Enright et al. (13). Performing 3 acceptable maneuvers with an FVC variability of 100 ml or less was rated "A"; a variability of 100–150 ml was rated "B"; variability between 150 and 200 ml was scored "C." A, B, or C grades were considered acceptable for analysis. Data were uploaded daily to a database, examined for incoherent data by the study supervisors and by the principal investigator. Quality control, based on the American Thoracic Society/European Respiratory Society criteria, was performed by a field supervisor at the filing center (12).

COPD was defined as a post-bronchodilator FEV_1/FVC ratio of <0.70, based on Global Initiative for Chronic Obstructive Lung Disease (GOLD) guidelines (14). The ratios of observed/predicted FEV_1 based on a nationwide study of reference values for spirometry in the Chinese population were used to stage the degree of obstruction: GOLD grade I ≥80% predicted, GOLD grade II 50–79% predicted, GOLD grade III 30–49% predicted, and GOLD grade IV <30% predicted (15). The lower limit of normal (LLN) of reference values was also used to define COPD in a sensitivity analysis based on GLI lung function equations for a South East Asian population (16). Awareness of COPD was defined as self-reported physician-diagnosed COPD among patients with COPD.

Exposure to household air pollution was defined as the use of wood, animal waste, or coal for cooking or heating during the previous 6 months or longer. Peripheral oxygen saturation was measured with a pulse-oximetry (PHILIPS DB12) before performing spirometry. Smoking status was categorized as: current smoker, former smoker, or never smoker. We defined current smokers as active smokers who had smoked more than 100 cigarettes in their life time; former smokers had smoked more than 100 cigarettes in their lifetime but had stopped smoking at least 12 months before the interview (17). The mean altitudes of the six study areas were obtained from the local administrative departments.

Statistical Analysis

Our study was designed to provide reliable estimates of the prevalence of COPD for both male and female from five age groups (15–29, 30–39, 40–49, 50–59, and ≥60 years) in rural and urban settings. The sample sizes were calculated separately for populations aged 15–39 and ≥40 years due to large differences in prevalence. Based on available data from previous studies, we assumed a COPD prevalence of 3.0% in the 15–39-year age group and 9.9% in the ≥40-year age group (18, 19). In addition, we used a design effect of 1.5 (the ratio of the variance of a statistic from a complex sample to the variance of the same statistic from a simple random sample of the same size) to account for the multistage cluster sampling design. The final sample sizes were 1,735 in the 15–39 years age group and 3,312 in the ≥40 years age group. Demographic data are expressed as mean ± SD for continuous variables, then compared by analysis of variance (ANOVA) or *t*-tests as appropriate. Data for categorical variables were presented as counts and proportions, and were compared by χ^2-tests. Multivariable logistic regression analyses were conducted to explore risk factors (sex, age, smoking status, region, altitude, educational level, household air pollution, history of tuberculosis, and exposure to dust or chemicals in the workplace) for COPD in all study participants. Differences with two-sided $P < 0.05$ were considered statistically significant. All statistical analyses were performed using SAS version 9.4 (SAS Institute Inc., Cary, North Carolina).

RESULTS

To meet the designed sample size, a total of 5,843 permanent residents were randomly selected and 5,647 participants were recruited. After excluding individuals with unreliable post-bronchodilator tests, 4,967 participants aged ≥15 years (2,415 male and 2,552 female) were included in the final analysis and completed the survey (**Figure 1**).

Table 1 summarizes the characteristics of individuals sorted by three different altitudes of residence: 2,100–3,000, 3,000–4,000, and >4,000 m. Educational level of men was higher than that of women for all subjects. Educational level was lower in subjects living at higher altitude. Proportion of current and former smokers was lower in men living at very high altitude (>4,000 m). Among male smokers, the proportion of heavy

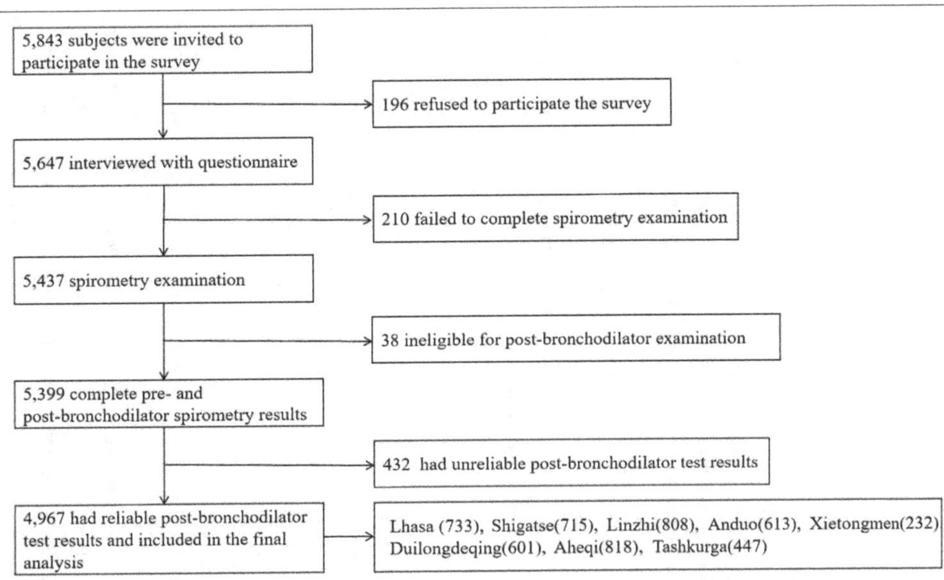

FIGURE 1 | Flow chart of study.

TABLE 1 | Demographic characteristics of high-altitude residents by altitude and gender: anthropometric data, education, smoking history, risk factors and results of pulmonary function tests.

Variables	Total (*n* = 4,967)				Men (*n* = 2,415)				Women (*n* = 2,552)			
	2,100–3,000 m (*n* = 1,626)	3,000–4,000 m (*n* = 1,895)	>4,000 m (*n* = 1,446)	*P-value*	2,100–3,000 m (*n* = 807)	3,000–4,000 m (*n* = 956)	>4,000 m (*n* = 652)	*P-value*	2,100–3,000 m (*n* = 819)	3,000–4,000 m (*n* = 939)	>4,000 m (*n* = 794)	*P-value*
Age, years												
15–39	898 (55.3%)	1,038 (54.7%)	723 (50.0%)	<0.0001	462 (57.2%)	605 (63.3%)	335 (51.4%)	<0.0001	436 (53.2%)	433 (46.1%)	388 (48.9%)	0.002
40–49	348 (21.4%)	382 (20.2%)	382 (26.4%)		162 (20.1%)	158 (16.5%)	175 (26.8%)		186 (22.7%)	224 (23.9%)	207 (26.1%)	
50–59	233 (14.3%)	271 (14.3%)	247 (17.1%)		104 (12.9%)	104 (10.9%)	105 (16.1%)		129 (15.8%)	167 (17.8%)	142 (17.9%)	
≥60	147 (9.0%)	204 (10.8%)	94 (6.5%)		79 (9.8%)	89 (9.3%)	37 (5.7%)		68 (8.3%)	115 (12.2%)	57 (7.2%)	
Body-mass index, kg/m²	23.4 (3.7)	23.7 (3.9)	24.0 (4.2)	<0.0001	23.3 (3.6)	23.5 (3.5)	24.0 (4.0)	0.001	23.4 (3.8)	23.9 (4.4)	24.0 (4.3)	0.022
Education level												
Primary school and lower	812 (49.9%)	863 (45.5%)	993 (68.7%)	<0.0001	332 (41.1%)	295 (30.9%)	421 (64.6%)	<0.0001	480 (58.6%)	568 (60.5%)	572 (72.0%)	<0.0001
Middle and high school	608 (37.4%)	473 (25.0%)	245 (16.9%)		341 (42.3%)	280 (29.3%)	126 (19.3%)		267 (32.6%)	193 (20.6%)	119 (15.0%)	
College and higher	206 (12.7%)	559 (29.5%)	208 (14.4%)		134 (16.6%)	381 (39.9%)	105 (16.1%)		72 (8.8%)	178 (19.0%)	103 (13.0%)	
Smoking status												
Never smoker	1,071 (65.9%)	1,371 (72.3%)	1,162 (80.4%)	<0.0001	317 (39.3%)	445 (46.5%)	471 (72.2%)	<0.0001	754 (92.1%)	926 (98.6%)	691 (87.0%)	<0.0001
Former smoker	112 (6.9%)	81 (4.3%)	107 (7.4%)		101 (12.5%)	76 (8.0%)	60 (9.2%)		11 (1.3%)	5 (0.5%)	47 (5.9%)	
Current smoker	443 (27.2%)	443 (23.4%)	177 (12.2%)		389 (48.2%)	435 (45.5%)	121 (18.6%)		54 (6.6%)	8 (0.9%)	56 (7.1%)	
Cigarette smoking, pack-year*												
0	1,071 (65.9%)	1,371 (72.5%)	1,162 (80.6%)	<0.0001	317 (39.4%)	445 (46.7%)	471 (72.6%)	<0.0001	754 (92.1%)	926 (98.7%)	691 (87.0%)	<0.0001
1–19	19 (1.2%)	50 (2.6%)	68 (4.7%)		17 (2.1%)	49 (5.1%)	47 (7.3%)		2 (0.2%)	1 (0.1%)	21 (2.6%)	
≥20	534 (32.9%)	470 (24.9%)	212 (14.7%)		471 (58.5%)	459 (48.2%)	130 (20.1%)		63 (7.7%)	11 (1.2%)	82 (10.3%)	
Risk factors for COPD												
Household air pollution*	1,356 (83.4%)	1,070 (56.5%)	944 (66.0%)	<0.0001	626 (77.6%)	472 (49.4%)	408 (63.6%)	<0.0001	730 (89.1%)	598 (63.7%)	536 (67.9%)	<0.0001
History of tuberculosis	82 (5.0%)	122 (6.4%)	50 (3.5%)	0.001	40 (5.0%)	52 (5.4%)	27 (4.1%)	0.497	42 (5.1%)	70 (7.5%)	23 (2.9%)	<0.0001
Exposure to dust or chemicals in the workplace*	14 (0.9%)	109 (5.9%)	15 (1.0%)	<0.0001	8 (1.0%)	54 (5.8%)	10 (1.5%)	<0.0001	6 (0.7%)	55 (6.0%)	5 (0.6%)	<0.0001
Spirometry,%												
Pre-BD FEV_1/FVC	79.34 (10.07)	84.38 (9.84)	84.56 (10.26)	<0.0001	79.10 (10.40)	84.61 (9.94)	84.36 (9.96)	<0.0001	79.58 (9.74)	84.16 (9.73)	84.72 (10.50)	<0.0001
Post-BD FEV_1/FVC	81.7 (10.0)	85.75 (9.30)	85.75 (9.47)	<0.0001	81.20 (10.41)	86.05 (9.23)	85.19 (10.14)	<0.0001	82.24 (9.57)	85.45 (9.37)	86.21 (8.86)	<0.0001
Pre-BD FVC %predicted	79.33 (10.08)	84.37 (9.84)	84.55 (10.26)	<0.0001	79.08 (10.40)	84.60 (9.94)	84.36 (9.96)	<0.0001	79.57 (9.75)	84.14 (9.73)	84.71 (10.51)	<0.0001
Post-BD FVC %predicted	82.07 (11.45)	85.88 (13.05)	86.25 (22.25)	<0.0001	81.75 (11.60)	86.43 (13.36)	85.00 (15.15)	<0.0001	82.38 (11.29)	85.33 (12.71)	87.28 (26.68)	<0.0001
Pre-BD FEV_1 %predicted	104.11 (13.47)	102.22 (15.02)	102.36 (24.07)	0.003	104.06 (13.68)	102.70 (16.51)	100.92 (14.76)	<0.0001	104.15 (13.26)	101.74 (13.32)	103.55 (29.56)	0.029
Post-BD FEV_1 %predicted	103.70 (11.74)	102.26 (12.30)	102.42 (15.76)	0.003	103.37 (11.74)	102.41 (12.67)	101.65 (13.80)	0.034	104.03 (11.75)	102.12 (11.93)	103.05 (17.19)	0.014
Oxyhemoglobin saturation, %	93.5 (3.3)	90.6 (5.1)	86.3 (4.5)	<0.0001	93.1 (3.1)	90.6 (4.9)	86.2 (4.6)	<0.0001	94.0 (3.3)	90.6 (5.3)	86.4 (4.4)	<0.0001

*Data are expressed as number (%) or mean (standard deviation, SD). COPD, chronic obstructive pulmonary disease; FVC, forced vital capacity; FEV1, forced expiratory volume in the first second; Pre-BD, pre-bronchodilator; Post-BD, post-bronchodilator. *assessed in Cigarette smoking with data missing for 10 participants, household air pollution with data missing for 15 participants and exposure to dust or chemicals in the workplace with data missing for 38 participants.*

smokers (≥20 pack-years) living at 2,100–3,000 m was more than twice that of those living above 4,000 m (58.5 vs. 20.1%). Exposure to household air pollution (3,370 subjects; 67.8%), was more important in the female population (73.0%) than in males (62.4%). Subjects living in rural regions (2,100–3,000 and >4,000 m) were more exposed to household air pollution. Conversely, participants living in cities (3,000–4,000 m) were more exposure to dust or chemicals in the workplace and had a higher prevalence of history of tuberculosis. As expected, oxyhemoglobin saturation (SpO_2) of participants decreased with altitude.

A total of 364 participants in the survey had an FEV_1/FVC ratio of <70% and were diagnosed with COPD (**Table 2**). The overall standardized prevalence of spirometry-defined COPD

TABLE 2 | Age-specific and age-standardized prevalence (%) of chronic obstructive pulmonary disease in the residents aged 15 years older living at high altitude.

Variables	Overall		Men		Women	
	Cases/total (*n*/*N*)	Prevalence of COPD (95%CI)	Cases/total (*n*/*N*)	Prevalence of COPD (95%CI)	Cases/total (*n*/*N*)	Prevalence of COPD (95%CI)
Prevalence	364/4,967	8.2% (7.4–8.9)	187/2,415	9.3% (8.2–10.4)	177/2,552	7.1% (6.1–8.2)
Age, year						
15–39	106/2,659	3.7% (2.9–4.4)	59/1,402	3.6% (2.5–4.6)	47/1,257	3.7% (2.6–4.7)
40–49	87/1,112	7.2% (5.6–8.9)	42/495	8.7% (6.1–11.2)	45/617	6.2% (4.1–8.3)
50–59	88/751	11.1% (8.7–13.6)	34/313	12.2% (8.5–15.8)	54/438	10.3% (7.0–13.5)
≥60	83/445	33.3% (29.3–37.3)	52/205	46.2% (39.3–53.1)	31/240	22.6% (18.0–27.1)
P for trend		<0.0001		<0.0001		<0.0001
Altitude, m						
2,100–3,000	170/1,626	12.1% (10.5–13.7)	95/807	13.9% (11.5–16.3)	75/819	10.1% (8.0–12.1)
3,000–4,000	119/1,895	6.9% (5.8–8.0)	52/956	6.7% (5.2–8.1)	67/939	7.0% (5.3–8.7)
>4,000	75/1,446	5.4% (4.2–6.6)	40/652	7.1% (5.2–8.9)	35/794	4.2% (2.8–5.7)
P for trend		<0.0001		<0.0001		<0.0001
Education level						
Primary school and lower	269/2,668	8.8% (7.5–10.0)	125/1,048	10.3% (8.2–12.4)	144/1,620	7.6% (6.2–9.1)
Middle and high school	55/1,326	6.3% (5.3–7.4)	38/747	8.4% (6.7–10.0)	17/579	2.6% (1.2–4.0)
College and higher	40/973	6.0% (4.7–7.2)	24/620	5.5% (3.9–7.0)	16/353	6.8% (4.6–9.0)
P for trend		<0.0001		<0.0001		<0.0001
Smoking status						
Never smoker	239/3,604	7.3% (6.5–8.1)	76/1,233	7.8% (6.4–9.2)	163/2,371	7.2% (6.1–8.2)
Former smoker	39/300	9.7% (5.6–13.7)	29/237	10.6% (6.2–15.1)	10/63	3.2% (2.6–3.9)
Current smoker	86/1,063	12.0% (10.3–13.7)	82/945	11.6% (9.7–13.5)	4/118	12.1% (8.8–15.5)
P for trend		0.001		0.002		0.006
Cigarette smoking*, pack-year						
0	239/3,604	7.3% (6.5–8.1)	76/1,233	7.8% (6.4–9.2)	163/2,371	7.2% (6.1–8.2)
1–19	8/137	9.8% (5.8–13.9)	4/113	4.2% (0.8–7.6)	4/24	25.3% (9.0–41.7)
≥20	117/1,216	10.4% (8.7–12.2)	107/1,060	11.2% (9.3–13.1)	10/156	5.0% (1.0–8.9)
P for trend		0.002		0.001		0.165
Household air pollution*						
Yes	288/3,370	9.0% (8.0–10.0)	145/1,506	10.7% (9.1–12.3)	143/1,864	7.7% (6.5–9.0)
No	76/1,582	6.2% (5.1–7.2)	42/899	6.4% (4.9–7.8)	34/683	5.6% (3.9–7.3)
P for difference		<0.0001		<0.0001		0.018
History of tuberculosis						
Yes	37/254	11.6% (6.9–16.3)	18/119	12.8% (5.8–19.8)	19/135	10.0% (3.7–16.4)
No	327/4,713	7.8% (7.0–8.5)	169/2,296	8.9% (7.8–10.0)	158/2,417	6.8% (5.8–7.8)
P for difference		<0.0001		0.002		0.001
Exposure in the workplace*						
Yes	15/138	8.2% (2.7–13.7)	9/72	9.9% (1.7–18.1)	6/66	5.5% (3.3–7.6)
No	346/4,791	8.2% (7.4–8.9)	176/2,325	3.8% (2.4–5.2)	170/2,466	7.1% (6.1–8.2)
P for difference		0.105		0.123		0.489

*COPD, chronic obstructive pulmonary disease. *Data missing for cigarette smoking (n = 10), household air pollution (n = 15) and exposure in the workplace (n = 38).*

(GOLD diagnostic criteria) was 8.2% (95% CI 7.4–8.9%); difference between genders was not significant. Prevalence increased with age (**Figure 2**); it reached 12.3% (10.9–13.7%; $P < 0.0001$ for age difference) among those aged ≥40 years. Conversely, as shown in **Figure 2**, prevalence of COPD decreased significantly with increasing altitude. **Supplementary Table 1** shows GOLD stage of the COPD population according to different altitudes. The prevalence of respiratory symptoms (i.e., cough, sputum, wheezing, and dyspnea) in patients with COPD is shown in the **Table 3**. Overall, more than a half of individuals with COPD had at least one respiratory symptom (57.9%), but 42.1% had no symptoms suggestive of COPD. The frequency of respiratory symptoms increased with GOLD severity stage. Among COPD with a completed CAT score (360), 87.2% had a score of 10 or higher. Only 1.1% of patients diagnosed with COPD were previously aware of their diagnosis. Of all patients with COPD, none had ever been tested by spirometry before the survey.

In a multivariable-adjusted analysis, being aged ≥40 years, living at a lower altitude, being exposed to household air pollution, having a lower educational level and a history of tuberculosis were significantly associated with a higher prevalence of COPD (**Table 4**).

We also performed a sensitivity analysis using age-specific LLN to define COPD. The overall prevalence of LLN-defined COPD was 11.0% (95% CI 10.1–11.9%): 10.5% (95% CI 9.3–11.7%) in males and 11.4% (95% CI 10.2–12.6%) in females. The prevalence of LLN-defined COPD by altitude was shown in **Figure 3**.

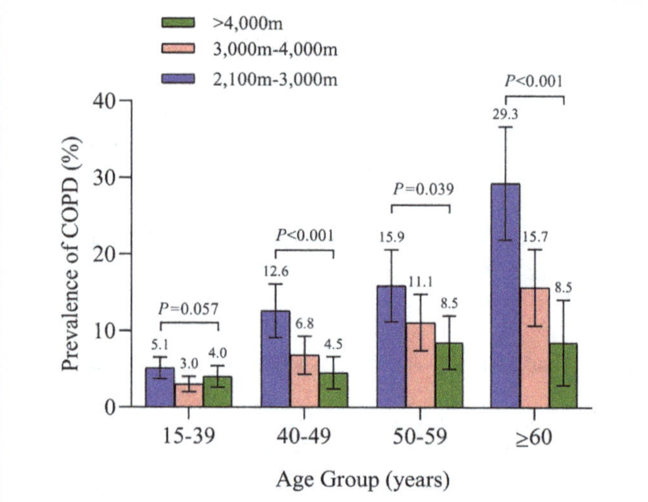

FIGURE 2 | Prevalence of Chronic Obstructive Pulmonary Disease in each age group according to altitude of residence.

DISCUSSION

This spirometry-based study in a representative sample of 4,967 residents shows that COPD is a major public health challenge at high altitudes (2,100–4,700 m): 8.2% of the high-altitude population aged more than 15 years had spirometry-defined COPD, making up for the gaps of region, altitude, and nationality. It also reveals that the majority of patients with COPD were unaware of their condition and that none of them had undergone previous pulmonary function testing. Finally, our data highlights exposure to household air pollution, history of pulmonary tuberculosis, and a low education level as major preventable risk factors for COPD in the high-altitude indigenous population.

Several cross-sectional surveys have reported the prevalence of COPD in various regions of the world below 1,500 m. The prevalence of spirometry-defined COPD in China in adults ≥40 years old is about 13.0%, with a 67% increase between 2004 and 2013 (6, 20, 21). In the BOLD study, the

TABLE 3 | Distributions of typical symptoms in the normal population and COPD patients by GOLD grades.

Symptoms	Status	Number (%)				
		Normal	**GOLD I**	**GOLD II**	**GOLD III-IV**	**Overall COPD**
Frequent cough	With	617 (13.6%)	53 (23.0%)	35 (31.0%)	7 (38.9%)	95 (26.3%)
	Without	3,907 (86.4%)	177 (77.0%)	78 (69.0%)	11 (61.1%)	266 (73.7%)
Sputum	With	572 (12.7%)	43 (18.7%)	34 (30.1%)	7 (38.9%)	84 (23.3%)
	Without	3,947 (87.3%)	187 (81.3%)	79 (69.9%)	11 (61.1%)	277 (76.7%)
Recurrent wheezing	With	221 (4.9%)	17 (7.4%)	17 (15.0%)	2 (11.1%)	36 (10.0%)
	Without	4,297 (95.1%)	213 (92.6%)	96 (85.5%)	16 (88.9%)	325 (90.0%)
Dyspnea in daily life	With	1,254 (27.7%)	104 (45.2%)	39 (34.5%)	8 (44.4%)	151 (41.8%)
	Without	3,271 (72.3%)	126 (54.8%)	74 (65.5%)	10 (55.6%)	210 (58.2%)
At least one of the above	With	1,771 (39.1%)	133 (57.8%)	64 (56.6%)	12 (66.7%)	209 (57.9%)
	Without	2,755 (60.9%)	97 (42.2%)	49 (43.4%)	6 (33.3%)	152 (41.8%)
CAT score	<10	1,045 (23.2%)	29 (12.6%)	17 (15.0%)	0	46 (12.8%)
	≥10	3,462 (76.8%)	201 (87.4%)	96 (85.0%)	17 (100%)	314 (87.2%)

GOLD stage I (mild COPD): FEV1 ≥80% predicted; GOLD stage II (moderate COPD): FEV1 ≥50% to <80% predicted; GOLD stage III (severe COPD): FEV1 ≥30% to <50% predicted; GOLD stage IV (very severe); GOLD stage III–IV were combined because of small numbers. GOLD, Global Initiative for Chronic Obstructive Lung Disease; COPD, chronic obstructive pulmonary disease; CAT, COPD assessment test.

TABLE 4 | Univariable-adjusted and multivariable-adjusted odds ratios of chronic obstructive pulmonary disease associated with risk factors.

Variables	Univariable-adjusted		Multivariable-adjusted	
	OR (95% CI)	P-value	OR (95% CI)	P-value
Male gender	1.12 (0.91–1.39)	0.275	1.25 (0.96–1.62)	0.095
Age, years				
15–39	1.00 (Reference)		1.00 (Reference)	
≥40	3.03 (2.40–3.82)	<0.0001	2.25 (1.72–2.95)	<0.0001
Altitude,m				
2,100–3,000	1.00 (Reference)		1.00 (Reference)	
3,000–4,000	0.57 (0.44–0.73)	<0.0001	0.61 (0.46–0.79)	<0.0001
>4,000	0.46 (0.35–0.62)	<0.0001	0.45 (0.33–0.61)	<0.0001
Education level				
Primary school and lower	1.00 (Reference)		1.00 (Reference)	
Middle and high school	0.38 (0.28–0.52)	<0.0001	0.49 (0.35–0.68)	<0.0001
College and higher	0.38 (0.27–0.53)	<0.0001	0.64 (0.43–0.95)	0.025
Pack-years of smoking				
0	1.00 (Reference)		1.00 (Reference)	
1–19	0.87 (0.42–1.80)	0.714	1.22 (0.58–2.57)	0.609
≥20	1.49 (1.18–1.88)	0.001	1.21 (0.91–1.60)	0.191
Household air pollution	1.82 (1.42–2.40)	<0.0001	1.34 (1.01–1.79)	0.043
History of tuberculosis	2.28 (1.58–3.29)	<0.0001	1.79 (1.23–2.61)	0.030
Exposure to dust or chemicals in the workplace	1.56 (0.90–2.70)	0.108	1.19 (0.67–2.10)	0.558

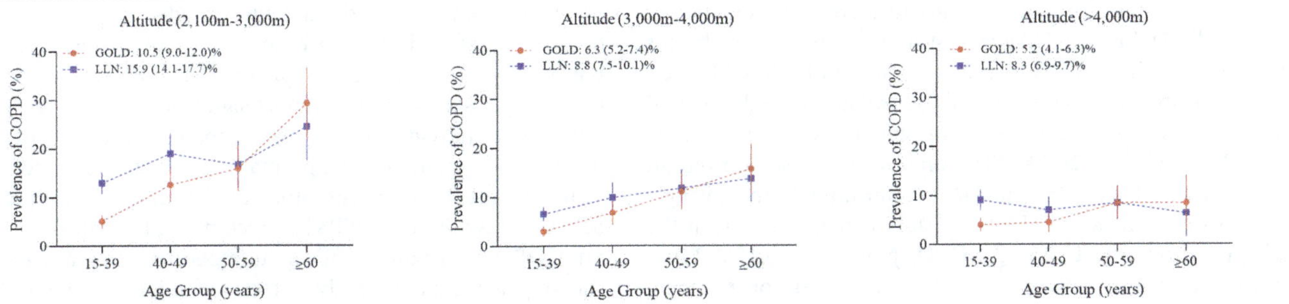

FIGURE 3 | Prevalence of COPD using Lower Limit of Normal or GOLD criteria by age group and altitude of residence.

prevalence of COPD in 12 different sites worldwide was 10.1% for GOLD stage II or greater (11.8% for men and 8.5% for women) (22). In the US, the prevalence of COPD in 2010 was 14.0% (23). Data from Mongolia, Kazakhstan and Japan report prevalence rates between 6.7 and 13.6% (24–26). However, very limited specific data exist concerning prevalence of COPD in high altitudes.

There are a few prior studies on prevalence of COPD at high altitude. Data from the Peruvian Altiplano (3,825 m above sea level) report a prevalence of COPD of 6.1% in Puno, and 9.9% in the rural Puno area (27). Estimated prevalence of COPD in Mexico city (2,240 m above sea level) (Latin American Project for the Investigation of Obstructive Lung Disease (PLATINO) study) was 7.8% [95% CI 5.9%–9.7%] (28). In the PREPOCOL study, prevalence of COPD in Bogotá (Columbia, 2,640 m) was 8.5% (29). Data from 27 Mexican cities located at >2,000 m above sea level yield a prevalence of 15.6% (30). However, these studies used smaller sample sizes, incorporated no post-bronchodilator testing, or were restricted to local occupational or urban cohorts. Furthermore, albeit for the data from the Peruvian altiplano, these studies included mainly subjects living at lower altitudes than the high-altitude population described in this study. The present study is to our knowledge the only one to describe the overall prevalence of spirometry-defined COPD among high altitude residents using a rigorous sampling design and quality control and also, the first time, residents over 4,000 m above sea level were included.

Studies about the relationship between the prevalence of COPD and altitude show conflicting results. The PREPOCOL study, conducted in four Peruvian regions, and studies from Columbia and Kyrgyztan found a higher prevalence of COPD at high-altitude (29–31). In a systematic review and meta-analysis of 10 studies analyzing the prevalence of COPD at high altitude, Xiong H et al. found that results differed according to continents studied, prevalence of COPD at high altitude being higher in Asia (Kyrgystan) than in Europe (Austria) or Latin America (Mexico, Colombia, Peru). However, altitude was not found to be an independent risk factor for developing COPD (32). Conversely, in the PLATINO study performed in five major Latin America cities [Sao Paulo (altitude: 800 m), Santiago (543 m), Mexico City (2,240 m), Montevideo (35 m), and Caracas (950 m)] COPD prevalence was lowest in Mexico City, and there was a clear negative adjusted correlation between prevalence and altitude (28). Another study covering 27 Mexican cities (altitude range: 1–2,680 m) found a weak but significant negative correlation between altitude and COPD prevalence (30). Our study also suggests that the prevalence of COPD decreases as altitude increases. Among possible explanations are changes in lung volumes as a physiological adaptation to altitude: we noted slightly higher values for FEV_1 and FVC (absolute and percent predicted) at higher altitudes, as well as an increase in FEV_1/FVC. In addition, the proportion of heavy smokers decreased with increasing altitude. Also, proportion of people exposed to HAP and with a history of TB was lower in high altitude areas. These factors may be contributive to the decrease of COPD prevalence at higher altitude.

Household Air Pollution (HAP) mainly refers to coal and biomass fuels (e.g., animal dung, wood, crop residues) used indoors, also known as solid fuels (33). Increasing evidence suggests that exposure to HAP leads to increased incidence of COPD (34, 35). In 2015, HAP was estimated to be responsible for 2.9 million deaths and 85.6 million lost years of healthy life (36). The proportion of subjects exposed to HAP in our study (67.8%) was higher than that reported in a previous nationwide survey of COPD in China (26.7%). The present data also showed an increase of 36% (OR: 1.36) with HAP, confirming the increasingly acknowledged impact of HAP on respiratory health. Given the high prevalence of HAP and COPD, prevention of HAP and use of alternative fuels are important strategies for reducing COPD, especially for high altitude regions. Systematic reviews have suggested that HAP leads to significant risk for COPD in women (37–39). Cooking and heating with solid fuels more than 6 months leads to significant level of lung damage. Lung pathological findings in HAP-exposed individuals demonstrate small airways fibrosis and emphysema. The lung damage mostly occurs in women, as women often prepare the meals close to the fire in poorly ventilated houses for several hours daily. The present study also showed that women were more exposed to household air pollution than men (73.0% of women vs. 62.4% of men), a potential explanation for the lack of gender difference in the prevalence of COPD in this population.

Cigarette smoking is the major risk factor for COPD. Surprisingly, our multivariable analyses found no relationship between smoking and COPD after adjusting for gender, age, altitude, educational level, exposure to household air pollution, and history of tuberculosis. This is probably explained by a much lower prevalence of smoking than exposure to household air pollution (27.4 vs. 67.8%). However, as expected, prevalence COPD of smokers, especially heavy smokers, is higher than in non-smokers. Smoking prevention and cessation remain among the major important strategies for reducing COPD.

Incidence of tuberculosis remains high in many low and middle-income countries. An estimated 10 million new onset cases of TB and 1.57 million TB-related deaths occurred in 2017 (40). Tuberculosis is a possibly neglected risk factor for COPD in developing countries. In high-altitude areas, our study found 254 subjects (5.1%) with a history of tuberculosis, which is about 9-fold the prevalence in other provinces of China (0.6%) (6). Tuberculosis is known as a cause, comorbidity, and aggravating factor for COPD, as mentioned in the 2017 GOLD guidelines (41). The BOLD study found that a self-reported history of tuberculosis was significantly associated with airflow obstruction and spirometry restriction (42). We also found a significant association between a positive history of tuberculosis and the presence of COPD in participants aged $\geq$15 years (OR 1.77 [95% CI 1.21–2.58]. Thus, effective measures for tuberculosis prevention are an important component for the prevention of COPD in this population.

In our study, 56, 39, and 5% of patients with COPD had mild, moderate, and severe or very severe disease, respectively. This distribution was similar to reports in the USA and in China (20, 23). Although around two-thirds of patients with COPD were asymptomatic below 1,500 m sea level, our findings show 41.8% of the high-altitude COPD population without at least one respiratory symptom. In our study, only 1.1% of COPD patients were previously aware of their diagnosis. High rates of unawareness of COPD at high altitudes may be influenced by low access to health care, low index of suspicion by local physicians, poor access to spirometry, and by the fact that these subjects may tend to report significantly fewer respiratory symptoms. Individuals with undiagnosed COPD, whether they were asymptomatic or symptomatic, have an increased risk of acute exacerbations, pneumonia, and death. The US Preventive Services Task Force (USPSTF) recommends against screening for COPD in asymptomatic adults because of scant evidence showing a benefit of early detection and treatment (43, 44). These findings highlight the real challenges of COPD detection, and prevention in the high-altitude areas, especially for those asymptomatic subjects.

One major finding of this study is the risk factors affect a different degree to the prevalence of COPD at high altitude. Household air pollution may be the most important factors for COPD patients, provided more useful information for policymakers to consider more stringent household air pollution control measures. Another advantage is that the study reveals that the respiratory symptoms of people in high altitude are obviously affected by altitude factors, so lung function is particularly important for COPD screening. Final strength is our data suggest that the prevalence of COPD decreases as altitude increases, although previous publications provide conflicting results. Our study findings have important public health implications for residents at high altitude. The harsh high-elevation environment and backward economy are very challenging for the provision of healthy living conditions. Increased exposure to household air pollution and high rate of tuberculosis aggravate the hazards to pulmonary health. Our results call for an increased focus on COPD awareness, diagnosis, and treatment for residents living at high altitude. Controlling household air pollution via the replacement of fuel sources, initiating programs for smoking cessation and progress in health services for tuberculosis prevention should be considered public health priorities.

Our study has several limitations. First, smoking status was self-reported and not validated biochemically using exhaled carbon monoxide or urinary cotinine. Secondly, outdoor $PM_{2.5}$ (particulate matter) was not analyzed in our study. We surmised that air quality at high altitudes has little effect on COPD prevalence because the outdoor $PM_{2.5}$ in Lhasa was 26 ug/m^3 from June 2015 to August 2016, much less than the national average level (45). Thirdly, we cannot eliminate the possibility that we misclassified people with asthma and other obstructive lung disorders as having COPD. Fourthly, the data covering subjects over 40 years of age were below estimated sample size.

In summary, our study documents the prevalence of COPD among a large sample of high altitude residents aged ≥15 years living at high altitude. Prevalence of COPD was inversely correlated with altitude. Furthermore, awareness of COPD was extremely low in this population. Increasing knowledge about COPD is important in this group. Household air pollution, a history of pulmonary tuberculosis and educational level were identified as major preventable risk factors for COPD.

AUTHOR CONTRIBUTIONS

YG, CW, and ZW conceived and designed the study. YG and CW supervised the study. SW, WM, and GS did the statistical analysis. YG and ZX drafted the manuscript. ZW, SW, and WM provide advices in the study and are listed in the acknowledgments. All authors contributed to acquisition, analysis, or interpretation of data, revised the report, and approved the final version before submission.

ACKNOWLEDGMENTS

We acknowledge the following investigators for their continuous support, assistance, and cooperation: Wang Miao from Beijing Anzhen Hospital, HongSheng Zhang, Xiaomeng Li, Xiaoming Tan, Mingming Pan, and Aonan Li from Beijing Hospital, Zengwu Wang, Linfeng Zhang, and Xin Wang from Fu Wai Hospital, Yundai Chen, and Bin Feng from Chinese PLA General Hospital, Sinan Wu, and Wenquan Liu form China-Japan Friendship Hospital.

REFERENCES

1. GBD 2016 Causes of Death Collaborators. Global, regional, and national age-sex specific mortality for 264 causes of death, 1980-2016: a systematic analysis for the Global Burden of Disease Study 2016. *Lancet.* (2017) 390:1151–210. doi: 10.1016/S0140-6736(17)32152-9
2. Adeloye D, Chua S, Lee C, Basquill C, Papana A, Theodoratou E, et al. Global and regional estimates of COPD prevalence: systematic review and meta-analysis. *J Glob Health.* (2015) 5:020415. doi: 10.7189/jogh.05.020415
3. GBD 2015 Chronic Respiratory Disease Collaborators. Global, regional, and national deaths, prevalence, disability-adjusted life years, and years lived with disability for chronic obstructive pulmonary disease and asthma, 1990-2015: a systematic analysis for the Global Burden of Disease Study 2015. *Lancet Respir Med.* (2017). 5:691–706. doi: 10.1016/S2213-2600(17)30293-X
4. Zhou M, Wang H, Zeng X, Zhou M, Bao L, Hatanpaa KJ, et al. Mortality, morbidity, and risk factors in China and its provinces, 1990-2017: a systematic analysis for the Global Burden of Disease Study 2017. *Lancet.* (2019) 394:1145–58. doi: 10.1016/S0140-6736(19)30427-1
5. GBD 2017 Disease and Injury Incidence and Prevalence Collaborators. Global, regional, and national incidence, prevalence, and years lived with disability for 354 diseases and injuries for 195 countries and territories, 1990-2017: a systematic analysis for the Global Burden of Disease Study 2017. *Lancet.* (2018) 392:1789–858. doi: 10.1016/S0140-6736(18)32279-7
6. Wang C, Xu J, Yang L, Xu Y, Zhang X, Bai C, et al. Prevalence and risk factors of chronic obstructive pulmonary disease in China (the China Pulmonary Health [CPH] study): a national cross-sectional study. *Lancet.* (2018) 391:1706–17. doi: 10.1016/S0140-6736(18)30841-9
7. Cohen JE, Small C. Hypsographic demography: the distribution of human population by altitude. *Proc Natl Acad Sci USA.* (1998) 5:14009–14. doi: 10.1073/pnas.95.24.14009
8. Burtscher M. Effects of living at higher altitudes on mortality: a narrative review. *Aging Dis.* (2014) 5:274–80. doi: 10.14336/AD.2014.0500274
9. Gilbert-Kawai ET, Milledge JS, Grocott MP, Martin DS. King of the mountains: Tibetan and Sherpa physiological adaptations for life at high altitude. *Physiology.* (2014) 29:388–402. doi: 10.1152/physiol.0001 8.2014
10. Huey RB. High altitude: an exploration of human adaptation. *Integrat Compar Biol.* (2002) 42:910. doi: 10.1093/icb/42.4.910
11. WHO. *Global Surveillance, Prevention and Control of Chronic Respiratory Diseases: A Comprehensive Approach.* Geneva: World Health Organization (2007).
12. Miller MR, Hankinson J, Brusasco V, Burgos F, Casaburi R, Coates A, et al. Standardisation of spirometry. *Euro Respir J.* (2005) 26:319–38. doi: 10.1183/09031936.05.00034805
13. Enright P. FEV1 and FVC repeatability goals when performing spirometry. *Primary Care Respir J.* (2010) 19:194. doi: 10.4104/pcrj.2010.00031
14. Singh D, Agusti A, Anzueto A, Barnes PJ, Bourbeau J, Celli BR. Global strategy for the diagnosis, management, and prevention of chronic obstructive lung disease: the GOLD science committee report 2019. *Eur Respir J.* (2019) 53:1900164. doi: 10.1183/13993003.00164-2019
15. Jian W, Gao Y, Hao C, Wang N, Ai T, Liu C, et al. Reference values for spirometry in Chinese aged 4-80 years. *J Thoracic Dis.* (2017) 9:4538–49. doi: 10.21037/jtd.2017.10.110
16. Quanjer PH, Stanojevic S, Cole TJ, Baur X, Hall GL, Culver BH, et al. Multi-ethnic reference values for spirometry for the 3-95-yr age range: the global lung function 2012 equations. *Eur Respir J.* (2012) 40:1324–43. doi: 10.1183/09031936.00080312
17. Ryan H, Trosclair A, Gfroerer J. Adult current smoking: differences in definitions and prevalence estimates-NHIS and NSDUH, (2008). *J Environ Public Health.* (2012) 2012:918368. doi: 10.1155/2012/918368
18. de Marco R, Accordini S, Marcon A, Cerveri I, Antó JM, Gislason T, et al. Risk factors for chronic obstructive pulmonary disease in a European cohort of young adults. *Am J Respir Crit Care Med.* (2011) 183:891–7. doi: 10.1164/rccm.201007-1125OC
19. Bao H, Fang L, Wang L. Prevalence of chronic obstructive pulmonary disease among community population aged ≥40 in China: a Meta-analysis on studies published between 1990 and 2014. *Zhonghua Liu Xing Bing Xue Za Zhi.* (2016) 37:119–24. doi: 10.1002/marc.201670007
20. Fang L, Gao P, Bao H, Tang X, Wang B, Feng Y, et al. Chronic obstructive pulmonary disease in China: a nationwide prevalence study. *Lancet Respir Med.* (2018) 6:421–30. doi: 10.1016/S2213-2600(18)30103-6
21. Zhong N, Wang C, Yao W, Chen P, Kang J, Huang S, et al. Prevalence of chronic obstructive pulmonary disease in China: a large, population-based survey. *Am J Respir Crit Care Med.* (2007) 176:753–60. doi: 10.1164/rccm.200612-1749OC

22. Buist AS, McBurnie MA, Vollmer WM, Gillespie S, Burney P, Mannino DM, et al. International variation in the prevalence of COPD (the BOLD Study): a population-based prevalence study. *Lancet.* (2007) 370:741–50. doi: 10.1016/S0140-6736(07)61377-4
23. Tilert T, Dillon C, Paulose-Ram R, Hnizdo E, Doney B. Estimating the U.S. prevalence of chronic obstructive pulmonary disease using pre- and post-bronchodilator spirometry: the National Health and Nutrition Examination Survey (NHANES) 2007-2010. *Respir Res.* (2013) 14:103. doi: 10.1186/1465-9921-14-103
24. Fukahori S, Matsuse H, Takamura N, Hirose H, Tsuchida T, Kawano T, et al. Prevalence of chronic obstructive pulmonary diseases in general clinics in terms of FEV1/FVC. *Int J Clin Pract.* (2009) 63:269–74. doi: 10.1111/j.1742-1241.2008.01873.x
25. Nakao M, Yamauchi K, Ishihara Y, Omori H, Solongo B, Ichinnorov D. Prevalence and risk factors of airflow limitation in a Mongolian population in Ulaanbaatar: cross-sectional studies. *PLOS ONE.* (2017) 12:e0175557. doi: 10.1371/journal.pone.0175557
26. Nugmanova D, Feshchenko Y, Iashyna L, Gyrina O, Malynovska K, Mammadbayov E, et al. The prevalence, burden and risk factors associated with chronic obstructive pulmonary disease in Commonwealth of Independent States (Ukraine, Kazakhstan and Azerbaijan): results of the CORE study. *BMC Pulm Med.* (2018) 18:26. doi: 10.1186/s12890-018-0589-5
27. Jaganath D, Miranda JJ, Gilman RH, Wise RA, Diette GB, Miele CH, et al. Prevalence of chronic obstructive pulmonary disease and variation in risk factors across four geographically diverse resource-limited settings in Peru. *Respir Res.* (2015) 16:40. doi: 10.1186/s12931-015-0198-2
28. Menezes AM, Perez-Padilla R, Jardim JR, Muiño A, Lopez MV, Valdivia G, et al. Chronic obstructive pulmonary disease in five Latin American cities (the PLATINO study): a prevalence study. *Lancet.* (2005) 366:1875–81. doi: 10.1016/S0140-6736(05)67632-5
29. Caballero A, Torres-Duque CA, Jaramillo C, Bolívar F, Sanabria F, Osorio P, et al. Prevalence of COPD in five Colombian cities situated at low, medium, and high altitude (PREPOCOL study). *Chest.* (2008) 133:343–9. doi: 10.1378/chest.07-1361
30. Laniado-Laborin R, Rendon A, Batiz F, Alcantar-Schramm JM, Bauerle O. High altitude and chronic obstructive pulmonary disease prevalence: a casual or causal correlation? *Arch de Bronconeumol.* (2012) 48:156–60. doi: 10.1016/j.arbr.2011.12.004
31. Brakema EA, Tabyshova A, Kasteleyn MJ, Molendijk E, van der Kleij RMJJ, van Boven JFM, et al. High COPD prevalence at high altitude: does household air pollution play a role? *Eur Respir J.* (2019) 53:1801193. doi: 10.1183/13993003.01193-2018
32. Xiong H, Huang Q, He C, Shuai T, Yan P, Zhu L, et al. Prevalence of chronic obstructive pulmonary disease at high altitude: a systematic review and meta-analysis. *Peer J.* (2020) 8:e8586. doi: 10.7717/peerj.8586
33. Bonjour S, Adair-Rohani H, Wolf J, Bruce NG, Mehta S, Prüss-Ustün A, et al. Solid fuel use for household cooking: country and regional estimates for 1980-2010. *Environ Health Perspect.* (2013) 121:784–90. doi: 10.1289/ehp.1205987
34. Smith KR, Pillarisetti A. *Household Air Pollution From Solid Cookfuels and Its Effects on Health.* Washington, DC: The International Bank for Reconstruction and Development / The World Bank(c) (2017) doi: 10.1596/978-1-4648-0522-6_ch7
35. Sood A, Assad NA, Barnes PJ, Churg A, Gordon SB, Harrod KS. ERS/ATS workshop report on respiratory health effects of household air pollution. *Eur Respir J.* (2018) 51:1700698. doi: 10.1183/13993003.00698-2017
36. GBD 2015 Risk Factor Collaborator. Global, regional, and national comparative risk assessment of 79 behavioural, environmental and occupational, and metabolic risks or clusters of risks, 1990-2015: a systematic analysis for the Global Burden of Disease Study 2015. *Lancet.* (2016) 388:1659–724. doi: 10.1016/S0140-6736(16)31679-8
37. Po JY, FitzGerald JM, Carlsten C. Respiratory disease associated with solid biomass fuel exposure in rural women and children: systematic review and meta-analysis. *Thorax.* (2011) 66:232–9. doi: 10.1136/thx.2010.147884
38. Sana A, Somda SMA, Meda N, Bouland C. Chronic obstructive pulmonary disease associated with biomass fuel use in women: a systematic review and meta-analysis. *BMJ Open Respir Res.* (2018) 5:e000246. doi: 10.1136/bmjresp-2017-000246
39. Raj TJ. Altered lung function test in asymptomatic women using biomass fuel for cooking. *J Clin Diagn Res.* (2014) 8:Bc01-3. doi: 10.7860/JCDR/2014/7253.4917
40. MacNeil A, Glaziou P, Sismanidis C, Maloney S, Floyd K. Global epidemiology of tuberculosis and progress toward achieving global targets - 2017. *MMWR Morbidity Mortality weekly Rep.* (2019) 68:263–6. doi: 10.15585/mmwr.mm6811a3
41. Vogelmeier CF, Criner GJ, Martinez FJ, Anzueto A, Barnes PJ, Bourbeau J, et al. Global strategy for the diagnosis, management, and prevention of chronic obstructive lung disease 2017. report: GOLD executive summary. *Eur Respir J.* (2017) 49:1700214. doi: 10.1164/rccm.201701-0218PP
42. Amaral AF, Coton S, Kato B, Tan WC, Studnicka M, Janson C, et al. Tuberculosis associates with both airflow obstruction and low lung function: BOLD results. *Eur Respir J.* (2015) 46:1104–12. doi: 10.1183/13993003.02325-2014
43. US Preventive Services Task Force (USPSTF). Screening for chronic obstructive pulmonary disease: US Preventive Services Task Force recommendation statement. *JAMA.* (2016) 315:1372–7. doi: 10.1001/jama.2016.2638
44. Press VG, Cifu AS, White SR. Screening for chronic obstructive pulmonary disease. *JAMA.* (2017) 318:1702–3. doi: 10.1001/jama.2017.15782
45. Ministry of Ecology and Environment of the People's Republic of China. (2016). http://www.mee.gov.cn/hjzl/dqhj/cskqzlzkyb/201609/P020160929519792904752.pdf (accessed December 20, 2018).

18

Chronic Obstructive Pulmonary Disease-Derived Circulating Cells Release IL-18 and IL-33 under Ultrafine Particulate Matter Exposure in a Caspase-1/8-Independent Manner

*Gianluigi De Falco[1], Chiara Colarusso[2,3,4], Michela Terlizzi[2,3], Ada Popolo[2,3], Michela Pecoraro[2,3], Mario Commodo[5], Patrizia Minutolo[5], Mariano Sirignano[1], Andrea D'Anna[1], Rita P. Aquino[2,3], Aldo Pinto[2,3], Antonio Molino[6] and Rosalinda Sorrentino[2,3]**

[1] Dipartimento di Ingegneria Chimica, dei Materiali e della Produzione Industriale, Università degli Studi di Napoli Federico II, Naples, Italy, [2] Department of Pharmacy, University of Salerno, Fisciano, Italy, [3] ImmunePharma s.r.l., University of Salerno, Fisciano, Italy, [4] Drug Discovery and Development Program, Department of Pharmacy, University of Salerno, Fisciano, Italy, [5] Institute for Research on Combustion (CNR), Naples, Italy, [6] Department of Respiratory Medicine, Respiratory Division, University of Naples Federico II, Naples, Italy

***Correspondence:**
Rosalinda Sorrentino
rsorrentino@unisa.it

Chronic obstructive pulmonary disease (COPD) is considered the fourth-leading causes of death worldwide; COPD is caused by inhalation of noxious indoor and outdoor particles, especially cigarette smoke that represents the first risk factor for this respiratory disorder. To mimic the effects of particulate matter on COPD, we isolated peripheral blood mononuclear cells (PBMCs) and treated them with combustion-generated ultrafine particles (UFPs) obtained from two different fuel mixtures, namely, pure ethylene and a mixture of ethylene and dimethylfuran (the latter mimicking the combustion of biofuels). UFPs were separated in two fractions: (1) sub-10 nm particles, named nano organic carbon (NOC) particles and (2) primarily soot particles of 20–40 nm and their agglomerates (200 nm). We found that both NOC and soot UFPs induced the release of IL-18 and IL-33 from unstable/exacerbated COPD-derived PBMCs. This effect was associated with higher levels of mitochondrial dysfunction and derived reactive oxygen species, which were higher in PBMCs from unstable COPD patients after combustion-generated UFP exposure. Moreover, lower mRNA expression of the repairing enzyme OGG1 was associated with the higher levels of 8-OH-dG compared with non-smoker and smokers. It was interesting that IL-18 and IL-33 release from PBMCs of unstable COPD patients was not NOD-like receptor 3/caspase-1 or caspase-8-dependent, but rather correlated to caspase-4 release. This effect was not evident in stable COPD-derived PBMCs. Our data suggest that combustion-generated UFPs induce the release of caspase-4-dependent inflammasome from PBMCs of COPD patients compared with healthy subjects, shedding new light into the biology of this key complex in COPD.

Keywords: combustion-generated ultrafine particles, inflammation, airway disease, chronic obstructive pulmonary disease, peripheral blood mononuclear cells

INTRODUCTION

Chronic obstructive pulmonary disease (COPD) is considered the fourth-leading causes of death worldwide, predicted to become the fifth ranked cause of disability worldwide (1). The development of COPD is caused by inhalation of noxious indoor and outdoor particles (2), especially cigarette smoke that represents the first risk factor for this respiratory disorder (3). Herein, chronic inflammatory pattern/s observed in the lung of COPD patients derives from the exposure of both cigarette smoke and air pollution, which affect lung resident and circulating cells (1, 3, 4). Although, the molecular mechanisms causing inflammatory patterns in COPD patients are still elusive; so far, an altered immune response followed by chronic inflammation has been described at the basis of COPD (1–3, 5, 6). Therefore, the main goal of our study was to understand the pro-inflammatory pattern induced by the exposure to ultrafine particles (UFPs) of human peripheral blood mononuclear cells (PBMCs) obtained from COPD patients, who are all former or current smokers. Over recent years, several papers demonstrated that oxidative stress due to cigarette smoking is critical for the activation of molecular mechanisms, such as NF-kB activation, that can lead to the release of pro-inflammatory mediators (3). In the milieu of pro-inflammatory mediators, IL-1-like cytokines have been detected in both sputum and bronchoalveolar lavage fluid of COPD patients (1) and of experimental murine models (7–9). It has been observed that biomass fuel smoke induces the activation of the inflammasome, a multimeric complex, that leads to the release of IL-1-like cytokines, which are responsible of early inflammation and that can result in a long-term chronic inflammation (10). Emerging evidence suggests that NOD-like receptor 3 (NLRP3) inflammasome may be involved in COPD pathogenesis (1). We previously demonstrated that ultrafine carbonaceous particulate matter (UFP) generated in very fuel-rich combustion conditions (mean sizes of 100 nm) triggered NLRP3/caspase-1-dependent inflammasome in smoker-derived PBMCs (11). To date, high levels of IL-1β are found in the lungs of patients with COPD after cigarette smoke exposure, implying the involvement of the inflammasome in this pathology. In support, several cigarette exposure COPD animal models showed that the genetic absence of both caspase-1, the enzyme involved in the canonical inflammasome complex, and NLRP3 reduced COPD-like features in mice (8, 9, 12), and this observation was further confirmed by neutralization of IL-1β (13). However, published experimental data on human samples from COPD patients are controversial in this regard (1). While several clinical studies have shown that IL-1-like cytokine levels are elevated in the lungs of patients with COPD (1), others found no correlation between NLRP3, caspase-1, and IL-1β responses when comparing stable COPD patients to smokers (14). Nevertheless, the latter study was performed on a cohort of stable COPD patients compared with healthy smokers. Di Stefano et al. proposed that, rather, the inflammasome complex could be relevant during COPD exacerbations (15).

In this article, we analyzed the effect of UFPs representative of those encountered in practical combustion conditions, including gasoline and diesel engines, and we found that PBMCs obtained from unstable/exacerbated COPD patients were able to solely release IL-18 and IL-33, but not IL-1α and IL-1β, when treated with combustion-formed UFPs. By contrast, PBMCs obtained from smoker and non-smoker healthy volunteers were less susceptible than unstable COPD-derived PBMCs to biofuel-like UFP exposure. Moreover, this effect was not dependent on NLRP3, caspase-1, and caspase-8, but rather on the release of caspase-4, implying the involvement of the non-canonical inflammasome pathway in PBMCs obtained from unstable/exacerbated COPD patients. By contrast, PBMCs obtained from stable COPD patients were not affected by the exposure to this particulate matter in terms of IL-18 and IL-33 release.

MATERIALS AND METHODS

Human Samples

Blood from COPD and non-COPD subjects were collected at the Hospital "Monaldi-Azienda Ospedaliera (AORN)-Ospedale dei Colli" in Naples, Italy, after signed informed consent. The experimental protocol was performed in accordance with the guidelines and regulations provided and accepted by the Ethical Committee of the "Monaldi-AORN-Ospedale dei Colli" Hospital (approval number 1254/2014). COPD and non-COPD subjects were 60 ± 10 (mean ± SEM) years of age. COPD subjects were smokers or former smokers; non-COPD subjects were divided in smokers and non-smokers. Blood was collected and used within 24 h.

Isolation of Human PBMCs

Mononuclear cells were isolated according to Ficoll's protocol as already reported (11). Briefly, blood (5 ml) was mixed with cell medium (5 ml) supplemented with sole antibiotics and Ficoll medium (Life Sciences, Italy). PBMC layer was collected, and platelets were separated by centrifugation at 150 *g* for 10 min. PBMCs were then collected in cell medium, plated (10^5 cells/well) and treated for 1, 3, or 5 h, accordingly. Treatment was performed in duplicate for each patient. Experimental time points were repeated for each patient.

Preparation of UFPs

Ultrafine particles were collected from laboratory premixed flames, which were run in fuel-rich conditions feeding ethylene/air and ethylene-2,5-dimethylfuran/air mixtures with an equivalence ratio of 2.0 and divided in two parts according to their sizes: sub-10 nm particles and larger soot particles (16).

Sub-10 nm particles were mostly constituted of organic carbon (17). They were stacks of few aromatic molecules, which had high-molecular mass and were constituted by four to six fused benzene rings with a dimension of about 1.2 nm connected by chain-like bridge (van der Waals interactions).

Larger soot particles were more graphitic carbon structures (17); they had sizes ranging from 20–40 nm, typical of the primary soot particles, to 100–200 nm typical of the chain-like aggregates of the primary particles: ultraviolet–visible and infrared spectroscopy and Raman spectroscopy were used for structural analysis of the carbon-network constituting the particles (18, 19). Soot particles appeared as a network of aromatic structures with few peripheral H atoms. Elemental analysis confirmed the low presence of H atoms in the soot particles, as the amount of C was approximately 95–98%, in mass, of the total material, and H was approximately 1–2%, with the rest being trace compounds, possibly oxygen.

Sub-10 nm particles and primary soot particles and aggregates were dispersed in bidistilled water to obtain a suspension with a concentration of 5 ppm (5 µg/ml). The mass concentrations were determined assuming a density of 1.2 and 1.8 g/cm^3 for sub-10 nm and soot particles, respectively. Here, we define NOC-E and NOC-ED the samples of sub-10 nm particles collected burning ethylene and the ethylene/dimethylfuran, whereas Soot-E and Soot-E/DMF the larger sizes soot particles collected burning ethylene and the ethylene/dimethylfuran, respectively. A summary of the particle characteristics is reported in **Table 1**.

Cytokine Measurements

IL-18 and IL-33 were measured in cell-free supernatants (75 × 10^4 cells/well) using commercially available ELISA kits (eBioscience, CA, USA). No differences in cytokine release were observed according to stage of COPD patients. 8-OH-dG was measured following manufacturer's instructions after 3 h of treatment (5 × 10^6 cells/well) (Elabscience, USA). The release of caspase-4 was analyzed by an ELISA kit patented by ImmunePharma s.r.l. (RM2014A000080 and PCT/IB2015/051262) (Department of Pharmacy, University of Salerno, Italy). According to the patent policy, and because it is still not commercially available, it is not at the moment possible to describe the technical approach to determine the release of caspase-4 by using the ImmunePharma's ELISA kit.

Calcium Measurement

Intracellular Ca^{2+} concentrations ([Ca^{2+}]i) were measured as previously reported after 1 h of treatment (5 × 10^3 cells/well) (20). Data were expressed as percentage of delta increase of fluorescence ratio (F340/F380 nm) induced by ionomycin (1 µM) or carbonyl cyanide p-trifluoromethoxy-phenylhydrazone (FCCP, 0.05 µM)—basal fluorescence/basal fluorescence ratio (F340/F380 nm).

TABLE 1 | Characteristics of the ultrafine particles (UFPs).

UFP characteristics					
Name	**Fuel**	**Particle size**	**H/C atomic**	**% O**	**Aromatic domain dimension**
NOC-E	Ethylene	sub-10 nm	0.6–0.8	n.d.	1.0–1.2 nm
NOC-ED	Ethylene/2,5 DMF (80/20 vol.%)	sub-10 nm	0.6–0.8	n.d.	1.0–1.2 nm
Soot-E	Ethylene	20–200 nm	0.2–0.3	<1%	1.2–1.4 nm
Soot-E/DMF	Ethylene/2,5 DMF (80/20 vol.%)	20–200 nm	0.2–0.3	<5%	1.2–1.4 nm

n.d., not detected; NOC, nano organic carbon; 2,5 DMF, 2,5 dimethylfuran.

Flow Cytometry

Peripheral blood mononuclear cells were stained for flow cytometry analysis (BD FACSCalibur Milan, Italy) using the following antibodies: CD14-PE and NLRP3-PeCy5.5. Healthy non-smoker-, smoker-, and COPD-derived PBMCs (2 × 10^5 cells/well) were stained for MitoSOX Mitochondrial Superoxide Indicator as indicated in the manufacturer's guide (Life Technologies, USA).

RT-PCR

Total RNA was isolated from PBMCs (10^7 cells/well) by using the RNA extraction kit (Qiagen, Milan, Italy). Reverse Transcription was performed by using first-strand cDNA synthesis kit (Qiagen, Milan, Italy) followed by PCR. Thermal cycling conditions were as follow:

1. 5 min at 95°C, followed by 40 cycles of 30 s at 95°C, 60 s at 54°C, 30 s at 60°C for OGG1.
2. 5 min at 95°C, followed by 40 cycles of 30 s at 95°C, 60 s at 58°C, 30 s at 68°C for caspase-4.

Primer pairs were as follow:
OGG1: Forward 5′-GACAAGACCCCATCGAATGC-3′
Reverse 5′-AGCTTCCTGAGATGAGCCTC-3′
CASPASE-4: Forward 5′-TCCCTGGGCAAAGATTTCCT-3′
Reverse 5′-GTCCAGCCTCCATATTCGGA-3′
β-actin: Forward 5′-ACTCTTCCAGCCTTCCTTCC-3′
Reverse 5′-CGTACAGGTCTTTGCGGATG-3′

Statistical Analysis

Data are reported as median ± interquartile range or as mean ± SEM. Statistical differences were assessed with one-way analysis of variance followed by Bonferroni's multiple comparison post test, and p values less than 0.05 were considered significant.

RESULTS

Combustion-Generated UFPs Induced the Release of IL-18 from Human PBMCs Obtained from Unstable COPD Patients

To mimic environmental pollution, PBMCs were isolated from smokers, non-smokers, and COPD patients, and then treated with two classes of combustion-generated UFPs for 5 h. **Figure 1** reports the release of IL-18 after the addition of Soot-E (A), Soot-E/DMF (B), NOC-E (C), and NOC-ED (D) at concentrations of 50 and 100 pg/ml. Clearly, UFPs induced the release of IL-18 from PBMCs obtained from unstable exacerbated COPD patients (black bars, **Figure 1**). To note, the release of IL-18 from PBMCs of unstable/exacerbated COPD patients was significantly higher than that observed from PBMCs of non-smoker (**Figure 1**, white bars) and smoker (**Figure 1**, dotted bars) volunteers. Noticeably, Soot-E (**Figure 1A**) and Soot-E/DMF (**Figure 1B**) did not induce IL-18 release from PBMCs obtained from non-smoker (**Figures 1A,B**, white bars) and smokers (**Figures 1A,B**, dotted bars), compared with the control (CTR)/basal levels.

Similarly, the same mass concentrations of NOC-E (**Figures 1C**) and NOC-ED (**Figure 1D**) increased the release of IL-18 from

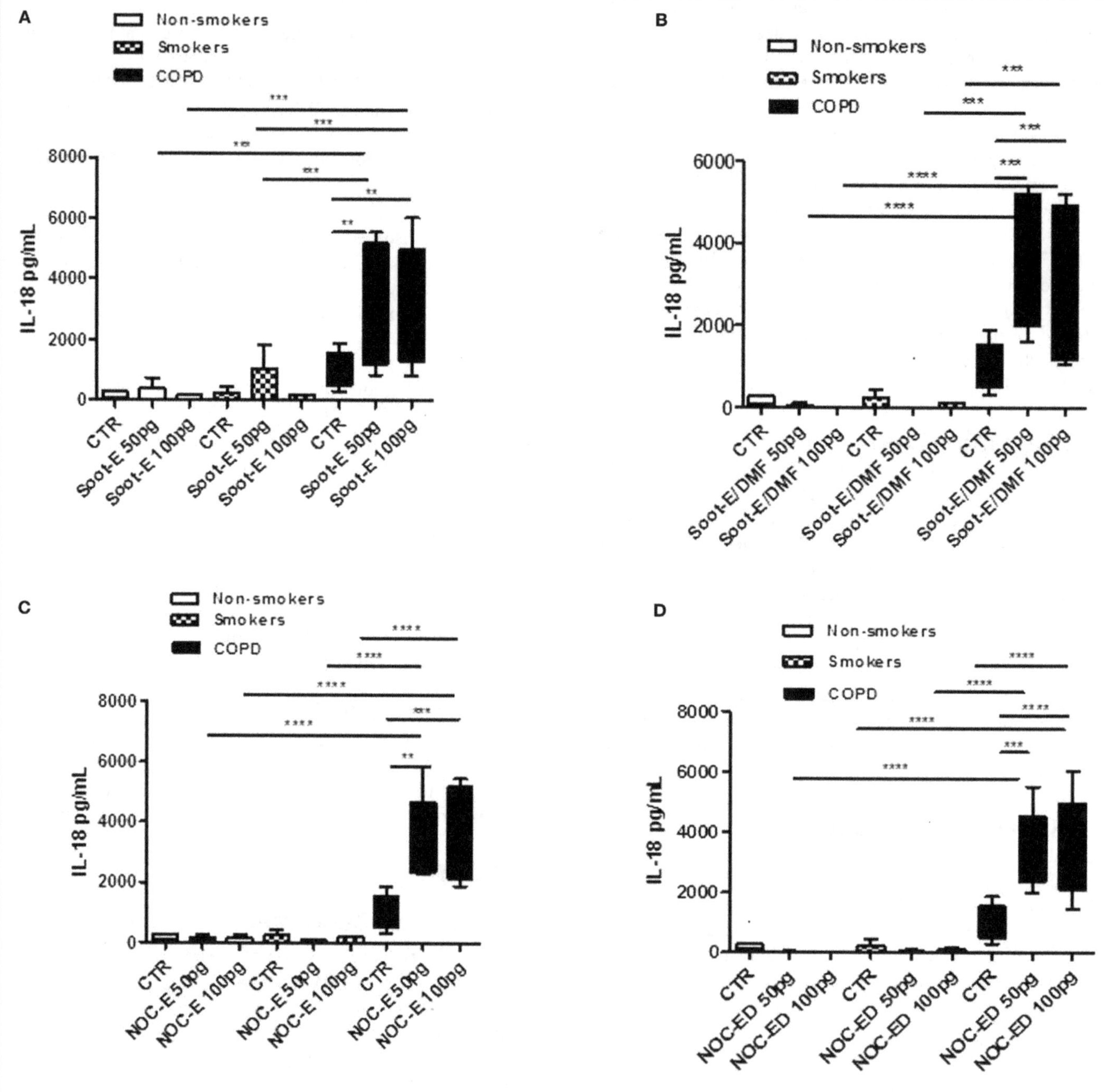

FIGURE 1 | The administration of combustion-generated ultrafine particles (UFPs) for 5 h induced the release of IL-18 by peripheral blood mononuclear cells (PBMCs) obtained from unstable/exacerbated chronic obstructive pulmonary disease (COPD) patients. Healthy non-smoker (white bars), smoker (dotted bars), and COPD (black bars)-derived PBMCs were treated with soot combustion-derived UFPs for 5 h. The addition of Soot-E **(A)**, Soot-E/DMF **(B)**, nano organic carbon (NOC)-E **(C)**, and NOC-ED **(D)** at the concentration of 50–100 pg/ml induced the release of IL-18. Control (CTR) represents untreated cells. Data are presented as median ± interquartile range (n = 7). Statistically significant differences were determined by one-way analysis of variance followed by Bonferroni's multiple comparison posttest. **, ***, and **** represent $p < 0.01$, $p < 0.0005$, and $p < 0.0001$, respectively.

PBMCs obtained from unstable COPD (**Figures 1C,D**, black bars) and were almost non-active at inducing IL-18 release from non-smoker- derived (white bars) and smoker-derived (dotted bars) PBMCs (**Figures 1C,D**).

The same mass concentrations of NOC and soot particles correspond to different surface area of the particles exposed to cells due to the different sizes of the particles. In particular, 100 pg/ml of soot have a surface area of 2.2E−4 cm^2/ml whereas the same amount of NOC has a surface area of 2E−3 cm^2/ml, implying that NOC particles expose higher surface area than soot particles, due to their lower size. To verify, whether the size of these sub-10 nm particles was a limitation, we treated cells with coronene and pyrene, polycyclic aromatic hydrocarbons with sizes comparable to those measured for the aromatic compounds that constitute the nanoparticles (1 pg/ml up to 1 ng/ml). As shown in Figures S1A–C in Supplementary Material, both coronene and pyrene (10 pg/ml) significantly increased IL-18 release from PBMCs of non-smokers (Figure S1A in Supplementary Material), smokers (Figure S1B in Supplementary Material), and unstable COPD (Figure S1C in Supplementary Material) at 10 pg/ml corresponding to 6E−4 cm^2, implying that the size of the particles was not as relevant as the nature of the particles. Moreover, similarly to NOC-E and NOC-ED particles, we observed that cells were more responsive to the lower concentrations than the higher (data not shown), reaching a plateau at 10 pg/ml. Interestingly, PBMCs from non-smokers (Figure S1A in Supplementary Material) and smokers (Figure S1B in Supplementary Material) were less responsive in terms of IL-18 release compared with PBMCs obtained from unstable COPD patients (Figure S1C in Supplementary Material), which instead showed a significant increase. These data underlie that the organic nature of UFPs, as well as soot and NOC, is of relevant importance for cell responsiveness in terms of IL-18 release.

Combustion-Generated UFPs Induced the Release of IL-33 from Human PBMCs Obtained from Unstable/Exacerbated COPD Patients

Similarly to what performed for IL-18, we treated PBMCs from the three cohorts with soot and NOC UFPs. The addition of Soot-E (**Figure 2A**), Soot-E/DMF (**Figure 2B**, black bars), NOC-E (**Figure 2C**, black bars), and NOC-ED (**Figure 2D**, black bars) significantly increased the release of IL-33 at the concentration of 50–100 pg/ml from PBMCs obtained from unstable/exacerbated COPD patients. Also in this case, we observed that IL-33 release reached a plateau at 50–100 pg/ml whereas at higher concentrations of these UFPs (>100 pg/ml up to 1 ng/ml, data not shown) no increasing effect was observed. However, it is to note that despite what happened for IL-18, no statistical increase of IL-33 release was observed comparing results among the groups represented by non-smokers (**Figure 2**, white bars) and smokers (**Figure 2**, dotted bars). Instead, the stimulation of PBMCs derived by unstable COPD patients with Soot-E (**Figure 2A**, black bars), Soot-ED (**Figure 2B**, black bars), NOC-E (**Figure 2C**, black bars), and NOC-ED (**Figure 2D**, black bars) increased the levels of IL-33. It is to note, though, that we observed a statistical difference in IL-33 basal levels that were higher in smokers than unstable COPD-derived PBMCs (**Figure 2**, dotted bars vs black bars).

Combustion-Generated UFPs Increased Oxidative Stress in Human PBMCs Obtained from Unstable/Exacerbated COPD Patients

In our previous study, we demonstrated that the release of IL-1-like cytokines after UFP exposure was caspase-1- and NLRP3 inflammasome dependent in PBMCs from healthy smokers (11). To understand the molecular mechanism underlying the release of IL-18 and IL-33 from unstable COPD patients after organic UFP exposure, we carried on evaluating the role of NLRP3 and mitochondrial-dependent oxidative stress. We observed that the expression of NLRP3 in $CD14^+$ PBMCs in basal conditions was significantly higher in COPD patients (**Figure 3A**, black bars) than non-smokers (**Figure 3A**, white bars) and smokers (**Figure 3A**, dotted bars). Similarly, mitochondrial-derived reactive oxygen species (mtROS) (identified as % Mitosox cells) were robustly higher in PBMCs from unstable/exacerbated COPD patients than non-smokers and smokers (**Figure 3B**). Starting from these observations and based on the concept that NLRP3 activation is strictly dependent on mtROS production (21), we measured mitochondria homeostasis under UFP treatment. The exposure to UFPs of PBMCs from non-smokers (**Figure 3C**, white bars) and smokers (**Figure 3C**, dotted bars) increased the release of calcium (Ca^{+2}) from mitochondria only after an external stimulus (carbonyl cyanide p-trifluoromethoxy-phenylhydrazone, FCCP) during the measurement/detection, implying that UFP treatment did not alter mitochondrial calcium stores. By contrast, the measurement of Ca^{+2} stores in the mitochondria of unstable COPD-derived PBMCs were lower (**Figure 3C**, black bars) than those observed in non-smokers and smokers (**Figure 3C**, white and dotted bars) after Soot-E, Soot-E/DMF, NOC-E, and NOC-ED (100 pg/ml) treatment. The above data imply that the stimulation of PBMCs with these particles had already induced the release of Ca^{+2} from the mitochondria in unstable COPD-derived PBMCs. Because the release of Ca^{+2} from the mitochondria is strictly correlated to the release of mtROS (20) and protein/DNA damage, the levels of 8-hydroxy-deoxyguanosine (8-OH-dG), a well-known marker for DNA damage derived from oxidative stress (22), were measured. Very interestingly, the addition of NOC-E and NOC-ED significantly increased the release of 8-OH-dG in non-smoker (**Figure 3D**, white bars) and smokers (**Figure 3D**, dotted bars). However, 8-OH-dG release was more pronounced in PBMCs from unstable/exacerbated COPD patients after the addition of Soot-E/DMF, NOC-E, and NOC-ED (100 pg/ml) (**Figure 3D**, black bars).

To note, we did not observe a significant increase in mtROS from non-smokers after the addition of all particle samples (Soot-E, Soot-E/DMF, NOC-E, and NOC-ED, each 100 pg/ml) compared with smokers and COPD PBMCs (data not shown). Therefore, we went on to analyze the levels of a repairing enzyme, 8-oxoguanine glycosylase, OGG1, highly important to avoid DNA damage following oxidative stress (23). The administration of all UFPs (100 pg/ml) significantly increased the levels of mRNA in PBMCs obtained from non-smokers (**Figure 3E**, white bars). By contrast, PBMCs from smokers did not show any increase compared with the basal levels of mRNA for OGG1 after all UFP (100 pg/ml) exposure (**Figure 3E**, dotted bars), but rather, a significant decrease was observed. Interestingly, PBMCs from unstable COPD patients showed no increase of OGG1 mRNA levels after Soot-E, Soot-E/DMF, NOC-E, and NOC-ED (100 pg/ml) exposure (**Figure 3E**, black bars).

These data imply that treatment of PBMCs obtained from unstable/exacerbated COPD patients with Soot-E, Soot-E/DMF, NOC-E, and NOC-ED leads to mitochondrial dysfunction in that

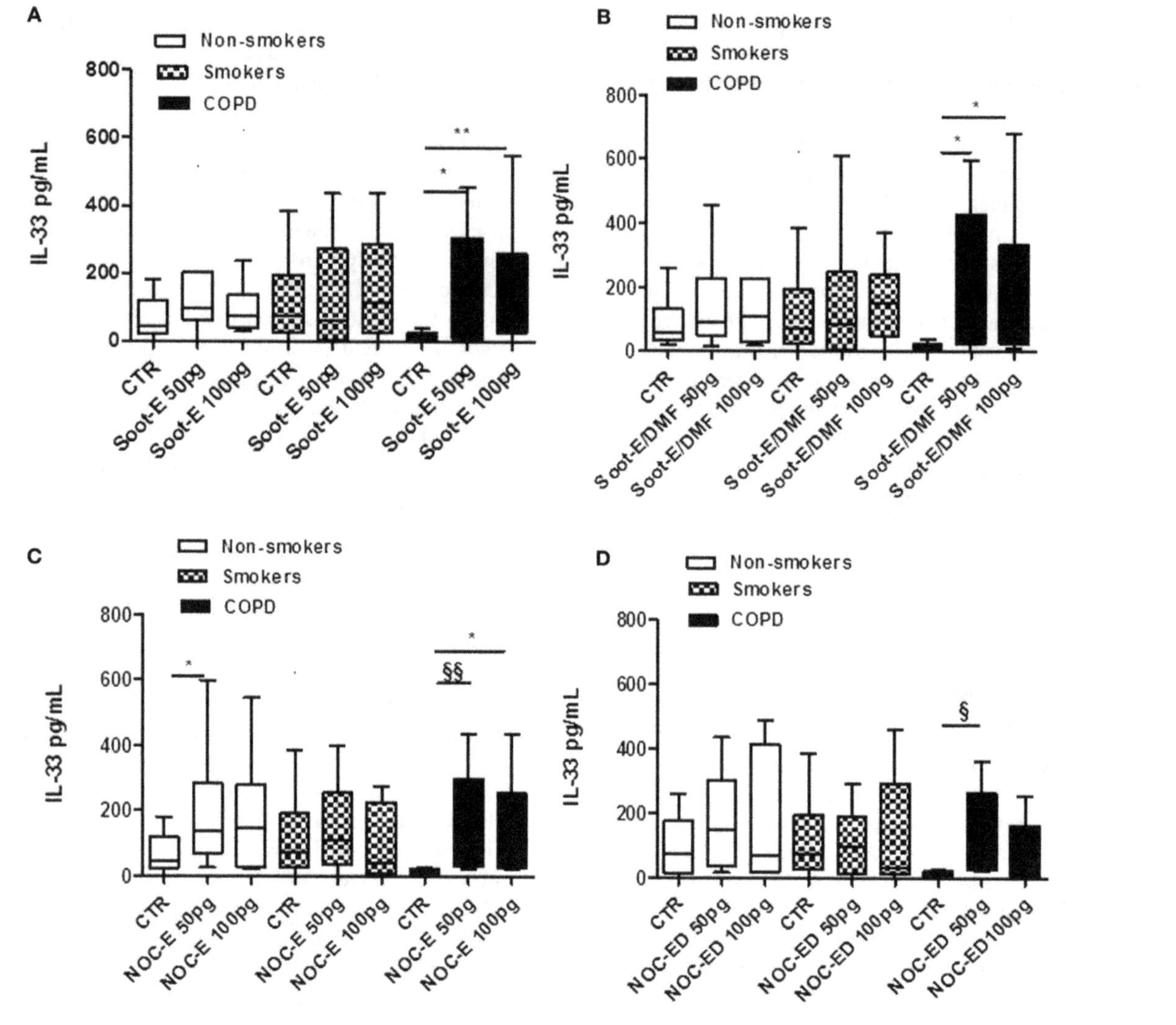

FIGURE 2 | The administration of combustion-generated ultrafine particles (UFPs) for 5 h induced the release of IL-33 by peripheral blood mononuclear cells (PBMCs) obtained from unstable/exacerbated chronic obstructive pulmonary disease (COPD) patients. Healthy non-smoker (white bars), smoker (dotted bars), and COPD (black bars)-derived PBMCs were treated with soot combustion-derived UFPs for 5 h. The addition of Soot-E **(A)**, Soot-E/DMF **(B)**, NOC-E **(C)**, and NOC-ED **(D)** at the concentration of 50–100 pg/ml induced the release of IL-33. Control (CTR) represents untreated cells. Data are presented as median ± interquartile range M ($n = 7$). Statistically significant differences were determined by one-way analysis of variance followed by Bonferroni's multiple comparison posttest. *, **, §, and §§ represent $p < 0.05$, $p < 0.01$, $p < 0.005$, and $p < 0.001$, respectively.

oxidative stress occurs. In this context, however, this effect is not countered by repairing enzymes, such as OGG1, establishing a pro-inflammatory/prooxidative cytoplasmic molecular pattern that leads to the release of IL-18 and IL-33 from PBMCs obtained from unstable/exacerbated COPD patients.

The Release of IL-18 and IL-33 from Unstable COPD-Derived PBMCs Is Not NLRP3/Caspase-1-Dependent after Combustion-Generated UFP Exposure

Because the release of mtROS and the presence of 8-OH-dG are able to induce the activation of NLRP3 inflammasome and because we found that NLRP3 protein levels are higher in unstable COPD patients, we went on by analyzing the molecular mechanism underlying the release of IL-18 and IL-33 from unstable COPD-derived PBMCs after combustion-generated UFP exposure. Therefore, unstable COPD-derived PBMCs were treated with pharmacological inhibitors for caspase-1, ac-Y-Vad (Y-Vad, 1 μg/ml) (20), for NLRP3, glybenclamide (Gly, 1 μM) (11, 20) and for caspase-8, z-IETD-fmk (IE, 0.5 μg/ml) (24, 25) together with combustion-generated UFPs.

The pharmacological inhibition of caspase-1 did not alter the levels of IL-18 from unstable COPD-derived PBMCs after Soot-E (**Figure 4A**), Soot-E/DMF (**Figure 4B**), NOC-E (**Figure 4C**), or NOC-ED (**Figure 4D**) exposure. In support, the inhibition of NLRP3 by means of Gly did not affect the levels of IL-18 from unstable COPD-derived PBMCs after Soot-E (**Figure 4A**),

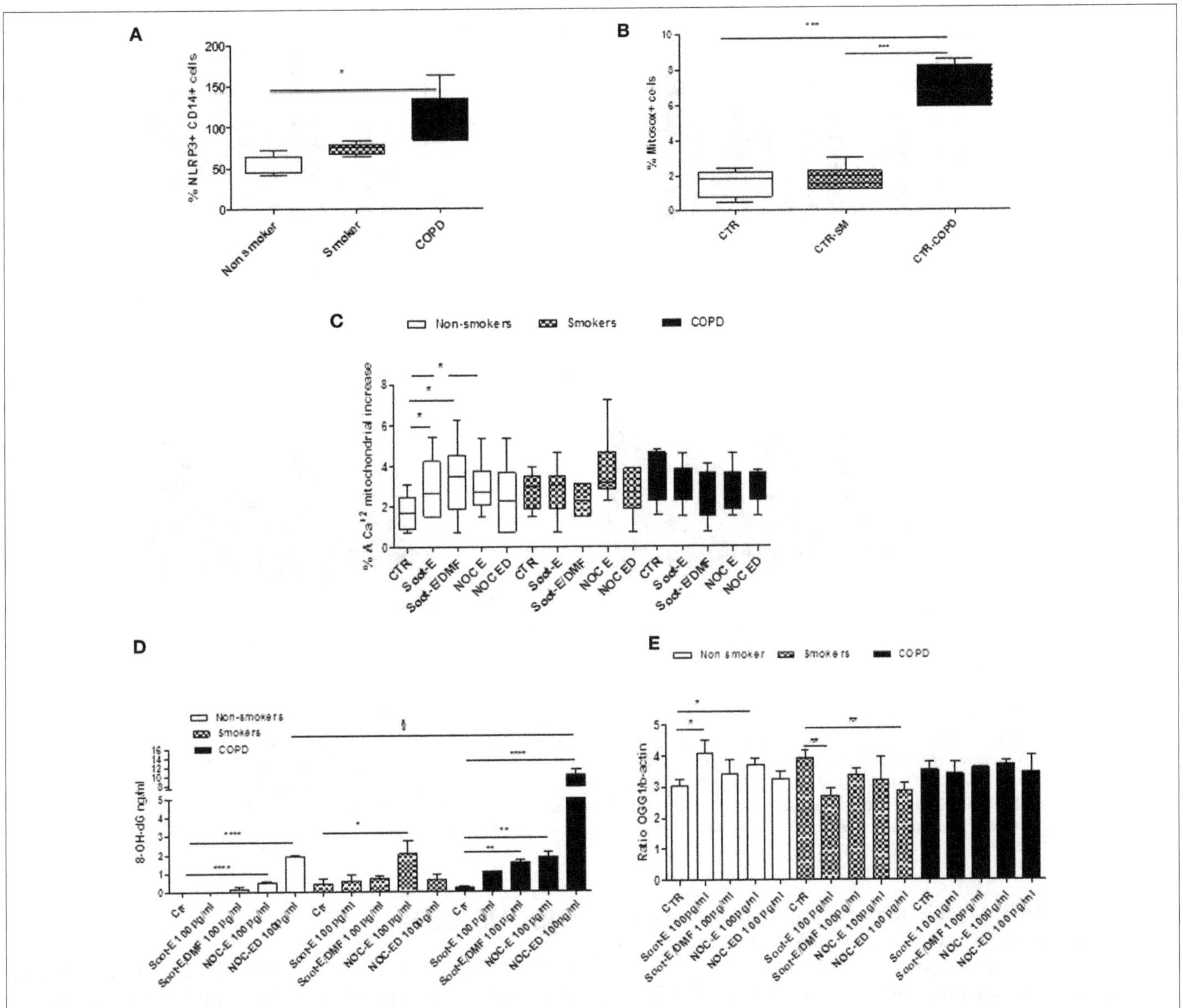

FIGURE 3 | The administration of combustion-generated ultrafine particles (UFPs) induced mitochondria-dependent oxidative stress. Healthy non-smoker (white bars), smoker (dotted bars), and chronic obstructive pulmonary disease (black bars)-derived peripheral blood mononuclear cells (PBMCs) were treated with soot combustion-derived UFPs for 5 h. Levels of NOD-like receptor 3 (NLRP3) inflammasome **(A)** in CD14+ PBMCs and mitochondria-derived reactive oxygen species (mtROS), identified as Mitosox+ cells determined by means of flow cytometry **(B)**. **(C)** Levels of mitochondrial Ca^{+2} stores after the addition of Soot-E, Soot-E/DMF, nano organic carbon (NOC)-E, and NOC-ED at the concentration of 100 pg/ml for 1 h. **(D)** Levels of cytoplasmic 8-OH-dG after 3 h of treatment of PBMCs with Soot-E, Soot-E/DMF, NOC-E, and NOC-ED at the concentration of 100 pg/ml. **(E)** Levels of mRNA levels of OGG1 after 3 h of treatment of PBMCs with Soot-E, Soot-E/DMF, NOC-E, and NOC-ED at the concentration of 100 pg/ml, determined by means of RT-PCR. Control (CTR) represents untreated cells. Data are presented as median ± interquartile range **(A,B)** and means ± SEM **(C–E)** ($n = 7$). Statistically significant differences were determined by one-way analysis of variance followed by Bonferroni's multiple comparison posttest. *, **, §, ***, and **** represent $p < 0.05$, $p < 0.01$, $p < 0.001$, $p < 0.0005$, and $p < 0.0001$, respectively.

Soot-E/DMF (**Figure 4B**), NOC-E (**Figure 4C**), or NOC-ED (**Figure 4D**) exposure. Moreover, the pharmacological inhibition of caspase-8, another enzyme involved in the non-canonical inflammasome-dependent pathway (26), did not alter IL-18 levels (**Figures 4A–D**).

The same results were obtained for IL-33, where we observed that neither the inhibition of caspase-1 (**Figures 5A–D**) nor the inhibition of NLRP3 and caspase-8 (**Figures 5A–D**) altered the levels of the cytokine released from PBMCs obtained from unstable COPD patients exposed to combustion-generated UFPs.

The Exposure of Unstable COPD-Derived PBMCs to Combustion-Generated UFPs Induced the Release of Caspase-4

Non-canonical inflammasome was also described as caspase-4-dependent in humans (caspase-11 in mice) (26). However,

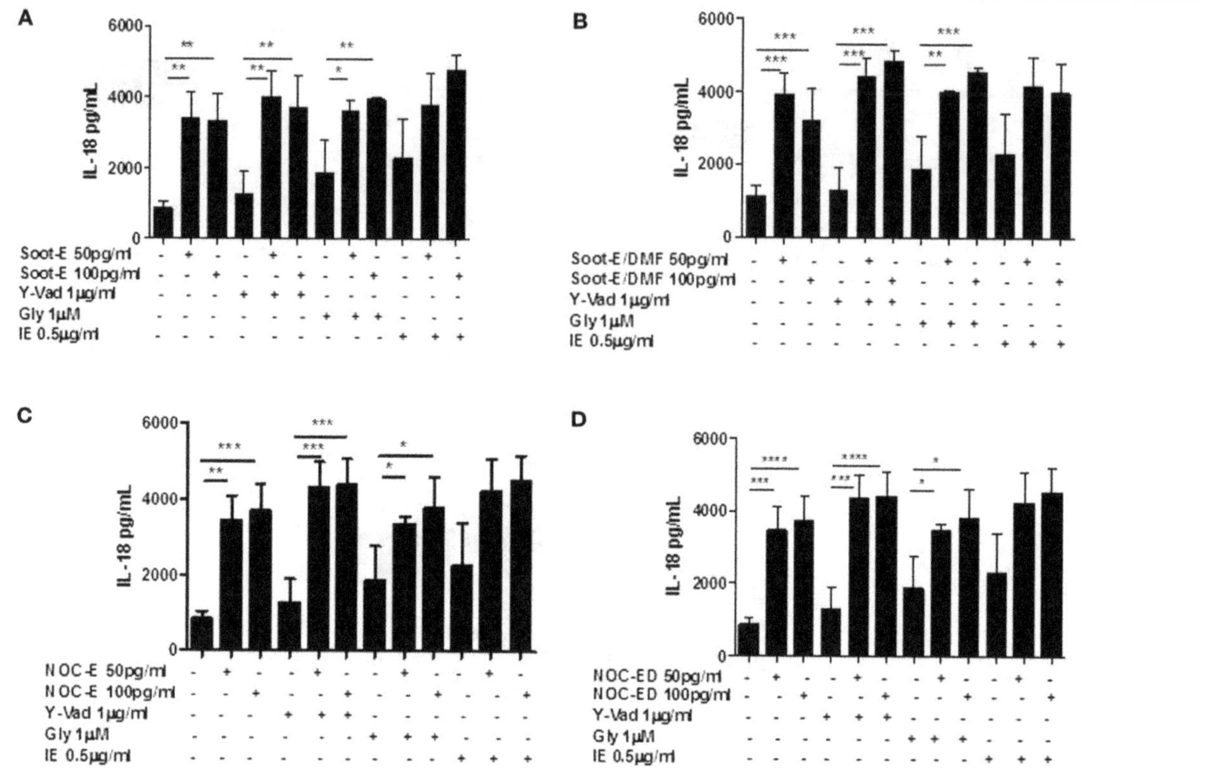

FIGURE 4 | The release of IL-18 from chronic obstructive pulmonary disease (COPD) peripheral blood mononuclear cells (PBMCs) treated with combustion-generated ultrafine particles (UFPs) was not NOD-like receptor 3 (NLRP3)/caspase-1 and caspase-8-dependent. COPD (black bars)-derived PBMCs were treated with soot combustion-derived UFPs for 5 h in the presence of y-Vad, caspase-1 inhibitor (1 µg/ml), glybenclamide (Gly), NLRP3 inhibitor (1 µM), and IE (0.5 µg/ml) a caspase-8 inhibitor. The levels of IL-18 after **(A)** Soot-E, Soot-E/DMF **(B)**, nano organic carbon (NOC)-E **(C)**, and NOC-ED **(D)** treatment was not reduced in the presence of Y-Vad, Gly, and IE. Data are presented as the means ± SEM ($n = 7$). Statistically significant differences were determined by one-way analysis of variance followed by Bonferroni's multiple comparison posttest. *, **, ***, and **** represent $p < 0.05$, $p < 0.01$, $p < 0.0005$, and $p < 0.0001$, respectively.

caspase-11 was defined as inducible, not constitutive, in mice (27). Therefore, we first analyzed the levels of mRNA for caspase-4 in PBMCs obtained from unstable COPD patients.

We found that caspase-4 mRNA levels were detectable in CTR cells and, interestingly, the treatment of cells with NOC-ED significantly increased caspase-4 mRNA levels (**Figure 6A**). To evaluate the potential involvement of caspase-4 in UFP effects, we used a patented ELISA kit (as described in Section "Materials and Methods"). Very interestingly, the addition of NOC-ED significantly increased the release of caspase-4 from PBMCs obtained by unstable COPD patients (**Figure 6B**). However, we were not able to reach a statistical difference when cells were treated with the other three UPFs samples, Soot-E or Soot-E/DMF or NOC-E (**Figure 6B**). Nevertheless, a potential increase was observed: 0.61 ± 0.32 ng/ml for Soot-E (100 pg/ml) vs 0.35 ± 0.09 ng/ml for CTR; 1.36 ± 0.74 ng/ml for NOC-E (100 pg/ml) vs 0.35 ± 0.09 ng/ml for CTR. Similar data were observed when COPD-derived PBMCs were treated with coronene (10 pg/ml; 1.74 ± 0.7 ng/ml).

Taken together, these data imply the extracellular release of caspase-4 and its involvement in IL-18 and IL-33 increase when PBMCs obtained from unstable COPD patients are treated with UFPs.

DISCUSSION

In this study, we found that combustion-generated UFPs induced mitochondrial-derived oxidative stress, which is not countered by the enzyme OGG1, deputed to repairing oxidative stress damage, leading to the release of IL-18 and IL-33 from PBMCs obtained from unstable/exacerbated COPD patients. Importantly, the release of IL-18 and IL-33 was not dependent on the activation of the canonical, caspase-1-dependent, and non-canonical, caspase-8-dependent, inflammasome pathway but rather on the release of the caspase-4, which activity still remains to be defined after UFP exposure. By contrast, PBMCs obtained from stable COPD patients were not affected by the exposure to this particulate matter in terms of IL-18 and IL-33 release.

Literature data report that high levels of IL-1β and IL-18 are usually found in the lungs of patients with COPD after cigarette smoke exposure, implying the involvement of the inflammasome in this pathology (1, 7, 13). In support, the adaptor protein ASC was found at high levels and in a speck-like form in the sputum of COPD patients (12). Experimental COPD animal models showed that the genetic absence of both caspase-1, the enzyme involved in the canonical inflammasome complex, and NLRP3 reduce COPD-like features in mice exposed to cigarette

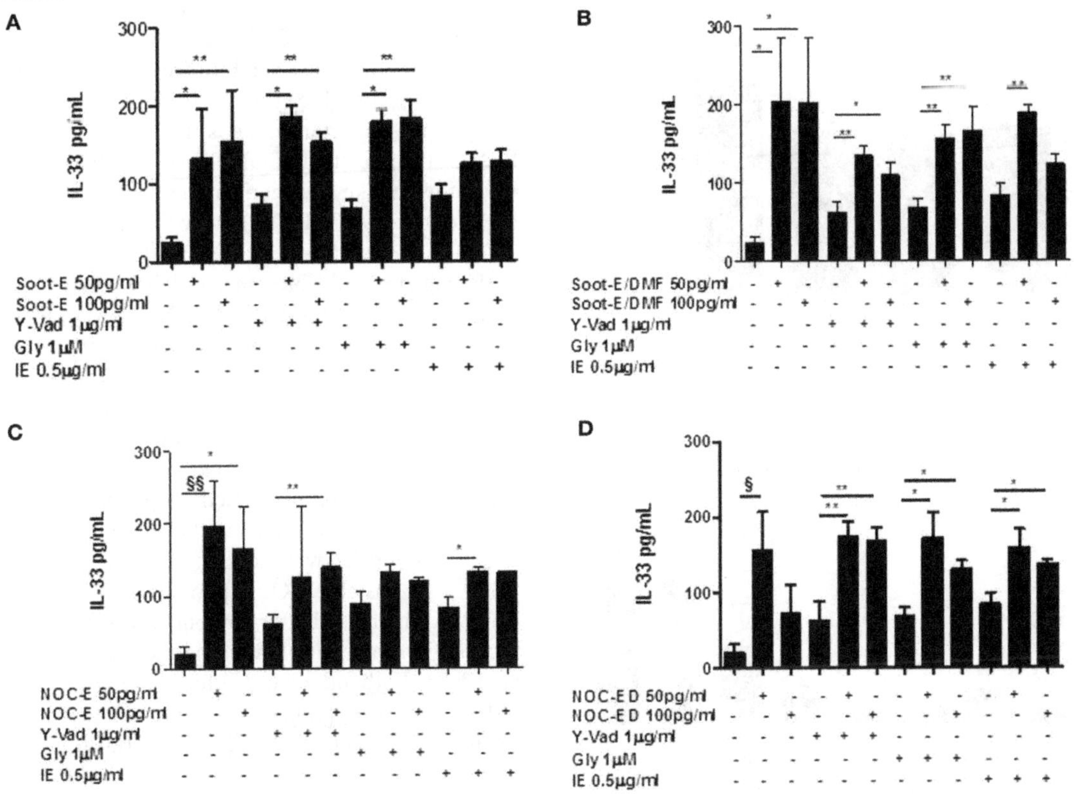

FIGURE 5 | The release of IL-33 from chronic obstructive pulmonary disease (COPD) peripheral blood mononuclear cells (PBMCs) treated with combustion-generated ultrafine particles (UFPs) was not NOD-like receptor 3 (NLRP3)/caspase-1 and caspase-8-dependent. COPD (black bars)-derived PBMCs were treated with soot combustion-derived UFPs for 5 h in the presence of y-Vad, caspase-1 inhibitor (1 μg/ml), glybenclamide (Gly), NLRP3 inhibitor (1 μM). and IE (0.5 μg/ml) a caspase-8 inhibitor. The levels of IL-33 after **(A)** Soot-E, Soot-E/DMF **(B)**, nano organic carbon (NOC)-E **(C)**, and NOC-ED **(D)** treatment was not reduced in the presence of Y-Vad, Gly, and IE. Data are presented as the means ± SEM (n = 7). Statistically significant differences were determined by one-way analysis of variance followed by Bonferroni's multiple comparison posttest. *, **, §, and §§ represent $p < 0.05$, $p < 0.01$, $p < 0.005$, and $p < 0.001$, respectively.

smoking (5, 9, 10, 12), further confirmed by neutralization of IL-1β. However, published data on human samples from COPD patients are controversial in that no correlation between NLRP3, caspase-1, and IL-1β responses was observed when comparing stable COPD patients with smokers (1). These data imply that the inflammasome is not triggered in these clinical conditions, probably explaining the discrepancy in literature and the unsuccessful randomized clinical trials performed on stable COPD patients subjected to canakinumab (monoclonal antibody against IL-1β) or an anti-P2X7 antagonist (1). To note, most of the human studies were performed on stable COPD-derived samples. In sharp contrast, our study was focused on PBMCs from unstable/exacerbated COPD patients, and we found that the sole IL-18 and IL-33, but not IL-1α and IL-1β (undetectable), were released after the exposure to combustion-generated UFPs. Instead, stable COPD-derived PBMCs were not responsive to combustion-generated UFPs in terms of IL-18 and IL-33 release (data not shown). This is, to the best of our knowledge, the first study showing that unstable COPD-derived PBMCs were able to release IL-1-like cytokines in a non-canonical inflammasome-dependent manner after combustion-generated UFPs exposure. In support, as proposed by Di Stefano et al., NLRP3, Caspase-1 and IL-1β responses in exacerbated/unstable COPD patients would be relevant (15). We found that although, the higher levels of NLRP3 in the PBMCs of these patients, it was not involved in the release of IL-18 and IL-33 after combustion-generated UFP exposure. However, in our previous study, we found that the stimulation of smoker-derived PBMCs with pyrolytic combustion-derived UFPs released higher IL-1-like cytokines in a NLRP3-dependent manner (11). Because all the PBMCs we used were obtained from smoking or former smoking COPD patients, we expected that NLRP3 inflammasome was most likely leading to the chronic inflammatory response typical of COPD after combustion-generated UFP exposure. Instead, we found that smokers were less responsive to combustion-generated UFPs than COPD patients, implying that the nature of air pollutants is of great relevance. Moreover, it is likely that although the higher levels, NLRP3 may be impaired in PBMCs of unstable COPD patients (11, 15), explaining the discrepancies in the literature. Indeed, the pharmacological inhibition of NLRP3 by means of Gly did not alter IL-18 and IL-33 levels. Similarly, we did not observe any inhibition of these cytokines when we inhibited caspase-1 and caspase-8, which underlie NLRP3 activation in a canonical and non-canonical manner, respectively (26). It is to note that although the inhibition of caspase-8 did not alter IL-18 production after UFPs addition (**Figures 4A–D**), we were not

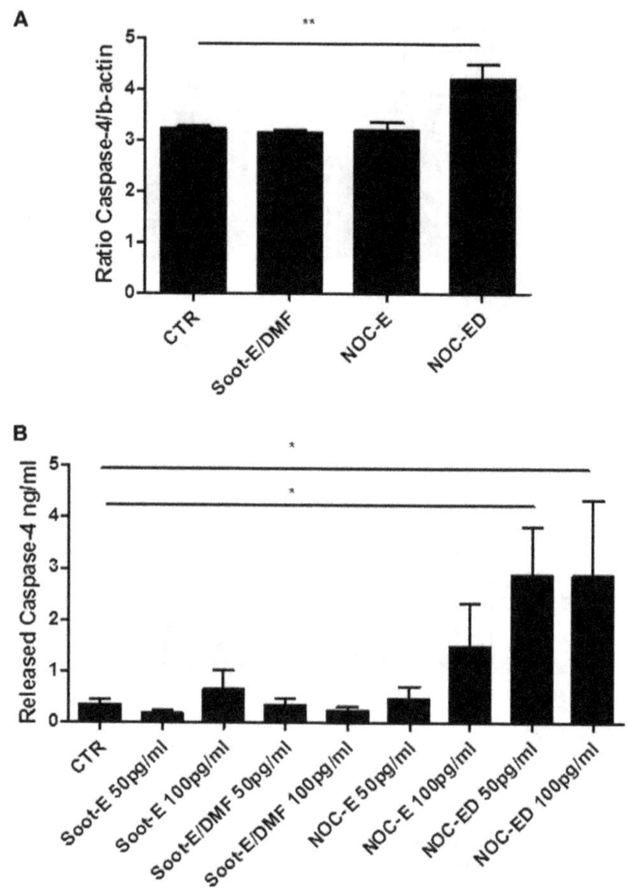

FIGURE 6 | The stimulation of unstable chronic obstructive pulmonary disease (COPD)-derived peripheral blood mononuclear cells (PBMCs) with combustion-generated ultrafine particles (UFPs) induced caspase-4 release. COPD (black bars)-derived PBMCs were treated with soot combustion-derived UFPs for 5 h. The levels of caspase-4 mRNA were determined **(A)** after Soot-E/DMF, nano organic carbon (NOC)-E, and NOC-ED treatment. The release of caspase-4 **(B)** was evaluated by means of a patented ImmunePharma's ELISA kit. Control (CTR) represents untreated cells. Data are presented as the means ± SEM **(A)** and **(B)** ($n = 7$). Statistically significant differences were determined by one-way analysis of variance followed by Bonferroni's multiple comparison posttest. * and ** represent $p < 0.05$ and $p < 0.01$, respectively.

able to reach a statistical difference between the basal levels when the sole caspase-8 inhibitor was added, versus the levels of the cytokine when the inhibitor and UFPs were added (**Figure 4D**). This effect was not observed for IL-33 (**Figure 5**).

By contrast, we found that caspase-4 release occurred after the exposure of PBMCs obtained from unstable COPD patients to combustion-generated UFPs, implying its involvement in IL-18 and IL-33 release. It is to point out, though, that we cannot assume by these data that caspase-4 was directly involved in IL-18 and IL-33 release due to the absence of a commercially available specific inhibitor of the sole caspase-4. Moreover, we have to highlight that stable COPD-derived PBMCs treated with combustion-generated UFPs did not induce caspase-4 release. Similarly we did not detect any difference compared with the basal conditions of release of IL-18 and IL-33 from PBMCs obtained from stable COPD patients treated with UFPs. These data further underlie the relevance of inflammasome-dependent mechanisms in stable vs unstable COPD patients.

Another important issue is the role of the oxidative stress in PBMCs from unstable COPD patients. Oxidative stress is a critical feature and key mechanism in many molecular processes during the onset of COPD (1). Mitochondrial dysfunction leads to excessive production of mtROS resulting in harmful effects, such as damage to lipids, proteins, and DNA. In this study, we found that unstable COPD-derived PBMCs exposed to combustion-generated UFPs had higher mitochondrial impairment in that higher levels of oxidized nucleic acids (i.e., 8-OH-dG, widely used as a marker), were found compared with non-smoker PBMCs. 8-OH-dG levels in unstable COPD-derived PBMCs were even higher than those observed in smoker-derived PBMCs after UFP exposure. This effect was strictly dependent on the expression of OGG1, an enzyme involved in the repair of DNA damage following mitochondrial dysfunction (23). OGG1 was not higher in the PBMCs of unstable COPD patients and even more important, it was not increased after combustion-generated UFP exposure, focusing on the clinical outcome/lifestyle of these patients when exposed to both indoor and outdoor pollution. Moreover, because of the strict correlation between NLRP3 activation and mtROS/oxidized DNA derivatives, it was obvious to believe that NLRP3 was involved. Instead, the pharmacological inhibition of NLRP3 did not show any correlation with IL-18 and IL-33 release after combustion-generated UFP exposure. In this context, though, we have to highlight that as reported by Shimada et al. (21), 8-OH-dG can bind to NLRP3 avoiding the activation of the inflammasome. Therefore, it is likely that NLRP3 is not involved in UFP-induced IL-18 and IL-33 release because of its inhibition by 8-OH-dG. More importantly, we found that caspase-4 is released into cell-free supernatant. The biological role of the released caspase-4 from unstable COPD-derived PBMCs is still under-investigated, and it still remains to investigate how caspase-4 is involved in IL-18 and IL-33 levels from PBMCs of unstable COPD patients.

In conclusion, our study highlights a novel molecular mechanism by which combustion-generated nanoparticles induce the release of the pro-inflammatory IL-18 and IL-33 in a non-canonical caspase-4-dependent inflammasome pathway from PBMCs of unstable/exacerbated COPD patients. Our study opens new perspectives in the field of the inflammasome in COPD during the exacerbation of clinical conditions, when the active form of caspase-4 is more relevant after cigarette smoke and air pollution exposure, paving the way for alternative pathways to be pharmacologically triggered in COPD pathogenesis.

AUTHOR CONTRIBUTIONS

GF, CC, MT, MS, MC, APinto, MP, AD, RA, PM, and RS designed the experimental protocol. GF, CC, MT, APopolo, and MP per formed the experiments. MC and MS prepared the soot particle samples. AD, RA, APinto, and RS interpreted the data and wrote the manuscript. All the authors read and approved the final manuscript.

SUPPLEMENTARY MATERIAL

FIGURE S1 | The stimulation of healthy non-smoker [white bars **(A)**], smoker [dotted bars **(B)**], and chronic obstructive pulmonary disease [black bars **(C)**] with coronene (10 pg/ml) or pyrene (10 pg/ml) induced the release of IL-18. Control (CTR) represents untreated cells. Data are presented as the means ± SEM ($n = 7$). Statistically significant differences were determined by one-way analysis of variance followed by Bonferroni's multiple comparison posttest. * represents $p < 0.05$.

REFERENCES

1. Colarusso C, Terlizzi M, Molino A, Pinto A, Sorrentino R. Role of the inflammasome in chronic obstructive pulmonary disease (COPD). *Oncotarget* (2017) 8:81813–24. doi:10.18632/oncotarget.17850
2. Tripple JW, McCracken JL, Calhoun WJ. Biologic therapy in chronic obstructive pulmonary disease. *Immunol Allergy Clin North Am* (2017) 37:345–55. doi:10.1016/j.iac.2017.01.009
3. Caramori G, Casolari P, Barczyk A, Durham AL, Di Stefano A, Adcock I. COPD immunopathology. *Semin Immunopathol* (2016) 38:497–515. doi:10.1007/s00281-016-0561-5
4. Raviv S, Hawkins KA, DeCamp MM, Kalhan R. Lung cancer in chronic obstructive pulmonary disease. *Am J Respir Crit Care Med* (2011) 183(9):1138–46. doi:10.1164/rccm.201008-1274
5. Kearley J, Silver JS, Sanden C, Liu Z, Berlin AA, White N, et al. Cigarette smoke silences innate lymphoid cell function and facilitates an exacerbated type I interleukin-33-dependent response to infection. *Immunity* (2015) 42:566–79. doi:10.1016/j.immuni.2015.02.011
6. Liew FY. Cigarette smoke resets the alarmin IL-33 in COPD. *Immunity* (2015) 42(3):401–3. doi:10.1016/j.immuni.2015.02.014
7. De Nardo D, De Nardo CM, Latz E. New insights into mechanisms controlling the NLRP3 inflammasome and its role in lung disease. *Am J Pathol* (2014) 184:42–54. doi:10.1016/j.ajpath.2013.09.007
8. Pauwels NS, Bracke KR, Dupont LL, Van Pottelberge GR, Provoost S, Vanden Berghe T, et al. Role of IL-1α and the Nlrp3/caspase-1/IL-1β axis in cigarette smoke-induced pulmonary inflammation and COPD. *Eur Respir J* (2011) 38:1019–28. doi:10.1183/09031936.00158110
9. Beckett EL, Stevens RL, Jarnicki AG, Kim RY, Hanish I, Hansbro NG, et al. A new short-term mouse model of chronic obstructive pulmonary disease identifies a role for mast cell tryptase in pathogenesis. *J Allergy Clin Immunol* (2013) 131:752–62. doi:10.1016/j.jaci.2012.11.053
10. Li C, Zhihong H, Wenlong L, Xiaoyan L, Qing C, Wenzhi L, et al. The nucleotide-binding oligomerization domain-like receptor family pyrin domain-containing 3 inflammasome regulates bronchial epithelial cell injury and proapoptosis after exposure to biomass fuel smoke. *Am J Respir Cell Mol Biol* (2016) 55(6):815–24. doi:10.1165/rcmb.2016-0051OC
11. De Falco G, Terlizzi M, Sirignano M, Commodo M, D'Anna A, Aquino RP, et al. Human peripheral blood mononuclear cells (PBMCs) from smokers release higher levels of IL-1-like cytokines after exposure to combustion-generated ultrafine particles. *Sci Rep* (2017) 7:43016. doi:10.1038/srep43016
12. Franklin BS, Bossaller L, De Nardo D, Ratter JM, Stutz A, Engels G, et al. The adaptor ASC has extracellular and 'prionoid' activities that propagate inflammation. *Nat Immunol* (2014) 15:727–37. doi:10.1038/ni.2913
13. Yang W, Ni H, Wang H, Gu H. NLRP3 inflammasome is essential for the development of chronic obstructive pulmonary disease. *Int J Clin Exp Pathol* (2015) 8(10):13209–16.
14. Pinkerton JW, Kim RY, Robertson AAB, Hirota JA, Wood LG, Knight DA, et al. Inflammasomes in the lung. *Mol Immunol* (2017) 86:44–55. doi:10.1016/j.molimm.2017.01.014
15. Di Stefano A, Caramori G, Barczyk A, Vicari C, Brun P, Zanini A, et al. Innate immunity but not NLRP3 inflammasome activation correlates with severity of stable COPD. *Thorax* (2014) 69(6):516–24. doi:10.1136/thoraxjnl-2012-203062
16. Sgro LA, D'Anna A, Minutolo P. On the characterization of nanoparticles emitted from combustion sources related to understanding their effects on health and climate. *J Hazard Mater* (2012) 211–212:420–6. doi:10.1016/j.jhazmat.2011.10.097
17. D'Anna A. Combustion-formed nanoparticles. *Proc Combust Inst* (2009) 32:593–613. doi:10.1016/j.proci.2008.09.005
18. Russo C, D'Anna A, Ciajolo A, Sirignano M. Analysis of the chemical features of particles generated from ethylene and ethylene/2,5 dimethyl furan flames. *Combust Flame* (2016) 167:268–73. doi:10.1016/j.combustflame.2016.02.003
19. Commodo M, De Falco G, Bruno A, Borriello C, Minutolo P, D'Anna A. Physicochemical evolution of nascent soot particles in a laminar premixed flame: from nucleation to early growth. *Combust Flame* (2015) 162:3854–63. doi:10.1016/j.combustflame.2015.07.022
20. Sorrentino R, Terlizzi M, Di Crescenzo VG, Popolo A, Pecoraro M, Perillo G, et al. Human lung cancer-derived immunosuppressive plasmacytoid dendritic cells release IL-1α in an AIM2 inflammasome-dependent manner. *Am J Pathol* (2015) 185:3115–24. doi:10.1016/j.ajpath.2015.07.009
21. Shimada K, Crother TR, Karlin J, Dagvadorj J, Chiba N, Chen S, et al. Oxidized mitochondrial DNA activates the NLRP3 inflammasome during apoptosis. *Immunity* (2012) 36:401–14. doi:10.1016/j.immuni.2012.01.009
22. Valavanidis A, Vlachogianni T, Fiotakis C. 8-hydroxy-2' -deoxyguanosine (8-OHdG): a critical biomarker of oxidative stress and carcinogenesis. *J Environ Sci Health C Environ Carcinog Ecotoxicol Rev* (2009) 27(2):120–39. doi:10.1080/10590500902885684
23. Tumurkhuu G, Shimada K, Dagvadorj J, Crother TR, Zhang W, Luthringer D, et al. Oggl-dependent DNA repair regulates NLRP3 inflammasome and prevents atherosclerosis. *Circ Res* (2016) 119(6):e76–90. doi:10.1161/CIRCRESAHA.116.308362
24. Terlizzi M, Colarusso C, Popolo A, Pinto A, Sorrentino R. IL-1α and IL-1β-producing macrophages populate lung tumor lesions in mice. *Oncotarget* (2016) 7:58181–92. doi:10.18632/oncotarget.11276
25. Terlizzi M, Di Crescenzo VG, Perillo G, Galderisi A, Pinto A, Sorrentino R. Pharmacological inhibition of caspase-8 limits lung tumour outgrowth. *Br J Pharmacol* (2015) 172:3917–28. doi:10.1111/bph.13176
26. Terlizzi M, Casolaro V, Pinto A, Sorrentino R. Inflammasome: cancer's friend or foe? *Pharmacol Ther* (2014) 143:24–33. doi:10.1016/j.pharmthera.2014.02.002
27. Kayagaki N, Wong MT, Stowe IB, Ramani SR, Gonzalez LC, Akashi-Takamura S, et al. Noncanonical inflammasome activation by intracellular LPS independent of TLR4. *Science* (2013) 341(6151):1246–9. doi:10.1126/science.1240248

19

A Refined View of Airway Microbiome in Chronic Obstructive Pulmonary Disease at Species and Strain-Levels

Zhang Wang[1†], Haiyue Liu[2†], Fengyan Wang[3†], Yuqiong Yang[3†], Xiaojuan Wang[1], Boxuan Chen[1], Martin R. Stampfli[4], Hongwei Zhou[2], Wensheng Shu[1], Christopher E. Brightling[5], Zhenyu Liang[3]* and Rongchang Chen[3,6]*

[1] Institute of Ecological Science, School of Life Sciences, South China Normal University, Guangzhou, China, [2] State Key Laboratory of Organ Failure Research, Microbiome Medicine Center, Division of Laboratory Medicine, Zhujiang Hospital, Southern Medical University, Guangzhou, China, [3] State Key Laboratory of Respiratory Disease, National Clinical Research Center for Respiratory Disease, Guangzhou Institute of Respiratory Health, The First Affiliated Hospital of Guangzhou Medical University, Guangzhou, China, [4] Department of Medicine, Firestone Institute for Respiratory Health at St. Joseph's Healthcare, McMaster University, Hamilton, ON, Canada, [5] Institute for Lung Health, NIHR Leicester Biomedical Research Centre, Department of Respiratory Sciences, University of Leicester, Leicester, United Kingdom, [6] Pulmonary and Critical Care Department, Shenzhen Institute of Respiratory Diseases, Shenzhen People's Hospital, Shenzhen, China

***Correspondence:**
Zhenyu Liang
490458234@qq.com
Rongchang Chen
chenrc@vip.163.com

[†] These authors have contributed equally to this work

Little is known about the underlying airway microbiome diversity in chronic obstructive pulmonary disease (COPD) at in-depth taxonomic levels. Here we present the first insights on the COPD airway microbiome at species and strain-levels. The full-length 16S rRNA gene was characterized from sputum in 98 COPD patients and 27 age-matched healthy controls, using the Pacific Biosciences sequencing platform. Individual species within the same genus exhibited reciprocal relationships with COPD and disease severity. Species dominant in health can be taken over by another species within the same genus but with potentially increasing pathogenicity in severe COPD patients. *Ralstonia mannitolilytica,* an opportunistic pathogen, was significantly increased in frequent exacerbators (fold-change = 4.94, FDR P = 0.005). There were distinct patterns of interaction between bacterial species and host inflammatory mediators according to neutrophilic or eosinophilic inflammations, two major airway inflammatory phenotypes in COPD. *Haemophilus influenzae*, *Moraxella catarrhalis, Pseudomonas aeruginosa,* and *Neisseria meningitidis* were associated with enhanced Th1, Th17 and pro-inflammatory mediators, while a group of seven species including *Tropheryma whipplei* were specifically associated with Th2 mediators related to eosinophilia. We developed an automated pipeline to assign strain-level taxonomy leveraging bacterial intra-genomic 16S allele frequency. Using this pipeline we further resolved three non-typeable *H. influenzae* strains PittEE, PittGG and 86-028NP with reasonable precision and uncovered strain-level variation related to airway inflammation. In particular, 86-028NP and PittGG strains exhibited inverse associations with Th2 chemokines CCL17 and CCL13, suggesting their abundances may inversely predict eosinophilic inflammation. A systematic comparison of 16S hypervariable regions indicated V1V3 instead of the commonly used V4 region was the best surrogate for airway microbiome. The full-length 16S data augmented the power of functional inference, which slightly better recapitulated the actual metagenomes. This led to the unique identification of butyrate-producing and nitrate reduction pathways as depleted in COPD. Our analysis uncovered finer-scale airway microbial diversity that was previously underappreciated, thus enabled a refined view of the airway microbiome in COPD.

Keywords: airway microbiome, COPD, full-length 16S sequencing, PacBio, airway inflammation

INTRODUCTION

Chronic obstructive pulmonary disease (COPD) is a heterogeneous lung disease characterized by airflow obstruction and persistent airway inflammation. The respiratory microbiome in COPD has been well studied in the last decade. The airway microbiome differs between health and COPD (Pragman et al., 2012; Sze et al., 2012; Zakharkina et al., 2013; Einarsson et al., 2016), shifts during acute exacerbations (Huang et al., 2014; Wang et al., 2016, 2018), associates with airway inflammation (Wang et al., 2016; Wang Z. et al., 2019) and predicts 1-year mortality of hospitalized exacerbation patients (Leitao Filho et al., 2018), all suggesting the implication of airway microbiome in COPD pathophysiology. Despite advances, the role of airway microbiome in COPD remains incompletely understood. An important knowledge gap is that our current view of airway microbiome is limited at most to its composition at bacterial genus-level, due to insufficient resolution of one or few hypervariable regions of 16S rRNA gene being sequenced in essentially all previous amplicon sequencing-based studies. In these studies, certain bacterial genera were often reported to be altered as a whole in disease and in relation to airway inflammation (Wang et al., 2016, 2018). However, from an ecological perspective, members of microbial community do not necessarily function according to their taxonomic groups, instead diversified species can act in the form of ecological "guilds" that co-adapt to altered environment (Zander, 2001; Zhao et al., 2018). Therefore, the aggregated genus-level associations can often be spurious or even misleading due to violation of basic ecological concepts. The inadequate depth of taxonomic profiling limits not only the accuracy of ecological inferences but also the ability to identify key bacterial species to use in follow-up experimental studies.

The recently advanced 'third-generation' sequencing technologies such as Pacific Biosciences (PacBio) and Nanopore is increasingly applied to microbiome studies (Goodwin et al., 2016; Levy and Myers, 2016). By generating long reads that extend tens of thousands of nucleotides, they offer the promise of increased taxonomic resolution by sequencing the full-length of 16S rRNA gene, thus serve as an attractive alternative for in-depth microbial taxonomic profiling (Wagner et al., 2016). In these applications, the 16S amplicon is circularized and read through multiple passes before circular consensus sequences (CCS) are generated, which greatly reduced the initial high error rate (~10%) of the long-read sequencing to that comparable to short-read sequencing (~0.5%) (Jiao et al., 2013; Hebert et al., 2018). Recent development of sophisticated denoising algorithms further enable accurate bacterial species identification at single-nucleotide resolution with near-zero error rate (Callahan et al., 2019). In some situations, strain-level identity can be further resolved utilizing information on the full complement of 16S rRNA gene alleles in bacterial genomes (Callahan et al., 2019; Johnson et al., 2019).

Here, we present the first analysis of the airway microbiome in COPD at species-level using PacBio sequencing. We also developed an automated pipeline to further resolve strain-level identity when possible. Our results uncovered additional diversity and heterogeneity in the airway microbiome at species-level and below, which was associated with patient clinical features and airway inflammation.

MATERIALS AND METHODS

Patient Inclusion and Exclusion Criteria

Sputum samples of 98 stable COPD patients and 27 age-matched healthy controls were collected in the First Affiliated Hospital of Guangzhou Medical University. The study was approved and supervised by the ethics committee of the First Affiliated Hospital of Guangzhou Medical University (reference number: No. 2017-22) and was registered in www.clinicaltrials.gov (NCT 03240315). All COPD patients met the diagnostic criteria according to GOLD guideline and were also assessed for symptoms and exacerbation frequency (**Table 1**). GOLD classification for disease severity (stage I-IV) was assigned to COPD patients based on pulmonary function test. For COPD patients, the inclusion criteria were: (1) age > 40 years; and (2) confirmed diagnosis of COPD according to the GOLD guideline (post-bronchodilator forced expiratory volume in 1s [FEV1]/forced vital capacity [FVC] ratio < 0.7). The exclusion criteria were: (1) physician-diagnosis of asthma or significant respiratory disease other than COPD; (2) COPD exacerbation within 4 weeks of enrollment; (3) history of lung surgery and tuberculosis; (4) diagnosis of cancer; (5) blood transfusion within 4 weeks of enrollment; (6) diagnosis of autoimmune diseases;

(7) enrollment in a blinded drug trial; and (8) short-term antibiotic usage within 4 weeks of enrollment. Informed consent was obtained from all patients.

Quality Control of Sputum Samples

Induced sputum were obtained for all subjects and quality-controlled upon collection. Briefly, sputum plugs which contained the most viscous material were picked up in a petri dish and isolated from saliva. The selected sputum plugs were prepared for cytology by dilution with 0.1% dithiothreitol (DTT) solution and filtered through 48 μm nylon-mesh filter according to standardized sputum processing protocol (Bafadhel et al., 2012). The numbers of total cells, squamous epithelial cells and leukocytes were counted and recorded. Sputum specimens with squamous epithelial cells: leukocytes < 1:2.5 were considered unlikely to be contaminated with oropharyngeal flora and acceptable for downstream experiments (Murray and Washington, 1975; Roson et al., 2000).

TABLE 1 | Major demographic and clinical characteristics of subjects.

Demographic and clinical features	Healthy (n = 27)	COPD (n = 98)	P-value
Age	65.4 (10.8)	66.2 (8.9)	0.67
Gender, n(M/F)	23/4	89/9	0.48
Current smoking, n(Y/N)	9/18	85/13	1.0e−4***
GOLD (1/2/3/4)	NA	24/33/32/9	NA
New GOLD (a/b/c/d)$	NA	39/38/4/17	NA
Frequent exacerbator (Y/N)$$	NA	20/78	NA
ICS usage (Y/N)	NA	58/40	NA
Long-term antibiotics (Y/N)	0/27	1/97	0.60
pre-FEV_1 (L)	2.8 ± 0.1	1.5 ± 0.1	5.1e−10***
pre-FVC (L)	3.4 ± 0.2	2.9 ± 0.1	0.01**
pre-FEV_1 (%)	100.0 ± 2.6	56.1 ± 2.7	1.0e−10***
pre-FEV_1/FVC	0.81 ± 0.01	0.49 ± 0.02	2.5e−13***
post-FEV_1 (L)	NA	1.6 ± 0.7	NA
post-FVC (L)	NA	3.1 ± 0.8	NA
post-FEV_1 (%)	NA	59.6 ± 2.6	NA
post-FEV_1/FVC	NA	0.5 ± 0.1	NA
CAT score	NA	4.0 ± 0.6	NA
mMRC	NA	0.4 ± 0.1	NA
Total sputum cells (cells × 10^9/L)	NA	20.4 ± 2.8	NA
Sputum neutrophils (%)	NA	86.2 ± 1.2	NA
Sputum eosinophils (%)	NA	5.3 ± 0.7	NA
Sputum lymphocyte (%)	NA	0.7 ± 0.1	NA
Sputum monocyte (%)	NA	7.9 ± 1.1	NA
Blood neutrophils (cells × 10^9/L)	NA	3.9 ± 0.1	NA
Blood eosinophils (cells × 10^9/L)	NA	0.3 ± 0.0	NA
Blood lymphocyte (cells × 10^9/L)	NA	1.8 ± 0.1	NA
Blood monocyte (cells × 10^9/L)	NA	0.5 ± 0.1	NA

*Continuous data are present as mean (range) or mean ± SEM. P-value was calculated using Fisher exact test for categorical variables and using Wilcoxon rank-sum test for continuous variables. ***P < 0.001; **P < 0.01; *P < 0.05 ICS: inhaled corticosteroids; FEV_1: forced expiratory volume in 1 s; FVC: forced vital capacity, CAT: COPD Assessment Test, mMRC: modified Medical Research Council. $The new GOLD classification based on mMRC, CAT and exacerbation frequency (2019) [Global Initiative for Chronic Obstructive Lung Disease (GOLD), 2019]. $$The frequent exacerbator was defined as exacerbation event > = 2/last year.*

Sputum Inflammatory Mediators

A panel of 47 sputum mediators (BLC, Eotaxin, Eotaxin-2, CXCL11, CXCL10, CCL2, CCL3, CCL4, CCL5, CCL13, CCL17, G-CSF, GM-CSF, I-309, ICAM-1, IFNg, IL-1a, IL-1ra, IL-1b, IL-2, IL-4, IL-5, IL-6, IL-6R, IL-7, IL-8, IL-10, IL-12p40, IL-12p70, IL-13, IL-15, IL-16, IL-17, IL-21, MCSF, MIG, MIP-1d, MMP-8, MMP-9, PDGF-AB, Procalcitonin, TNFa, TNFb, TNFRI, TNFRII, TIMP-1, TIMP-2) were measured in a subset of 59 patients with available sputum samples using custom antibody microarray (Human Cytokine Antibody Microarray slides; RayBiotech Inc., Norcross, GA, United States) (Wang F. et al., 2019).

The Full-Length 16S Sequencing and Analysis

Bacterial genomic DNA was extracted from selected sputum plugs using Qiagen DNA Mini kit. Negative controls for extraction (no sputum) and PCR amplification (no DNA template, ddH2O only) were included and sequenced together with all samples. The full-length (V1V9) bacterial 16S rRNA gene sequences were amplified using barcoded 27F (AGRGTTYGATYMTGGCTCAG) and 1492R (RGYTACCTTGTTACGACTT) primers. Library construction was performed using Pacific Biosciences (PacBio) SMRTbell^{TM} Template Prep Kit V1 on normalized pooled PCR products, and was sequenced using PacBio Sequel platform.

Circular consensus sequences reads were generated using the *ccs* application in SMRTLink 5.1 with minPasses = 5 and minPredictedAccuracy = 0.90. The demultiplexed CCS were analyzed using DADA2 v1.12.1 customized for the PacBio full-length 16S sequencing data (Callahan et al., 2016, 2019). Briefly, primers were removed from the CCS sequences using the *removePrimers* function. Sequences without primer matches were discarded. The remaining CCS sequences were filtered using the *filterAndTrim* function with parameters: minLen = 1000, maxLen = 1600, maxN = 0, maxEE = 2, and minQ = 3. Sequences were dereplicated and used for learning the dataset-specific error model using the *learnErrors* function with parameter errorEstimationFunction = dada2:PacBioErrfun. Sequences were denoised using the error model and Amplicon Sequence Variants (ASVs) were identified using the *dada* function. Taxonomy up to the genus-level was assigned using the *assignTaxonomy* function based on the silva_nr_v128_train_set sequence database. ASVs were further assigned to species if they had exact unambiguous sequence match to species in the silva_species_assignment_v132 sequence database using the *addSpecies* function[1]. For the remaining ASVs, an additional step of BLASTn search was performed against the local NCBI

[1]https://benjjneb.github.io/dada2/assign.html

nt database to make possible species-level calls based on exact unambiguous sequence match. Chimera sequences were removed using the *removeBimeraDenovo* function.

For comparison with the DADA2 approach, we performed two different clustering-based analyses that were previously used for full-length 16S amplicon sequences. First, we used the MCSMRT pipeline developed by Earl et al. for PacBio full-length 16S sequences ($-e = 2$), which clustered sequences into 97% operational taxonomic units (OTUs) and assigned taxonomy using a utax classifier on a custom-built full-length 16S database (Earl et al., 2018). Second, we performed a *de novo* clustering using the quality-filtered CCS reads into OTUs at 99% sequence identity using USEARCH (v11.0.667) (Edgar, 2010), according to Johnson et al. (2019). A custom Naïve Bayes classifier was trained on the Greengenes 13_8 99% OTUs using full-length 16S sequences obtained with 27F and 1492R primers, and applied to assign taxonomy for the representative sequence of each OTU using QIIME2 (Bolyen et al., 2018).

For downstream analyses, when analyzing microbiomes at the community level (i.e., alpha/beta diversity, functional inference), all ASVs were included irrespective of their taxonomic assignments. For differential analysis and correlation analyses with host mediators, we only focused on ASVs with species-level assignment, in order to identify species-level markers that were biologically interpretable. The ASV profile was rarefied to 3,119 reads per sample (**Supplementary Figure S1**).

Metagenomic Sequencing and Analysis

To assess the precision of functional inference based on full-length 16S data, we randomly selected sputum samples from 10 healthy controls and 10 COPD patients for shotgun metagenomic sequencing as benchmark. Shotgun metagenomic library was prepared using the extracted genomic DNA and sequenced using Illumina NovaSeq platform. Quality filtering of the metagenomic reads was performed using Cutadapt v1.18 ($-q = 20$) (Marcel, 2011). Host reads were removed by mapping the quality-filtered reads to human reference genome hg38 using bowtie2 (Langmead and Salzberg, 2012). The remaining reads were subject to functional profiling using HUMANn2 (Franzosa et al., 2018). An average of 1.3 million reads per sample can be putatively assigned to KO genes (range 188,636–6,882,594 reads). The HUMANn2 profile was downsized to 188,636 reads per sample only when performing correlation analysis on gene features across all samples, to eliminate variations influenced by sequencing depth. The raw Fastq data of this study has been deposited in the Chinese National Gene Bank (CNGB) Nucleotide Sequence Archive (CNSA) under accession code CNP0000837.

Strain-Level Identification Pipeline

Callahan et al. (2019) described a method for strain-level identification by hand using full-length 16S data leveraging the full complement of 16S rRNA alleles in bacterial genomes. In principle, a strain can be confidently assigned if all intra-genomic 16S sequence variants of that strain are recovered in integral ratios according to its genuine allelic variants. In extension to this approach, we designed an automated pipeline to assign strain-level ASV bins in four steps below. (1) All copies of 16S sequences were retrieved from 14,062 complete bacterial genomes in Genbank (assessed May 3, 2019) and the intra-genomic 16S copy number ratios were calculated. (2) All species-level ASVs were BLASTn-searched against the 16S database in step 1. ASVs with exact match to the same bacterial genome were assigned to the same initial bins. (3) The ASVs within each initial bin were subject to pairwise correlation, to generate refined bins by identifying ASVs with co-occurrence pattern (Pearson's $R > 0.7$). (4) For each refined bin, the copy number ratio of ASVs were determined based on linear regression slope, and reconciled with the genuine copy number ratio of the 16S alleles in the corresponding bacterial genomes. The ASVs in integral copy number ratio with the genuine ratio ($\pm$ 0.3) were retained in the final bins and assigned with strain-level taxonomy. The non-unique BLASTn matches (i.e., multiple genome-bins for the same set of ASVs) were resolved in this step using the genuine copy number ratio, when possible. The genomic abundances of each strain in each sample was calculated as the average abundances of ASVs normalized by their copy numbers in the genome. The curated intra-genomic 16S copy number ratio for all complete bacterial genomes and the code for the pipeline are available at GitHub[2].

Statistical Analysis

Differential microbiome features between COPD and healthy controls were identified using a linear discriminant analysis (LDA) effect size (LEfSe) method with a threshold of logarithmic LDA score 2.0 (Segata et al., 2011). Random forest analysis was performed using genus and species-level microbiome features selected by LEfSe (LDA > 2.0) using Weka 3.8 with 7-fold cross-validation (Frank et al., 2016). Area under receiver operative characteristic curve (AUC) were assessed to evaluate the performance of the random forest models. Statistical comparison of AUCs was performed using pROC package in R (Robin et al., 2011). Co-occurrence analysis of microbiome was performed using SparCC (Friedman and Alm, 2012). Functional inference of microbiome was performed using PICRUSt2 (Douglas et al., 2020). The false discovery rate (FDR) method was used to adjust *P*-values.

To identify microbiome-mediator associations independent of patient demographic factors, we performed a residualized correlation analysis (Lloyd-Price et al., 2019). All microbiome features and the 47 sputum mediators were first residualized using a general linear model adjusting for patient demographic covariates including age, gender, smoking history, exacerbation frequency and ICS usage. An all-against all correlation analysis was performed on the residues of microbiome features and sputum mediators using HAllA (Hierarchical All-against-All association testing) (Lloyd-Price et al., 2019), a computational tool to identify pairs of statistically significant associations in a hierarchical manner (FDR $P < 0.05$). A two-way hierarchical clustering analysis was performed on the microbiome-mediator correlation matrix using Ward's method, in which microbiome features and mediators were both clustered. The mediators were

[2]https://github.com/wangzlab/Strain_ID_FL16S

clustered into three groups based on dendrogram and termed based on their inflammatory classes (Group 1: Th2-related, Group 2: Th1/Th17/Pro-inflammatory-related, Group 3: Others). The microbiome features were clustered into four groups based on dendrogram. The four microbiome groups were termed according to their association patterns with the three groups of mediators ("Pro-inflammatory," "Neutrophilic," "Eosinophilic," and "Anti-inflammatory"). The "Neutrophilic" microbiome group had specific association pattern with Th1/Th17/Pro-inflammatory mediators. The "Eosinophilic" microbiome group had specific association pattern with Th2 mediators. The "Pro-inflammatory" and "Anti-inflammatory" microbiome groups had overall consistent positive or negative association pattern with the broad panel of inflammatory mediators. Patients were further stratified into eosinophilic-high and eosinophilic-low subgroups based on established criteria on sputum eosinophilic percentage (eosinophilic-high: sputum eosinophil > = 3%, eosinophilic-low: sputum eosinophil < 3%) (Bafadhel et al., 2011).

Individual partitions of 16S rRNA gene sequences were generated by truncating different hypervariable regions (V1V2, V1V3, V2, V3, V3V4, V3V5, V4, V6V8, and V6V9) from the full-length 16S sequences according to established primer sets using Cutadapt v2.6 (Marcel, 2011). The same DADA2 analysis as described above was performed on each individual partition. Mantel test was performed to assess the similarity in compositional and functional profiles generated using the full-length 16S sequences as well as using individual sub-regions.

Quantitative PCR Assays

To validate our results for species identification and quantification, quantitative PCR assays were performed on a subset of 87 subjects with sufficient sputum genomic DNA (76 COPD patients and 11 controls). We designed species-specific primers for *Haemophilus influenzae, Haemophilus parainfluenzae,* and *Ralstonia mannitolilytica.* Species-specific genes were first identified using a BLASTp search of all protein-coding genes from each species against an in-house database of protein-coding genes from 2,764 complete bacterial genomes, to identify genes present in at least 90% of genomes of that species but absent in all other bacterial genomes. Primers were designed on the species-specific genes using Primer 3[3] and were checked for primer-dimer and binding specificity to the bacterial genomes. We also identified strain-specific protein coding genes for *Haemophilus influenzae* strains PittEE, PittGG and 86-028NP using similar strategies as above, and designed primers based on these genes. The primer sequences for *Trophyrema whipplei* were adopted from the study of Lozupone et al. (2013), based on the *hsp65* gene sequence. To make standard curves for absolute quantification, an initial qPCR was performed on one of the sputum samples with sufficient quantity to amplify the PCR products using all primers. The PCR products were verified by Sanger sequencing and subject to standard *Escherichia coli* transformation procedure to obtain DNA templates with absolute copy numbers. The primers and their targeting genes for each species and sub-species were listed in **Supplementary Table S1**.

[3]http://primer3.ut.ee

For validation of functional inference, we performed qPCR assays on butyryl-CoA:acetate CoA-transferase gene (EC:2.8.3.8) using the validated broad-spectrum primers reported by Vital et al. (2013) (but_3F: GHATYGGIGSTA TGCC, but_3R: AAGTCWAAYTGWCCRCC). The universal marker *rpoB* gene was used as the internal control in the qPCR assays (F: GGYTWYGAAGTNCGHGACGTDCA, R: TGACGYTGCATGTTBGMRCCCATMA). The fold change of the *but* gene between COPD and healthy controls was calculated using the $2^{-\Delta\Delta Ct}$ approach.

All qPCR assays were performed using 96-well MicroAmp Fast Optical 96-Well Reaction Plate on the Applied Biosystems StepOnePlus™ Real-Time System. The 20 μl reaction mixture contained 10 μl of SYBR® Select Master Mix (2×), 6 μl of microbial-free water, 2 μl DNA templates, and 1 μl forward and reverse primer each. The following cycling parameters were used: initial cycle of 95°C for 10 min; 40 cycles of 95°C for 15 s; 60°C for 1 min. All qPCR templates were run in duplicate. For standard curve calculation, each plate run included a decimal serial dilution of the corresponding double-stranded DNA templates as obtained above from 1E8 to 1E3 copies per μl. For qPCR of the functional gene (EC:2.8.3.8) using broad-spectrum primers, a high $MgCl_2$ concentrations of 3mM was used and thermocycling was performed as follows: 95°C for 2 min; 95°C for 45 s, 54°C for 45 s, 72°C for 45 s (× 40); 10 min at 72°C, according to the original publication (Vital et al., 2013).

RESULTS

Overview of the Species-Level Airway Microbiome Profile

A total of 1,317,570 high-quality CCS reads were obtained for 98 stable COPD patients and 27 healthy controls (**Table 1**). The average number of passes on the 16S gene was 34.9 for all CCS reads (5-270 passes), equivalent to a low error rate of ~0.48% based on previous sequencing runs on a mock community (Johnson et al., 2019). A total of 2,868 non-singleton ASVs were identified using the DADA2 approach. Seven ASVs were present in reagent controls totaling 106 reads and were subtracted from the samples (**Supplementary Table S2**). At the community level, there were significant shifts in COPD patients versus controls (**Figures 1A,B**, Adonis, $P = 0.004$). There were no significant community shifts between smokers and non-smokers within COPD patients or healthy controls, between patients with and without inhaled corticosteroid usage, and between the patients that were frequent and non-frequent exacerbators (frequent exacerbators defined as exacerbation events > = 2/last year, **Supplementary Figures S2A,B**).

Of the 2,868 ASVs, 795 ASVs constituting 52.1% of all CCS reads were putatively assigned to 228 bacterial species in 92 genera (**Supplementary Figure S3A**). In comparison, using the MCSMRT pipeline, 499 out of 2,121 non-singleton OTUs constituting 44.8% reads were assigned to 164 bacterial species in 88 genera (**Supplementary Table S3**). Using the

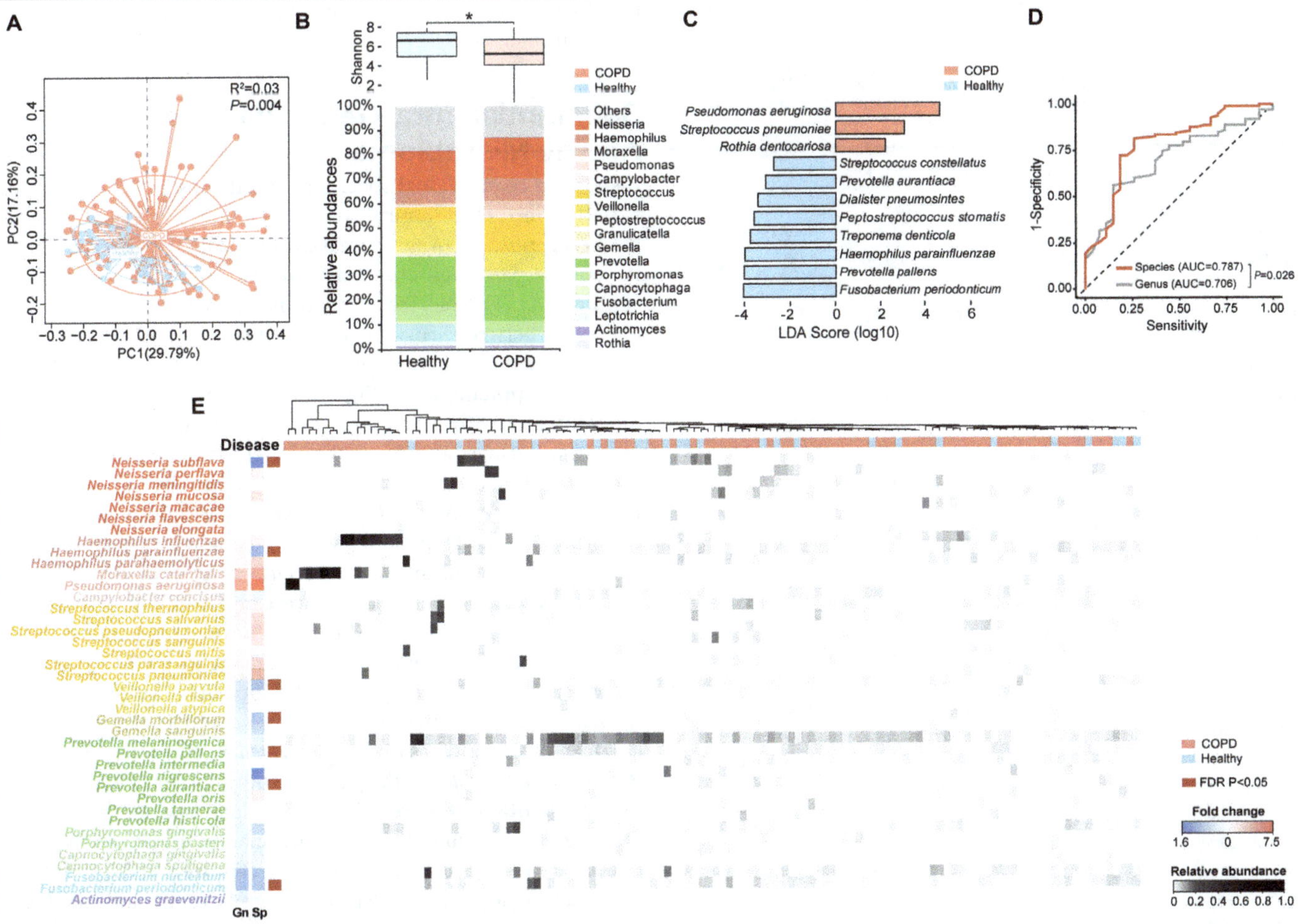

FIGURE 1 | The overview of species-level profile of the airway microbiome in COPD patients and healthy controls. **(A)** Principal coordinate analysis based on weighted UniFrac distance on sputum samples from 98 COPD patients and 27 healthy controls. **(B)** The Shannon diversity and relative abundances of major genera (relative abundance > 0.005) in COPD patients and healthy controls. **(C)** The 11 top discriminatory species-level taxa between COPD and controls as identified from LEfSe analysis (LDA > 2.0). **(D)** The receiver operating characteristic curves for the Random Forest analyses using the 11 species-level and 9 genus-level discriminatory taxa (LDA > 2.0) to segregate COPD patients from controls. **(E)** The heatmap for the species-level microbiome profile. The major species-level taxa (relative abundance > 0.001) within each genus in panel **(B)** were shown. The fold change of each species (Sp) and its corresponding genus (Gn) in COPD patients versus controls were shown beside the taxonomy. * Wilcoxon test, $P < 0.05$.

99% OTU-based clustering approach, 681 out of 2,159 non-singleton OTUs constituting 39.0% reads were assigned to 110 bacterial species in 60 genera (**Supplementary Table S3**). The DADA2 approach outperformed the clustering-based approaches for our data in terms of the number of species and the proportion of reads assigned to species, and was chosen for downstream analyses. Twenty species had an average relative abundance greater than 0.005 (**Table 2**). The number of species capable of being detected increased by 3.26 folds compared to a re-analysis of all previous COPD airway microbiome studies using similar pipeline (**Supplementary Table S4**). *Streptococcus, Prevotella,* and *Neisseria* had the highest numbers of 26, 18 and 12 species identified (**Supplementary Figure S3B**). LEfSe analysis identified 11 discriminatory species-level taxa between COPD and controls (**Figure 1C**, LDA > 2.0). Random forest analysis using these 11 species yielded increased precision in classifying patients, compared to that using 9 genera obtained with the same criteria (LDA > 2.0) (**Figure 1D** and **Supplementary Figure S3C**, AUC: 0.787 versus 0.706, $P = 0.026$). **Figure 1E** showed an overview of species-level airway microbiome profile.

Among the species-level taxa, *Haemophilus parahaemolyticus* was significantly increased in COPD smokers versus COPD non-smokers (fold-change = 6.40, FDR $P = 0.02$, **Supplementary Figure S2C**). *Ralstonia mannitolilytica*, an opportunistic pathogen, was significantly increased in frequent exacerbators, a subgroup of COPD patients that experienced more frequent acute exacerbation events than others (fold-change = 4.94, FDR $P = 0.005$, **Supplementary Figure S2C**). The increase of *R. mannitolilytica* was further confirmed by qPCR (**Supplementary Figure S2D**).

There was an overall decreased alpha diversity (Shannon index) and non-significantly increased relative abundance of *Haemophilus* in patients with increased severity measured

TABLE 2 | The major species-level taxa identified in this study (average relative abundance > 0.005).

Species	All average	COPD average	Healthy average	Fold change	FDR *P*-value
Prevotella intermedia	0.005	0.006	0.005	1.191	0.319
Prevotella melaninogenica	0.060	0.057	0.071	0.801	0.342
Prevotella pallens	0.013	0.012	0.017	0.700	0.0140*
Streptococcus pseudopneumoniae	0.017	0.020	0.004	5.667	0.222
Streptococcus salivarius	0.013	0.015	0.004	3.664	0.277
Streptococcus thermophilus	0.027	0.030	0.014	2.228	0.809
Haemophilus influenzae	0.043	0.052	0.008	6.779	0.617
Haemophilus parahaemolyticus	0.009	0.010	0.004	2.564	0.204
Haemophilus parainfluenzae	0.012	0.009	0.020	0.474	0.0074**
Neisseria meningitidis	0.009	0.009	0.008	1.044	0.128
Neisseria mucosa	0.007	0.008	0.002	4.452	0.785
Neisseria perflava	0.011	0.012	0.005	2.391	0.742
Neisseria subflava	0.017	0.012	0.036	0.330	0.0415*
Fusobacterium nucleatum	0.016	0.013	0.027	0.495	0.139
Fusobacterium periodonticum	0.014	0.012	0.022	0.531	0.0199*
Pseudomonas aeruginosa	0.016	0.020	0.000	NA	0.105
Moraxella catarrhalis	0.030	0.038	0.001	28.947	0.275
Veillonella parvula	0.005	0.004	0.010	0.439	0.208
Porphyromonas gingivalis	0.010	0.009	0.015	0.570	0.282
Campylobacter concisus	0.006	0.006	0.007	0.902	0.233

*P-value was calculated using Wilcoxon rank-sum test. ***FDR P < 0.001; **P < 0.01; *P < 0.05.*

using both spirometry-based GOLD I-IV and new GOLD A-D classification scheme based on exacerbation frequency, CAT and mMRC scores [Global Initiative for Chronic Obstructive Lung Disease (GOLD), 2019], consistent with previous findings (Mayhew et al., 2018; Dicker et al., 2020) (**Supplementary Figures S4A,B**). No species-level taxa reached statistical significance in association with GOLD classification, CAT or mMRC scores (FDR $P < 0.05$). *Fusobacterium periodontium* exhibited significant positive correlation with pre-FEV_1 (FDR $P < 0.05$, **Supplementary Figure S4C**).

In our study, 58 out of 98 patients were administered long-term ICS. We classified the 58 patients into subgroups based on their daily ICS doses (500 ug/day [$n = 5$], 320 ug/day [$n = 15$], 250 ug/day [$n = 14$], 160 ug/day [$n = 17$], and less than 160 ug/day [$n = 7$]). All five groups have comparable alpha diversity (**Supplementary Figure S5A**). No clear clustering was observed for these groups in principal coordinate analysis based on Bray-Curtis dissimilarity (**Supplementary Figure S5B**). No genus or species-level taxa were significantly different across these groups. There was a non-significant increase of *Moraxella* and *Pseudomonas* in the higher dose groups (500 ug and 320 ug groups, **Supplementary Figure S5A**), consistent with the notion that higher dose of ICS may increase pathogenic bacterial load (Contoli et al., 2017).

Substantial Intra-Genus Variation in the Airway Microbiome

Inspection of individual species revealed substantial intra-genus variation in their relationships with COPD. For example, while *Neisseria mucosa* was increased in COPD versus controls, its counterpart *Neisseria subflava* was significantly depleted (**Figure 2A**). The reciprocal relationships with COPD were also observed between *Haemophilus influenzae* and *Haemophilus parainfluenzae*, and between *Prevotella oris* and other *Prevotella* species (**Supplementary Figure S6**). The species also altered differentially with enhanced disease severity. For example, *H. parainfluenzae* and *N. subflava* were the most predominant species within the respective genera in healthy subjects, while *H. influenzae* and *N. meningitidis* were over-dominant in GOLD IV class of COPD patients with the highest disease severity (**Figure 2A**). Within *Streptococcus*, *Streptococcus salivarius* and *Streptococcus thermophilus* were most highly abundant in GOLD I patients, whereas *Streptococcus pseudopneumoniae* and *Streptococcus pneumoniae* were dominant in GOLD II and IV patients, respectively (**Figure 2A**). Opposite relationships were further observed between *H. influenzae* and *H. parainfluenzae* (**Figure 2B**), and between *Prevotella melaninogenica* and *Prevotella denticola* with patient sputum neutrophilic levels (**Supplementary Figure S7**). Individual species within the same genus exhibited disproportionately more co-exclusive than co-occurrence relationships (**Figure 2C**), indicating potential ecological interference. These results indicated that there was substantial intra-genus heterogeneity in the airways possibly resulting from interspecific competition. qPCR using primers designed on species-specific genes showed overall concordance between the absolute count and relative abundance of *H. influenzae* and *H. parainfluenzae* (**Figure 2D**), although the qPCR results showed better sensitivity at lower abundances.

Major Airway Inflammatory Phenotypes Shaped Species-Level Microbiome-Host Interactions

To investigate how the intra-genus heterogeneity was related to airway inflammation, we performed an all-against-all correlation analysis between the species-level microbiome features and a panel of 47 sputum inflammatory mediators measured in a subset of 59 COPD patients. We used residualized correlation to identify microbiome-mediator correlations independent of patient demographic co-factors (Lloyd-Price et al., 2019). Unsupervised two-way hierarchical clustering based on the microbiome-mediator correlation profile revealed four clusters of bacterial species that each had distinct association patterns with three groups of mediators (Group 1–3, **Figure 3**). Four pathogens, *Moraxella catarrhalis, Pseudomonas aeruginosa, N. meningitidis* and *H. influenzae*, exhibited negative associations with a group of 11 mediators mostly Th2-related (i.e., IL-5, IL-13, CCL17), while they were positively correlated with

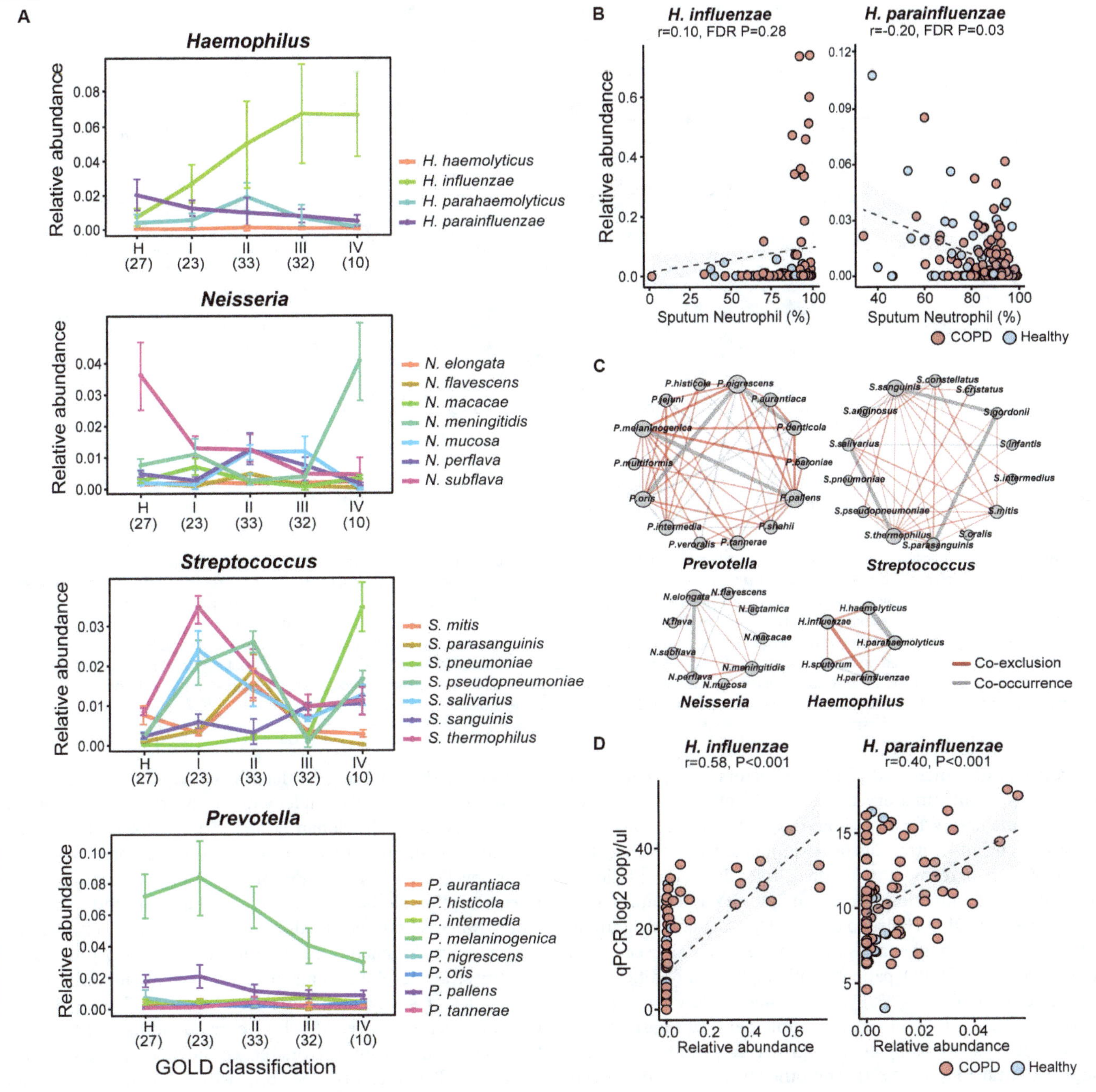

FIGURE 2 | The intra-genus heterogeneity of the airway microbiome. **(A)** The alternation of major species in *Haemophilus*, *Neisseria*, *Streptococcus*, and *Prevotella* between healthy controls and COPD patients with increasing disease severity based on GOLD classification (spirometry-based). The average relative abundance and standard deviation of each species in each group were shown. The number of subjects in each subgroup was indicated in the parenthesis. **(B)** The reciprocal relationship between *H. influenzae* and *H. parainfluenzae* with sputum neutrophilic percentage. **(C)** The species-level co-occurrence network showed more pervasive co-exclusive than co-occurrence relationships between major species-level taxa within *Prevotella*, *Streptococcus*, *Neisseria* and *Haemophilus*. Each node represents a species-level taxon and each edge represents a correlation between paired taxa. Only significant correlations were shown in the networks (SparCC, $P < 0.05$). The size of the node is proportional to its degree of connectivity. The width of the edge is proportional to the absolute correlation coefficient. Co-exclusion relationships were colored in red, whereas co-occurrence relationships were colored in gray. **(D)** qPCR assays using species-specific primers showed concordance between absolute counts and relative abundances of *H. influenzae* and *H. parainfluenzae*.

a group of 21 mediators mostly Th1, Th17-related or pro-inflammatory (i.e., IL-8, IL-17, MMP-8), and had mixed relationships with the remaining mediators. By contrast, another seven species, *Prevotella aurantiaca, Fusobacterium nucleatum, Leptotrichia buccalis, Prevotella histicola, Porphyromonas gingivalis, N. mucosa* and *Tropheryma whipplei,* were specifically

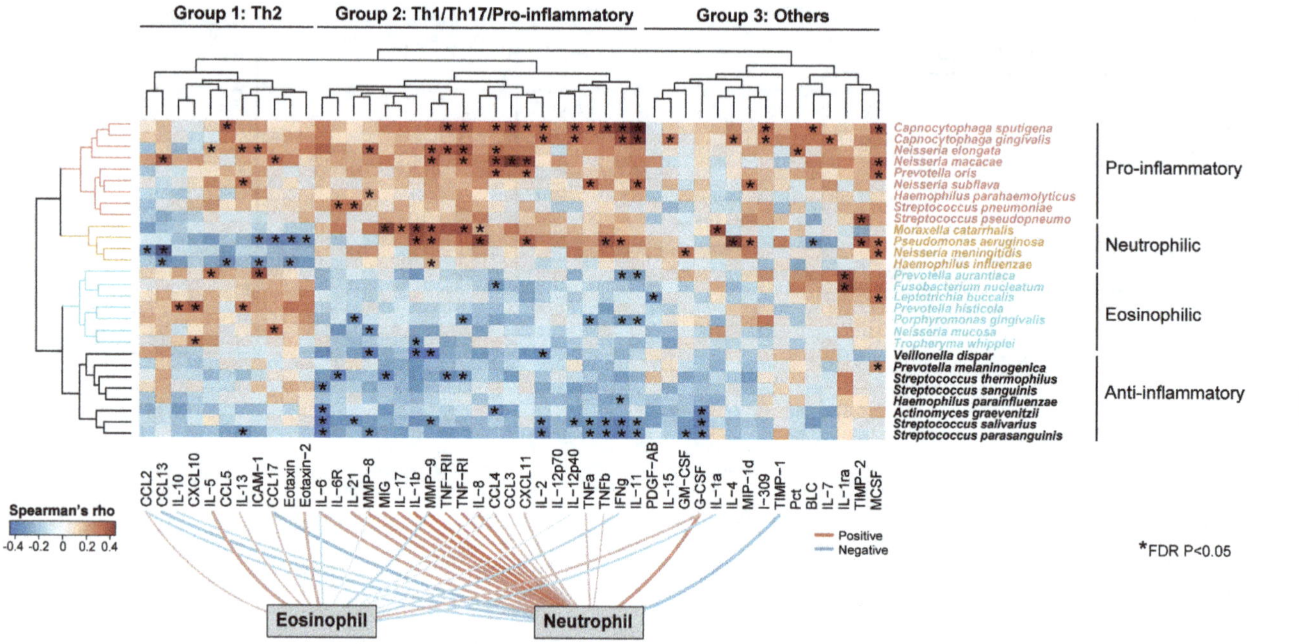

FIGURE 3 | Species-specific association of airway microbiome with inflammatory phenotypes. Unsupervised two-way hierarchical clustering analysis on an all-against-all correlation profile between species-level microbiome features and 47 sputum mediators from a subset of 59 COPD patients (Ward's method), in which microbiome features and mediators were both clustered. The species were shown if they had relative abundance > 0.001 and were significantly associated with at least one of the 47 sputum mediators (HAllA, FDR $P < 0.05$). The mediators were clustered into three groups and termed based on their classes and associations with airway eosinophils or neutrophils (Group 1: Th2-related, Group 2: Th1/Th17/Pro-inflammatory-related, Group 3: Others). The microbiome features were clustered into four groups based on their association patterns with the three groups of mediators (termed "Pro-inflammatory," "Neutrophilic," "Eosinophilic," and "Anti-inflammatory"). The significant associations were indicated in asterisks. Significant positive and negative associations between sputum mediators and neutrophilic and eosinophilic percentages were shown on bottom of the heatmap (FDR $P < 0.05$).

associated with increased Th2 mediators and decreased Th1/Th17/pro-inflammatory mediators. Members of these two groups of mediators further showed specific correlations with increased sputum neutrophils or eosinophils, respectively (FDR $P < 0.05$), in agreement with their roles in neutrophilic or eosinophilic inflammation, the two major airway inflammatory phenotypes in COPD (Balzano et al., 1999; Saha and Brightling, 2006). Correspondingly, all seven species were increased in the subgroup of COPD patients with high eosinophilic levels (sputum eosinophil > = 3%) versus those with low eosinophilic levels (sputum eosinophil < 3%, **Supplementary Figure S8A**). The increase of *T. whipplei* was further confirmed by qPCR (**Supplementary Figure S8B**). The other two groups of species in general showed consistent positive or negative associations with the broad panel of inflammatory mediators (denoted as 'Pro-inflammatory' or 'Anti-inflammatory' in **Figure 3**). Such phenotype-specific clustering pattern was not observed at the genus-level (**Supplementary Figure S9**), indicating that airway microbiome interacted with host in a species-specific manner, which was shaped by major airway inflammatory phenotypes.

An Automated Pipeline for Strain-Level Identification in the Airway Microbiome

We further explored possible strain-level diversity in the airway microbiome. Recent studies showed that it is possible to resolve strain-level identity using full-length 16S sequences by leveraging the power of the full complement of 16S rRNA alleles within bacterial genomes (Callahan et al., 2019; Johnson et al., 2019). Callahan et al. introduced a simple rule to manually assign strain-level taxonomy by examining ASVs according to 16S integral ratio, similar taxonomy assignments and consistent patterns across samples (Callahan et al., 2019). In extension to this rule, we designed a pipeline to automate this process and identify strain-level ASV bins in a large-scale. Using this pipeline with a set of stringent criteria (see methods, **Figure 4A**), we identified genome-level ASV bins corresponding to 14 different bacterial strains with reasonable confidence (**Supplementary Table S5**). This included ASV bins with sequence identical and in integral copy number ratio to the 16S rRNA gene alleles of three non-typeable *H. influenzae* (NTHi) strains PittEE, PittGG and 86-028NP, although the major 16S allele of 86-028NP was not detected (**Figures 4B–D**). All three strains increased in COPD versus controls. The three strains were associated with distinct groups of mediators, implicating that they likely provoked different types of host inflammatory response (**Figure 4E**). In particular, 86-028NP and PittGG exhibited inverse associations with Th2 chemokines such as CCL17 and CCL13 related to eosinophilic inflammation. qPCR using strain-specific primers showed moderate concordance for PittEE and PittGG (**Figure 4F**), although the strain detection rate by sequencing was lower than that using

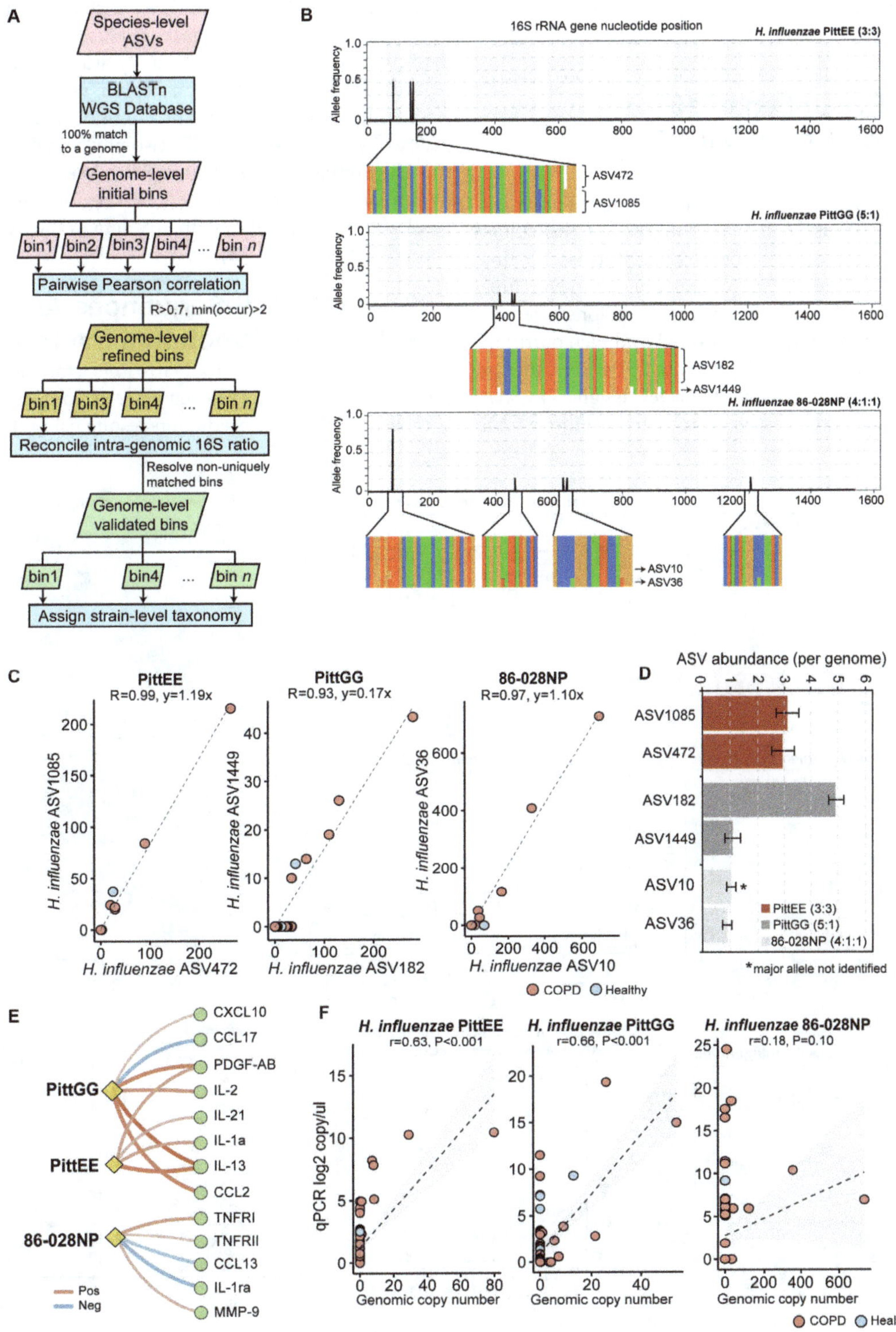

FIGURE 4 | Strain-level identification in the airway microbiome. **(A)** The designed pipeline for identifying strain-level ASV bins. **(B)** The polymorphism in the 16S rRNA gene sequences for *H. influenzae* PittEE, PittGG and 86-028NP strains. The position and frequency of substitution in the full-length 16S sequences of the three strains were shown. The magnified regions showed respective positions in the alignment of all six copies of 16S gene in the corresponding *H. influenzae* genomes. The genuine ratios of 16S allelic variants in the three genomes are: 3:3, 5:1 and 4:1:1. **(C)** The correlation pattern between the counts for pairs of ASVs assigned to the strains PittEE, PittGG and 86-028NP (Pearson's $R > 0.93$). **(D)** The copy number of the highly-correlated ASVs are in integral ratio with the genuine allelic frequency of the 16S rRNA genes within the genome. The major 16S allele of the 86-028NP strain was not detected. **(E)** Significant associations between the three *H. influenzae* strains with sputum mediators (Spearman, FDR $P < 0.05$). **(F)** qPCR results using strain-specific primers for the three *H. influenzae* strains in relation to their relative abundances in the sequencing data.

qPCR. qPCR for 86-028NP yield positive but non-significant correlation (**Figure 4F**).

A Systematic Evaluation of 16S Sub-Regions for Airway Microbiome Profiling

The full-length 16S sequences can serve as a benchmark for a systematic evaluation on the performance of individual hypervariable regions for airway microbiome studies. To this end, we created partitions of 16S sequences from the full-length data according to nine hypervariable regions used in previous COPD microbiome studies, and analyzed each partition separately. Among all sub-regions, V1V3 and V3V4 were among the highest in terms of the number of species assigned as well as the proportion of sequences assigned to species (**Figure 5A**). In addition, the V1V3 and V3V4 regions captured the greatest microbial beta diversity measured using pairwise Bray-Curtis dissimilarity, whereas the diversity was the lowest for the V4 region (**Figure 5A**). The V4 region was particularly poor in classifying Proteobacteria and Actinobacteria, with 79.8 and 90.9% of sequences from these two phyla unable to be assigned to species (**Supplementary Figure S10**). Mantel test for Bray-Curtis dissimilarity showed that the V1V3 region also bear the highest similarity with the full-length 16S data in the overall community composition (**Figure 5B**).

Full-Length 16S Sequences Augmented the Power of Functional Inference

PICRUSt is a useful tool to infer functional capacity of microbiome based on 16S sequences (Douglas et al., 2020). We compared PICRUSt2 prediction results using the full-length 16S

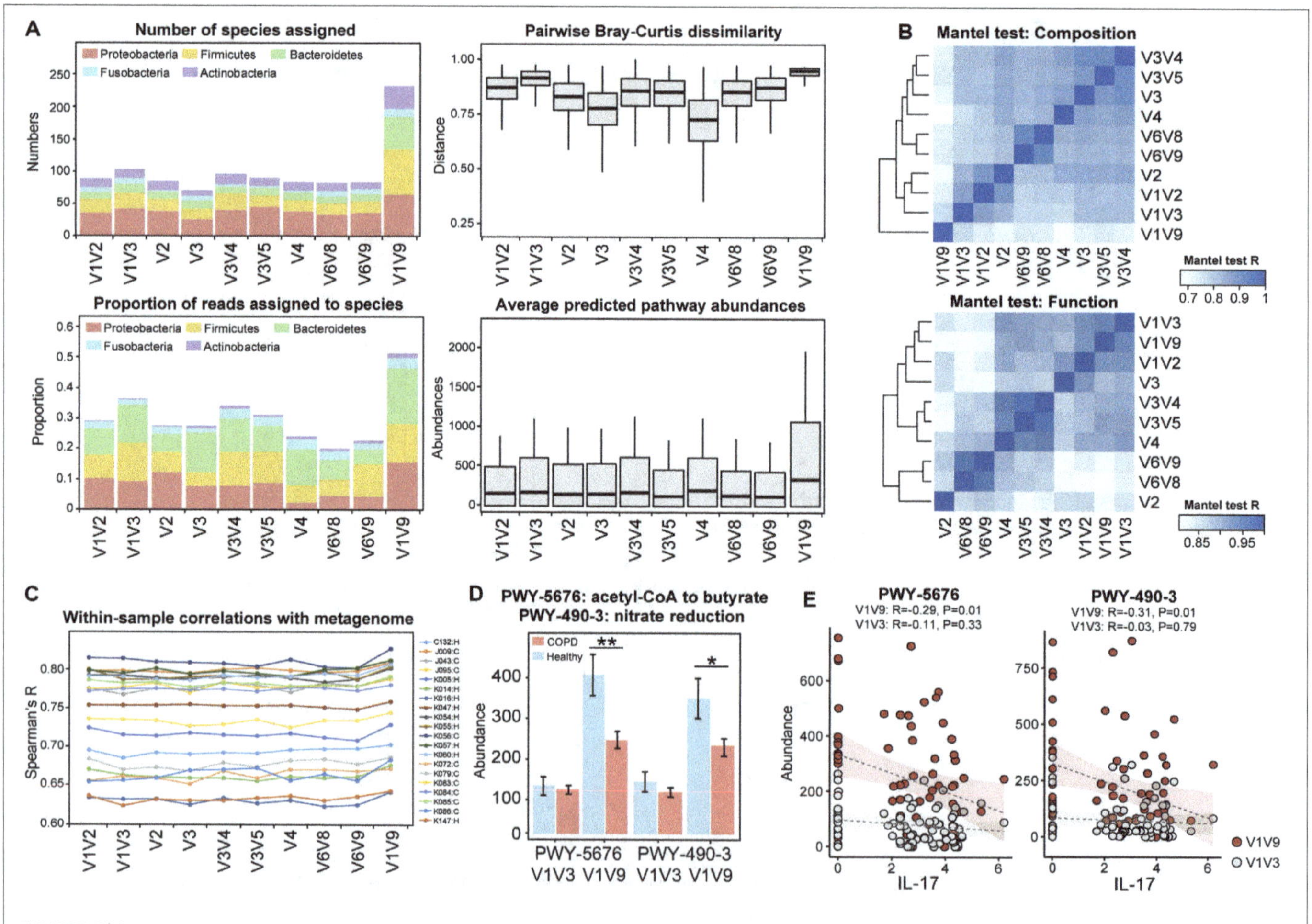

FIGURE 5 | Systematic comparison of full-length 16S data and sub-region data for taxonomic diversity and functional inference. **(A)** Comparisons between the full-length 16S data and the sub-region data, in terms of (1) the number of species-level taxa assigned, (2) the proportion of reads that can be assigned to species, (3) the pairwise Bray-Curtis dissimilarity across all samples, and (4) the average abundances of pathways predicted by PICRUSt2. **(B)** Heatmap showing similarity in compositional and functional profiles between the full-length 16S data and data for individual 16S sub-regions. Mantel test for Bray-Curtis dissimilarity was performed to assess the profile-level correlations. **(C)** The correlation between PICRUSt2-inferred genes and the same genes in the actual metagenome, within each of the 20 samples. The sample IDs and their corresponding groups (COPD: **C**, Healthy: **H**) were indicated. **(D)** The PICRUSt2-inferred abundances of the two pathways 'PWY-5676: acetyl-CoA fermentation to butyrate' and 'PWY-490-3: nitrate reduction' in COPD and controls using the full-length (V1V9) and V1V3 data (** FDR $P < 0.01$, * FDR $P < 0.05$). **(E)** The two pathways showed negative correlations with IL-17, which was more pronounced when inferred from full-length 16S sequences than V1V3 sequences.

sequences and sequences from the nine hypervariable regions. PICRUSt analysis using the full-length 16S data greatly enhanced the power of functional inference by increasing the copy number abundances of the predicted pathways by an average 1.83-fold compared to individual sub-regions. Again, V1V3 were the next best in terms of the predicted pathway abundances (**Figure 5A**). The same sub-region also showed the highest similarity with the full-length 16S data in the inferred functional profile (Mantel test, **Figure 5B**).

To further assess the precision of functional inference using the full-length 16S data, we characterized the airway metagenome for a randomly selected set of 10 COPD patients and 10 controls as benchmark. We performed correlation analysis between genes in the actual metagenome and PICRUSt2-inferred metagenome using the full-length 16S data as well as sub-region data. When examining each sample, there was an overall correlation pattern between the PICRUSt2-inferred genes and those from the metagenomic data (**Figure 5C, Supplementary Figure S11, Supplementary Table S5**, Spearman's R: 0.624–0.818). The correlations were notably centric to the abundant genes, whereas genes with less abundance showed more random patterns (**Supplementary Figure S11**). This suggested that PICRUSt2 better predicted the more abundant genes in the metagenome. PICRUSt2 inference based on full-length 16S sequences yielded slightly better per-sample correlations with metagenome than those based on sub-region sequences (i.e., Spearman's R: 0.750 ± 0.06 for full-length data versus 0.736 ± 0.06 for V1V3 data, **Figure 5C, Supplementary Table S6**), as well as a higher resemblance to the sample-wise metagenome profiles based on Mantel test for Bray-Curtis dissimilarity (**Supplementary Table S6**). When examining each individual gene, PICRUSt2 inference using full-length 16S data generated more genes that showed correlations with metagenome across all samples, compared to the inferences using sub-region data (305 KO genes versus 248.2 ± 18.8 genes, Spearman's $R > 0.5$, **Supplementary Table S6**).

At the pathway level, PICRUSt2 inference based on full-length 16S sequences led to slightly different set of pathways differentially abundant in COPD versus controls (FDR $P < 0.05$, **Supplementary Table S7**). This included the identification of 9 pathways that were uniquely associated with COPD when inferred using the full-length 16S data (**Supplementary Table S8**). Of interest are two pathways 'acetyl-CoA fermentation to butyrate' and 'nitrate reduction,' both inferred as significantly depleted in COPD (FDR $P < 0.05$, **Figure 5D, Supplementary Figure S12**). Both pathways were also decreased in COPD versus controls in the subset metagenomic data (log2 fold-change = −1.608 and −2.502 respectively, **Supplementary Table S8**). qPCR using validated broad-spectrum primers on butyryl-CoA:acetate-CoA-transferase gene (Vital et al., 2013) in the butyrate pathway further supported the finding by showing a 4.32-fold decrease of the gene in COPD versus controls (**Supplementary Table S9**). Furthermore, the two pathways showed inverse correlations with sputum inflammatory marker IL-17, which were more pronounced when inferred from full-length 16S data than from sub-regions (**Figure 5E**).

DISCUSSION

Here, we provided the first insights on the COPD airway microbiome at the species and strain-levels. By applying the 'third-generation' PacBio sequencing to the full-length 16S rRNA gene, we uncovered diversity and complexity in the airway microbiome at in-depth taxonomic levels that were previously underappreciated. In light of our results, many aspects of our understanding of the airway microbiome need to be refined.

Our results showed that there were substantial intra-genus variations in the airway microbiome in relation to patient clinical outcomes. Individual species within the same genus often altered differentially in COPD and with enhanced clinical severity. The species predominant in healthy state can be taken over by another species within the same genus but with potentially increasing pathogenicity in severe COPD patients. Understanding such variation is a prerequisite in precisely identifying and targeting key microbial species at play at different clinical stages of COPD. All previous studies by reporting the aggregated genus-level associations failed to capture such phenomenon. Thus those results by neglecting the species-level variations only represent an attenuated signal by the mixed effects of individual species within, and should be interpreted with caution.

Unsupervised clustering analysis demonstrated clear species-level microbiome-host interaction patterns according to neutrophilic or eosinophilic inflammation, the two major inflammatory phenotypes in COPD (Balzano et al., 1999; Saha and Brightling, 2006). The neutrophil-specific bacterial species included known respiratory pathogens including *H. influenzae*, *M. catarrhalis*, *N. meningitidis*, and *P. aeruginosa* in Proteobacteria that provoked pro-inflammatory host response (Sethi and Murphy, 2001). There is increasing evidence showing that airway microbiome is associated with inflammatory phenotypes of COPD patients. Several studies have showed that airway microbiome differs between exacerbation phenotypes in particular between bacterial-associated and eosinophilic exacerbations, with reduced microbial diversity and increased Proteobacteria in the former group (Wang et al., 2016, 2018; Mayhew et al., 2018). In this regard, our results are consistent and extend these findings by showing that specific Proteobacteria species may be key members contributing to enhanced neutrophilic over eosinophilic inflammations. The respiratory pathogens can frequently colonize and be persistent in the airways despite innate host immunity through various evasive pathogenic mechanisms. For example, non-typeable *H. influenzae* evades host immune recognition and clearance by neutrophil extracellular traps (NETs) through invading host epithelial cells, forming biofilms, altering gene expression and displaying surface antigenic variation (Ahearn et al., 2017). *P. aeruginosa* is able to modify its motility, alginate production, biofilm formation or susceptibility to host anti-microbial defenses to establish niches of persistent infection (Skopelja-Gardner et al., 2019). *N. meningitidis* can be resistant against NETs through a series of mechanisms including modification of LPS and escape from NET-mediated nutritional immunity (Lappann et al., 2013). A recent study showed that *M. catarrhalis* achieved its persistent colonization in COPD patients through regulating major adhesin Hag/MID (Murphy et al., 2019). Our data showed significant positive correlations between *M. catarrhalis* and *P. aeruginosa* with NET-triggering inflammatory mediators such as CXCL8, IL-1b and TNFa, supporting possible involvement of NETs in COPD host-microbiome interactions (Dicker et al., 2018). Further studies are warranted to investigate association between the species or strain-level airway microbiome with NETopathic inflammation in COPD (Uddin et al., 2019).

The eosinophil-specific species included *T. whipplei*, a clinically important species reported to be implicated in pneumonia (Bousbia et al., 2010), HIV infection (Lozupone et al., 2013) and eosinophilic, corticosteroid-resistant asthma (Goleva et al., 2013; Simpson et al., 2016). Thus the association between *T. whipplei* and eosinophilic inflammation may be a common signature across airway diseases. Such phenotype-specific host-microbiome interaction pattern was not detected at the broader genus-level, which supports the notion that phylogenetically diversified airway bacterial species may act as ecological "guilds" in response to specific types of environmental stimuli (here being the different types of host inflammations). The species delineation enabled an ecologically coherent view of airway microbiome according to host inflammatory phenotypes.

The full-length 16S sequencing is capable of resolving subtle nucleotide substitutions that exist between 16S gene copies within a bacterial genome. It has been shown that such intra-genomic variations, when properly accounted for, can aid in strain-level identification (Johnson et al., 2019). Callahan et al. introduced an approach by manually obtaining ASV copy number ratios and reconciling with the genuine 16S ratio of their corresponding bacterial genomes (Callahan et al., 2019). By curating the intra-genomic 16S variations for all complete bacterial genomes, we show that this process can be made fully automated and applied in real, complex microbial communities. We detected three NTHi clinical strains PittEE, PittGG and 86-028NP in the airway microbiome with reasonable confidence, and suggested that even within the pathogenic species there may be variations between strains in their relationships with airway inflammations (Chin et al., 2005). All three strains were initially isolated from otitis media patients (Harrison et al., 2005; Hogg et al., 2007; Arce et al., 2009). It has been shown that the PittGG strain, by possessing an extra cluster of 339 genes and a Hif-type pili structure, conveyed greater virulence than PittEE (Arce et al., 2009). qPCR assays based on *alpA* gene on this extra locus confirmed our results in PittGG quantification. While all three strains were related to increased Th1/Th17 mediators, 86-028NP and PittGG were further associated with decreased Th2-related CCL13 and CCL17, indicating their abundances may inversely predict eosinophilic inflammation. The microbiome species or strains may be suitable markers for airway inflammatory phenotypes.

We identified *Ralstonia mannitolilytica* as significantly increased in a subgroup of COPD patients that experienced more frequent acute exacerbations than others, a clinically important phenotype in COPD for which the underlying pathophysiology was not completely understood (Wedzicha et al., 2013). *R. mannitolilytica* is an opportunistic pathogen that has been recovered from cystic fibrosis airways (Coenye et al., 2002). In a previous report, the same species was isolated from one COPD exacerbation patient in western China with extreme symptoms and acute respiratory failure (Zong and Peng, 2011). *Ralstonia* spp. rarely cause infection in healthy individuals but can be a severe pathogen especially in immunosuppressed patients (Basso et al., 2019). Therefore, the presence of *R. mannitolilytica* in stable COPD patients may be a risk factor in predisposing patients to recurrent infection and exacerbations.

There is emerging evidence showing that airway microbiome is associated with clinical outcome and mortality of COPD patients. Leitao Filho et al. found that microbiome dysbiosis, in particular the presence of *Staphylococcus* and absence of *Veillonella*, was associated with increased 1-year mortality for hospitalized AECOPD patients (Leitao Filho et al., 2018). *Staphylococcus* spp. were barely detected in our patients (3 out of 98 COPD patients) so their association with clinical outcomes were unable to be assessed in our cohort. A key difference between our study and Leitao Filho et al. is that only patients with severe exacerbations that required hospitalization were included in their study, whereas we captured mild, moderate and severe patients at clinical stability. Nevertheless, both our results (increased *Ralstonia mannitolilytica* in frequent exacerbators) and those of Leitao Filho et al. supported the notion that identification of rare opportunistic pathogens may be associated with worse clinical outcome and prognosis of COPD patients. A recent study by Dicker et al. showed that *Haemophilus* dominance at COPD clinical stability was linked to increased severity, frequent exacerbations and increased mortality (Dicker et al., 2020). This is also consistent with our finding that increased relative abundance of *Haemophilus*, in particular *H. influenzae* species, was observed in patients with enhanced GOLD status.

The systematic comparison of individual 16S sub-regions indicated that V1V3 region performed the best in terms of the species-level microbial alpha and beta diversity, the power of functional inference, as well as the profile resemblance with full-length 16S data in terms of both microbiome composition and function. Our results based on real sequencing data on natural microbial communities are consistent with the *in silico* analysis by Johnson et al. based on existing 16S databases (Johnson et al., 2019), and should guide future studies that sequencing V1V3 may be a surrogate for airway microbiome when sequencing the full-length 16S gene is not available. Conversely, sequencing the V4 region alone, despite its wide usage in previous airway microbiome studies, might not provide sufficient resolution for in-depth taxonomic profiling in particular in Proteobacteria and Actinobacteria.

The full-length 16S sequences yielded increased abundances for genes and pathways capable of being predicted, possibly due to the higher precision of full-length 16S sequences in hidden state prediction in the PICRUSt2 algorithm[24]. The augmented power led to better concordance with the actual metagenomes in a subset of 20 samples, thereby also increased the accuracy of functional inference. With better power, we inferred butyrate-producing and nitrate reduction pathways as uniquely depleted in COPD using the full-length 16S data. The decreases of these pathways were supported by the subset of samples with metagenomic data as well as some preliminary qPCR results. Butyrate is a well-characterized microbial metabolite with anti-inflammatory effects in human gut (Cait et al., 2018), whereas its role in the airways remains unclear. Nitric oxide, the end product of nitrate reduction, may have possible disease-ameliorating effects by suppressing NLRP3 inflammasome activation in the airways (Mao et al., 2013; Lee et al., 2016). The mechanistic roles of these pathways in COPD remain to be determined.

There are several caveats to our study. First, the study design is single-centered and cross-sectional so the temporal stability of the airway microbiome is unable to be tracked. Nevertheless, the major microbiome composition in our cohort, as well as the associations between key microbiome taxa and neutrophilic and eosinophilic inflammations, were generally consistent with previous findings on European and US cohorts, suggesting that there may be a common core airway flora and microbiome-host interactions despite geographical differences. Additional multi-centered cohorts preferably across continents (i.e., similar as the design in Mac Aogain et al., 2018) with longitudinal follow-up are needed to test this hypothesis and further validate our findings. Second, despite multiple approaches and databases employed, only about half of all CCS reads in our data can be confidently assigned to bacterial species-level taxa. This was also reflected by the lower sensitivity for species and strains detection based on sequencing compared to that based on qPCR. This is an important caveat due to inherently limited power of 16S sequences for species or strain resolution, its sensitivity to potential sequencing errors and incompleteness of current reference databases. Therefore even the full-length 16S gene survey may still underrepresent the true microbial species diversity in the airways. Third, despite efforts made in quality control and careful selection of sputum plugs from saliva, potential sources of oral contamination cannot be fully excluded. Comparative studies with concurrent oral rinse sampling are needed to distinguish bacterial species and strains originated from oral cavity and airways. Fourth, we lack sufficient data to explore species-specific relationships with other COPD etiological factors such as viral infections.

In summary, we present a finer-scale taxonomic analysis on the COPD airway microbiome. We showed there were substantial microbial diversity and heterogeneity at species-level and below, which was associated with patient clinical outcome and host inflammation. Sequencing the full-length 16S rRNA gene enabled a refined view on the composition and function of the airway microbiome in COPD, and should see a wider applicability in airway microbiome studies in future.

AUTHOR'S NOTE

This manuscript has been released as a pre-print at BioRxiv (Wang et al., 2020).

AUTHOR CONTRIBUTIONS

ZW conceived and designed the study. HL, FW, YY, and ZL coordinated the collection of sputum samples and clinical data. HL, XW, and BC processed the sputum samples, performed the DNA extraction, and library preparation. ZW performed all data analysis. MS, CB, and WS provided key insights to the work. RC and HZ supervised the study. ZW wrote the manuscript. All authors provided critical comments and approved the final version of the manuscript.

REFERENCES

1. Ahearn, C. P., Gallo, M. C., and Murphy, T. F. (2017). Insights on persistent airway infection by non-typeable *Haemophilus influenzae* in chronic obstructive pulmonary disease. *Pathog. Dis.* 75:ftx042. doi: 10.1093/femspd/ft x042
2. Arce, F. T., Carlson, R., Monds, J., Veeh, R., Hu, F. Z., Stewart, P. S., et al. (2009). Nanoscale structural and mechanical properties of nontypeable *Haemophilus influenzae* biofilms. *J. Bacteriol.* 191, 2512–2520. doi: 10.1128/JB.01596-08
3. Bafadhel, M., McCormick, M., Saha, S., McKenna, S., Shelley, M., Hargadon, B., et al. (2012). Profiling of sputum inflammatory mediators in asthma and chronic obstructive pulmonary disease. *Respiration* 83, 36–44. doi: 10.1159/000330667
4. Bafadhel, M., McKenna, S., Terry, S., Mistry, V., Reid, C., Haldar, P., et al. (2011). Acute exacerbations of chronic obstructive pulmonary disease: identification of biologic clusters and their biomarkers. *Am. J. Respir. Crit. Care Med.* 184, 662–671. doi: 10.1164/rccm.201104-05 97OC
5. Balzano, G., Stefanelli, F., Iorio, C., De Felice, A., Melillo, E. M., Martucci, M., et al. (1999). Eosinophilic inflammation in stable chronic obstructive pulmonary disease. Relationship with neutrophils and airway function. *Am. J. Respir. Crit. Care Med.* 160(5 Pt 1), 1486–1492. doi: 10.1164/ajrccm.160.5.9810105
6. Basso, M., Venditti, C., Raponi, G., Navazio, A. S., Alessandri, F., Giombini, E., et al. (2019). A case of persistent bacteraemia by *Ralstonia mannitolilytica* and *Ralstonia pickettii* in an intensive care unit. *Infect. Drug Resist.* 12, 2391–2395. doi: 10.2147/IDR.S206492
7. Bolyen, E., Rideout, J. R., Dillon, M. R., Bokulich, N. A., Abnet, C., Al-Ghalith, G. A., et al. (2018). QIIME 2: reproducible, interactive, scalable, and extensible microbiome data science. *PeerJ Preprints* 6:e27295v2.
8. Bousbia, S., Papazian, L., Auffray, J. P., Fenollar, F., Martin, C., Li, W., et al. (2010). *Tropheryma whipplei* in patients with pneumonia. *Emerg. Infect. Dis.* 16, 258–263. doi: 10.3201/eid1602.090610
9. Cait, A., Hughes, M. R., Antignano, F., Cait, J., Dimitriu, P. A., Maas, K. R., et al. (2018). Microbiome-driven allergic lung inflammation is ameliorated by short-chain fatty acids. *Mucosal. Immunol.* 11, 785–795. doi: 10.1038/mi.20 17.75
10. Callahan, B. J., McMurdie, P. J., Rosen, M. J., Han, A. W., Johnson, A. J., and Holmes, S. P. (2016). DADA2: high-resolution sample inference from Illumina amplicon data. *Nat. Methods* 13, 581–583. doi: 10.1038/nmeth.3869
11. Callahan, B. J., Wong, J., Heiner, C., Oh, S., Theriot, C. M., Gulati, A. S., et al. (2019). High-throughput amplicon sequencing of the full-length 16S rRNA gene with single-nucleotide resolution. *Nucleic Acids Res.* 47:e103. doi: 10.1093/ nar/gkz569
12. Chin, C. L., Manzel, L. J., Lehman, E. E., Humlicek, A. L., Shi, L., Starner, T. D., et al. (2005). *Haemophilus influenzae* from patients with chronic obstructive pulmonary disease exacerbation induce more inflammation than colonizers. *Am. J. Respir. Crit. Care Med.* 172, 85–91. doi: 10.1164/rccm.200412-1687OC
13. Coenye, T., Vandamme, P., and LiPuma, J. J. (2002). Infection by *Ralstonia* species in cystic fibrosis patients: identification of *R. pickettii* and *R. mannitolilytica* by polymerase chain reaction. *Emerg. Infect. Dis.* 8, 692–696.

doi: 10.3201/eid0807. 010472

14. Contoli, M., Pauletti, A., Rossi, M. R., Spanevello, A., Casolari, P., Marcellini, A., et al. (2017). Long-term effects of inhaled corticosteroids on sputum bacterial and viral loads in COPD. *Eur. Respir. J.* 50:1700451. doi: 10.1183/13993003.00451-2017
15. Dicker, A. J., Crichton, M. L., Pumphrey, E. G., Cassidy, A. J., Suarez-Cuartin, G., Sibila, O., et al. (2018). Neutrophil extracellular traps are associated with disease severity and microbiota diversity in patients with chronic obstructive pulmonary disease. *J. Allergy Clin. Immunol.* 141, 117–127. doi: 10.1016/j.jaci.2017.04.022
16. Dicker, A. J., Huang, J. T., Lonergan, M., Keir, H. R., Fong, C. J., Tan, B., et al. (2020). The sputum microbiome, airway inflammation and mortality in chronic obstructive pulmonary disease. *J. Allergy Clin. Immunol.* (in press). doi: 10. 1016/j.jaci.2020.02.040
17. Douglas, G. M., Maffei, V. J., Zaneveld, J. R., Yurgel, S. N., Brown, J. R., Taylor, C. M., et al. (2020). PICRUSt2 for prediction of metagenome functions. *Nat. Biotechnol.* 38, 685–688.
18. Earl, J. P., Adappa, N. D., Krol, J., Bhat, A. S., Balashov, S., Ehrlich, R. L., et al. (2018). Species-level bacterial community profiling of the healthy sinonasal microbiome using Pacific Biosciences sequencing of full-length 16S rRNA genes. *Microbiome* 6:190. doi: 10.1186/s40168-018-0569-2
19. Edgar, R. C. (2010). Search and clustering orders of magnitude faster than BLAST. *Bioinformatics* 26, 2460–2461. doi: 10.1093/bioinformatics/btq461
20. Einarsson, G. G., Comer, D. M., McIlreavey, L., Parkhill, J., Ennis, M., Tunney, M. M., et al. (2016). Community dynamics and the lower airway microbiota in stable chronic obstructive pulmonary disease, smokers and healthy non-smokers. *Thorax* 71, 795–803. doi: 10.1136/thoraxjnl-2015- 207235
21. Frank, E., Hall, M., and Witten, I. (2016). *The WEKA Workbench. Online Appendix for "Data Mining: Practical Machine Learning Tools and Techniques"*, 4 Edn. Burlington, MA: Morgan Kaufmann.
22. Franzosa, E. A., McIver, L. J., Rahnavard, G., Thompson, L. R., Schirmer, M., Weingart, G., et al. (2018). Species-level functional profiling of metagenomes and metatranscriptomes. *Nat. Methods* 15, 962–968. doi: 10.1038/s41592-018-0176-y
23. Friedman, J., and Alm, E. J. (2012). Inferring correlation networks from genomic survey data. *PLoS Comput. Biol.* 8:e1002687. doi: 10.1371/journal.pcbi.1002687 Global Initiative for Chronic Obstructive Lung Disease (GOLD) (2019). *Pocket Guide to COPD Diagnosis, Management and Prevention. A Guide for Health Care Professionals. 2019 Report*. Available online at: www.goldcopd.com (June 25, 2020).
24. Goleva, E., Jackson, L. P., Harris, J. K., Robertson, C. E., Sutherland, E. R., Hall, C. F., et al. (2013). The effects of airway microbiome on corticosteroid responsiveness in asthma. *Am. J. Respir. Crit. Care Med.* 188, 1193–1201. doi: 10.1164/rccm.201304-0775OC
25. Goodwin, S., McPherson, J. D., and McCombie, W. R. (2016). Coming of age: ten years of next-generation sequencing technologies. *Nat. Rev. Genet.* 17, 333–351. doi: 10.1038/nrg.2016.49
26. Harrison, A., Dyer, D. W., Gillaspy, A., Ray, W. C., Mungur, R., Carson, M. B., et al. (2005). Genomic sequence of an otitis media isolate of nontypeable *Haemophilus influenzae*: comparative study with *H. influenzae* serotype d, strain KW20. *J. Bacteriol.* 187, 4627–4636. doi: 10.1128/JB.187.13.4627-4636.2005
27. Hebert, P. D. N., Braukmann, T. W. A., Prosser, S. W. J., Ratnasingham, S., deWaard, J. R., Ivanova, N. V., et al. (2018). A sequel to sanger: amplicon sequencing that scales. *BMC Genomics* 19:219. doi: 10.1186/s12864-018- 4611-3
28. Hogg, J. S., Hu, F. Z., Janto, B., Boissy, R., Hayes, J., Keefe, R., et al. (2007). Characterization and modeling of the *Haemophilus influenzae* core and supragenomes based on the complete genomic sequences of Rd and 12 clinical nontypeable strains. *Genome Biol.* 8:R103. doi: 10.1186/gb-2007-8-6-r103
29. Huang, Y. J., Sethi, S., Murphy, T., Nariya, S., Boushey, H. A., and Lynch, S. V. (2014). Airway microbiome dynamics in exacerbations of chronic obstructive pulmonary disease. *J. Clin. Microbiol.* 52, 2813–2823. doi: 10.1128/JCM.00035-14
30. Jiao, X., Zheng, X., Ma, L., Kutty, G., Gogineni, E., Sun, Q., et al. (2013). A benchmark study on error assessment and quality control of CCS reads derived from the PacBio RS. *J. Data Mining Genomics Proteomics* 4:16008. doi: 10.4172/ 2153-0602.1000136
31. Johnson, J. S., Spakowicz, D. J., Hong, B. Y., Petersen, L. M., Demkowicz, P., Chen, L., et al. (2019). Evaluation of 16S rRNA gene sequencing for species and strain- level microbiome analysis. *Nat. Commun.* 10:5029. doi: 10.1038/s41467-019- 13036-1
32. Langmead, B., and Salzberg, S. L. (2012). Fast gapped-read alignment with Bowtie 2. *Nat. Methods* 9, 357–359. doi: 10.1038/nmeth.1923
33. Lappann, M., Danhof, S., Guenther, F., Olivares-Florez, S., Mordhorst, I. L., and Vogel, U. (2013). In vitro resistance mechanisms of *Neisseria meningitidis* against neutrophil extracellular traps. *Mol. Microbiol.* 89, 433–449. doi: 10.1111/ mmi.12288
34. Lee, S., Suh, G. Y., Ryter, S. W., and Choi, A. M. (2016). Regulation and function of the nucleotide binding domain leucine-rich repeat- containing receptor, pyrin domain-containing-3 inflammasome in lung disease. *Am. J. Respir. Cell Mol. Biol.* 54, 151–160. doi: 10.1165/rcmb.2015- 0231TR
35. Leitao Filho, F. S., Alotaibi, N. M., Ngan, D., Tam, S., Yang, J., Hollander, Z., et al. (2018). Sputum microbiome is associated with 1-year mortality following COPD hospitalizations. *Am. J. Respir. Crit. Care Med.* 199, 1205–1213. doi: 10.1164/rccm.201806-1135OC
36. Levy, S. E., and Myers, R. M. (2016). Advancements in next-generation sequencing. *Annu. Rev. Genomics Hum. Genet.* 17, 95–115. doi: 10.1146/annurev-genom- 083115-022413
37. Lloyd-Price, J., Arze, C., Ananthakrishnan, A. N., Schirmer, M., Avila-Pacheco, J., Poon, T. W., et al. (2019). Multi-omics of the gut microbial ecosystem in inflammatory bowel diseases. *Nature* 569, 655–662. doi: 10.1038/s41586-019-1237-9
38. Lozupone, C., Cota-Gomez, A., Palmer, B. E., Linderman, D. J., Charlson, E. S., Sodergren, E., et al. (2013). Widespread colonization of the lung by *Tropheryma whipplei* in HIV infection. *Am. J. Respir. Crit. Care Med.* 187, 1110–1117. doi: 10.1164/rccm.201211-2145OC
39. Mac Aogain, M., Chandrasekaran, R., Lim, A. Y. H., Low, T. B., Tan, G. L., Hassan, T., et al. (2018). Immunological corollary of the pulmonary mycobiome in bronchiectasis: the CAMEB study. *Eur. Respir. J.* 52:1800766. doi: 10.1183/ 13993003.00766-2018
40. Mao, K., Chen, S., Chen, M., Ma, Y., Wang, Y., Huang, B., et al. (2013). Nitric oxide suppresses NLRP3 inflammasome activation and protects against LPS-induced septic shock. *Cell Res.* 23, 201–212. doi: 10.1038/cr.2013.6
41. Marcel, M. (2011). Cutadapt removes adapter sequences from high-throughput sequencing reads. *EMBnet J.* 17, 10–12. doi: 10.14806/ej.17.1.200
42. Mayhew, D., Devos, N., Lambert, C., Brown, J. R., Clarke, S. C., Kim, V. L., et al. (2018). Longitudinal profiling of the lung microbiome in the AERIS study demonstrates repeatability of bacterial and eosinophilic COPD exacerbations. *Thorax* 73, 422–430. doi: 10.1136/thoraxjnl-2017-210408
43. Murphy, T. F., Brauer, A. L., Pettigrew, M. M., LaFontaine, E. R., and Tettelin, H. (2019). Persistence of *Moraxella* catarrhalis in chronic obstructive pulmonary disease and regulation of the Hag/MID Adhesin. *J. Infect. Dis.* 219, 1448–1455. doi: 10.1093/infdis/jiy680
44. Murray, P. R., and Washington, J. A. (1975). Microscopic and baceriologic analysis of expectorated sputum. *Mayo Clin. Proc.* 50, 339–344.
45. Pragman, A. A., Kim, H. B., Reilly, C. S., Wendt, C., and Isaacson, R. E. (2012). The lung microbiome in moderate and severe chronic obstructive pulmonary disease. *PLoS One* 7:e47305. doi: 10.1371/journal.pone.0047305
46. Robin, X., Turck, N., Hainard, A., Tiberti, N., Lisacek, F., Sanchez, J. C., et al. (2011). pROC: an open-source package for R and S+ to analyze and compare ROC curves. *BMC Bioinformatics* 12:77. doi: 10.1186/1471-2105-12-77
47. Roson, B., Carratala, J., Verdaguer, R., Dorca, J., Manresa, F., and Gudiol, F. (2000). Prospective study of the usefulness of sputum Gram stain in the initial approach to community-acquired pneumonia requiring hospitalization. *Clin. Infect. Dis.* 31, 869–874. doi: 10.1086/318151
48. Saha, S., and Brightling, C. E. (2006). Eosinophilic airway inflammation in COPD. *Int. J. Chron. Obstruct. Pulmon. Dis.* 1, 39–47. doi: 10.2147/copd.2006.1.1.39 Segata, N., Izard, J., Waldron, L., Gevers, D., Miropolsky, L., Garrett, W. S., et al. (2011). Metagenomic biomarker discovery and explanation. *Genome Biol.* 12:R60. doi: 10.1186/gb-2011-12-6-r60
49. Sethi, S., and Murphy, T. F. (2001). Bacterial infection in chronic obstructive pulmonary disease in 2000: a state-of-the-art review. *Clin. Microbiol. Rev.* 14, 336–363. doi: 10.1128/CMR.14.2.336-363.2001
50. Simpson, J. L., Daly, J., Baines, K. J., Yang, I. A., Upham, J. W., Reynolds, P. N., et al. (2016). Airway dysbiosis: *Haemophilus influenzae* and *Tropheryma* in poorly controlled asthma. *Eur. Respir. J.* 47, 792–800. doi: 10.1183/13993003.00405-2015
51. Skopelja-Gardner, S., Theprungsirikul, J., Lewis, K. A., Hammond, J. H., Carlson, K. M., Hazlett, H. F., et al. (2019). Regulation of *Pseudomonas aeruginosa*- mediated neutrophil extracellular traps. *Front. Immunol.* 10:1670. doi: 10.3389/ fimmu.2019.01670
52. Sze, M. A., Dimitriu, P. A., Hayashi, S., Elliott, W. M., McDonough, J. E., Gosselink, J. V., et al. (2012). The lung tissue microbiome in chronic

obstructive pulmonary disease. *Am. J. Respir. Crit. Care Med.* 185, 1073–1080. doi: 10.1164/ rccm.201111-2075OC

53. Uddin, M., Watz, H., Malmgren, A., and Pedersen, F. (2019). NETopathic inflammation in chronic obstructive pulmonary disease and severe asthma. *Front. Immunol.* 10:47. doi: 10.3389/fimmu.2019.00047
54. Vital, M., Penton, C. R., Wang, Q., Young, V. B., Antonopoulos, D. A., Sogin, M. L., et al. (2013). A gene-targeted approach to investigate the intestinal butyrate-producing bacterial community. *Microbiome* 1:8. doi: 10.1186/2049- 2618-1-8
55. Wagner, J., Coupland, P., Browne, H. P., Lawley, T. D., Francis, S. C., and Parkhill, J. (2016). Evaluation of PacBio sequencing for full-length bacterial 16S rRNA gene classification. *BMC Microbiol.* 16:274. doi: 10.1186/s12866-016-0891-4
56. Wang, F., Liang, Z., Yang, Y., Zhou, L., Guan, L., Wu, W., et al. (2019). Reproducibility of fluid-phase measurements in PBS-treated sputum supernatant of healthy and stable COPD subjects. *Int. J. Chron. Obstruct. Pulmon. Dis.* 14, 835–852. doi: 10.2147/COPD.S187661
57. Wang, Z., Bafadhel, M., Haldar, K., Spivak, A., Mayhew, D., Miller, B. E., et al. (2016). Lung microbiome dynamics in COPD exacerbations. *Eur. Respir. J.* 47, 1082–1092. doi: 10.1183/13993003.01406-2015
58. Wang, Z., Liu, H., Wang, F., Yang, Y., Wang, X., Chen, B., et al. (2020). A Refined view of airway microbiome in chronic obstructive pulmonary disease at species and strain-levels. *bioRxiv* [Preprint]. doi: 10.1101/2020.01.18.908624
59. Wang, Z., Maschera, B., Lea, S., Kolsum, U., Michalovich, D., Van Horn, S., et al. (2019). Airway host-microbiome interactions in chronic obstructive pulmonary disease. *Respir. Res.* 20:113.
60. Wang, Z., Singh, R., Miller, B. E., Tal-Singer, R., Van Horn, S., Tomsho, L., et al. (2018). Sputum microbiome temporal variability and dysbiosis in chronic obstructive pulmonary disease exacerbations: an analysis of the COPDMAP study. *Thorax* 73, 331–338. doi: 10.1136/thoraxjnl-2017-210741
61. Wedzicha, J. A., Brill, S. E., Allinson, J. P., and Donaldson, G. C. (2013). Mechanisms and impact of the frequent exacerbator phenotype in chronic obstructive pulmonary disease. *BMC Med.* 11:181. doi: 10.1186/1741-7015-11-181
62. Zakharkina, T., Heinzel, E., Koczulla, R. A., Greulich, T., Rentz, K., Pauling, J. K., et al. (2013). Analysis of the airway microbiota of healthy individuals and patients with chronic obstructive pulmonary disease by T-RFLP and clone sequencing. *PLoS One* 8:e68302. doi: 10.1371/journal.pone.0068302
63. Zander, C. D. (2001). The guild as a concept and a means in ecological parasitology. *Parasitol. Res.* 87, 484–488. doi: 10.1007/s004360100386
64. Zhao, L., Zhang, F., Ding, X., Wu, G., Lam, Y. Y., Wang, X., et al. (2018). Gut bacteria selectively promoted by dietary fibers alleviate type 2 diabetes. *Science* 359, 1151–1156. doi: 10.1126/science.aao5774
65. Zong, Z. Y., and Peng, C. H. (2011). Ralstonia mannitolilytica and COPD: a case report. *Eur. Respir. J.* 38, 1482–1483. doi: 10.1183/09031936.0004 6011

20

Role of Proteases in Chronic Obstructive Pulmonary Disease

Kailash C. Pandey[1]*, *Sajal De*[2] *and Pradyumna K. Mishra*[3]

[1] Department of Biochemistry, National Institute for Research in Environmental Health (ICMR), Bhopal, India, [2] Department of Pulmonary Medicine, National Institute for Research in Environmental Health (ICMR), Bhopal, India, [3] Department of Molecular Biology, National Institute for Research in Environmental Health (ICMR), Bhopal, India

***Correspondence:**
Kailash C. Pandey
kailash.pandey.nireh@gov.in

Chronic obstructive pulmonary disease (COPD) is generally associated with progressive destruction of airways and lung parenchyma. Various factors play an important role in the development and progression of COPD, like imbalance of proteases, environmental and genetic factors and oxidative stress. This review is specifically focused on the role of proteases and their imbalance in COPD. There are three classes (serine, mettalo, and cysteine) of proteases involved in COPD. In serine proteases, neutrophil elastase, cathepsin G, and proteinase-3 are involved in destruction of alveolar tissue. Matrix-mettaloproteinase-9, 12, 13, plays an influential role in severity of COPD. Among cysteine proteases, caspase-3, caspases-8 and caspase-9 play an important role in controlling apoptosis. These proteases activities can be regulated by inhibitors like α-1-antitrypsin, neutrophil elastase inhibitor, and leukocyte protease inhibitor. Studies suggest that neutrophil elastase may be a therapeutic target for COPD, and specific inhibitor against this enzyme has potential role to control the disease. Current study suggests that Dipeptidyl Peptidase IV is a potential marker for COPD. Since the expression of proteases and its inhibitors play an important role in COPD pathogenesis, therefore, it is worth investigating the role of proteases and their regulation. Understanding the biochemical basis of COPD pathogenesis using advanced tools in protease biochemistry and aiming toward translational research from bench-to-bedside will have great impact to deal with this health problem.

Keywords: COPD, cysteine protease, mettaloproteinase, degradation, oxidative stress, apoptosis, caspase, protease-antiprotease imbalance

GENERAL INTRODUCTION AND PATHOLOGY

Chronic obstructive pulmonary disease (COPD) is enhanced inflammatory response of airways as well as lung parenchyma to harmful particles or gases. In COPD, airways are obstructed by loss of alveolar attachments, mucosal inflammation, and mucous obstruction of lumen (**Figure 1**).

The inflammation causes structural damage, narrowing of airways, and the destruction of lung parenchyma (emphysema) (Demedts et al., 2006). The airflow obstruction in COPD is not fully reversible and usually progressive. Besides inflammation, the other processes involved in the pathogenesis of COPD are (i) an imbalance between proteases and anti-proteases, (ii) imbalance between oxidants and antioxidants (Demedts et al., 2006). COPD broadly encompasses two pathologic entities i.e., emphysema and chronic bronchitis. Emphysema is defined by alveolar wall destruction and irreversible enlargement of the air spaces distal to the terminal bronchioles and without evidence of fibrosis (Murray and Lopez, 1999).

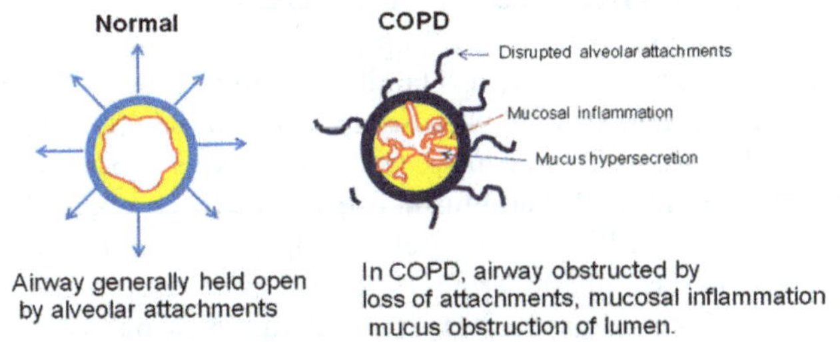

FIGURE 1 | Air flow in Normal vs. COPD. The airway in normal condition is distended by alveolar attachments at the time of expiration. But in COPD these alveolar attachments are mainly disrupted due to emphysema, therefore contributing to airway closure during expiration, and hyperinflation due to air trap in the alveoli. Inflammation, fibrosis and mucus secretions further obstructed and distorted the peripheral airways and consequently create the poor mucociliary clearance (Barnes, 2004).

These components vary in proportion among COPD patients. A clinical diagnosis of COPD is considered in any patient with dyspnea, chronic cough, sputum production as well as history of exposure to the disease. As defined by the National Institute for Clinical Excellence (NICE), a diagnosis of COPD is based on the ratio of forced expiratory volume/second (FEV1)/ forced vital capacity (FVC) is <0.7 in spirometry analysis suspect the presence of airflow limitation and thus of COPD (Murray and Lopez, 1999). Unfortunately, COPD is undiagnosed until there are clinical symptoms and the disease is moderately advanced, therefore a mild condition may go unnoticed in the community. It is estimated that about 3 million deaths were caused by this disease in 2015, globally. A current epidemiological estimation predicted by 2020, COPD may become the third leading cause of death worldwide (Murray and Lopez, 1999; Peto et al., 1999). A major risk factor for the development of COPD is tobacco smoking (Peto et al., 1999; Vestbo et al., 2014). Other risk factors are air pollution (both indoor and outdoor), occupation exposure to dust and chemicals, and frequent respiratory tract infections in childhood. There are available drugs for COPD based on anti-cholinergics, beta-2-agonist, phosphodiesterase-4-inhibitors and corticosteroids (Prakash et al., 2013). Despite intensive research all over the world, the biochemical, cellular, and molecular mechanisms underlying COPD pathobiology are not yet well understood. Therefore, the scientific community needs to investigate this important health problem with modern tools.

An important question is the identification of factors which interact with smoking and causes more rapid decline in FEV1 as well as the development of COPD. These may be caused by either additional environmental factors or susceptibility of genes (Murray and Lopez, 1999). Analyzing these factors into detail will provide new avenues to prevent the development of this disease and target potential pathways that can reduce disease progression. Published literature regarding sputum proteomic analysis suggests that changes in various proteins are associated with the development of Acute Exacerbation COPD (AECOPD), caused by heavy smoking (Uh et al., 2012; Faner et al., 2014). A serum surfactant protein D (SP-D) has been suggested as a marker in patients with AECOPD, but unfortunately cannot distinguish between COPD and AECOPD (Lomas et al., 2009; Koutsokera et al., 2013). A recent study suggested that microfibrillar-associated protein 4 (MFAP4), a matricellular glycoprotein that co-localizes with elastic fibers expressed in the lung tissues, is associated with the severity in COPD (Kishore et al., 2006; Johansson et al., 2014). Other marker, a C-reactive protein (CRP) binds to bacteria, oxidized lipids, and apoptotic cells, consequently facilitates their clearance via innate immune system. Therefore, act as an inflammatory marker for heart and lung diseases, including COPD, but it is not specific marker for COPD, and its role in COPD is not yet established (Bircan et al., 2008). Among environmental factors, tobacco smoking is the most important risk factor for the development of COPD (Peto et al., 1999). Oxidative stress is another factor contributes to COPD, generally occurs when reactive oxygen species are produced in excess (Barnes, 2004). The genetic variations (deficiencies of α-antitrypsin) have also been linked to COPD associated pathogenesis (Perlmutter, 1996). This review will specifically focus on the role of proteases in COPD.

INDIAN PROSPECTIVE

The prevalence of COPD varies from 3–8% among Indian males and approximately 2.5–4.5% in Indian females (Bhome, 2012). It is estimated that by the end of 2016, more than 5.7 million people are suffering from COPD in India, and the estimated economic burden of COPD (2010–2011) was more than six billion USD (Kalkana et al., 2016). The Indian study on epidemiology of asthma, respiratory symptoms and chronic bronchitis in adults involved a total of 85,105 men, 84,470 women from 12 urban and 11 rural sites (Jindal et al., 2012). This study has shown that the overall prevalence of chronic bronchitis in adults >35 years was around 3.5% (Jindal et al., 2012). There are wide variations in the occurrence of COPD in Indian subcontinent (Kalkana et al., 2016). Based on these studies, the national burden of chronic bronchitis was estimated around 14 to 14.5 million (Jindal et al., 2012; Salvi and Agarwal, 2012; Vijayan, 2013). A long term epidemiological study on the health effect of toxic gas in Bhopal, was carried out by ICMR-National Institute for Research in Environmental Health, revealed that the highest percentage (22%) of people in the toxic gas exposed cohort suffered from various respiratory morbidities including COPD (NIREH, 2014).

Previously a multicentric study based on epidemiology of COPD and its relationship with tobacco smoking and environmental tobacco smoke exposure was studied (Jindal et al., 2006). A total 35295 subjects were included in this study, 4.1% COPD cases diagnosed with male and female ratio of 1.5: 1, and smoker to non- smoker ratio of 2.6:1. This study also indentified the prevalence among Bidi (filled with crude tobacco flake and mainly wrapped in a *Piliostigma racemosum* leaf) and cigarette smokers was 8.2 and 5.9%, respectively (Jindal et al., 2006). A recent cross sectional study was conducted among twelve hundred adults in Delhi, India (Sinha et al., 2017). This study suggested the prevalence of COPD was 10%, and the tobacco smoking adults were the strongest risk factor with this disease. The old smoker had 63 % lesser risk as compare to current smokers (Sinha et al., 2017). Further, environmental smoke, occupational exposure, age factor, and biomass fuel are the others important factors which influence this health problem (Sinha et al., 2017). Due to heterogeneity, limited numbers of studies and further their unsuitability for meta-analysis, these discussed figures are most unlikely to apply for all subpopulations in India. Therefore, the general prevalence of COPD from all across the country largely remains unknown.

Role of Proteases and Their Association with COPD

Proteases cleave proteins into smaller fragments and classified according to their catalytic site. Proteases associated with COPD pathology has been divided into three main classes; serine protease, matrix-mettaloproteinase, cysteine protease (**Figure 2**; Barnes, 2004).

Proteases are involved in pathogenesis of various diseases such as arthritis, osteoporosis, AIDS, immune-related diseases, atherosclerosis, cancer, and for a wide variety of parasitic diseases e.g., malaria, amebiasis, chagas disease, leishmaniasis, or African sleeping sickness, therefore act as potential targets (Lecaille et al., 2002; Pandey et al., 2005; Gills et al., 2007; Salminen-Mankonen et al., 2007; Verma et al., 2016). Targeting proteases in COPD still need to be explored in great detail.

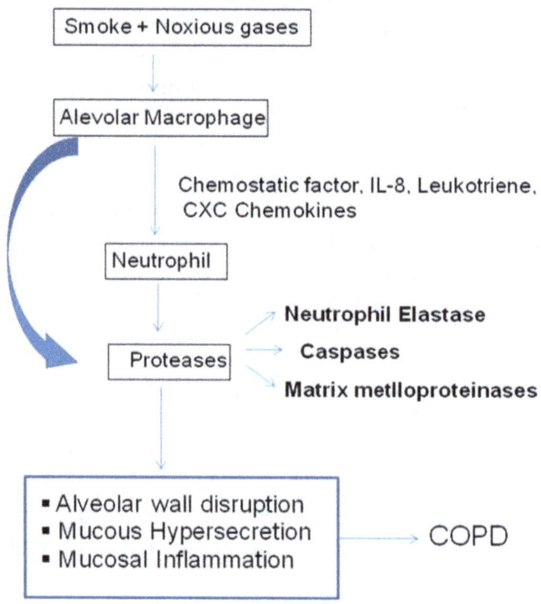

FIGURE 2 | Inflammatory mechanism in COPD. Cigarette smoke or other toxic particles activates the macrophage in the respiratory tract and release neutrophil chemotactic factors like IL-8, leukotrine, CXC chemokines. These cells further release proteases of different classes, which break down connective tissue in the lung parenchyma resulting COPD (Barnes, 2004).

Role of Serine Protease in COPD

Seine proteases (or serine endopeptidases) belongs to a PA clan and S1 (trypsin/chymotrypsin) family of proteolytic enzymes. S1 family include neutrophil elastase (NE), protinase-3, cathepsin G. Studies suggest that these enzymes are synthesized as pro-enzymes in the ER and further processed by cleavage of the signal peptide and finally removal of a dipeptide by cathepsin C (Belaaouaj et al., 1998). Serine proteases have been reported to be located in blood monocytes, mast cells and neutrophils, act as potent mucus stimulants (Qiu et al., 2003). Neutrophil elastase, a serine proteases play as potent secretor, therefore mucus might aggravate airflow obstruction in COPD (Lee et al., 2015). This enzyme is mainly involved in the destruction of alveolar tissue (Qiu et al., 2003). The mice model study suggested that elastase play important role in emphysema (Belaaouaj et al., 1998), further study suggest that NE has a role in pathogenesis of COPD by enhancing inflammation and apoptosis (Belaaouaj et al., 1998; Qiu et al., 2003). NE is released by activated neutrophils and macrophages, which induce small airway and alveolar epithelial cell apoptosis using intrinsic pathway (Lee et al., 2015). These reactions slow down a serine/threonine protein kinase phosphorylation and activate proteinase activated receptor-1 (PAR) and finally proceed for apoptosis pathway by caspase-3(Qiu et al., 2003; Lee et al., 2015). The potent NE inhibitors with nM ranges of IC_{50}, have been identified (Tsai and Hwang, 2015). These inhibitors including, pyrimidinone, tetra-hydro-pyrrolo-pyrimidinedione, pyrazinone, benzoxazinone, and uracil derivatives have been indentified (Tsai and Hwang, 2015). Using templates of these existing inhibitors and detail kinetic study of NE, we believe that in the future more potential compounds with efficient therapeutic NE inhibitors will become available for clinical applications. Some of the potential drugs against NE will be discussed in the section entitled targeting neutrophil elastase.

ROLE OF DIPEPTIDYL PEPTIDASE IV

Dipeptidyl Peptidase IV (DPPIV) is a serine expopeptide that catalyzes the release of an N-terminal dipeptide. DPPIV is present as a homo dimer on the cell surface and catalytically active protease. DPPIV is a multifunctional cell surface protein express in cell types including T lymphocytes (Javidroozi et al., 2012). DPPIV present in the serum as soluble truncated form of enzyme without transmenbrane and intracellular domains. It has already been established that DPPIV plays an important role in tumor biology as a suppressor in the development of cancer, therefore a useful biomarker for different cancers (Schade et al., 2008; Cordero et al., 2009; Javidroozi et al., 2012; Larrinaga et al., 2012). In addition, DPPIV also plays an important role in glucose metabolism, e.g., DPPIV is responsible for the degradation of glucagon-like peptide-1 (Somborac-Bačura et al., 2012). But interestingly, DPPIV also plays an important role in the inflammatory response in the lungs, therefore it is worth to mention with related to lung biology (Somborac-Bačura et al., 2012). In fact, recently, it has been shown that the serum containing DPPIV activity in patients with stable COPD (722–1,037 ng/ml) is significantly lower than healthy people (1,080–1,620 ng/ml) (Holst and Deacon, 2005). Further, the level of this enzyme is not affected by smoking, age, and other factors (Holst and Deacon, 2005). Study systematically investigated the correlation between serum level of DPPIV and types of COPD, including stable COPD, AECOPD, measuring serum concentrations of DPPIV with ELISA, followed by a comprehensive analysis of the relationships between a set of parameters of COPD and different forms of COPD using statistical analysis methods (Holst and Deacon, 2005; Chang et al., 2016). The above mentioned study suggested that DPPIV was signifintely decreased in both stable COPD (722–1,037 ng/ml) and AECOPD (610–966 ng/ml) compare to healthy people (1,080–1,620 ng/ml). Therefore, DPPIV may be a predictor in patients having COPD and seems to be a valuable serologic biomarker. However, detail study with larger number of patients and the role of this enzyme in COPD are indeed required to further strengthen the preliminary data.

Role of Matrix Mettaloproteinase in COPD

Matrix mettaloproteinase (MMPs) are a family of matrix degrading enzymes which degenerate the protein components of extracellular matrix (Finlay et al., 1997). MMPs are believed to be important for the development, tissue remodeling and repairing of damaged tissue. MMPs are produced by inflammatory cells e.g., neutrophils and alveolar macrophage (Finlay et al., 1997). The MMPs are divided into different subgroups according to their primary substrates like collagenases which include MMP-1 and MMP-13. Using MALDI-TOF MS analysis, Lee et al., showed that the expression of matrix metalloproteinase-13 (MMP-13) was increased in lung tissues of COPD patients (Lee et al., 2009). MMP-13, a major proteolytic enzyme believes to be implicated in tissue damage and remodeling, which is predominantly expressed in alveolar macrophages and type II pneumocytes (Chaudhuri et al., 2012). Presence of MMP-12 in sputum and activity in patients with COPD are directly associated with the extent of emphysema measured by means of lung function and computed tomography (Chaudhuri et al., 2012). Further Haq et al. suggested that a single nucleotide polymorphisms reduce the enzyme activity of MMP-12 and consequently protect from emphysema in COPD (Haq et al., 2010, 2011). The genetic and animal studies have suggested MMP-12 in the pathogenesis of COPD (Haq et al., 2010, 2011). MMP-12 SNP affects the enzyme activity, and protects against emphysema in COPD (Jormsjo et al., 2000; Haq et al., 2010). It has previously been shown that individuals with homozygous for the A/A allele of rs652438 in MMP-12, are prone to suffer with severe COPD (Jormsjo et al., 2000; Haq et al., 2010). Study also implicated that rs652438 SNP changes the MMP-12 activity and increased macrophage infiltration and emphysema in the lungs of COPD patients (Jormsjo et al., 2000; Haq et al., 2011).

MMP-2 and MMP-9 mainly degrade basal membrane components like fibronectin; elastin, and these proteases have a broad spectrum of extra cellular membrane as targets. MMP-9 plays an important role in COPD, it is 92–96 kD in size, the sources of MMP-9 have been keratinocytes, monocytes, leukocytes, macrophages, and fibroblasts (Emjabbar et al., 1999; Johnson, 2016). It plays an important role in the cellular invasion of the basement membrane by mononuclear phagocytes, synovial fibroblasts. MMP-9 has been considered to play a major role in cell migration and airway inflammatory response in COPD. Studies including *in vitro* and *in vivo* suggested that MMP-9 may play an important role during eosinophil migration and influence the severity of COPD (Van den Steen et al., 2002; Linder et al., 2015). A population-based cross-sectional study demonstrated that in serum of COPD, MMP-9 concentration is higher compare to non-COPD, and production of cough and decreasing FEV1 were associated with MMP-9 in COPD (Legrand et al., 1999; Linder et al., 2015). An increase of ~10 to 100 folds concentrations of MMP-9 and MMP-3 in the epithelial lining fluid of the patients with respiratory problem suggests that they may involved in COPD (Legrand et al., 1999). MMP-9 controls the migration of repairing human bronchial epithelial cells by remodeling the provisional extracellular matrix, remodeling is facilitates by wound healing, angiogenesis, establishment of more stable fibronectin-containing contacts in the central part of the cell (Legrand et al., 1999; Linder et al., 2015). MMP-9 (or Type IV collagenase) is abundant in various lung diseases e.g.. asthma, idiopathic pulmonary fibrosis, and COPD, while their levels are reportedly low in normal human lungs. Its role in matrix remodeling makes it an important candidate during fibrosis that occurs in COPD.

Role of Cysteine Proteases

Increasing number of data suggests that cysteine proteases; caspase-3, caspases-8 and caspase-9 play important roles in COPD (Muzio et al., 1998; Yasuda et al., 1998; Demedts et al., 2006; Abboud and Vimalanathan, 2008). These caspases are involved in COPD by controlling the mechanism of apoptosis. The death of structural cells in the lung possibly is an important event in the pathogenesis of COPD (Hirata et al., 1998; Muzio et al., 1998). Published literature suggested that there is an increase in apoptotic alveolar epithelial and endothelial cells in the lungs of COPD patients (Hirata et al., 1998). The above mentioned caspases mRNA expression were higher in COPD cells (Hirata et al., 1998). This study suggests that in COPD, the apoptosis is mediated by the receptor mediated extrinsic pathway by activation of caspase-8 (Hirata et al., 1998). The enhanced p53 (cell cycle regulatory protein) levels can stimulate the induction of caspase-8 resulting in apoptosis of bronchial epithelial cell in COPD (Yasuda et al., 1998). Inflammatory response and oxidative stress signals in COPD, are mediated by binding of members of the tumor necrosis factor family (Fas ligand, TNF-α). Consequently, formation of the death induce signal complex (DISC), which is made up of multiple adaptor molecules such as the Fas associated death domain (FADD). Yasuda et al. also suggested a significant increase in death receptor (Fas) in the plasma of COPD patients (Yasuda et al., 1998). A death receptor recruits procaspase-8 and leads to the autolytic activation to caspase-8, and finally start apoptosis using caspase-3 (Hirata et al., 1998; Muzio et al., 1998; Yasuda et al., 1998). In summary, it is suggested that in case of COPD pathogenesis, caspase-9, caspase-8, caspase-3 play crucial role in apoptosis (Kidokoro et al., 1977; Perlmutter, 1996; Churg and

Wright, 2005; Gogebakan et al., 2014). Further, using TUNEL-staining in lung cells of mice with COPD suggested that an increase in apoptotic cells compare to normal cells (Demedts et al., 2006) (**Figure 3**). Those mediators involved in apoptosis could be interesting targets to prevent the development of COPD. Therefore, it is important to explore the role of caspases in COPD.

PROTEASE-ANTIPROTEASE IMBALANCE IN COPD PATHOGENESIS

Published literature using human and animal studies support the evidence that protease-anti-proteases imbalance may play crucial role in the pathogenesis of COPD (Gadek and Pacht, 1990; Muzio et al., 1998; Churg and Wright, 2005; Demedts et al., 2006; Abboud and Vimalanathan, 2008; Gogebakan et al., 2014). Excess neutrophils accumulation and activation disrupt the protease-antiprotease balance and trigger lung destruction process in COPD (Churg and Wright, 2005; Gogebakan et al., 2014; Demedts et al., 2006). The endogenous secretory neutrophils elastase inhibitors neutralize the proteolytic activity of neutrophil elastase, and these inhibitors are abundant in the respiratory tract which controls the activity of neutrophil elastase (Kidokoro et al., 1977; Abboud and Vimalanathan, 2008). A protease inhibitor, α-1-antitrypsin plays an important role in controlling proteases activities. This inhibitor exerts potent control over the proteolytic activity of neutrophil elastase, proteinase-3, cathepsin G, and neutrophils serine protease-4 (Perlmutter, 1996). The deficiency of α-1-antitrypsin results in emphysema, which can be successfully treated via exogenous supplementation of α-1-antitrypsin (Perlmutter, 1996). Study suggests that the treatment of COPD patients with α-1-antitrypsin deficiency, reduce mortality and slow the progression of emphysema (Perlmutter, 1996). A molecule like secretory leukocyte protease inhibitor (SLPI) and elafin, members of the chelonianin family, are also able to inhibit NE and control the proteolytic activity (Tsai and Hwang, 2015). Since SLPI and elafin are primarily produced by respiratory tract epithelial cells, it seems they may play an important role in COPD.

The balance of protease-antiprotease may be affected by a low level of α-1-antitrypsin or insufficient production of α-1-antitrypsin because of genetic defects or the inactivation of α-1-antitrypsin by smoking-induced oxidants. The genetic variations (deficiencies of α-1-antitrypsin) have also been linked to COPD associated pathogenesis (Perlmutter, 1996). The deficiency of α-1-antitrypsin causes non-regulation and over expression of neutrophil elastase that result in lung parenchymal destruction. The critical role of neutrophil elastase in anti-trypsin-deficient COPD is supported by the correlation of increased leukocyte elastase concentration (Perlmutter, 1996). Beside gene deficiency, environmental toxin and smoking may cause a protease-anti-protease imbalance in the lung by reducing the functional activity of α-1-antitrypsin in the lung interstitium and "alveolar" lining fluid by increasing the amount of elastolytic proteases released in the lung (Perlmutter, 1996; Hirata et al., 1998; Demedts et al., 2006). Literature further suggested that oxidative stress also impair the function of anti-proteases such as α-1-antitrypsin and SLPI and thereby accelerates the breakdown of elastin in lung parenchyma (Perlmutter, 1996; Hirata et al., 1998). Since expression of proteases and its inhibitors play significant role in COPD pathogenesis, therefore, it is worth to investigate the role of proteases and their regulation.

TARGETING NEUTROPHIL ELASTASE

In normal condition, neutrophil elastase express on the cellular membrane, and only 4–5% being released into the extracellular (Tsai and Hwang, 2015). But in COPD, neutrophil elastase is much more available extracellularly because of the increased concentration of necrotic neutrophils (Kidokoro et al., 1977). In COPD patients, the airway leads to neutrophil necrosis which promote to an excessive and uncontrolled secretion of enzyme (Kidokoro et al., 1977). The highest NE activity was found in BAL fluid of severe COPD patients (Kidokoro et al., 1977; Demedts et al., 2006), which can damage the tissue by degradation of TIMP-1 and activation of pro-MMP-9. In addition, NE is a very potent inducer of mucous gland hyperplasia, one of the characteristics of emphysema (Kidokoro et al., 1977). Excessive NE activity as well as indirect burden of this enzyme can be restricted by using specific inhibitors. Other approach is to decrease neutrophil accumulation by inhibiting dipeptide peptide activity (or cathepsin C), since cathepsin C post-translationally process inactive NE into an active enzyme

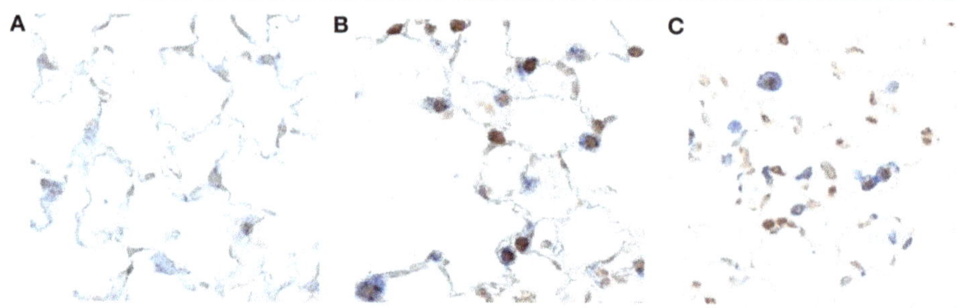

FIGURE 3 | Visualization of apoptotic cells in the lung of mice with COPD. TUNEL-staining demonstrates an increase in apoptotic cells (dark brown nuclei) in the lungs of mice exposed to cigarette smoke **(B,C)** compared to air-exposed animals **(A)**. This figure has been adapted from Demedts et al. (2006).

(Demedts et al., 2006). This strategy indirectly decreased total NE activity and believes to be advantageous in COPD. The literature has increasingly implicated the role of NE in the pathogenesis of COPD, however only few inhibitors have been validated for therapeutic use in clinical settings. Sivelestat is the only NE synthetic inhibitor in clinical market currently approved in Japan and South Korea to treat systemic inflammatory response syndrome (Vandivier et al., 2002). There are some effective inhibitors against NE, which need to study in great detail.

INHIBITOR BASED ON NEUTROPHIL ELASTASE

There are peptide based inhibitors have been developed against NE, which tend to inhibit NE activity (Iba et al., 2006; Wada et al., 2006). The inhibitory concentrations of these peptides for NE are approximately 0.094 mM, e.g., H-L-Arg-Phg-L-Val-Phg-OH. Comparing with linear peptide, a template fixed beta hairpin peptidomimetics are cyclic peptides, which provide more stability and structural rigidity in physiological conditions duo to their macrolactam cysteine knot scaffold (Kawabata et al., 1991). For example, hPhe-Cys-Thr-Ala-Ser-OctG, Pro-Pro-Gln-Cys-Tyr is a peptide based on fixed beta hairpin with IC_{50} is 6.0 nM, but non-peptide hetrocyclic based inhibitors are more common due to potential target for NE. The heterocyclic NE inhibitors are small molecular mass, structurally diverse and act as reversible competitive inhibitors. A pyrimidine moiety with significant characteristic of heterocyclic nitrogen, believe to be potential target for NE, which is applied for pharmaceutical designs (Kawabata et al., 1991). Since pyrimidine derivatives exhibit therapeutic properties such as, antifungal, calcium-blocking and anti-inflammatory activities, they are also been used to inhibit NE activity. The other class of hetrocyclic NE inhibitor is dihydropyrimidinones, which act as calcium channel modulators and antagonist of α 1A adrenoreceptor. The derivatives of these compounds have been found to be potent NE inhibitors, therefore proposed as potential therapeutics for COPD (Hansen et al., 2011; Von Nussbaum et al., 2012). Study suggested that dihydropyrimidinone derivatives are claimed to be potential NE inhibitors and IC_{50} value for most of these compounds are in the range of pM to nM (Hansen et al., 2011). Pyrimidinone, pyrimidinedione, and pyrimidine derivatives were revealed to have IC_{50} values for NE in the ranges of 0.2–1.0 nM (**Figure 4**).

The dihydropyrimidinones groups of inhibitor function as calcium channel modulators as well as selective α 1a-adrenoceptor antagonist. Hansen et al. (2011), suggested that the derivatives of these compounds have been found to be potent human NE inhibitors and have thus been proposed as potential COPD therapeutics (Kawabata et al., 1991). Using these inhibitors, NE selectivity assays showed selectivity ranging from 1- to > 300-fold for various proteases and demonstrated desirable human NE inhibitory activity in an NE-induced lung hemorrhage model in rats, and there has been no noticeable side effect reported in these study (Kawabata et al., 1991). The protective effects of these compounds were also confirmed in human NE and lipopolysaccharide (LPS) induced rat lung injury models (Hsieh et al., 2010). The tetrahydropyrrolo-pyrimidinediones display human NE inhibitory activity in the range of 1–50 nM, and they were shown to protect rat lungs in a human NE-induced acute lung injury model (Bergstrom et al., 2011). 2-pyrazinones derivative displayed IC_{50} values for human NE activity in the nano molar range. These compounds generally administered orally or as dry powder for inhalination without any noticeable side effect (Ray et al., 2010). A benzoxazinone groups exhibited inhibitory activity on human NE in the <15–150 nM range. The beneficial effect of benzoxazinone was tested in a rat LPS induced acute lung injury model, a heterocyclic acylating moiety of those compounds inhibited human NE via a mechanism involving the formation of an acyl enzyme intermediate (Hsieh et al., 2010).

The current information suggests that Sivelestat (**Figure 4**) is a NE inhibitor approved in Japan and South Korea for acute lung injury, acute respiratory distress syndrome in patients with systemic inflammatory response. In non-clinical studies, Sivelestat seems to show benefit in lung injury without inhibiting the host immune defense. The available evidence suggests that Sivelestat may show some benefit in the treatment of acute lung injury/acute respiratory distress syndrome, but large and randomized controlled trials are need to be done in specific pathophysiological conditions to explore the potential benefits in case of COPD.

SUMMARY AND FUTURE DIRECTION

Many proteases are involved in the inflammatory process of COPD and responsible for the destruction of elastin fibers in the lung parenchyma, therefore, identification of those enzymes and other inflammatory mediators as well as understanding their interactions are important for the development of anti-inflammatory treatments for this disease. Redundancy among protease functions and the multiple beneficial effects of MMPs at different sites make those classes of proteases a challenging task to use in the field. Despite of published evidences there are challenges to consider the complexity of proteases and their inhibitors networks. No single molecule could be proposed yet for wide use in clinical practice, therefore, there is a need of basic study to look into detail with modern tools of biochemistry and molecular biology. The current approach of targeting specific pathways/ or processes of these proteases, but only after detail evaluation and the mechanism of these targets are likely to be a safer and more practical approach. The invention of novel NE inhibitors with high potency and low toxicity are the requirement of present time as in the future it may be used for patient therapy. To find out the cause of destruction of lung tissue in patients, it would be worth to study the role of proteases and their imbalance between proteolytic and anti-proteolytic activities and related oxidative stress in great details. The clinical diagnosis of COPD cases could be strengthened by adopting translational bench-to-bedside approach applying proteases biochemistry to biological samples obtained from clinically diagnosed patients. The complexity of COPD will definitely require a multi-target therapeutic approach. Therefore, other targets beside proteases would be beneficial to consider in COPD.

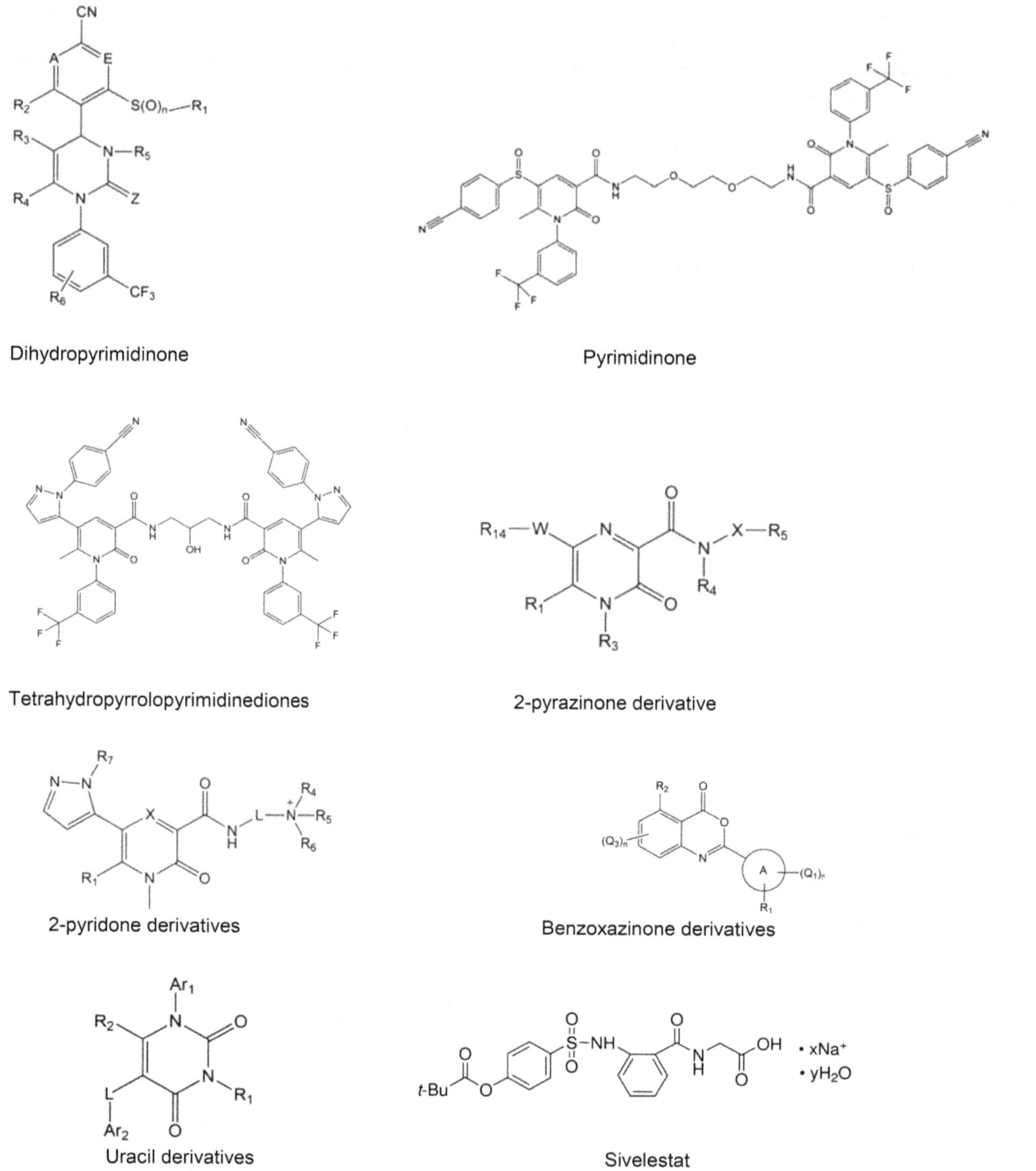

FIGURE 4 | Neutrophil elastase based inhibitors; Pyrimidinone, Pyrimidinedione, and Pyrimidine derivatives are act as NE inhibitors. The IC_{50} values of dihydropyrimidinone (0.3 nM), pyrimidinone (0.61 nM), tetra hydro pyrrolo pyrimidinediones (0.20 nM), 2-pyrazinone derivative (0.33 nM), 2-pyridone derivatives (3.5 nM), benzoxazinone derivatives (15 nM), uracil derivatives (3.5 nM) (Gadek and Pacht, 1990; Vandivier et al., 2002; Iba et al., 2006), sivelestat (46 nM), indicate that above derivatives are potential inhibitors (Ainge et al., 2010; Hsieh et al., 2010; Ray et al., 2010; Bergstrom et al., 2011; Von Nussbaum et al., 2012). Abbreviation used in the figures A and E both represent $C-R_7$ or one of the two ring members A and E represents N and the other represents $C-R_7$, in which R_7 represents in each case hydrogen, fluorine or chlorine, Z represents O or S, *n* represents the number 0, 1, or 2. W represents a 5-membered heterocyclic ring comprising at least one ring heteroatom selected from nitrogen, oxygen, and sulphur. X represents unsubstituted C1-C2 alkylene, L represents C2-C4 alkylene, wherein A is a 5–10 membered heterocyclyl or heteroaryl ring connected to the benzoxazine core by a carbon atom of the heterocyclyl or heteroaryl ring, Q1, Q2, Q3 are halo, pseudohalo, hydroxy, oxo, thia, nitrile, nitro, formyl etc. Ar1 and Ar2 independently represent a 5- to 6-membered aromatic ring group which may contain 1–3 hetero atoms. In the last structure, x indicates number of sodium ions and y is number of water molecules.

AUTHOR CONTRIBUTIONS

KP is an expert in Protease Biochemistry and generate ideas and wrote the review, SD is an expert in Pulmonary Medicine and help in writing process, and PM is an expert in Environmental toxicology and help in writing process.

ACKNOWLEDGMENTS

We thank Indian Council of Medical Research (ICMR) for grant (No. 65/02/KP/NIREH/2016-NCD-II), and we would like to acknowledge Chaitanya for critically reading the manuscript.

REFERENCES

1. Abboud, R. T., and Vimalanathan, S. (2008). Pathogenesis of COPD. Part, I. The role of protease-antiprotease imbalance in emphysema. *Int. J. Tuberc. Lung Dis.* 12, 361–367.
2. Ainge, D., Chapman, D., Lindsjo, M., Lonn, H., Lundkvist, M., Munck, M., et al. (2010). *2-Pyrazinone Derivatives and their Use as Inhibitors of Neutrophil Elastase.* US0280048A1.
3. Barnes, P. J. (2004). Mediators of chronic obstructive pulmonary disease. *Pharmacol. Rev.* 56, 515–548. doi: 10.1124/pr.56.4.2
4. Belaaouaj, A., McCarthy, R., Baumann, M., Gao, Z., Ley, T. J., Abraham, S. N., et al. (1998). Mice lacking neutrophil elastase reveal impaired host defense against gram negative bacterial sepsis. *Nat. Med.* 4, 615–618. doi: 10.1038/nm05 98-615
5. Bergstrom, L., Lonn, H., Lundkvist, M., and Sjo, P. (2011). *Multimeric Heterocyclic Compounds Useful as Neutrophil Elastase Inhibitors.* US0003858A1; 70.
6. Bhome, A. B. (2012). COPD in India: Iceberg or volcano? *J. Thorac. Dis.* 4, 298–309. doi: 10.3978/j.issn.2072-1439.2012.03.15
7. Bircan, A., Gokirmak, M., Kilic, O., Ozturk, O., and Ak- kaya, A. (2008). C-reactive protein levels in patients with chronic obstructive pulmonary disease: role of infection. *Med. Princ. Pract.* 17, 202–208. doi: 10.1159/000117793
8. Chang, X-Y., Yang, Y., Jia, X-Q., Wang, Y., Peng, L-N., Ai, X-H., et al. (2016). Expression and clinical significance of serum dipeptidyl peptidase IV chronic obstructive pulmonary disease. *Am. J. Med. Sci.* 351, 244–252. doi: 10.1016/j.amjms.2015.12.011
9. Chaudhuri, R., McSharry, C., Brady, J., Donnelly, I., Grierson, C., McGuinness, S., et al. (2012). Sputum matrix metalloproteinase-12 in patients with chronic obstructive pulmonary disease and asthma: relationship to disease severity. *J. Allergy Clin. Immunol.* 129, 655.e8–663.e8. doi: 10.1016/j.jaci.2011.12.996
10. Churg, A., and Wright, J. L. (2005). Proteases and emphysema. *Curr. Opin. Pulm. Med.* 11, 153–159. doi: 10.1097/01.mcp.0000149592.51761.e3
11. Cordero, O. J., Salgado, F. J., and Nogueira, M. (2009). On the origin of serum CD26 and its altered concentration in cancer patients. *Cancer Immunol. Immunother.* 58, 1723–1747. doi: 10.1007/s00262-009-0728-1
12. Demedts, I. K., Demoor, T., Bracke, K. R., Joos, G. F., and Brusselle, G. G. (2006). Role of apoptosis in the pathogenesis of COPD and pulmonary emphysema. *Respir. Res.* 7:53. doi: 10.1186/1465-9921-7-53
13. Emjabbar, H., Gosset, P., and Lamblin, C. (1999). Contribution of 92 KD gelatinase/type IV collagenase in bronchial inflammation during status asthmaticus. *Am. J. Respir. Crit. Care Med.* 159, 1298–1307. doi: 10.1164/ajrccm.159.4.9708080
14. Faner, R., Tal-Singer, R., Riley, J. H., Celli, B., Vestbo, J., MacNee, W., et al. (2014). ECLIPSE study investigators. Lessons from ECLIPSE: a review of COPD biomarkers. *Thorax* 69, 666–672. doi: 10.1136/thoraxjnl-2013-204778
15. Finlay, G. A., O'Driscoll, L. R., Russell, K. J., D'Arcy, E. M., Masterson, J. B., FitzGerald, M. X., et al. (1997). Matrix metalloproteinase expression and production by alveolar macrophages in emphysema. *Am. J. Respir. Crit. Care Med.* 156, 240–247. doi: 10.1164/ajrccm.156.1.9612018
16. Gadek, J. E., and Pacht, E. R. (1990). The protease antiprotease balance within the human lung: implications for the pathogenesis of emphysema. *Lung* 168(Suppl.), 552–564. doi: 10.1007/BF02718178
17. Gills, J. J., Lopiccolo, J., Tsurutani, J., Shoemaker, R. H., Best, C. J., Abu- Asab, M. S., et al. (2007). Nelfinavir, A lead HIV protease inhibitor, is a broad-spectrum, anticancer agent that induces endoplasmic reticulum stress, autophagy, and apoptosis *in vitro* and *in vivo*. *Clin. Cancer Res.* 135, 183–194. doi: 10.1158/1078-0432.CCR-07-0161
18. Gogebakan, B., Bayraktar, R., Ulaslı, M., Oztuzcu, S., Tasdemir, D., and Bayram, H. (2014). The role of bronchial epithelial cell apoptosis in the pathogenesis of COPD. *Mol. Biol. Rep.* 1, 5321–5327. doi: 10.1007/s11033-014-3403-3
19. Hansen, G., Gielen-Haertwig, H., Reinemer, P., Schomburg, D., Harrenga, A., and Niefind, K. (2011). Unexpected active-site flexibility in the structure of human neutrophil elastase in Complex with a new dihydropyrimidone inhibitor. *J. Mol. Biol.* 409, 681–691. doi: 10.1016/j.jmb.2011.04.047
20. Haq, I., Chappell, S., Johnson, S. R., Lotya, J., Daly, L., Morgan, K., et al. (2010). Association of *MMP-12* polymorphisms with severe and very severe COPD: a case control study of *MMPs 1, 9* and *12* in a European population. *BMC Med. Genet.* 11:7. doi: 10.1186/1471-2350-11-7
21. Haq, I., Lowrey, G. E., Kalsheker, N., and Johnson, S. R. (2011). Matrix metalloproteinase-12 (MMP-12) SNP affects MMP activity, lung macrophage infiltration and protects against emphysema in COPD. *Thorax* 66, 970–976. doi: 10.1136/thx.2011.159087
22. Hirata, H., Takahashi, A., Kobayashi, S., Yonehara, S., Sawai, H., Okazaki, T., et al. (1998). Caspases are activated in a branched protease cascade and control distinct downstream processes in Fas-induced apoptosis. *J. Exp. Med.* 187, 587–600. doi: 10.1084/jem.187.4.587
23. Holst, J. J., and Deacon, C. F. (2005). Glucagon-likepeptide-1mediatesthetherapeutic actions of DPP-IV inhibitors. *Diabetologia* 48, 612–615. doi: 10.1007/s00125-005-1705-7
24. Hsieh, P. W., Yu, H. P., Chang, Y. J., and Hwang, T. L. (2010). Synthesis evaluation of benzoxazinone derivatives on activity of human neutrophil elastase and on hemorrhagic shock-induced lung injury in rats. *Eur. J. Med. Chem.* 45, 3111–3115. doi: 10.1016/j.ejmech.2010.03.046
25. Iba, T., Kidokoro, A., Fukunaga, M., Takuhiro, K., Yoshikawa, S., Sugimotoa, K., et al. (2006). Pre-treatment of sivelestat sodium hydrate improves the lung microcirculation and alveolar damage in lipopoly saccharide induced acute lung inflammation in hamsters. *Shock* 26, 95–98. doi: 10.1097/01.shk.0000223126.34017.d9
26. Javidroozi, M., Zucker, S., and Chen, W. T. (2012). Plasma DPP4 levels as markers of disease and prognosis in cancer. *Dis. Mark.* 32, 309–320. doi: 10.1155/2012/706745
27. Jindal, S. K., Aggarwal, A. N., Chaudhry, K., Chhabra, S. K., D'Souza, G. A., Gupta, D., et al. (2006). A multicentric study on epidemiology of chronic obstructive pulmonary disease and its relationship with tobacco smoking and environmental tobacco smoke exposure. *Indian J. Chest Dis. Allied Sci.* 48, 23–29.
28. Jindal, S. K., Aggarwal, A. N., Gupta, D., Agarwal, R., Kumar, R., Kaur, T., et al. (2012). Indian study on epidemiology of asthma, respiratory symptoms and chronic bronchitis in adults (INSEARCH). *Int. J. Tuberc. Lung Dis.* 16, 1270–1277. doi: 10.5588/ijtld.12.0005
29. Johansson, S. L., Roberts, N. B., Schlosser, A., et al. (2014). Microfibrillar-associated protein 4: A potential biomarker of chronic obstructive pulmonary disease. *Respir. Med.* 108, 1336–1344. doi: 10.1016/j.rmed.2014.06.003
30. Johnson, S. R. (2016). Untangling the protease web in COPD: metalloproteinases in the silent zone, *Thorax* 71, 105–106. doi: 10.1136/thoraxjnl-2015-208204 Jormsjö, S., Ye, S., Walter, D. H., Moritz, J., Dimmeler, S., Zeiher, A. M., et al. (2000). Allele-specific regulation of matrix metalloproteinase-12 gene activity is associated with coronary artery luminal dimensions in diabetic patients with manifest coronary artery disease. *Circ. Res.* 86, 998–1003. doi: 10.1161/01.RES.86.9.998
31. Kalkana, T., Moitra, S., Jindal, S. K., and Moitra, S. (2016). Increasing burden of COPD in rural India: an example why India warrants primary healthcare reforms. *ERJ Open Res.* 13:2. doi: 10.1183/23120541.00032-2016
32. Kidokoro, Y., Kravis, T. C., Moser, K. M., Taylor, J. C., and Crawford, I. P. (1977). Relationship of leukocyte elastase concentration to severity of emphysema in homozygous alpha1-antitrypsin-deficient persons. *Am. Rev. Respir. Dis.* 115, 793–803.
33. Kishore, U., Greenhough, T. J., Waters, P., Shrive, A. K., Ghai, R., Kamran, M. F., et al. (2006). Surfactant proteins SP-A and SP-D: structure, function and receptors. *Mol. Immunol.* 43, 1293–1315. doi: 10.1016/j.molimm.2005.08.004
34. Koutsokera, A., Kostikas, K., Nicod, L. P., and Fitting, J.-W. (2013). Pulmonary Somborac-Bacˇura, A., Buljevicˇb, S., Rumora, L., Cˇ ulic´, O., Dijana, D.,

biomarkers in COPD exacerbations: a systematic review. *Respir. Res.* 14:111. doi: 10.1186/1465-9921-14-111
35. Kawabata, K., Suzuki, M., Sugitani, M., Imaki, K., Toda, M., and Miyamoto, T. (1991). ONO-5046, a novel inhibitor of human neutrophil elastase. *Biochem. Biophys. Res.* 177, 814–820.
36. Larrinaga, G., Blanco, L., Sanz, B., Perez, I., Gil, J., Unda, M., et al. (2012). The impact of peptidase activity on clear cell renal cell carcinoma survival. *Am. J. Physiol. Renal Physiol.* 303, F1584–F1591. doi: 10.1152/ajprenal.00477.2012
37. Lecaille, F., Kaleta, J., and Brömme, D. (2002). Human parasitic papain-like cysteine proteases: their role in physiology and pathology and recent developments in inhibitor design. *Chem. Rev.* 102, 4459–4488. doi: 10.1021/cr0101656
38. Lee, E. J., In, K. H., Kim, J. H., Lee, S. Y., Shin, C., Shim, J. J., et al. (2009). Proteomic analysis in lung tissue of smokers and COPD patients. *Chest* 135, 344–352. doi: 10.1378/chest.08-1583
39. Lee, K.-H., Lee, C.-H., Jeong, J., Jang, A.-H., and Yoo, C.-G. (2015). Neutrophil elastase differentially regulates IL-8 and VEGF production by cigarette smoke extract. *J. Biol. Chem.* 290, 28438–28445. doi: 10.1074/jbc.M115.6 63567
40. Legrand, C., Gilles, C., Zahm, J. M., Polette, M., Buisson, A. C., Kaplan, H., et al. (1999). Airway epithelial cell migration dynamics: MMP-9 Role in Cell–extracellular matrix remodeling. *J. Cell Biol.* 146, 517–529. doi: 10.1083/jcb.146.2.517
41. Linder, R., Rönmark, E., Pourazar, J., Behndig, A., Blomberg, A., and Lindberg, A. (2015). Serum metalloproteinase-9 is related to COPD severity and symptoms - cross-sectional data from a population based cohort-study. *Respir. Res.* 16, 28. doi: 10.1186/s12931-015-0188-4
42. Lomas, D. A., Silverman, E. K., Edwards, L. D., Locantore, N. W., Miller, B. E., Horstman, D. H., et al. (2009). Serum surfactant protein D is steroid sensitive and associated with exacerbations of COPD. *Eur. Respir. J.* 34, 95–102. doi: 10.1183/09031936.00156508
43. Murray, C. J. L., and Lopez, A. D. (1999). *Global Burden of Disease and Injury Series: Global Health Statistics: A Compendium of Incidence, Prevalence, and Mortality Estimates for Over 200 Conditions,* Vol. 2. Cambridge, MA: Harvard School of Public Medicine.
44. Muzio, M., Stockwell, B. R., Stennicke, H. R., and Salvesen, G. S. (1998). Dixit VM: an induced proximity model for caspase-8 activation. *J. Biol. Chem.* 273, 2926–2930. doi: 10.1074/jbc.273.5.2926
45. NIREH (2014). *NIREH, Annual Report, 2013-14: 13-14.* NIREH.
46. Pandey, K. C., Wang, S. X., Sijwali, P. S., Lau, A. L., McKerrow, J. H., and Rosenthal,
47. P. J. (2005). The Plasmodium falciparum cysteine protease falcipain-2 captures its substrate, hemoglobin, via a unique motif. *Proc. Natl. Acad. Sci. U.S.A.* 102, 9138–9143. doi: 10.1073/pnas.0502368102
48. Perlmutter, D. H. (1996). Alpha-1-antitrypsin deficiency: biochemistry and clinical manifestations. *Ann. Med.* 28, 385–394. doi: 10.3109/07853899608999097
49. Peto, R., Chen, Z.-M., and Boreham, J. (1999). Tobacco—the growing epidemic. *Nat. Med.* 5, 15–17. doi: 10.1038/4691
50. Prakash, A., Babu, K. S., and Morjaria, J. B. (2013). Novel anti-cholinergics in COPD drug discovery today. 18, 1117–1126. doi: 10.1038/bjp.2008.284
51. Qiu, Y., Zhu, J., Bandi, V., Atmar, R. L., Hattotuwa, K., Guntupalli, K. K., et al. (2003). Biopsy neutrophilia, neutrophil chemokine and receptor gene expression in severe exacerbations of chronic obstructive pulmonary disease. *Am. J. Respir. Crit. Care Med.* 168, 968–975. doi: 10.1164/rccm.200208-794OC
52. Ray, N. C., Finch, H., Edwards, C., and O'Connor, E. (2010). *Tetrahydropyrrolo-Pyrimidinediones and their Use as Human Neutrophil Elastase Inhibitors.* EP2024367B1.
53. Salminen-Mankonen, H. J., Morko, J., and Vuorio, E. (2007). Role of cathepsin K in normal joints and in the development of arthritis. *Curr. Drug Targets* 8, 315–323. doi: 10.2174/138945007779940188
54. Salvi, S., and Agarwal, A. (2012). India needs a national COPD prevention and control program. *J. Assoc. Phys. India* 60(Suppl.), 5–7.
55. Schade, J., Stephan, M., Schmiedl, A., Wagner, L., Niestroj, A. J., Demuth, H.-U., et al. (2008). Regulation of expression and function of dipeptidyl peptidase4 (DP4),DP8/9,and DP10 in allergic responses of the lung in rats. *J. Histochem. Cytochem.* 56, 147–155. doi: 10.1369/jhc.7A7319.2007
56. Sinha, B., Vibha., Singla, R., Chowdhury, R. (2017). An epidemiological profile of chronic obstructive pulmonary disease: a community-based study in Delhi. *J. Post Grad. Med.* 63, 29–35. doi: 10.4103/0022-3859.194200
57. Somborac-Ba˘cura, A., Buljevi˘cb, S., Rumora, L., ˘ Culi´c, O., Dijana, D., et al. (2012). Decreasedsoluble dipeptidyl peptidase IV activity as a potential serum biomarker for COPD. *Clin. Biochem.* 45, 1245–1250. doi: 10.1016/j.clinbiochem.2012.04.023
58. Tsai, Y.-F., and Hwang, T.-L. (2015). Neutrophil elastase inhibitors: a patent review and potential applications for inflammatory lung diseases (2010 – 2014). *Expert Opin. Ther. Pat.* 25, 1145–1158. doi: 10.1517/13543776.2015.10 61998
59. Uh, S.-T., Ko, S. A., Jang, A. S., Park, S. W., Kim, Y.-H., Paik, Y.- K., et al. (2012). Comparison of protein profiles in sputum between COPD and acute exacerbation of COPD. *Open J. Respir. Dis.* 2, 25–30. doi: 10.4236/ojrd.2012.22004
60. Van den Steen, P. E., Dubois, B., Nelissen, I., Rudd, P. M., Dwek, R. A., and Opdenakker, G. (2002). Biochemistry and molecular biology of gelatinase B or matrix metalloproteinase-9 (MMP-9). *Crit. Rev. Biochem. Mol. Biol.* 37, 375–536. doi: 10.1080/10409230290771546
61. Vandivier, R. W., Fadok, V. A., Hoffmann, P. R., Bratton, D. L., Penvari, C., Brown, K. K., et al. (2002). Elastase-mediated phosphatidylserine receptor cleavage impairs apoptotic cell clearance in cystic fibrosis and bronchiectasis. *J. Clin. Invest.* 109, 661–670. doi: 10.1172/JCI0213572
62. Verma, S., Dixit, R., and Pandey, K. C. (2016). Cysteine proteases: modes of activation and future prospects as pharmacological targets. *Front. Pharmacol.* 7:107. doi: 10.3389/fphar.2016.00107
63. Vestbo, J., Agusti, A., Wouters, E. F., Bakke, P., Calverley, P. M., Celli, B., et al. (2014). Evaluation of COPD longitudinally to identify predictive surrogate endpoints (ECLIPSE) study investigators. Should we view COPD differently after ECLIPSE? A clinical perspective from the study team. *Am. J. Respir. Crit. Care Med.* 189, 1022–1030. doi: 10.1164/rccm.201311- 2006PP
64. Vijayan, V. K. (2013). Chronic obstructive pulmonary disease. *Indian J. Med. Res.* 137, 251–269.
65. Von Nussbaum, F., Karthaus, D., Anlauf, S., Delbeck, M., Volkhart Min-Jian, L., Daniel, M., et al. (2012). *4-(4-Cyano-2-Thioaryl) Dihydropyrimidinones and their Use.* US8288402B2.
66. Wada, Y., Yoshida, K., Hihora, J., Konishi, K., Tanabe, K., Ukon, K., et al. (2006). Sivelestat, a specific neutrophil elastase inhibitor, suppresses the growth of gastric carcinoma cells by preventing the release of transforming growth factor-Alfa. *Cancer Sci.* 97, 1037–1043. doi: 10.1111/j.1349-7006.2006.00278.x
67. Yasuda, N., Gotoh, K., Minatoguchi, S., Asano, K., Nishigaki, K., Nomura, M., et al. (1998). Fujiwara H: an increase of soluble Fas, an inhibitor of apoptosis, associated with progression of COPD. *Respir. Med.* 92, 993–999.

21

Herbal Medicine Compared to Placebo for Chronic Obstructive Pulmonary Disease

Chan-Young Kwon[1†]*, Boram Lee*[2†]*, Beom-Joon Lee*[3]*, Kwan-Il Kim*[3*] *and Hee-Jae Jung*[3*]

[1]*Department of Oriental Neuropsychiatry, Dong-eui University College of Korean Medicine, Busan, South Korea,* [2]*Department of Clinical Korean Medicine, Graduate School, Kyung Hee University, Seoul, South Korea,* [3]*Division of Allergy, Immune and Respiratory System, Department of Internal Medicine, College of Korean Medicine, Kyung Hee University, Seoul, South Korea*

***Correspondence:**
Kwan-Il Kim
myhappy78@naver.com
Hee-Jae Jung
hanfish@khmc.or.kr

†*These authors have contributed equally to this work and share first authorship*

Chronic obstructive pulmonary disease (COPD) is a respiratory disease characterized by irreversible airflow limitation. Many COPD patients use complementary and alternative modalities, including herbal medicines (HMs). This systematic review investigated the effectiveness and safety of HM in managing COPD symptoms compared to placebo. Nine electronic databases were searched to identify relevant randomized controlled trials (RCTs) up to February 12, 2021. The Cochrane risk of bias tool was used to assess the methodological qualities of the included studies. Primary outcomes were lung function parameters and exercise capacity. A meta-analysis was conducted to determine the effect size for homogeneous outcomes. Fourteen studies were included. There was low to very low quality evidence that HM significantly improved forced expiratory volume in 1 s (FEV1) (L), FEV1 (%) and 6-minute walk distance, as well as moderate quality evidence that HM significantly improved forced vital capacity (FVC) (L) compared to placebo. However, according to low quality evidence, there was no significant difference in FEV1/FVC (%) or vital capacity (L) between the groups. Low to moderate evidence suggests that HM has the potential to help improve some respiratory functions, COPD symptoms, and some aspects of quality of life in COPD patients compared to placebo. However, these findings are challenged by the poor methodological quality of the included studies, the heterogeneity of HMs used, and potential publication bias. Therefore, the findings could be significantly influenced by further larger, more rigorous RCTs on this topic. Moreover, it may also be recommended to develop standardized HMs focused on some individual herbs that are frequently used or expected to play an important role in patients with COPD, and to elucidate the underlying mechanisms.

Keywords: COPD, east asian traditional medicine, chronic bronchitis, emphysema, systematic review

---

Abbreviations: AECOPD, acute exacerbation of chronic obstructive pulmonary disease; CAT, chronic obstructive pulmonary disease assessment test; CI, confidence interval; COPD, chronic obstructive pulmonary disease; EATM, East Asian traditional medicine; FEV1, forced expiratory volume in 1 s; FVC, forced vital capacity; GRADE, grading of recommendations assessment development and evaluations; HM, herbal medicine; IL, interleukin; MD, mean difference; mMRC, the modified Medical Research Council; PRISMA, preferred reporting items for systematic reviews and meta-analyses; RCT, randomized controlled trial; RR, risk ratio; SGRQ, St. George respiratory questionnaire; TER, total effective rate; TGF, transforming growth factor; TNF, tumor necrosis factor; VC, vital capacity; WHOQOL-BREF, World Health Organization quality of life instruments-abbreviated version; 6MWD, 6-min walk distance.

INTRODUCTION

Chronic obstructive pulmonary disease (COPD), including chronic bronchitis and emphysema, is a respiratory disease characterized by irreversible airflow limitation that causes symptoms like chronic cough, phlegm, and dyspnea (Singh et al., 2019). COPD is relatively more common in men than in women, and its prevalence is estimated to be approximately 16% in men and 10% in women worldwide (Varmaghani et al., 2019). The most common risk factor for COPD is smoking, with toxic chemicals, air pollution, and chronic bronchitis being the other causes contributing to damage to the airways and lung parenchyma by chronic inflammation (Singh et al., 2019). In addition, older age, being underweight or obese, and low economic and social status are considered to be relevant risk factors (Osman et al., 2017).

Treatment of COPD can be broadly classified into the initial and follow-up phases (Singh et al., 2019). Pharmacological treatments include long-acting bronchodilators, long-acting muscarinic antagonists, inhaled corticosteroids, long-acting β2-agonist, or their combination, depending on respiratory ability and frequency of exacerbation (Singh et al., 2019). Moreover, quitting smoking is an important lifestyle modification to prevent exacerbations in COPD patients (Ambrosino and Bertella, 2018). Comorbidities, such as cardiovascular disease, osteoporosis, poor sleep quality, and depression, can adversely affect the health of COPD patients; therefore, these conditions should be treated concurrently (Recio Iglesias et al., 2020).

The main treatment for COPD involves bronchodilators, which can improve patients' respiratory symptoms and quality of life, and prevent exacerbation; however, this therapeutic strategy alone is not effective enough and does not cure the underlying etiology. Therefore, pulmonary rehabilitation, long-term oxygen therapy, and phosphodiesterase-4 inhibitors be additionally used (Candela et al., 2019). In this respect, herbal medicine (HM) can also be considered an effective adjuvant therapy for COPD. The various active ingredients contained in HM, particularly flavonoid derivatives, have the potential to exert therapeutic effects on the underlying pathology of COPD by reducing inflammation in the lungs (Kim et al., 2017). Moreover, a systematic review published in 2014 concluded that HM can improve the clinical symptoms and quality of life of patients with COPD based on 15 high quality studies (Chen et al., 2014). However, evidence in this area is not yet established, and the authors conclude that, in particular, double-blind randomized controlled trials (RCTs) are needed (Chen et al., 2014).

A well-designed placebo control is needed for successful double-blind RCTs using HM. Unlike chemical drugs, HM can be described by its characteristics of taste and aroma, which poses a challenge for successful blinding of participants. However, there has not yet been a comprehensive review of the effectiveness and safety of HM for COPD compared to placebo from this perspective. Therefore, this systematic review and meta-analysis was conducted to investigate the effectiveness and safety of HM in managing COPD symptoms compared to placebo.

METHODS

The protocol of this study was pre-registered with OSF registries (10.17605/OSF.IO/3EJD2). This systematic review complied with the Preferred Reporting Items for Systematic Reviews and Meta-Analyses (PRISMA) 2010 statement (**Supplementary File S1**) (Moher et al., 2009).

Data Sources and Search Strategy

One researcher (BL) searched nine electronic databases, including three core ones (Medline via PubMed, EMBASE *via* Elsevier, and Cochrane Central Register of Controlled Trials), one database related to complementary and alternative medicine (Allied and Complementary Medicine Database), two Korean databases (Korean Studies Information Service System and Korea Citation Index), and three Chinese databases (China National Knowledge Database, WanFang data, and VIP). The search date was February 12, 2021. All relevant studies published up to the search date were considered without language and publication status limitations. Grey literature consisting of dissertations and conference papers was also included. In addition, the bibliographic list of the relevant articles was reviewed and missing data related to the potentially relevant studies were collected through manual searches on Google Scholar. Finally, the search strategy was confirmed through sufficient discussions with experts on systematic reviews and clinical experts on COPD. The search strategies and results from each database are listed in **Supplementary File S2**.

Eligibility Criteria

The inclusion criteria for this review were as follows. **1) Type of study:** Only RCTs were included in this review. **2) Types of participants:** Adult patients (over 18 years of age) diagnosed with COPD were included, regardless of sex, COPD stage, and status of exacerbations. Patients with COPD and other pathological conditions were excluded from the study. Studies including people with COPD and other respiratory diseases (e.g., asthma COPD overlap syndrome) were also excluded. **3) Types of interventions:** Only oral HM based on East Asian traditional medicine (EATM) theory was considered. There were no restrictions on the dosage form of HM. It was allowed when usual care or other active interventions for COPD were applied to the treatment and control groups at the same time. Studies that used a single herb or an ingredient extracted from one herb as their intervention or used HM not based on the EATM theory were excluded. **4) Types of controls:** We only allowed oral placebo HM as a control. In this review, placebo HM refers to a substance in which the difference in taste, aroma, and texture from active HM cannot be discerned. Studies that did not describe a similarity between placebo and original HM in taste or aroma as well as visual characteristics were excluded. **5) Types of outcomes:** Primary outcomes included lung function parameters (e.g., forced expiratory volume in 1 s [FEV1], forced vital capacity [FVC], FEV1/FVC, or vital capacity [VC]) and exercise capacity (6-min walk distance [6MWD]). Secondary outcomes included severity of dyspnea (e.g., the modified Medical Research Council [mMRC] dyspnea scale, or other assessment tools such as patient-reported measures, self-assessment, questionnaires, etc.), quality of life (COPD assessment test [CAT], other assessment tools such as the St. George respiratory questionnaire [SGRQ]), and adverse events or safety measurements. Studies that did not report outcomes of interest, especially those that did not report respiratory function or respiratory symptoms, were excluded.

Study Selection

After removing duplicate studies, two researchers (CYK and BL) independently screened the titles and abstracts of the searched studies to check for eligibility. Then, the full-texts of the screened studies were reviewed by two researchers (CYK and BL) for inclusion in this review. Discrepancies were resolved by discussion with a third researcher (KIK). EndNote X8 (Clarivate Analytics, Philadelphia, United States) was used to manage the bibliographic information.

Data Extraction

The extracted data from the eligible studies by two researchers (CYK and BL) were entered into a pre-defined Microsoft Excel file. Microsoft Excel 2016 (Microsoft, Redmond, WA, United States) was used for the data extraction. The following items were extracted: name of the first author, publication year, publication country, study setting, sample size and withdrawals, details of participants, details of treatment and control interventions, outcome measures, safety data, information for assessment of the risk of bias, and funding sources. Discrepancies were resolved by discussion of the researchers (CYK and BL), or if needed, with a third researcher (KIK).

Risk of Bias Assessment

The Cochrane risk of bias tool was used to assess the methodological quality of the included RCTs. In this tool, the methodological quality of RCTs is evaluated in terms of risk of bias, including random sequence generation, allocation concealment, blinding of participants, personnel and outcome assessors, completeness of outcome data, selective reporting, and other biases (Higgins et al., 2011). Each bias item is evaluated as "low risk," "unclear risk," or "high risk" (10). Quality assessment was performed by two independent researchers (CYK and BL). Discrepancies were resolved by discussion with a third researcher (KIK).

Data Analysis and Synthesis

All included studies were descriptively analyzed. If enough homogeneous data existed, meta-analysis was performed using RevMan 5.4 (The Cochrane Collaboration, London, England). Dichotomous data were presented as risk ratios (RRs) with 95% confidence intervals (CIs) while continuous data were reported as mean difference (MD) with 95% CIs. Heterogeneity between the studies in terms of effect measures was assessed using both the χ^2 test and the I^2 statistic. I^2 values ≥50% and ≥75% were considered indicative of substantial and considerable heterogeneity, respectively. Meta-analysis was performed using a random-effects model if the included studies had significant heterogeneity (I^2 value ≥50%). When the heterogeneity was not significant or the number of studies included in the meta-analysis was very small, in which the estimate of the between-study variance had poor precision, a fixed-effect model was used (Graves, 2002). Subgroup analysis was conducted by classifying COPD patients according to the condition, including stable COPD, acute exacerbation of COPD (AECOPD), and treatment duration (≤ 4 weeks or ≥2 months). In addition, a sensitivity analysis was conducted, excluding studies that did not properly conduct the blinding of participants and personnel.

Dealing With Missing Data

The authors contacted the corresponding author via email regarding unclear information in the study. If data were still insufficient after contacting the corresponding author or if contact was impossible, only the available data were included in the analysis.

Publication Bias

If the number of studies included in the meta-analysis was 10 or more, a funnel plot was used to assess potential publication bias.

Quality of Evidence

Two researchers (CYK and BL) assessed the quality of evidence for the main findings using the Grading of Recommendations, Assessment, Development and Evaluations (GRADE) approach (Balshem et al., 2011). The risk of bias of the studies included in each meta-analysis, imprecision, inconsistency, indirectness of the results, and relevant publication bias were evaluated for each finding. The quality of evidence is categorized into four categories, as follows: "high," "moderate," "low," or "very low."

RESULTS

Study Selection

Of the 1,643 documents searched initially, titles and abstracts of 1,112 were screened, excluding duplications. Consequently, 148 potentially relevant papers were selected. Upon reviewing the full-text of these studies, one RCT not using placebo, one conference proceeding without detailed research data, one secondary analysis of RCT, one using a single herb rather than complex HM, 124 with unclear differences between active HM and placebo without obvious differences in taste or aroma (e.g., using caramel placebo), one using duplicated data, and five with unavailable full-texts were excluded (**Supplementary File S3**). Finally, 14 RCTs were included in this systematic review and meta-analysis (**Figure 1**) (Li et al., 2011; Liu, 2011; Guo et al., 2014; Liu et al., 2014; Wang et al., 2014; Chen, 2015; Shi, 2016; Gao et al., 2017; Hong, 2018; Huang et al., 2019; Jin et al., 2019; Luo et al., 2019; Hu et al., 2020).

Study Characteristics

The included studies were published between 2011 and 2020, all of which were conducted in China. Eight (Liu, 2011; Sun, 2013; Guo et al., 2014; Wang et al., 2014; Shi, 2016; Hong, 2018; Jin et al., 2019; Hu et al., 2020) involved patients with stable COPD, while four (Li et al., 2011; Liu et al., 2014; Huang et al., 2019; Luo

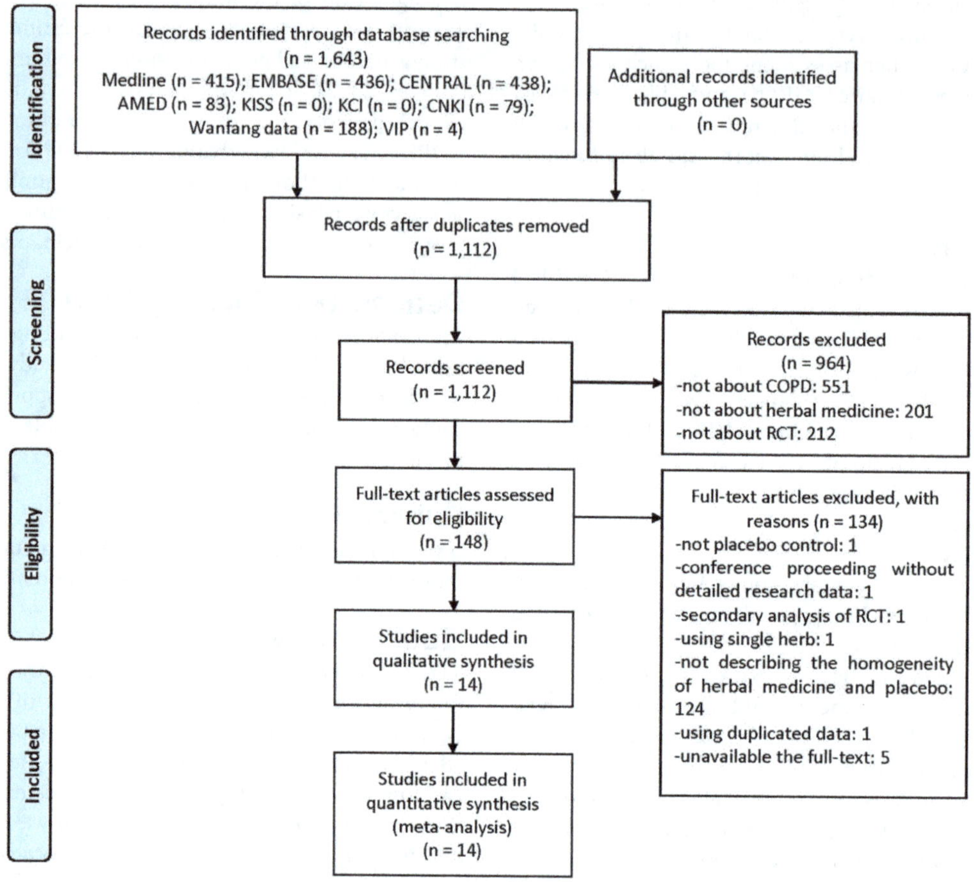

FIGURE 1 | A PRISMA flow diagram of the literature screening and selection process. AMED, Allied and Complementary Medicine Database; CENTRAL, Cochrane Central Register of Controlled Trials; CNKI, China National Knowledge Infrastructure; COPD, chronic obstructive pulmonary disease; KCI, Korea Citation Index; KISS, Koreanstudies Information Service System; RCT, randomized controlled trial.

et al., 2019) involved patients with AECOPD. For the other two RCTs (Chen, 2015; Gao et al., 2017), the subjects' COPD status were unclear. In one study, Wang et al. (2014) compared two HMs and one placebo in a three-arm clinical trial. Therefore, we separated and extracted the effects of the two HMs used in this study into Wang 2014(A) and Wang 2014(B). In all studies, the study setting was a hospital, and eight studies (Li et al., 2011; Liu, 2011; Guo et al., 2014; Liu et al., 2014; Wang et al., 2014; Chen, 2015; Huang et al., 2019; Jin et al., 2019; Luo et al., 2019; Hu et al., 2020) that identified the source of funding were supported by national or provincial funding. All studies performed conventional therapies, such as health education and Western medication therapy, including inhaled albuterol and long-acting bronchodilators, to all participants. Eight studies (Guo et al., 2014; Liu et al., 2014; Wang et al., 2014; Chen, 2015; Hong, 2018; Huang et al., 2019; Jin et al., 2019; Hu et al., 2020) were approved by the institutional review board prior to study initiation, and 12 studies (Liu, 2011; Sun, 2013; Guo et al., 2014; Liu et al., 2014; Wang et al., 2014; Chen, 2015; Shi, 2016; Hong, 2018; Huang et al., 2019; Jin et al., 2019; Luo et al., 2019; Hu et al., 2020) received informed consent from participants. The published articles did not confirm whether other studies were approved by the institutional review board or an informed consent was received from the participants. Twelve studies (Sun, 2013; Guo et al., 2014; Liu et al., 2014; Wang et al., 2014; Chen, 2015; Shi, 2016; Gao et al., 2017; Hong, 2018; Huang et al., 2019; Jin et al., 2019; Luo et al., 2019) recruited participants according to specific pattern identification, of which deficiency of specific organs was the most common, seen in five studies (Sun, 2013; Wang et al., 2014; Chen, 2015; Shi, 2016; Jin et al., 2019); phlegm-heat or phlegm-turbidity obstructing the lungs in three studies (Liu et al., 2014; Gao et al., 2017; Luo et al., 2019); blood stasis in two studies (Li et al., 2011; Huang et al., 2019); and deficiency of the lung, spleen, and kidney with retention of phlegm and blood stasis in two studies (Guo et al., 2014; Hong, 2018). Nine studies (Liu, 2011; Sun, 2013; Guo et al., 2014; Liu et al., 2014; Wang et al., 2014; Chen, 2015; Shi, 2016; Hong, 2018; Hu et al., 2020) reported the occurrence of adverse events during the clinical trial period. Detailed study characteristics of the included studies are summarized in **Supplementary Table S1.**

Details of HM Used

A wide variety of HMs were used in the included studies. With regard to dosage type, decoction was the most common in six studies (Sun, 2013; Chen, 2015; Shi, 2016; Gao et al., 2017; Huang et al., 2019; Jin et al., 2019), followed by granules in five studies (Li et al., 2011; Liu, 2011; Guo et al., 2014; Liu et al., 2014; Hong, 2018). In general, *Poria cocos (Schw.) Wolf [*Polyporaceae; *Poria(Hoelen)*] and *Citrus unshiu Markovich [*Rutaceae; *Citri unshius pericarpium]* were the most frequently used herbs in six studies, followed by *Codonopsis pilosulae (Fr.) Nannf [*Campanulaceae; *Codonopsis pilosulae radix], Atractylodes macrocepha-la Koidz [*Asteraceae; *Atractylodis rhizoma alba],* and *Glycyrrhiza uralensis Fisch [*Leguminosae; *Glycyrrhizae radix]* in five studies each. To evaluate stable COPD, *Codonopsis pilosulae (Fr.) Nannf [*Campanulaceae; *Codonopsis pilosulae radix]* was used the most in five studies, followed by *Atractylodes macrocepha-la Koidz [*Asteraceae; *Atractylodis rhizoma alba], Poria cocos (Schw.) Wolf [*Polyporaceae; *Poria(Hoelen)*], *Cornus officinalis Sieb. et Zucc [*Cornaceae; *Corni fructus], Rehmannia glutinosa (Gaertner) Libosch [*Scrophulariaceae; *Rehmanniae radix preparat], Citrus unshiu Markovich [*Rutaceae; *Citri unshius pericarpium]*, and *Astragalus membranaceus Bunge [*Leguminosae; *Astragali radix]* in three studies each. Herbs were not commonly used in more than three studies on AECOPD. Instead, *Paeonia lactiflora Pallas [*Paeoniaceae; *Paeoniae radix], Prunus persica (L.) Batsch [*Rosaceae; *Persicae semen], Rheum palmatum L [*Polygonaceae; *Rhei radix et rhizoma], Prunus armeniaca L.* var. *ansu Maxim [*Rosaceae; *Armeniacae semen], Pinellia ternata (Thunb.) Breit [*Araceae; *Pinelliae rhizoma], Poria cocos (Schw.) Wolf [*Polyporaceae; *Poria(Hoelen)*], and *Citrus unshiu Markovich [*Rutaceae; *Citri unshius pericarpium]* were used in two studies. In three studies (Li et al., 2011; Chen, 2015; Gao et al., 2017), herbs were added to the basic HM prescription according to specific symptoms or pattern identification. The period of HM administration varied widely from day 10–180. In particular, studies on AECOPD had relatively short treatment periods ranging from 10 to 14 days. Four studies (Liu, 2011; Guo et al., 2014; Wang et al., 2014; Hu et al., 2020) performed follow-up after the completion of HM administration, and the duration varied from 4 months to 1 year (**Supplementary Table S2**).

Risk of Bias Assessment

Ten studies (Li et al., 2011; Liu, 2011; Guo et al., 2014; Liu et al., 2014; Wang et al., 2014; Gao et al., 2017; Hong, 2018; Huang et al., 2019; Jin et al., 2019; Hu et al., 2020) using appropriate random number generation methods, such as random number tables, were evaluated as having a low risk of bias in the random sequence generation domain. Three studies (Liu et al., 2014; Hong, 2018; Hu et al., 2020) using opaque sealed envelopes to conceal allocation were evaluated as having a low risk of bias in the allocation concealment domain. Eight (Li et al., 2011; Liu, 2011; Guo et al., 2014; Liu et al., 2014; Wang et al.; Chen, 2015; Hong, 2018; Jin et al., 2019) and two studies (Liu, 2011; Liu et al., 2014) properly blinded participants and personnel as well as outcome assessors, respectively. Four studies (Liu, 2011; Guo et al., 2014; Wang et al., 2014; Hong, 2018) that performed only per-protocol analysis were evaluated as having a high risk of attrition bias, and one study (Jin et al., 2019) that presented only the total effective rate (TER) without raw data was evaluated as having a high risk of reporting bias (**Figure 2**).

Effectiveness and Safety of HM for COPD

Lung Function (Primary Outcome)

Post-treatment, there were significant differences between the HM and placebo groups in FEV1 (L) (eight studies; MD 0.14, 95% CI 0.03 to 0.24; I^2 = 79%), FEV1 (%) (10 studies; MD 4.46, 95% CI 1.93 to 6.99; I^2 = 54%), and FVC (L) (four studies; MD 0.22, 95% CI 0.12 to 0.31; I^2 = 16%). In subgroup analysis, however, the significant benefits of HM were observed in FEV1 (L) and FEV1 (%) only for AECOPD when the treatment duration was ≤ 4 weeks. They were not observed for stable COPD when the treatment duration was ≥2 months. The significant benefits of FVC (L) were maintained according to the COPD status and treatment duration, regardless of the subgroup. In FEV1/FVC (%) (seven studies; MD 1.91, 95% CI −0.72 to 4.55; I^2 = 58%), and VC (L) (two studies; MD 0.00, 95% CI −0.18 to 0.18; I^2 = 0%), significant difference was not observed according to COPD status and treatment duration, regardless of the subgroup. In the sensitivity analysis excluding studies not properly conducting blinding of participants and personnel, the significant effect on FEV1 (L) (five studies; MD 0.11, 95% CI −0.02 to 0.24; I^2 = 77%) and FEV1 (%) (seven studies; MD 3.49, 95% CI −0.10 to 7.08; I^2 = 63%) disappeared, and the results of the remaining outcomes were not significantly affected (**Supplementary Table S3**) (**Figures 3A–E**).

Exercise Capacity (Primary Outcome)

At post-treatment, HM group showed significantly better 6MWD (m) (six studies; MD 35.82, 95% CI 15.26 to 56.38; I^2 = 78%). In subgroup analysis, however, the significant benefits of 6MWD of HM remained for AECOPD and unclear COPD when the treatment duration was ≤ 4 weeks, but not for stable COPD when the treatment duration was ≥2 months. In the sensitivity analysis excluding studies not properly conducting blinding of participants and personnel, the significant effect on 6MWD remained (four studies; MD 38.48, 95% CI 22.52 to 54.45; I^2 = 85%) (**Supplementary Table S3**) (**Figure 3F**).

Symptom Severity (Secondary Outcome)

At post-treatment, the HM group showed significantly lower mMRC scores (two studies; MD −1.13, 95% CI, −1.21 to −1.05; I^2 = 94%). In subgroup analysis, however, the significant benefits on the mMRC score of HM remained for AECOPD, but not for stable COPD. In stable COPD patients, the frequency of acute exacerbation at the 1-year follow-up was significantly lower in the HM group than in the placebo group (two studies; MD −0.60, 95% CI −0.69 to −0.51; I^2 = 0%). In the sensitivity analysis, excluding studies not properly conducting blinding of participants and personnel, the significant effect on the frequency of acute exacerbation in the 1-year follow-up remained (one study; MD −0.60, 95% CI −0.69 to −0.51). The HM group showed significantly higher TER based on clinical symptoms (10 studies; RR 1.26, 95% CI 1.11 to 1.44; I^2 = 76%). The significant benefits of TER were maintained according to COPD status and treatment duration, regardless of the subgroup.

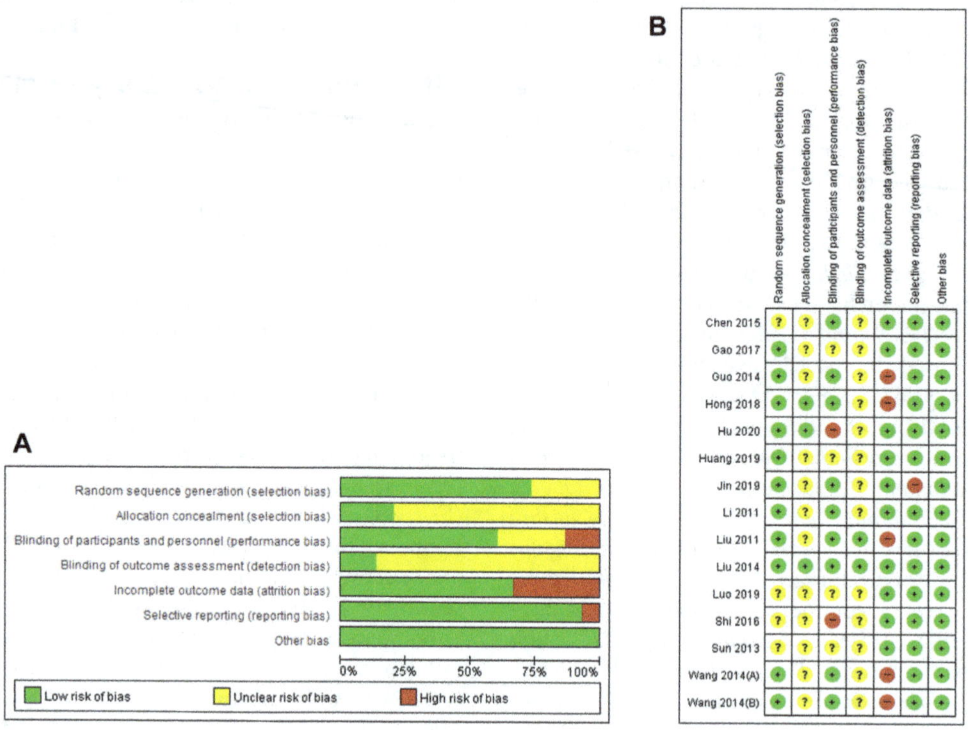

FIGURE 2 | Risk of bias for all included studies. Low, unclear, and high risk, respectively, are represented with the following symbols: "+," "?" and "–".

However, in the sensitivity analysis excluding studies not properly conducting blinding of participants and personnel, the significant effect of HM on TER disappeared on stable COPD (three studies; RR 1.80, 95% CI 0.88 to 3.65; I^2 = 95%) and AECOPD (one study; RR 1.08, 95% CI 0.92–1.27) (**Supplementary Table S3**).

Quality of Life (Secondary Outcome)

Post-treatment, the HM group showed significantly lower CAT scores (five studies; MD −3.78, 95% CI −5.73 to −1.83; I^2 = 78%) and SGRQ scores (six studies; MD −7.56, 95% CI −14.4 to −0.72; I^2 = 93%) than the placebo group. In the subgroup analysis, however, the significant benefits on CAT score of HM remained for stable COPD and AECOPD, but not for unclear COPD. In addition, the significant benefits of the SGRQ score of HM were not retained for both stable COPD and AECOPD. In the World Health Organization quality of life instruments-abbreviated version (WHOQOL-BREF), the psychological domain was significantly higher in the HM group (three studies; MD 0.99, 95% CI 0.35 to 1.64; I^2 = 66%). Subgroup analysis according to COPD status and treatment duration showed a significant difference between groups only in AECOPD when the treatment duration was ≤ 4 weeks, but not in stable COPD when the treatment duration was ≥2 months. The social relationships domain of WHOQOL-BREF was significantly lower in the HM group (one study; MD −0.83, 95% CI −1.55 to −0.11). However, there were no differences in physical health (one study; MD 0.46, 95% CI −0.23 to 1.15) and in the environment domain (one study; MD −0.04, 95% CI −0.72 to 0.64). There was no significant difference detected in the sensitivity analysis excluding studies that did not properly conduct blinding of participants and personnel (**Supplementary Table S3**).

Safety Data

There were no significant differences between the HM and placebo groups in the incidence of adverse events (eight studies; RR 1.08, 95% CI 0.51 to 2.28; I^2 = 22%). This non-significance was maintained according to COPD status and treatment duration, regardless of the subgroup. In addition, in the sensitivity analysis excluding studies that did not properly conduct blinding of participants and personnel, this non-significance still remained (**Supplementary Table S3**). The adverse events reported in the HM group were cold limbs (1 case), lip color turning red (1 case), glycosuria (1 case), diarrhea (1 case), and proteinuria (1 case) in one study (Liu, 2011) and sweating (1 case) in another study (Shi, 2016). Hong (2018) reported a case in the HM group in which the color of the sputum changed from thick white to light yellow. Two studies (Liu et al., 2014; Hu et al., 2020) reported adverse reactions in six cases and diarrhea in two cases in the HM group.

Impact of HM on Inflammation-Related Parameters

Despite the lack of pre-defined outcomes of interest, some studies have reported an effect of HM on inflammation-related parameters in COPD patients. A study by Guo et al. (2014), in

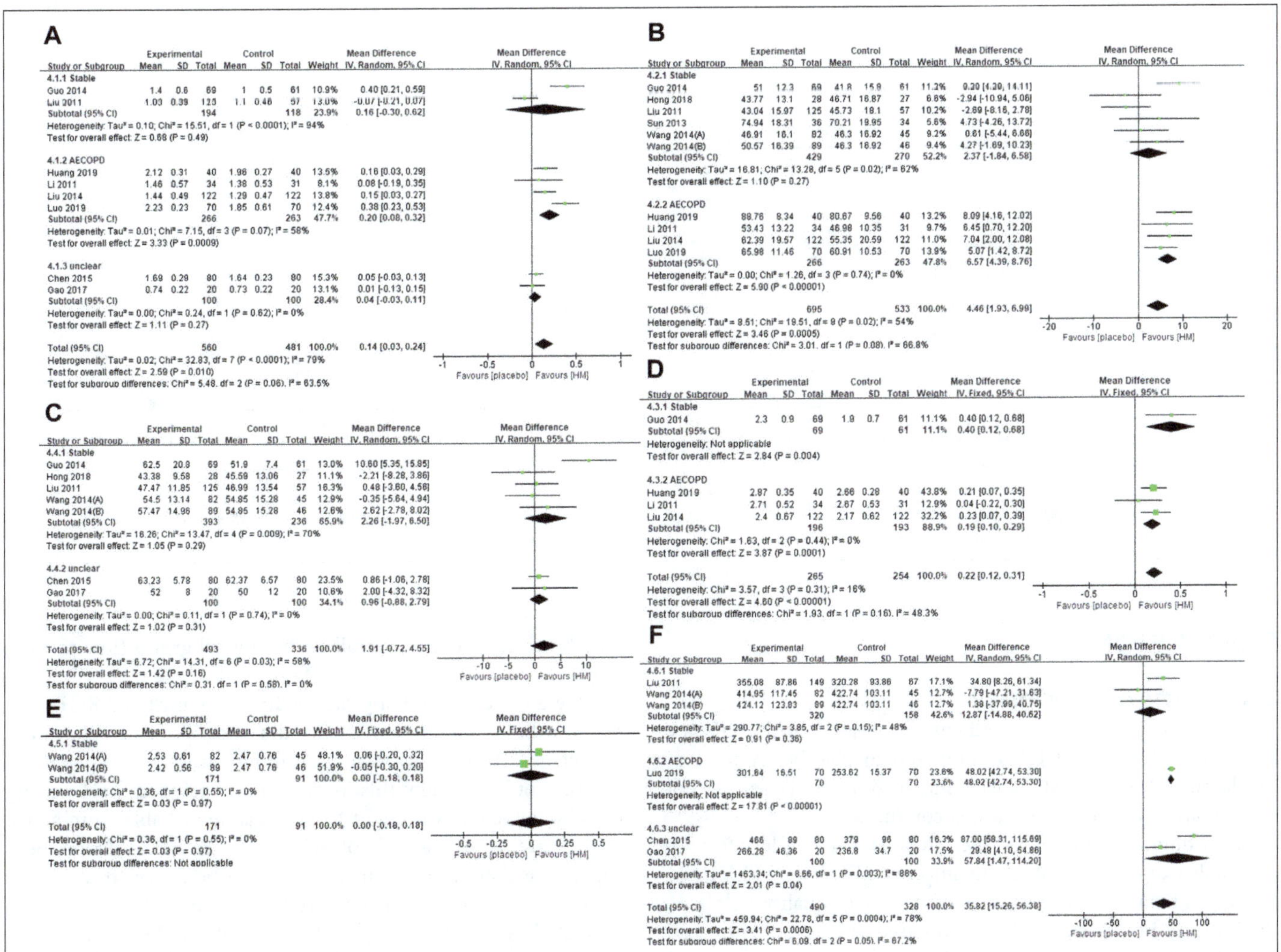

FIGURE 3 | Forest plots of **(A)** FEV1 (L), **(B)** FEV1 (%), **(C)** FEV1/FVC (%), **(D)** FVC (L), **(E)** VC (L), and **(F)** 6MWD. AECOPD, acute exacerbations of chronic obstructive pulmonary disease; FEV1, forced expiratory volume in one second; FVC, forced vital capacity; VC, vital capacity; 6MWD, 6-min walking distance.

which patients with stable COPD were administered Bufei granules for 12 weeks reported that serum interleukin (IL)-6, IL-8, tumor necrosis factor (TNF)-α, and transforming growth factor (TGF)-β1 after treatment were not significantly different between the two groups ($p > 0.05$). However, IL-8, TNF-α, and TGF-β1 decreased significantly only in the HM group ($p < 0.05$). A study by Sun (2013), in which patients with stable COPD were administered Sijunzi-tang combined with Jinkui Shenqi pills for 4 weeks, serum IL-8 levels in the HM group after treatment were significantly lower than those in the placebo group ($p < 0.05$). However, there was no significant difference in serum TNF-α levels between the groups ($p > 0.05$). In a study by Wang et al. (2014), in which patients with stable COPD were administered Bushen Yiqi granules or Bushen Fangchaun tablets for 180 days, serum IL-17 levels in the two HM groups were significantly lower than those in the placebo group (both, $p < 0.05$). However, there were no significant differences in other parameters, including serum IL-6, IL-8, IL-10, IL-1β, TGF-β1, TNF-α, and cortisol between groups (all, $p > 0.05$). In a study by Huang et al. (2019), in which patients with AECOPD were administered Mengshiguntan-wan for 2 weeks, levels of IL-17 and 8-iso-prostaglandins in exhaled breath condensates were significantly lower than those in the placebo group (both, $p < 0.05$), while the levels of IL-10 in exhaled breath condensates were significantly higher than those in the placebo group ($p < 0.05$).

Publication Bias

Funnel plot evaluation was possible only for FEV1 (%) and TER based on clinical symptoms. All of them showed obvious asymmetries, suggesting a potential publication bias (**Figures 4A,B**).

Quality of Evidence

The quality of evidence for the main results was mostly "very low" to "moderate". The reason for downgrading was the high risk of bias of the included studies, inconsistency of results due to high heterogeneity, and imprecision of results due to wide CIs and small sample sizes (**Supplementary Table S3**).

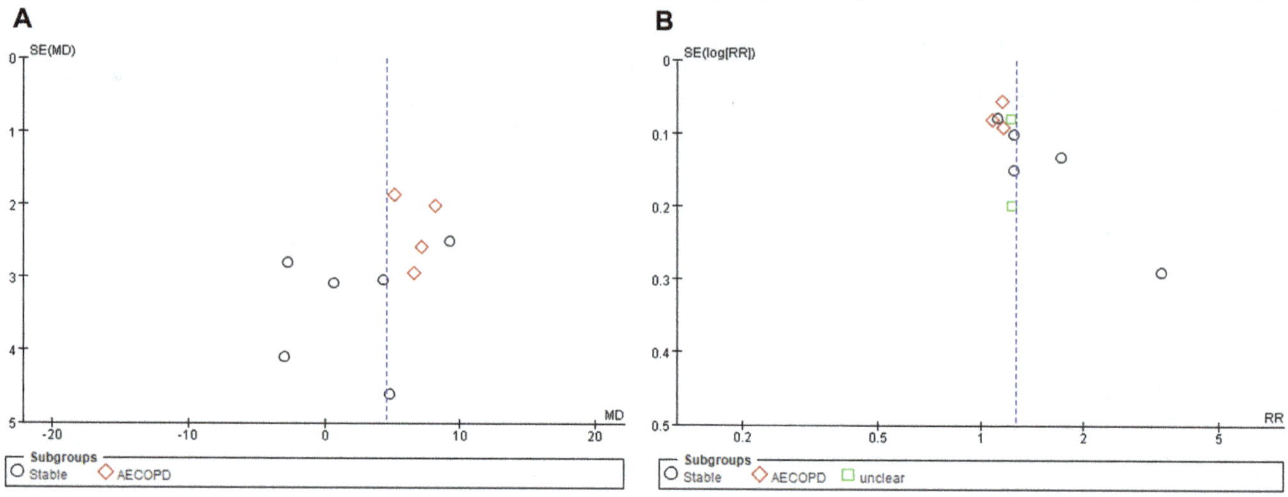

FIGURE 4 | Funnel plots of **(A)** FEV1 (%) and **(B)** TER based on clinical symptoms. AECOPD, acute exacerbations of chronic obstructive pulmonary disease; FEV1, forced expiratory volume in one second; TER, total effective rate.

DISCUSSION

Summary of Evidence

This systematic review comprehensively evaluated the efficacy and safety of HM in COPD compared to placebo. A total of 14 placebo-controlled RCTs were included in this review, and a meta-analysis of 16 outcomes was conducted.

According to the findings, there was evidence of low to very low quality that HM significantly improved FEV1 (L), FEV1 (%) and 6MWD, as well as evidence of moderate quality that HM significantly improved FVC (L) compared to placebo. However, according to evidence of low quality, there was no significant difference in FEV1/FVC (%) or VC (L) between the groups. Interestingly, in subgroup analysis according to COPD status and treatment duration, significant improvements in the use of HM in AECOPD patients were observed when the treatment duration was ≤ 4 weeks, but not for stable COPD when the treatment duration was ≥2 months. HM significantly reduced the severity of dyspnea evaluated by mMRC in AECOPD patients (high quality), but not in stable COPD patients (low quality), compared to placebo. The HM group showed significantly better TER (low quality; high quality) and CAT (low quality; high quality) than the placebo group in both stable COPD and AECOPD, regardless of the treatment duration. In addition, HM significantly lowered the frequency of acute exacerbations in patients with stable COPD compared to placebo (moderate quality). HM showed significant improvement in SGRQ compared to placebo in the total sample (low quality), but no significant improvement in stable COPD (very low quality) or AECOPD (moderate quality) in the subgroup analysis. Regarding quality of life, HM significantly improved the psychological domain evaluated by WHOQOL-BREF compared to placebo in AECOPD (high quality), but the opposite was seen in terms of social relationships (high quality). Regarding adverse events, no significant differences were observed between the HM and placebo groups, either overall or in any subgroup (low to high quality).

Overall, the methodological quality of the included RCTs was not the best, and in particular, the description of allocation concealment and assessor blinding was inadequate or insufficient. Although this review only included RCTs using placebo, which was thought to be indistinguishable from active HM, there is still a risk of selection bias or detection bias, suggesting that skewed conclusions may be drawn from actual results. In addition, most of the results of the quality of evidence evaluated as GRADE were low to moderate, and the evidence of high quality was insufficient. Therefore, the findings of this review are likely to be significantly affected by the subsequent implementation of larger RCTs with higher methodological quality. At the same time, however, the findings of this review show that low or moderate levels of evidence revealed that HM is likely to improve respiratory function in COPD patients, especially AECOPD patients; reduce acute exacerbation in patients with stable COPD; and improve COPD symptoms compared to placebo.

Clinical Implications

Research shows that many COPD patients prefer complementary and alternative medicine (CAM) modalities (Abadoglu et al., 2008; Şahin and Şahin 2013). HM is a representative CAM modality, but in terms of evidence-based medicine, high quality evidence is needed to draw conclusions about its use for COPD (Chen et al., 2014). The findings in this review show that HM has the potential to help improve some respiratory functions, COPD symptoms, and some aspects of quality of life in COPD patients compared to placebo. Moreover, although not our outcome of interest, some RCTs included provided biological outcomes suggesting the anti-inflammatory effects of HM in COPD patients. This is consistent with recent findings suggesting the underlying mechanism of HM in COPD

(Santana et al., 2016; Kim et al., 2017; Yang et al., 2020). In addition, flavonoids, alkaloids, and terpenoids, which are major components of several HMs, have the potential to positively affect COPD through various mechanisms, such as lessening of inflammation and oxidative stress, inhibition of cellular senescence, restoration of corticosteroid sensitivity, and improvement of pulmonary histology as well as pulmonary function (Santana et al., 2016; Yang et al., 2020). The possible underlying therapeutic mechanisms of HM shared with conventional medicine for COPD may raise expectations for a positive synergistic effect in treating COPD, but, conversely, may raise concerns about herb-drug interactions (Pao et al., 2012). Although our review suggests that HM has the potential to improve some outcomes of COPD patients prior to placebo, in clinical settings, it may not only have synergistic effects with conventional medicine for COPD, but may also have potentially negative herb-drug interaction which should be further studied before making recommendations regarding the use of HM in COPD patients. Moreover, the findings in this review suggest that HM may improve some aspects of respiratory function, especially in AECOPD patients. Given that conventional medicine could be a major treatment strategy in AECOPD patients, studies regarding herb-drug interactions could further encourage or hinder the use of HM in this population. However, the effect of HM in reducing acute exacerbation in stable COPD patients seem to be steadily garnering much research attention.

Strengths and Limitations

The strength of this systematic review is that it was comprehensive and was conducted without limiting the participants' COPD status. It was also a critical review conducted only on studies using placebo interventions that could be recognized as meaningful. However, due to the following limitations, the findings of this review should be interpreted with caution:

First, the methodological quality of the included studies was not the best. Although this review included only RCTs with placebo HM, in which the difference in taste, aroma, and texture from active HM cannot be discerned, most included RCTs were still not free from the risk of selection bias and detection bias. **Second**, all included studies were conducted in China. Considering that HM based on EATM theory is mostly implemented in East Asian countries such as China, Japan, Korea, and Taiwan, this is not a strange result, but regionally uneven publication hinders generalization of the results. In addition, visual asymmetry was observed in the funnel plot of the two outcomes, suggesting potential publication bias. This suggests that a pre-registered, larger, more rigorous RCT is needed for this topic in the future, which ideally should be evenly distributed regionally, ethnically, and racially. **Third**, the HMs used in the included studies were heterogeneous, suggesting the necessity of developing and using standardized HM. In recent years, for example, standardized HMs such as PM014 have been developed, and further clinical research is expected (Jung et al., 2013). Moreover, some frequently used herbs for treating COPD, including *Poria cocos (Schw.) Wolf* [Polyporaceae; *Poria(Hoelen)*] and *Citrus unshiu Markovich [*Rutaceae; *Citri unshius pericarpium]* found in this review, can be considered in the development of standardized HMs, such as PM014. Moreover, some herbs that were frequently used in studies on stable and unclear COPD including *Codonopsis pilosulae (Fr.) Nannf* [Campanulaceae; *Codonopsis pilosulae radix]*, *Atractylodes macrocepha-la Koidz* [Asteraceae; *Atractylodis rhizoma alba]*, *Cornus officinalis Sieb. et Zucc* [Cornaceae; *Corni fructus]*, *Rehmannia glutinosa (Gaertner) Libosch* [Scrophulariaceae; *Rehmanniae radix preparat]*, and *Astragalus membranaceus Bunge* [Leguminosae; *Astragali radix]* were not used in studies on AECOPD. *Codonopsis pilosulae (Fr.) Nannf.* [Campanulaceae; *Codonopsis pilosulae radix]* was the most frequently used herb only in studies on stable COPD. In contrast, *Carthamus tinctorius L.* [Asteraceae; *Carthami flos]*, *Pheretima aspergillum (E. Perrier)* [Lumbricidae; *Lumbricus corpus]*, *Sinapis alba L* [Brassicaceae; *Sinapis semen]*, and *Raphanus sativus L.* [Brassicaceae; *Raphani semen]* were the only herbs used in studies on AECOPD. The differential use of these herbs may be considered clinically for COPD and the development of standardized HMs. Further, small number of studies were included and the use of HM was heterogeneous; therefore, it was difficult to analyze the effect of each of these herbs on the individual symptoms of COPD. The heterogeneity of the HM may be due to the broad intervention criteria established in this review. Future research may try to further analyze focused on frequently used HMs, HMs containing specific important herbs, or standardized HMs. It is expected that the findings of this review can be used as a reference in this further research. **Fourth**, among the included studies, most have specified the status of COPD, such as stable COPD or AECOPD, but there were also studies that did not. However, these two conditions differ pathologically, and it is likely that some of the outcomes may show differences in the treatment responsiveness of HM according to our results. Thus, future studies should require a clear description of the participants' COPD status. **Fifth**, we included studies describing the similarity between placebo and original HM with regard to taste or aroma as well as visual characteristics for only high-quality trials having a minimal relevant performance bias. However, studies might not fully explain the homogeneity of HM and placebo, resulting in the exclusion of a significant number of large-scale studies from the study selection process. Therefore, the inclusion of these studies may have affected the results of this study. **Sixth**, in the 14 trials, three of them used HMs with additional components; however, reports were not found on how they and the corresponding placebo were manufactured and blinded. Emails were sent to the authors to confirm this; however, no response was received. Therefore, caution is needed when interpreting the results of these studies. **Finally**, most of the included studies described the quality control of the used HM, but only a study by Wang et al. (2014) reported chemical analysis of HM. However, the included studies are HMs composed of multiherbs, and chemical analysis such as high performance liquid chromatography needs to be performed and reported to explore its potential mechanism. In future studies, it is highly recommended not only to standardize the composition of HM, but also to report the component analysis results.

CONCLUSION

According to the results of this systematic review, very low to moderate evidence suggests that HM has the potential to help improve some COPD patients' respiratory functions, especially those with AECOPD; COPD symptoms; and quality of life compared to placebo. However, these findings are challenged by the poor methodological quality of the included studies, the heterogeneity of HMs used, and potential publication bias. Therefore, the findings could be significantly influenced by further larger, more rigorous RCTs on this topic. Moreover, it may also be recommended to develop standardized HMs focused on some individual herbs that are frequently used or expected to play an important role in patients with COPD, and to elucidate the underlying mechanisms.

assessment were conducted by C-YK and BL. The manuscript was drafted by C-YK and BL and revised by K-IK, B-JL, and H-JJ. All authors have read and approved the final manuscript.

REFERENCES

1. Abadoglu, O., Cakmak, E., and Kuzucu Demir, S. (2008). The View of Patients with Asthma or Chronic Obstructive Pulmonary Disease (COPD) on Complementary and Alternative Medicine. *Allergol. Immunopathol (Madr)* 36, 21–25. doi:10.1157/13115667
2. Ambrosino, N., and Bertella, E. (2018). Lifestyle Interventions in Prevention and Comprehensive Management of COPD. *Breathe (Sheff)* 14, 186–194. doi:10.1183/20734735.018618
3. Balshem, H., Helfand, M., Schünemann, H. J., Oxman, A. D., Kunz, R., Brozek, J., et al. (2011). GRADE Guidelines: 3. Rating the Quality of Evidence. *J. Clin. Epidemiol.* 64, 401–406. doi:10.1016/j.jclinepi.2010.07.015
4. Candela, M., Costorella, R., Stassaldi, A., Maestrini, V., and Curradi, G. (2019). Treatment of COPD: the Simplicity Is a Resolved Complexity. *Multidiscip. Respir. Med.* 14, 18. doi:10.1186/s40248-019-0181-8
5. Chen, H. Y., Ma, C. H., Cao, K.-J., Chung-Man Ho, J., Ziea, E., Wong, V. T., et al. (2014). A Systematic Review and Meta-Analysis of Herbal Medicine on Chronic Obstructive Pulmonary Diseases. *Evid. Based Complement. Alternat. Med.* 2014, 925069. doi:10.1155/2014/925069
6. Chen, R. M. (2015). Clinical Trial Study on Treatment of Chronic Obstructive Pulmonary Disease (Lung Qi Deficiency Type) by Lifei Yishen Decoction. *Chin. Traditional Patent Med.* 37, 2565–2567. doi:10.3969/j.issn.1001-1528.2015.11.055
7. Gao, X., Shen, Y., and Gong, X. Y. (2017). Clinical Study on Modified Dingchuan Decoction in Treating 40 Cases of Chronic Obstructive Pulmonary Disease. *Asia-Pacific Traditional Med.* 13, 148–149. doi:10.11954/ytctyy.201702065
Graves, R. S. (2002). Users' Guides to the Medical Literature: a Manual for Evidence-Based Clinical Practice. *J. Med. Libr. Assoc.* 90, 483.
8. Guo, S., Sun, Z., Liu, E., Feng, J., Fu, M., Li, Y., et al. (2014). Effect of Bufei Granule on Stable Chronic Obstructive Pulmonary Disease: a Randomized, Double Blinded, Placebo-Controlled, and Multicenter Clinical Study. *J. Tradit. Chin. Med.* 34, 437–444. doi:10.1016/s0254-6272(15)30043-1
9. Higgins, J. P. T., Altman, D. G., and Sterne, J. A. C. (2011). "Chapter 8: Assessing Risk of Bias in Included Studies,," in *Cochrane Handbook for Systematic Reviews of Interventions Version 5.1.0.* Editors J. P. T. Higgins and S. Green (London: The Cochrane Collaboration).
10. Hong, M. L. (2018). *Study on TCM Syndrome Elements Distribution and Miscellaneous Characteristics and Effects of Yufeining Prescription on TCM Syndrome Elements in Patients with Stable COPD.* Dissertation. Fuzhou: Fujian University of Traditional Chinese Medicine.
11. Hu, W. P., Wu, X. D., Li, Z. Z., and Zhang, J. (2020). Preventive Effects of Qingfei Yihuo Capsules () on Air Pollution Associated Exacerbation of Chronic Obstructive Pulmonary Disease: a Single-Blind, Randomized, Controlled Trial. *Chin. J. Integr. Med.* 26, 806–811. doi:10.1007/s11655-020-3321-2
12. Huang, M. R., Yang, Y. P., Xu, Z. B., and He, F. (2019). Effect of Pengshi Guntan Pills on IL-17, IL-10, 8-Iso-PG of Exhaled Air Condensate in Patients with Acute Exacerbation of Chronic Obstructive Pulmonary Disease. *Traditional Chin. Med. J.* 18 (18), 40–43. doi:10.14046/j.cnki.zyytb2002.2019.02.016
13. Jin, J., Li, F. S., Li, Z., Xu, D., Jing, J., and Wang, J. (2019). Effects of Yiqi Gubiao Pills on Expressions of miRNA of Low FFMI COPD Patients. *China J. Inf. TCM* 26, 16–22. doi:10.3969/j.issn.1005-5304.2019.05.004
14. Jung, K. H., Haam, K. K., Park, S., Kim, Y., Lee, S. R., Lee, G., et al. (2013). The Standardized Herbal Formula, PM014, Ameliorated Cigarette Smoke-Induced Lung Inflammation in a Murine Model of Chronic Obstructive Pulmonary Disease. *BMC Complement. Altern. Med.* 13, 219. doi:10.1186/1472-6882- 13-219
15. Kim, H. P., Lim, H., and Kwon, Y. S. (2017). Therapeutic Potential of Medicinal Plants and Their Constituents on Lung Inflammatory Disorders. *Biomol. Ther. (Seoul).* 25, 91–104. doi:10.4062/biomolther.2016.187
16. Li, J. S., Li, B., Yu, X. Q., Chen, P., Hou, Z. K., Li, S. Y., et al. (2011). Clinical Effect Evaluation on Herbs for Promoting Blood Circulation and Removing Blood
17. Stasis (活血化瘀) in Treatment of Acute Exacerbation of Chronic Obstructive Pulmonary Disease with Blood Stasis Syndrome (血瘀证). *Chin. J. TCM. WM. Crit. Care* 18, 9–13.
18. Liu, M., Zhong, X., Li, Y., Zheng, F., Wu, R., Sun, Y., et al. (2014). Xuan Bai Cheng Qi Formula as an Adjuvant Treatment of Acute Exacerbation of Chronic Obstructive Pulmonary Disease of the Syndrome Type Phlegm-Heat Obstructing the Lungs: a Multicenter, Randomized, Double-Blind, Placebo-Controlled Clinical Trial. *BMC Complement. Altern. Med.* 14, 239. doi:10.1186/1472-6882-14-239
19. Liu, Y. (2011). Chronic Obstructive Pulmonary Disease Stabilization Traditional Chinese Medicine Combined Efficacy Evaluation Model of the Preliminary Discussion. Master's thesis. Guangzhou: Guangzhou University of Chinese Medicine.
20. Luo, G., Mo, C., Yuan, G., Yang, Z., and Chen, Y. (2019). Effect of Modified Sanzi Yangqin Decoction on IL-32 Expression in Patients with Acute Exacerbation of Chronic Obstructive Pulmonary Disease. *China Mod. Doctor* 57, 13–15. , 20.
21. Moher, D., Liberati, A., Tetzlaff, J., and Altman, D. G. (2009). Preferred Reporting Items for Systematic Reviews and Meta-Analyses: the PRISMA Statement. *Plos Med.* 6, e1000097. doi:10.1371/journal.pmed.1000097
22. Osman, S., Ziegler, C., Gibson, R., Mahmood, R., and Moraros, J. (2017). The Association between Risk Factors and Chronic Obstructive Pulmonary Disease in Canada: a Cross-Sectional Study Using the 2014 Canadian Community Health Survey. *Int. J. Prev. Med.* 8, 86. doi:10.4103/ijpvm.IJPVM_330_17
23. Pao, L. H., Hu, O. Y., Fan, H. Y., Lin, C. C., Liu, L. C., and Huang, P. W. (2012). Herb- drug Interaction of 50 Chinese Herbal Medicines on CYP3A4 Activity *In Vitro* and *In Vivo*. *Am. J. Chin. Med.* 40, 57–73. doi:10.1142/S0192415X1250005X
24. Recio Iglesias, J., Díez-Manglano, J., López García, F., Díaz Peromingo, J. A., Almagro, P., and Varela Aguilar, J. M. (2020). Management of the COPD Patient with Comorbidities: an Experts Recommendation Document. *Int. J. Chron. Obstruct. Pulmon. Dis.* 15, 1015–1037. doi:10.2147/COPD.S242009
25. Şahin, Z. A., and Şahin, M. (2013). The View of Patients with Choronic Obstructive Pulmonary Disease (COPD) on Complementary and Alternative Medicine (CAM) in Eastern Turkey. *Afr. J. Tradit. Complement. Altern. Med.* 10, 116–121. doi:10.4314/ajtcam.v10i4.19
26. Santana, F. P. R., Pinheiro, N. M., Mernak, M. I. B., Righetti, R. F., Martins, M. A., Lago, J. H. G., et al. (2016). Evidences of Herbal Medicine-Derived Natural Products Effects in Inflammatory Lung Diseases. *Mediators Inflamm.* 2016, 2348968. doi:10.1155/2016/2348968
27. Shi, S. Q. (2016). *Yiqi Yangxin Dingzhi Fixed Determination Method to Improve the State of the Anxiety of Patients with Chronic Obstructive Pulmonary Disease Clinical Research.* Beijing: China Academy of China Medical Sciences. master's thesis.
28. Singh, D., Agusti, A., Anzueto, A., Barnes, P. J., Bourbeau, J., Celli, B. R., et al. (2019). Global Strategy for the Diagnosis, Management, and Prevention of Chronic Obstructive Lung Disease: the GOLD Science Committee Report 2019. *Eur. Respir. J.* 53, 1900164. doi:10.1183/13993003.00164-2019
29. Sun, Q. (2013). *Strengthening the Spleen and Invigorating the Kidney in Patients with Chronic Obstructive Pulmonary Disease in Stable Period the Influence of the Content IL-8and TNF-α.* master's thesis. Chengdu: Chengdu University of Traditional Chinese Medicine.
30. Varmaghani, M., Dehghani, M., Heidari, E., Sharifi, F., Moghaddam, S. S., and

Farzadfar, F. (2019). Global Prevalence of Chronic Obstructive Pulmonary Disease: Systematic Review and Meta-Analysis. *East. Mediterr. Health J.* 25, 47–57. doi:10.26719/emhj.18.014

31. Wang, G., Liu, B., Cao, Y., Du, Y., Zhang, H., Luo, Q., et al. (2014). Effects of Two Chinese Herbal Formulae for the Treatment of Moderate to Severe Stable Chronic Obstructive Pulmonary Disease: a Multicenter, Double-Blind, Randomized Controlled Trial. *PLoS One* 9, e103168. doi:10.1371/journal.pone.0103168
32. Yang, Y., Jin, X., Jiao, X., Li, J., Liang, L., Ma, Y., et al. (2020). Advances in Pharmacological Actions and Mechanisms of Flavonoids from Traditional Chinese Medicine in Treating Chronic Obstructive Pulmonary Disease. *Evid. Based Complement. Alternat. Med.* 2020, 8871105. doi:10.1155/2020/ 8871105

22

Subjective and Objective Outcomes in Patients with COPD after Pulmonary Rehabilitation – The Impact of Comorbidities

Maria Charikiopoulou[1,2], Pantelis Theodoros Nikolaidis[3], Beat Knechtle[4], Thomas Rosemann[4], Aggeliki Rapti[1,2] and Georgia Trakada[5]*

[1] Pulmonary Rehabilitation Department, General Hospital for Chest Diseases of Athens "SOTIRIA", Athens, Greece, [2] 2nd Pulmonary Department, General Hospital for Chest Diseases of Athens "SOTIRIA", Athens, Greece, [3] Exercise Physiology Laboratory, Nikaia, Greece, [4] Institute of Primary Care, University of Zurich, Zurich, Switzerland, [5] Division of Pulmonology, Department of Clinical Therapeutics, School of Medicine, Alexandra Hospital, National and Kapodistrian University of Athens, Athens, Greece

***Correspondence:**
Beat Knechtle
beat.knechtle@hispeed.ch

Background: Chronic obstructive pulmonary disease (COPD) is a heterogeneous disease with multiple systemic manifestations and comorbidities, which contribute independently to its total morbidity and mortality. Pulmonary rehabilitation is an evidence-based intervention that is indicated for COPD patients who remain symptomatic, despite optimal pharmacological therapy. Although it is well documented in pure COPD, the role of pulmonary rehabilitation is uncertain in coexisting comorbidities. The aim of the present study was to clarify the effect of a pulmonary rehabilitation program in COPD patients with concomitant comorbidities.

Methods: Thirty two patients with COPD were evaluated before and after a comprehensive pulmonary rehabilitation program, in terms of dyspnea, quality of life (QOL), pulmonary function tests and exercise capacity. The patients were also divided into two groups, according to the presence or the absence of comorbidities. Patients with none or only one comorbidity (Group 1, $n = 11$) were compared to those who had two or more comorbidities (Group 2, $n = 21$).

Results: All patients significantly improved in dyspnea, as expressed by modified Medical Research Council scale and the COPD assessment Test ($p < 0.001$), QOL as assessed by the St. George respiratory questionnaire ($p < 0.001$) and exercise tolerance in six minute walking test ($p < 0.001$). Peak oxygen uptake relatively increased and body mass decreased in Group 1 compared to Group 2 ($p < 0.05$).

Conclusion: Pulmonary rehabilitation in COPD seems to be beneficial for all patients, independently of the presence, the number or the nature of their comorbidities. Thus, the presence of comorbidities must not represent an exclusion criterion for patients that are referred to pulmonary rehabilitation programs.

Trial Registration: Current controlled trials ISRCTN14648515 Retrospectively registered 15 February 2018.

Keywords: dyspnea, quality of life, six minute walking test, cardiopulmonary exercise test, lung disease

INTRODUCTION

Chronic obstructive pulmonary disease (COPD) is a progressive disease associated with significant morbidity and mortality. The latest Global Initiative for Obstructive Lung Disease (GOLD) defines the disease as: "A common preventable and treatable disease, characterized by persistent airflow limitation that is usually progressive and associated with an enhanced chronic inflammatory response in the airways and the lung to noxious particles or gases. Exacerbations and comorbidities contribute to the overall severity in individual patients" (Global strategy for the diagnosis, management and prevention of COPD, global initiative for chronic obstructive lung disease (GOLD), 2016).

Several studies demonstrate that 86–98% of COPD patients have at least one comorbidity, with the average number per individual varying between from 1.2 to 4.0 (Putcha et al., 2013, 2015). Comorbidities often contribute to dyspnea, limitation of exercise capacity, deterioration of quality of life (QOL), increased healthcare utilization and cost, and increased exacerbation and mortality risk (Patel and Hurst, 2011). COPD patients are more likely to die from a comorbid disease than COPD itself, as "only 40% of the deaths are definitely or probably related to COPD, with the remainder being mostly unrelated to COPD (50%) or unknown (9%)" (McGarvey et al., 2007). Based on this evidence, current guidelines for the management of COPD, besides treating chronic airflow limitation with traditional pharmacological therapy, adopt a more holistic approach by incorporating the assessment and appropriate treatment of comorbid diseases in order to ameliorate the health status and the prognosis of the patients (GOLD Global strategy for the diagnosis, management and prevention of COPD, global initiative for chronic obstructive lung disease (GOLD), 2016).

Common comorbidities in patients with COPD include cardiovascular disease (CVD) (such as arterial hypertension, systemic venous thromboembolism (VTE), stroke, heart failure, coronary heart disease, arrhythmias and pulmonary hypertension), lung cancer and other cancers, psychiatric diseases (such as anxiety and depression disorders), metabolic conditions (such as malnutrition, obesity, diabetes mellitus, dyslipidemia), anemia, osteoporosis, musculoskeletal dysfunction, sleep disorders and gastroesophageal reflux (Patel and Hurst, 2011). Some of these comorbidities (pulmonary artery disease and malnutrition) are directly caused by COPD (secondary to COPD), whereas others share common risk factors, such as lifestyle factors (e.g., smoking), environmental exposures (place of work, air pollution etc.), and genetic susceptibility, and are associated with similar pathophysiological mechanisms, like airway and systemic inflammation, lung hyperinflation and endothelial dysfunction and oxidative stress (Patel and Hurst, 2011).

Pulmonary rehabilitation is an evidence-based intervention that is indicated for COPD patients who remain symptomatic – despite optimal pharmacological therapy – to reduce dyspnea, increase exercise capacity and improve QOL (Spruit et al., 2013). Exercise training is the best available way of improving muscle function and exercise tolerance in patients with COPD (Wu et al., 2017). Moreover, regular physical activity is recommended and is beneficial for patients with CVD, musculoskeletal disease, obesity, diabetes mellitus and most other chronic medical conditions (Ciolac, 2013). However, a review on this topic concluded inconsistent data about pulmonary rehabilitation outcomes in COPD patients with comorbidities (Franssen and Rochester, 2014). For instance, patients with multiple comorbidities would present limited benefits from their participation in pulmonary rehabilitation (Crisafulli et al., 2008), whereas most comorbidities were not related to rehabilitation outcomes (Crisafulli et al., 2010). In most studies reported in the abovementioned review, outcomes were evaluated with functional exercise capacity as measured by six minute walking test (6MWT) and not with peak oxygen uptake (VO_2peak) as measured during incremental exercise. Some studies proved worse outcomes in patients with cardiovascular, metabolic or psychological comorbid conditions, whereas others did not confirm this or reported opposite effects (Franssen and Rochester, 2014). Such knowledge would be of great practical value for practitioners working with COPD as it would allow them prescribing optimal pulmonary rehabilitation programs.

Therefore, the aim of our study was to further clarify pulmonary rehabilitation outcomes in stable COPD patients with coexisting comorbidities, in terms of specific diseases and total number. The principal end points were QOL, degree of dyspnea and aerobic capacity. We assessed exercise capacity using both 6MWT and VO_2peak, in order to evaluate possible differences in results between the two methods.

MATERIALS AND METHODS

Thirty two patients with COPD (25 men and 7 women, age 66 ± 6 years, body mass index (BMI) 27.14 ± 4.88 kg/m^2) (**Table 1**), sample of convenience, were selected for the present study from our outpatient clinics in the Division of Pulmonology, to the Department of Clinical Therapeutics of the National and Kapodistrian University of Athens School of Medicine, at Alexandra Hospital of Athens. COPD was diagnosed by history, physical examination, and standard pulmonary function tests according to GOLD criteria (Global strategy for the diagnosis, management and prevention of COPD, global initiative for chronic obstructive lung disease (GOLD), 2016). Also, at baseline each patient underwent detailed general medical history – including the number, the type and the medications of other coexisting diseases. Finally, each patient signed a written informed consent and the study protocol was approved by the Ethical Committee of our hospital. The study adheres to the CONSORT criteria (**Figure 1**). All data are available in the **Supplementary Material**.

Eligible participants were 25 men and 7 women, with mean age 66 ± 6 years-old (range: 49–76) who met the following inclusion criteria: (1) COPD diagnosis of any stage (A, B, C, D), (2) stable

---

Abbreviations: 6MWT, six minute walking test; ATS, American Thoracic Society; BMI, body mass index; CAT, COPD assessment test; COPD, chronic obstructive pulmonary disease; CPR, cardiopulmonary resuscitation; CVD, cardiovascular disease; GOLD, global initiative for obstructive lung disease; MRC, medical research council; QOL, quality of life; SGRQ, St. George respiratory questionnaire; VO_2peak, Peak oxygen uptake; VTE, systemic venous thromboembolism.

TABLE 1 | Baseline characteristics of participants.

Parameters	Total (n = 32)	Group 1 (n = 11)	Group 2 (n = 21)
Patients (number (%), males/females)	25 (78%)/7 (22%)	10 (91%)/1 (9%)	15 (71%)/6 (29%)
Age (years)	66.03 ± 6.03	64.36 ± 5.45	66.91 ± 6.26
BMI (kg/m^2)	27.14 ± 4.88	25.36 ± 4.73	28.07 ± 4.81
FEV_1 (L)	1.297 ± 0.605	1.09 ± 0.53	1.40 ± 0.63
FEV_1 (% predicted)	43.08 ± 15.07	35.78 ± 14.12	48.02 ± 15.16*
FEV_1/FVC (%)	51.67 ± 10.25	45.43 ± 6.93	54.94 ± 10.30*
RV/TLC (%)	54.87 ± 19.68	68.20 ± 28.98	47.76 ± 5.73*
TLCO (% predicted)	38.2 ± 22.8	21.7 ± 18.0	61.8 ± 20.0*
MRC	2.5 ± 0.9	2.5 ± 1.0	2.5 ± 0.9
CAT	16.9 ± 9.3	15.6 ± 5.7	17.5 ± 10.8
SGRQ	47.3 ± 19.0	41.1 ± 16.2	50.5 ± 20.0
GOLD Severity (number, A/B/C/D)	1/9/14/8	0/2/4/5	1/7/10/3
6MWT (m)	280 ± 81	297 ± 95	271 ± 74
Workload (W)	58.4 ± 31.5	56.1 ± 29.6	59.5 ± 33.1
VO_2peak (mL min^{-1} kg^{-1})	13.2 ± 4.1	16.9 ± 5.0	11.9 ± 3.7*

*BMI: Body Mass Index, FEV_1: Forced Expiratory Volume in 1 s, FVC: Forced Vital Capacity, RV: Residual Volume, TLC: Total Lung Capacity, TLCO: Diffusing Capacity, MRC: modified Medical Research Council scale, CAT: COPD Assessment Test, SGRQ: St. George Respiratory Questionnaire, GOLD: Global Strategy for the diagnosis, management, and prevention of COPD, 6MWT: 6 min Walking Test, VO_2peak: Peak Oxygen Uptake. *$p < 0.05$.*

condition, (3) optimal bronchodilation therapy, (4) optimal therapy of comorbidities, (5) reduced exercise capacity, and (6) completed successfully all parts of experimental intervention. Stable COPD was defined as no history of exacerbation in last 2 months prior to the study (Biswas et al., 2017).

The patient population was divided in two groups, according to the presence or the absence of comorbidities. The comorbidities were both self-reported and confirmed in the medical records of the patients. Patients with none or only one comorbidity (n = 11, Group 1) were compared to those who had two or more comorbidities (n = 21, Group 2), in terms of dyspnea, QOL and exercise capacity, before and after a pulmonary rehabilitation program. The characteristics of each group were presented in **Table 1**. The experimental intervention was administered twice a week, for 13 weeks between 1 November 2012 and 31 December 2014 at the Division of Pulmonology, Department of Clinical Therapeutics of the National and Kapodistrian University of Athens School of Medicine, at Alexandra Hospital of Athens. Comorbidities were assessed using patient-report of a physician diagnosis.

At baseline, each patient underwent clinical examination, arterial blood gases analysis (GEM Premier 3500, United States), and Pulmonary Function Tests (PFTs) (Master screen Diffusion, Jaeger, Germany): spirometry (pre/post-bronchodilation), diffusing capacity and static lung volumes. Dyspnea was assessed by both the modified Medical Research Council (MRC) scale (Simsic et al., 2018) and the COPD Assessment Test (CAT) (Jo et al., 2018). QOL was assessed by the St. George Respiratory Questionnaire (SGRQ) (Oliveira and Marques, 2017). BMI was calculated using patient's weight in kilograms (kg) divided by his or her height in meters squared.

Six minute walking test (Reychler et al., 2016) and standard cardiopulmonary exercise test (Ergoline Variable 500, Viasys Health Care, Jaeger, Germany) were also carried out, while breathing room air. Expiratory oxygen and carbon dioxide fractions, work rate, airflow, cardiac frequency and oxygen saturation were continuously recorded. The results were obtained (1) at rest, (2) after 1 min of unloaded exercise, and (3) during incremental exercise. The incrementation rate was 25 W per minute. The pedaling frequency was constant at 60 revolutions per min. Each patient exercised against progressive workloads up to symptom-limited, maximum exercise capacity. All indications to stop the test were known by the personnel involved in the testing. The procedure was performed under the supervision of a physician trained in conducting exercise tests and in advanced cardiopulmonary resuscitation (CPR). Full CPR equipment was available in the laboratory.

After the initial assessment, each patient started an individualized rehabilitation program, at the Pulmonary Rehabilitation Department of Sotiria Hospital, twice a week, for a period of 13 weeks (**Table 2**). The program included (1) interval, endurance exercise training using cycle ergometer to 100% of WRmax of each patient, switching between exercise and rest, for 40 min, (2) continuous endurance exercise training using treadmill for 10–20 min, (3) lower and upper extremity strengthening exercise training-conditioning using mainly weight lifting for 5–15 sets, (4) breathing retraining (pursed lips breathing technique) and (5) respiratory muscle training. Education, diet and psychological support were provided by specialized personnel during the experimental period. Other important therapeutic modalities that were stressed during the program included smoking cessation, oxygen therapy, and use of bronchodilators and antibiotics. At the end of the 13 weeks period of training, the patients were reassessed using the same testing protocol.

The values of all functional parameters were expressed as mean and standard deviation (M ± SD). An independent t-test examined differences between the two experimental groups. A between-within subjects analysis of variance examined the main effect of time and the time × group interaction on QOL, dyspnea and exercise tolerance. The magnitude of the differences between experimental groups was examined using effect size eta square (η^2) and was evaluated as following: small ($0.010 < \eta^2 \leq 0.059$), moderate ($0.059 < \eta^2 \leq 0.138$) and large ($\eta^2 > 0.138$) (Cohen, 1988). The correlations among the pre-post changes in exercise tolerance, dyspnea or QOL, and the baseline COPD stage were examined using the Spearman correlation coefficient *rho*. The acceptable type I error was set at $p < 0.05$.

RESULTS

The presence of comorbidities was very common (n = 28, 87.5% of patients) and included cardiovascular, diabetes mellitus, osteoporosis, psychological, and sleep disorders and cancers (**Table 3**). The two more frequently observed comorbidities

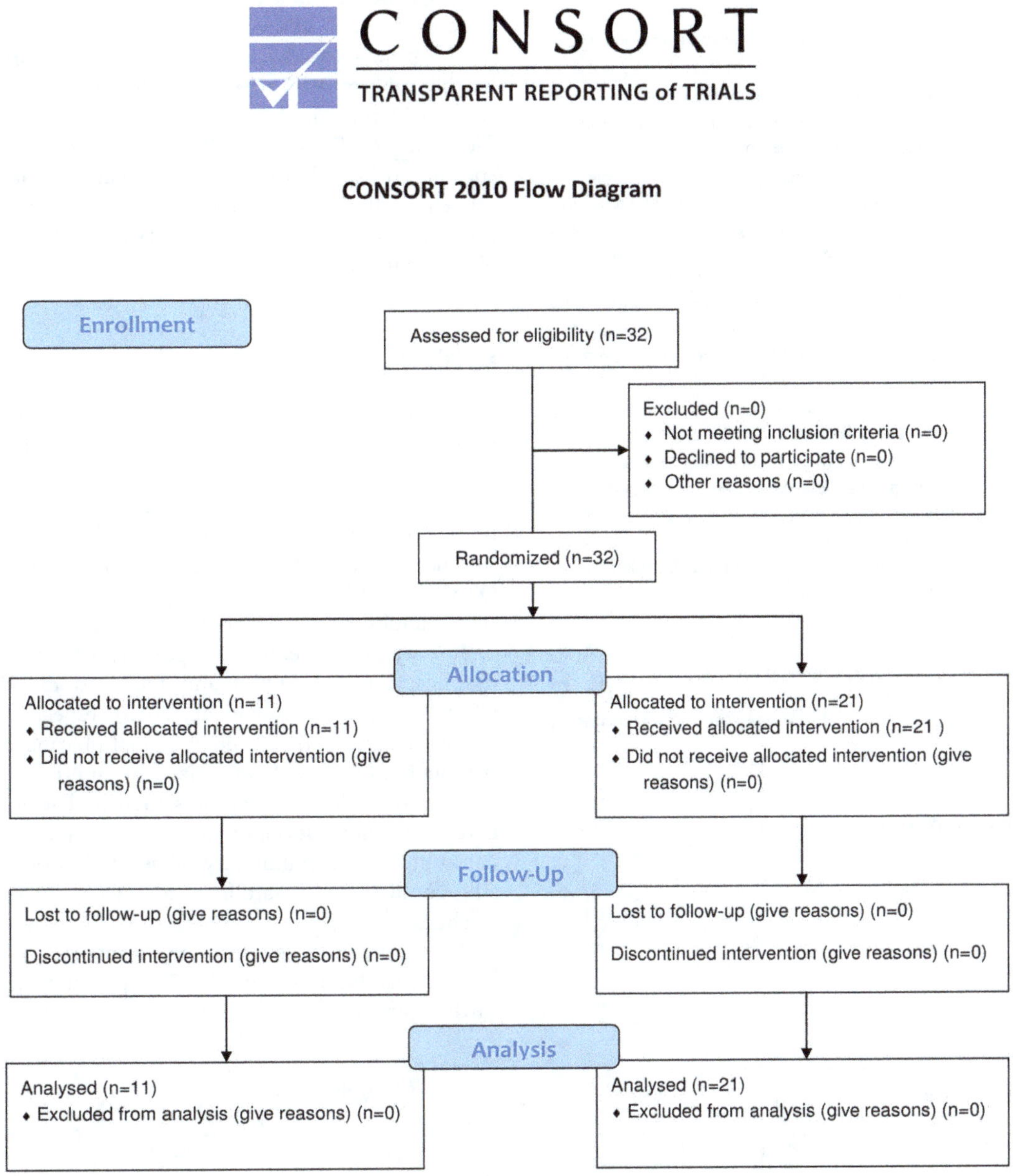

FIGURE 1 | CONSORT flow graph showing the enrollment, allocation, follow-up and analysis of participants.

were CVD and diabetes mellitus (n = 22, 68.8% and n = 17, 53.1%, respectively).

No statistically significant differences in performing the program were observed between the two groups. A large main effect of time was observed in MRC ($p < 0.001$, $\eta^2 = 0.665$), CAT ($p < 0.001$, $\eta^2 = 0.621$), SGRQ ($p < 0.001$, $\eta^2 = 0.457$), which decreased, and in 6MWT ($p < 0.001$, $\eta^2 = 0.608$), which increased across time (**Figures 2, 3**). No main effect of time was shown in body mass ($p = 0.313$, $\eta^2 = 0.035$), BMI ($p = 0.251$, $\eta^2 = 0.045$), FEV_1 ($p = 0.626$, $\eta^2 = 0.009$) and VO_2peak ($p = 0.074$, $\eta^2 = 0.159$). A large time * group interaction was found in body mass ($p = 0.012$, $\eta^2 = 0.198$) with decrease in group 1 compared to group 2 and VO_2peak ($p = 0.025$, $\eta^2 = 0.238$) with increase in group 1 compared to group 2. No time * group interaction was observed in BMI ($p = 0.249$, $\eta^2 = 0.046$), MRC ($p = 0.859$, $\eta^2 = 0.001$), CAT ($p = 0.279$, $\eta^2 = 0.039$), SGRQ ($p = 0.983$, $\eta^2 < 0.001$), 6MWT ($p = 0.888$, $\eta^2 = 0.001$) and FEV_1 ($p = 0.783$, $\eta^2 = 0.003$). In summary, the indices of dyspnea (MRC and CAT), QOL (SGRQ) and aerobic capacity (6MWT) improved across time. The combined effect of group and time was shown only in body mass and VO_2peak.

The severity of the disease was not significantly associated with any of the observed changes after the rehabilitation program (rho ≤ 0.23, $p \geq 0.205$). Only the reduction of dyspnea tended to be less – but not statistically significant – in severe and very severe

TABLE 2 | Characteristics of pulmonary rehabilitation program.

General approach	The program was multimodal and evolutionary for each participant.
Overall sessions	Twenty-five sessions for each participant.
Content	Each session consisted by both physical therapy modalities for the respiratory system and exercise.
	Exercise included both aerobic (treadmill, cycle ergometer and arm crank ergometer) and resistance training (3 set × 10–15 repetitions for 6–8 exercises of main muscle groups). Oxygen supply was provided continuously to maximize effort and exercise intensity maintaining hemoglobin saturation higher than 90%.
	Physical therapy included relaxation techniques for dyspnea, pursed lips breathing technique, exercise of diaphragm/respiratory muscles and effective cough.
Personnel	Participants were instructed by physical therapists under the guidance of physician and nurse.
Frequency	Two sessions weekly (Monday and Thursday morning). The participants were encouraged and guided to perform an additional session by their own.
Exercise intensity	Dyspnea was continuously monitored during each session using Borg scale and was considered to regulate exercise intensity.

TABLE 3 | Prevalence of selected comorbidities in participants.

Comorbidity	Frequency (*n*)	Percentage (%)
Cardiovascular	22	68.8
Diabetes mellitus	17	53.1
Sleep apnoea and other lung diseases	5	15.6
Osteoporosis	4	12.5
Lung cancer	1	3.1
Other cancers	5	15.6
Psychiatric	3	9.4
Chronic kidney failure	1	3.1
Gastrointestinal reflux	0	0

COPD patients when compared to mild and moderate COPD patients (DMRC: 33% vs. 50%).

VO_2peak showed a significant percentage increase of 25.7% in the subgroup of patients with none or one comorbidity (Group 1) compared to the subgroup of patients with two or more comorbidities (Group 2). However, the total number or/and specific comorbidities (CVD and diabetes mellitus) were not related to the general outcomes of pulmonary rehabilitation program, according to the correlation analysis. No harm was observed in participants.

DISCUSSION

Our prospective study demonstrated that all COPD patients improved, after a 13 week pulmonary rehabilitation program, in terms of dyspnea (MRC and CAT), QOL (SGRQ) and exercise tolerance in 6MWT, independently of the presence, the number or the nature of their comorbidities. We did not observe significant responses in FEV_1 or VO_2peak. To the best of our knowledge, this is the first study that evaluates the results of a rehabilitation program by both 6MWT and CPET.

It is well documented that pulmonary rehabilitation reduces dyspnea, improves QOL and increases exercise capacity in COPD patients (Spruit et al., 2013), especially in those who remain symptomatic despite maximal pharmacological therapy. Although COPD is characterized by multi – morbidity, which leads to worse disease symptoms, increased health care utilization and significant mortality, available data about the effect of comorbidities on pulmonary rehabilitation outcomes in COPD still conflicting (Crisafulli et al., 2008, 2010; Franssen and Rochester, 2014).

Most previous studies, that reported worse response after rehabilitation, in COPD patients with co-existing cardiovascular or metabolic diseases, were retrospective

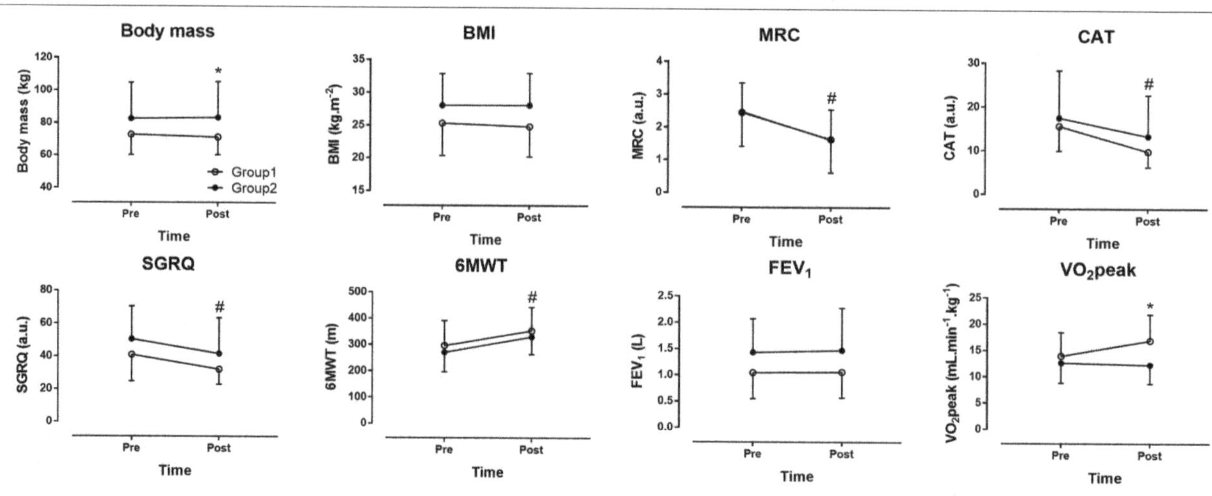

FIGURE 2 | The effect of pulmonary rehabilitation on dyspnea, quality of life (QOL) and aerobic capacity. Group 1 = patients with none or only one comorbidity, Group 2 = patients with two or more comorbidities, BMI = body mass index, FEV_1 = forced expiratory volume in 1 s, MRC = modified Medical Research Council scale, CAT = COPD assessment test, SGRQ = St. George respiratory questionnaire, GOLD = global strategy for the diagnosis, management, and prevention of COPD, 6MWT = 6 min walking test, VO_2peak = peak oxygen uptake. *group × time interaction at $p < 0.05$, #main effect of time at $p < 0.05$.

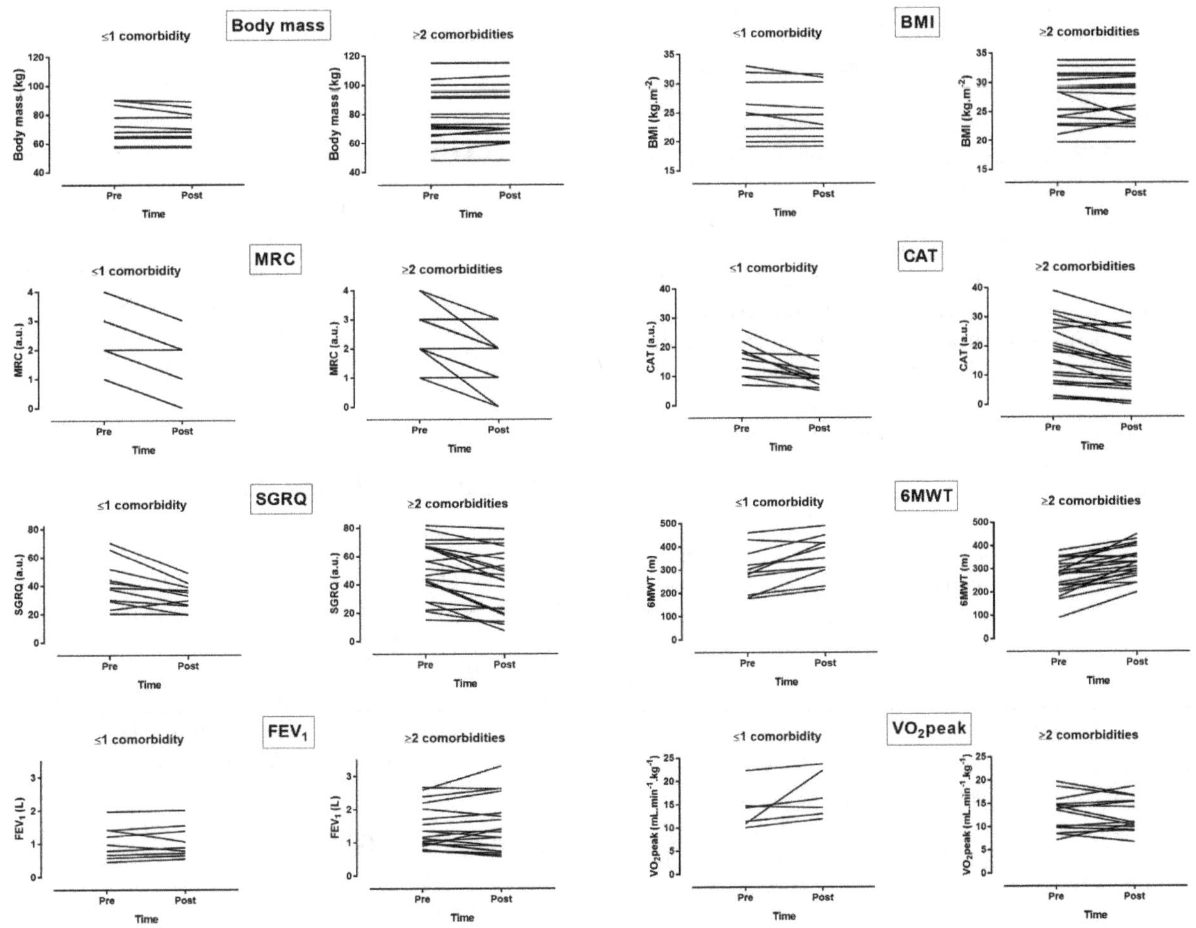

FIGURE 3 | Inter-individual variability in changes of dyspnea, QOL and aerobic capacity following pulmonary rehabilitation. BMI = body mass index, FEV_1 = forced expiratory volume in 1 s, MRC = modified Medical Research Council scale, CAT = COPD assessment test, SGRQ = St. George respiratory questionnaire, GOLD = global strategy for the diagnosis, management, and prevention of COPD, 6MWT = 6min walking test, VO_2peak = peak oxygen uptake.

(Crisafulli et al., 2008; Vagaggini et al., 2009; Carreiro et al., 2013). In some studies, health status and/or 6MWT were negatively influenced by the presence of cardiac or metabolic diseases (Crisafulli et al., 2008; Vagaggini et al., 2009; Carreiro et al., 2013). On the contrary, another retrospective study, reported better response in 6MWT in COPD patients with metabolic diseases (Walsh et al., 2013). BMI > 25 kg m^{-2} was an independent predictor of improvement in 6MWT, but not in SGRQ, in one study (Vagaggini et al., 2009), whereas other studies did not observe any difference between obese and non-obese patients (Ramachandran et al., 2008; Greening et al., 2012). Psychological symptoms led to reduced improvement in dyspnea (Carreiro et al., 2013) and increased risk of drop-out of the program (Garrod et al., 2006).

Our study was prospective and our data were in partial accordance with previous studies. All COPD patients, independently of the number or the nature of comorbidities, achieved less dyspnea and better QOL after the rehabilitation program. The level of dyspnea was higher and tended to ameliorate less – but not statistically significant – in severe and very severe COPD patients, compared to moderate and mild patients. Probably more severe patients have more dyspnea and a significant degree remains even after the intervention. Cardiovascular or metabolic comorbidities were not associated with the outcomes of the rehabilitation program.

The objective performance of participants was measured by both 6MWT and CPET. All patients improved in 6MWT, but not in workload or VO_2peak. In previous studies the most commonly assessed test was the 6MWT. It is reliable, simple, and of low cost. Furthermore, 6MWT resembles daily activities, as patients use to walk and not to cycle. However, changes in the 6MWT are not significantly correlated to changes in other indices of exercise performance (Ong et al., 2004), as it only measures a narrow range of the physical performance spectrum. Also, the 6MWT appears to be less sensitive to intervention than the CPET (Fotheringham et al., 2015). Group 1 achieved significantly better VO_2peak compared to Group 2, after the rehabilitation program. This was in accordance with a previous study which showed that the improvement in exercise capacity was significantly greater in patients without significant comorbidities (Crisafulli et al., 2008).Probably patients with better baseline condition have greater possibility for improvement.

The amelioration of symptoms and exercise capacity, as expressed by 6MWT, in the whole population – independently of coexisting comorbidities – can be explained by the fact that physical activity and regular exercise are beneficial not only for patients with COPD, but also for patients with CVD, musculoskeletal disease, obesity, diabetes mellitus and most other chronic medical conditions (Franssen and Rochester, 2014). Moreover, in patients with heart failure or diabetes mellitus type 2, prescribed exercise, involving aerobic and resistance training modalities, is also evidence-based treatment (McMurray et al., 2012). Thus, pulmonary rehabilitation is beneficial for individuals with COPD and comorbidities, as it has positive effects on both.

The major limitation of our study is the small number of the patients. Besides, the severity of their comorbidities is not quantified and we considered only the number of presented comorbidities (i.e., none or one versus two to nine). Also, a major point of discussion is whether the results suggest real pathophysiologic differences in the response to pulmonary rehabilitation or are due to a greater deconditioning in chronic illness patients. On the other hand, strength of the study was its novelty as limited information existed so far about the role of the number of comorbidities on the effectiveness of a rehabilitation program for COPD (Negewo et al., 2015). Considering the high prevalence of COPD (Sobrino et al., 2017) and the key role of comorbidities (Koskela et al., 2014), the findings of the present study were of great practical importance for practitioners working with COPD.

CONCLUSION

We conclude that all COPD patients benefit from a pulmonary rehabilitation program, independently of comorbidities. More severe patients and patients with ≥ 2 comorbidities have inferior outcomes when compared to moderate or to patients with 0–1 comorbidity. More studies are required to evaluate the effects of this intervention in the natural history of COPD and comorbidities.

AUTHOR CONTRIBUTIONS

MC, AR, and GT acquired and analyzed the data. PN, BK, and TR interpreted the data for the work. All authors made substantial contributions to the conception or design of the work, drafted the work or revised it critically for important intellectual content, provided final approval of the version to be published, and agreed to be accountable for all aspects of the work in ensuring that questions related to the accuracy or integrity of any part of the work are appropriately investigated and resolved.

ACKNOWLEDGMENTS

We gratefully acknowledge the participation of all volunteers.

REFERENCES

1. Biswas, D., Mukherjee, S., Chakroborty, R., Chatterjee, S., Rath, S., Das, R., et al. (2017). Occurrence of anxiety and depression among stable copd patients and its impact on functional capability. *J. Clin. Diagn. Res.* 11, OC24–OC27. doi: 10.7860/jcdr/2017/24203.9393
2. Carreiro, A., Santos, J., and Rodrigues, F. (2013). Impact of comorbidities in pulmonary rehabilitation outcomes in patients with chronic obstructive pulmonary disease. *Rev. Port. Pneumol.* 19, 106–113. doi: 10.1016/j.rppneu.2012.12.004
3. Ciolac, E. G. (2013). Exercise training as a preventive tool for age-related disorders: a brief review. *Clinics* 68, 710–717. doi: 10.6061/clinics/2013(05)20
4. Cohen, J. (1988). *Statistical Power Analysis for the Behavioral Sciences.* Hillsdale, NJ: Lawrence Erlbaum Associates.
5. Crisafulli, E., Costi, S., Luppi, F., Cirelli, G., Cilione, C., Coletti, O., et al. (2008). Role of comorbidities in a cohort of patients with COPD under- going pulmonary rehabilitation. *Thorax* 63, 487–492. doi: 10.1136/thx.2007. 086371
6. Crisafulli, E., Gorgone, P., Vagaggini, B., Pagani, M., Rossi, G., Costa, F., et al. (2010). Efficacy of standard rehabilitation in COPD outpatients with comorbidities. *Eur. Respir. J.* 36, 1042–1048. doi: 10.1183/09031936.002 03809
7. Fotheringham, I., Meakin, G., Punekar, Y. S., Riley, J. H., Cockle, S. M., and Singh, S. J. (2015). Comparison of laboratory- and field-based exercise tests for COPD: a systematic review. *Int. J. Chron. Obstruct. Pulmon. Dis.* 10, 625–643. doi: 10.2147/copd.s70518
8. Franssen, F. M., and Rochester, C. L. (2014). Comorbidities in patients with COPD and pulmonary rehabilitation: do they matter? *Eur. Respir. Rev.* 23, 131–141. doi: 10.1183/09059180.00007613
9. Garrod, R., Marshall, J., Barley, E., and Jones, P. W. (2006). Predictors of success and failure in pulmonary rehabilitation. *Eur. Respir. J.* 27, 788–794. doi: 10. 1183/09031936.06.00130605
10. Global strategy for the diagnosis, management and prevention of COPD, global initiative for chronic obstructive lung disease (GOLD) (2016). Available at: https://goldcopd.org/global-strategy-diagnosis-management-prevention-co pd-2016
11. Greening, N. J., Evans, R. A., Williams, J. E., Green, R. H., Singh, S. J., and Steiner, M. C. (2012). Does body mass index influence the outcomes of a waking-based pulmonary rehabilitation programme in COPD? *Chron. Respir. Dis.* 9, 99–106. doi: 10.1177/1479972312439317
12. Jo, Y. S., Yoon, H. I., Kim, D. K., Yoo, C. G., and Lee, C. H. (2018). Comparison of COPD assessment test and clinical COPD questionnaire to predict the risk of exacerbation. *Int. J. Chron. Obstruct. Pulmon. Dis.* 13, 101–107. doi: 10.2147/ copd.s149805
13. Koskela, J., Kilpelainen, M., Kupiainen, H., Mazur, W., Sintonen, H., Boezen, M., et al. (2014). Co-morbidities are the key nominators of the health related quality of life in mild and moderate COPD. *BMC Pulm. Med.* 14:102. doi: 10.1186/ 1471-2466-14-102
14. McGarvey, L. P., John, M., Anderson, J. A., Zvarich, M., and Wise, R. A. (2007). Ascertainment of cause-specific mortality in COPD: operations of the TORCH clinical endpoint committee. *Thorax* 62, 411–415. doi: 10.1136/thx.2006.072348 McMurray, J. J., Adamopoulos, S., Anker, S. D., Auricchio, A., Bohm, M., Dickstein, K., et al. (2012). ESC guidelines for the diagnosis and treatment of acute and chronic heart failure 2012: the task force for the diagnosis and treatment of acute and chronic heart failure 2012 of the european society of cardiology. Developed in collaboration with the heart failure association (HFA) of the ESC. *Eur. J. Heart Fail.* 14, 803–869. doi: 10.1093/eurjhf/hfs105
15. Negewo, N. A., Gibson, P. G., and McDonald, V. M. (2015). COPD and its comorbidities: impact, measurement and mechanisms. Respirology 20, 1160–1171. doi: 10.1111/resp.12642
16. Oliveira, A. L., and Marques, A. S. (2017). Outcome measures used in pulmonary

rehabilitation in patients with acute exacerbation of chronic obstructive pulmonary disease: a systematic review. Phys. Ther. 98, 191–204. doi: 10.1093/ptj/pzx122

17. Ong, K. C., Chong, W. F., Soh, C., and Earnest, A. (2004). Comparison of different exercise tests in assessing outcomes of pulmonary rehabilitation. Respir. Care 49, 1498–1503. doi: 10.1378/chest.126.4_MeetingAbstracts.767S-b
18. Patel, A. R., and Hurst, J. R. (2011). Extrapulmonary comorbidities in chronic obstructive pulmonary disease: state of the art. Expert Rev. Respir. Med. 5, 647–662. doi: 10.1586/ers.11.62
19. Putcha, N., Drummond, M. B., Wise, R. A., and Hansel, N. N. (2015). Comorbidities and chronic obstructive pulmonary disease: prevalence, influence on outcomes, and management. Semin. Respir. Crit. Care Med. 36, 575–591. doi: 10.1055/s-0035-1556063
20. Putcha, N., Puhan, M. A., Hansel, N. N., Drummond, M. B., and Boyd, C. M. (2013). Impact of co-morbidities on self-rated health in self-reported COPD: an analysis of NHANES 2001-2008. COPD 10, 324–332. doi: 10.3109/15412555.2012.744963
21. Ramachandran, K., McCusker, C., Connors, M., Zuwallack, R., and Lahiri, B. (2008). The influence of obesity on pulmonary rehabilitation outcomes in patients with COPD. Chron. Respir. Dis. 5, 205–209. doi: 10.1177/1479972308096711
22. Reychler, G., Debatisse, M., Lebecque, P., Pieters, T., Liistro, G., and Gohy, S. (2016). Variability of gait speed during six minutes walking test in COPD and cystic fibrosis patients. Gait Posture 49, 36–40. doi: 10.1016/j.gaitpost.2016.06.007
23. Simsic, A. A., Yorke, J., Regueiro, E. G., Di Lorenzo, V. P., and Baddini- Martinez, J. (2018). Validation of the dyspnoea-12 Scale into portuguese speaking COPD patients. Clin. Respir. J. 12, 1942–1948. doi: 10.1111/crj. 12762
24. Sobrino, E., Irazola, V. E., Gutierrez, L., Chen, C. S., Lanas, F., Calandrelli, M., et al. (2017). Estimating prevalence of chronic obstructive pulmonary disease in the southern cone of latin america: how different spirometric criteria may affect disease burden and health policies. BMC Pulm. Med. 17:187. doi: 10.1186/ s12890-017-0537-9
25. Spruit, M. A., Singh, S. J., Garvey, C., ZuWallack, R., Nici, L., Rochester, C., et al. (2013). An official american thoracic society/european respiratory society statement: key concepts and advances in pulmonary rehabilitation. Am. J. Respir. Crit. Care Med. 188, e13–e64. doi: 10.1164/rccm.201309-1 634ST
26. Vagaggini, B., Costa, F., Antonelli, S., De Simone, C., De Cusatis, G., Martino, F., et al. (2009). Clinical predictors of the efficacy of a pulmonary rehabilitation programme in patients with COPD. Respir. Med. 103, 1224–1230. doi: 10.1016/ j.rmed.2009.01.023
27. Walsh, J. R., McKeough, Z. J., Morris, N. R., Chang, A. T., Yerkovich, S. T., Seale, H. E., et al. (2013). Metabolic disease and participant age are independent predictors of response to pulmonary rehabilitation. J. Cardiopulm. Rehabil. Prev. 33, 249–256. doi: 10.1097/HCR.0b013e31829501b7
28. Wu, W., Guan, L., Zhang, X., Li, X., Yang, Y., Guo, B., et al. (2017). Effects of two types of equal-intensity inspiratory muscle training in stable patients with chronic obstructive pulmonary disease: a randomised controlled trial. Respir. Med. 132, 84–91. doi: 10.1016/j.rmed.2017.10.001

Permissions

All chapters in this book were first published by Frontiers; hereby published with permission under the Creative Commons Attribution License or equivalent. Every chapter published in this book has been scrutinized by our experts. Their significance has been extensively debated. The topics covered herein carry significant findings which will fuel the growth of the discipline. They may even be implemented as practical applications or may be referred to as a beginning point for another development.

The contributors of this book come from diverse backgrounds, making this book a truly international effort. This book will bring forth new frontiers with its revolutionizing research information and detailed analysis of the nascent developments around the world.

We would like to thank all the contributing authors for lending their expertise to make the book truly unique. They have played a crucial role in the development of this book. Without their invaluable contributions this book wouldn't have been possible. They have made vital efforts to compile up to date information on the varied aspects of this subject to make this book a valuable addition to the collection of many professionals and students.

This book was conceptualized with the vision of imparting up-to-date information and advanced data in this field. To ensure the same, a matchless editorial board was set up. Every individual on the board went through rigorous rounds of assessment to prove their worth. After which they invested a large part of their time researching and compiling the most relevant data for our readers.

The editorial board has been involved in producing this book since its inception. They have spent rigorous hours researching and exploring the diverse topics which have resulted in the successful publishing of this book. They have passed on their knowledge of decades through this book. To expedite this challenging task, the publisher supported the team at every step. A small team of assistant editors was also appointed to further simplify the editing procedure and attain best results for the readers.

Apart from the editorial board, the designing team has also invested a significant amount of their time in understanding the subject and creating the most relevant covers. They scrutinized every image to scout for the most suitable representation of the subject and create an appropriate cover for the book.

The publishing team has been an ardent support to the editorial, designing and production team. Their endless efforts to recruit the best for this project, has resulted in the accomplishment of this book. They are a veteran in the field of academics and their pool of knowledge is as vast as their experience in printing. Their expertise and guidance has proved useful at every step. Their uncompromising quality standards have made this book an exceptional effort. Their encouragement from time to time has been an inspiration for everyone.

The publisher and the editorial board hope that this book will prove to be a valuable piece of knowledge for researchers, students, practitioners and scholars across the globe.

List of Contributors

Simin Li, Wanchen Ning, Wei Wang, Shaohong Huang and Hui Xiao
Stomatological Hospital, Southern Medical University, Guangzhou, China

Dirk Ziebolz and Gerhard Schmalz
Department of Cariology, Endodontology and Periodontology, University Leipzig, Leipzig, Germany

Aneesha Acharya
Dr. D. Y. Patil Dental College and Hospital, Dr. D. Y. Patil Vidyapeeth, Pune, India

Jianjiang Zhao
Shenzhen Stomatological Hospital, Southern Medical University, Shenzhen, China

Chih-Ru Lin and Beata Kosmider
Department of Microbiology, Immunology, and Inflammation, Temple University, Philadelphia, PA, United States
Center for Inflammation and Lung Research, Temple University, Philadelphia, PA, United States

Karim Bahmed
Center for Inflammation and Lung Research, Temple University, Philadelphia, PA, United States
Department of Thoracic Medicine and Surgery, Temple University, Philadelphia, PA, United States

Yi-xing Wu, Yi-hui Zuo, Wei-ping Hu and Jing Zhang
Department of Pulmonary and Critical Care Medicine, Zhongshan Hospital, Fudan University, Shanghai, China

Qi-jian Cheng
Department of Respiratory Medicine, Ruijin North Hospital, School of Medicine, Shanghai Jiao Tong University, Shanghai, China

Yi Huang
Department of Pulmonary and Critical Care Medicine, Changhai Hospital of Shanghai, Second Military Medical University, Shanghai, China

Zhi-yao Bao
Department of Respiratory Medicine, Ruijin Hospital, School of Medicine, Shanghai Jiao Tong University, Shanghai, China

Xiao-yan Jin and Wei-qin Wang
Department of Respiratory Medicine, Tongren Hospital, School of Medicine, Shanghai Jiao Tong University, Shanghai, China

Xi-wen Gao
Department of Respiratory Medicine, Central Hospital of Minhang District, Shanghai, Fudan University, Shanghai, China

Chun-lin Tu
Department of Respiratory Medicine, Central Hospital of Jiading District, Shanghai, Fudan University, Shanghai, China

Jing-qing Hang and Feng-ying Zhang
Department of Respiratory Medicine, Shanghai Putuo District People's Hospital, Shanghai, China

Peijun Li, Jian Li, Yingqi Wang and Jun Xia
Department of Sports Rehabilitation, Shanghai University of Sport, Shanghai, China

Xiaodan Liu
School of Rehabilitation Science, Shanghai University of Traditional Chinese Medicine, Shanghai, China
Institute of Rehabilitation Medicine, Shanghai University of Traditional Chinese Medicine, Shanghai, China

Francesca Polverino
Asthma and Airway Disease Research Center, University of Arizona, Tucson, AZ, United States

Farrah Kheradmand
Baylor College of Medicine, Houston, TX, United States

Nicholas G. Norwitz
Department of Nutrition, Harvard Medical School, Boston, MA, United States

Russell Winwood
Respiratory Network, Ministry of Health Agency for Clinical Innovation, St Leonards, NSW, Australia

Brianna J. Stubbs
Buck Institute for Research on Aging, Novato, CA, United States

Dominic P. D'Agostino
Morsani College of Medicine, University of South Florida, Tampa, FL, United States
Institute for Human and Machine Cognition, Pensacola, FL, United States

Peter J. Barnes
National Heart and Lung Institute, Imperial College, London, United Kingdom

Fen Dong
Institute of Clinical Medical Sciences, China–Japan Friendship Hospital, Beijing, China
Department of Pulmonary and Critical Care Medicine, China-Japan Friendship Hospital, Beijing, China
National Clinical Research Center for Respiratory Diseases, Beijing, China
Institute of Respiratory Medicine, Chinese Academy of Medical Science, Beijing, China

Xiaoxia Ren, Ke Huang and Ting Yang
Department of Pulmonary and Critical Care Medicine, China-Japan Friendship Hospital, Beijing, China
National Clinical Research Center for Respiratory Diseases, Beijing, China
Institute of Respiratory Medicine, Chinese Academy of Medical Science, Beijing, China

Yanyan Wang
Department of Medical Records, China–Japan Friendship Hospital, Beijing, China

Jianjun Jiao
Department of Medical Administration, China–Japan Friendship Hospital, Beijing, China

Zhu-Xia Tan
Second Affiliated Hospital, Anhui Medical University, Hefei, China
Department of Toxicology, Anhui Medical University, Hefei, China

Lin Fu, Wen-Jing Wang, Ping Zhan and Hui Zhao
Second Affiliated Hospital, Anhui Medical University, Hefei, China

Hua Wang and De-Xiang Xu
Department of Toxicology, Anhui Medical University, Hefei, China

Xiao-Yue Chen
Graduate Institute of Medical Sciences, College of Medicine, Taipei Medical University, Taipei, Taiwan
School of Respiratory Therapy, College of Medicine, Taipei Medical University, Taipei, Taiwan

Yi-Ying Chen
School of Respiratory Therapy, College of Medicine, Taipei Medical University, Taipei, Taiwan

Willie Lin, Chien-Han Chen and Yu-Chieh Wen
Meridigen Biotech Co., Ltd., Taipei, Taiwan

Ta-Chih Hsiao
Graduate Institute of Environmental Engineering, National Taiwan University, Taipei, Taiwan

Hsiu-Chu Chou
Department of Anatomy and Cell Biology, School of Medicine, College of Medicine, Taipei Medical University, Taipei, Taiwan

Kian Fan Chung
National Heart and Lung Institute, Imperial College London, London, United Kingdom

Hsiao-Chi Chuang
School of Respiratory Therapy, College of Medicine, Taipei Medical University, Taipei, Taiwan
Division of Pulmonary Medicine, Department of Internal Medicine, Shuang Ho Hospital, Taipei Medical University, New Taipei City, Taiwan
Cell Physiology and Molecular Image Research Center, Wan Fang Hospital, Taipei Medical University, Taipei, Taiwan

Xuanqi Liu, Haiyan Ge and Huili Zhu
Department of Respiratory and Critical Care Medicine, Huadong Hospital, Fudan University, Shanghai, China

Xiumin Feng
Department of Respiratory and Critical Care Medicine, Changji Branch of First Affiliated Hospital of Xinjiang Medical University, Xinjiang, China

Jingqing Hang and Fengying Zhang
Department of Respiratory Medicine, Putuo People's Hospital, Shanghai, China

Xiaoyan Jin
Department of Respiratory Medicine, Tongren Hospital, Shanghai Jiaotong University School of Medicine, Shanghai, China

Hong Bao
Department of Respiratory Medicine Shanghai Pudong Hospital, Fudan University Pudong Medical Center, Shanghai, China

Min Zhou
Department of Respiratory and Critical Care Medicine, Ruijin Hospital, Shanghai Jiaotong University School of Medicine, Shanghai, China

Fengfeng Han
Department of Respiratory Medicine, Xinhua Hospital, Shanghai Jiaotong University School of Medicine, Shanghai, China

Shengqing Li
Department of Respiratory and Critical Care Medicine, Huashan Hospital, Fudan University, Shanghai, China

Yechang Qian
Baoshan District Hospital of Integrated Traditional Chinese and Western Medicine Hospital, Shanghai, China

Zhijun Jie
Department of Respiratory Medicine, Shanghai Fifth's Hospital, Fudan University, Shanghai, China

Wenchao Gu
Department of Respiratory Medicine, Pudong New District People's Hospital, Shanghai, China

Beilan Gao
Department of Respiratory Medicine, Shanghai Pulmonary Hospital, Tongji University, Shanghai, China

Li Yu
Department of Pulmonary and Critical Care Medicine, Tongji Hospital, Tongji University School of Medicine, Shanghai, China

Jian Wang
Department of Respiratory Medicine, Shanghai Ninth's Hospital, Shanghai Jiaotong University School of Medicine, Shanghai, China

Haiying Ji
Department of Respiratory and Critical Care Medicine, Zhongshan Hospital, Fudan University, Shanghai, China

Jingxi Zhang
Department of Respiratory and Critical Care Medicine, Changji Branch of First Affiliated Hospital of Xinjiang Medical University, Xinjiang, China
Department of Respiratory and Critical Care Medicine, Changhai Hospital Affiliated to Navy Military Medical University, Shanghai, China

Nguyen Thanh Tung
International Ph.D. Program in Medicine, College of Medicine, Taipei Medical University, Taipei, Taiwan
Otorhinolaryngology Department, Cho Ray Hospital, Ho Chi Minh City, Vietnam

Shu-Chuan Ho and Hsiao-Yun Kou
School of Respiratory Therapy, College of Medicine, Taipei Medical University, Taipei, Taiwan

Yueh-Hsun Lu
Department of Radiology, Shuang Ho Hospital, Taipei Medical University, New Taipei City, Taiwan
Department of Radiology, School of Medicine, College of Medicine, Taipei Medical University, Taipei, Taiwan

Tzu-Tao Chen and Kuan-Yuan Chen
Division of Pulmonary Medicine, Department of Internal Medicine, Shuang Ho Hospital, Taipei Medical University, New Taipei City, Taiwan

Kang-Yun Lee and Sheng-Ming Wu
Division of Pulmonary Medicine, Department of Internal Medicine, Shuang Ho Hospital, Taipei Medical University, New Taipei City, Taiwan
Division of Pulmonary Medicine, Department of Internal Medicine, School of Medicine, College of Medicine, Taipei Medical University, Taipei, Taiwan

Chih-Da Wu
Department of Geomatics, National Cheng Kung University, Tainan City, Taiwan
National Institute of Environmental Health Sciences, National Health Research Institutes, Miaoli, Taiwan

Han-Pin Kuo
Division of Pulmonary Medicine, Department of Internal Medicine, School of Medicine, College of Medicine, Taipei Medical University, Taipei, Taiwan

Huynh Nguyen Xuan Thao
Otorhinolaryngology Department, Ho Chi Minh City University of Medicine and Pharmacy, Ho Chi Minh City, Vietnam

Hoang Ba Dung
Otorhinolaryngology Department, Cho Ray Hospital, Ho Chi Minh City, Vietnam

Tran Phan Chung Thuy
Otorhinolaryngology Department, Faculty of Medicine, Vietnam National University Ho Chi Minh City, Ho Chi Minh City, Vietnam

Yueh-Lun Lee
Department of Microbiology and Immunology, School of Medicine, College of Medicine, Taipei Medical University, Taipei, Taiwan

Yueying Wu and Ning Li
Yunnan Provincial Key Laboratory of Molecular Biology for Sinomedicine, Kunming, China
First Clinical School of Medicine, Yunnan University of Chinese Medicine, Kunming, China

Hui Meng, Bo Qiao, Wenqing Jia, Haijing Xing, Yuqing Li, Jiali Yuan and Zhongshan Yang
Yunnan Provincial Key Laboratory of Molecular Biology for Sinomedicine, Kunming, China

Qiang Zhang
Basic Medical School, Shanghai University of Chinese Medicine, Shanghai, China

Paolo Solidoro and Carlo Albera
Division of University Respiratory Medicine, Cardiovascular and Thoracic Department, AOU Città della Salute e della Scienza di Torino, Turin, Italy
Department of Medical Sciences, University of Turin, Turin, Italy

Fulvia Ribolla and Michela Bellocchia
Division of University Respiratory Medicine, Cardiovascular and Thoracic Department, AOU Città della Salute e della Scienza di Torino, Turin, Italy

Luisa Brussino
Department of Medical Sciences, University of Turin, Turin, Italy
Allergy and Clinical Immunology Unit, AO Ordine Mauriziano Hospital, Turin, Italy

Filippo Patrucco
Division of Respiratory Diseases, Medical and Specialistic Department, AOU Maggiore della Carità, Novara, Italy
Translational Medicine Department, University of Piemonte Orientale, Novara, Italy

Yanfei Guo
National Clinical Research Center for Respiratory Diseases, Beijing, China
Department of Respiratory and Critical Care Medicine, Beijing Hospital, Beijing, China
National Center of Gerontology, Beijing, China

Zhenzhen Xing, Yuxia Wang, Yali Ma, Yaqi Tong, Yilin Huang and Yang Cao
Department of Respiratory and Critical Care Medicine, Beijing Hospital, Beijing, China
National Center of Gerontology, Beijing, China

Guangliang Shan
School of Basic Medicine, Institute of Basic Medical Sciences, Peking Union Medical College, Chinese Academy of Medical Sciences, Beijing, China

Jean-Paul Janssens
Division of Pulmonary Diseases, Department of Medicine, Geneva University Hospitals, Geneva, Switzerland

Tieying Sun
National Clinical Research Center for Respiratory Diseases, Beijing, China
Department of Respiratory and Critical Care Medicine, Beijing Hospital, Beijing, China
National Center of Gerontology, Beijing, China

Di Chai
Department of Respiratory and Critical Care Medicine, Beijing Hospital, Beijing, China

Weiming Liu
Department of Intensive Care Medicine, Beijing Boai Hospital, Beijing, China
Rehabilitation Research Center, Beijing, China

Chen Wang
National Clinical Research Center for Respiratory Diseases, Beijing, China
Department of Pulmonary and Critical Care Medicine, Center of Respiratory Medicine, China-Japan Friendship Hospital, Beijing, China
Chinese Academy of Medical Sciences and Peking Union Medical College, Beijing, China
Department of Respiratory Medicine, Capital Medical University, Beijing, China
WHO Collaboration Center for Tobacco Cessation and Respiratory Diseases Prevention, Beijing, China

Gianluigi De Falco, Mariano Sirignano and Andrea D'Anna
Dipartimento di Ingegneria Chimica, dei Materiali e della Produzione Industriale, Università degli Studi di Napoli Federico II, Naples, Italy

Chiara Colarusso
Department of Pharmacy, University of Salerno, Fisciano, Italy
ImmunePharma s.r.l., University of Salerno, Fisciano, Italy
Drug Discovery and Development Program, Department of Pharmacy, University of Salerno, Fisciano, Italy

Michela Terlizzi, Ada Popolo, Michela Pecoraro, and Rosalinda Sorrentino, Rita P. Aquino and Aldo Pinto
Department of Pharmacy, University of Salerno, Fisciano, Italy
ImmunePharma s.r.l., University of Salerno, Fisciano, Italy

Mario Commodo and Patrizia Minutolo
Institute for Research on Combustion (CNR), Naples, Italy

Antonio Molino
Department of Respiratory Medicine, Respiratory Division, University of Naples Federico II, Naples, Italy

Zhang Wang, Xiaojuan Wang, Boxuan Chen and Wensheng Shu
Institute of Ecological Science, School of Life Sciences, South China Normal University, Guangzhou, China

Haiyue Liu and Hongwei Zhou
State Key Laboratory of Organ Failure Research, Microbiome Medicine Center, Division of Laboratory Medicine, Zhujiang Hospital, Southern Medical University, Guangzhou, China

Fengyan Wang, Yuqiong Yang and Zhenyu Liang
State Key Laboratory of Respiratory Disease, National Clinical Research Center for Respiratory Disease, Guangzhou Institute of Respiratory Health, The First Affiliated Hospital of Guangzhou Medical University, Guangzhou, China

Martin R. Stampfli
Department of Medicine, Firestone Institute for Respiratory Health at St. Joseph's Healthcare, McMaster University, Hamilton, ON, Canada

Christopher E. Brightling
Institute for Lung Health, NIHR Leicester Biomedical Research Centre, Department of Respiratory Sciences, University of Leicester, Leicester, United Kingdom

Rongchang Chen
State Key Laboratory of Respiratory Disease, National Clinical Research Center for Respiratory Disease, Guangzhou Institute of Respiratory Health, The First Affiliated Hospital of Guangzhou Medical University, Guangzhou, China
Pulmonary and Critical Care Department, Shenzhen Institute of Respiratory Diseases, Shenzhen People's Hospital, Shenzhen, China

Kailash C. Pandey
Department of Biochemistry, National Institute for Research in Environmental Health (ICMR), Bhopal, India

Sajal De
Department of Pulmonary Medicine, National Institute for Research in Environmental Health (ICMR), Bhopal, India

Pradyumna K. Mishra
Department of Molecular Biology, National Institute for Research in Environmental Health (ICMR), Bhopal, India

Chan-Young Kwon
Department of Oriental Neuropsychiatry, Dong-eui University College of Korean Medicine, Busan, South Korea

Boram Lee
Department of Clinical Korean Medicine, Graduate School, Kyung Hee University, Seoul, South Korea

Beom-Joon Lee, Kwan-Il Kim and Hee-Jae Jung
Division of Allergy, Immune and Respiratory System, Department of Internal Medicine, College of Korean Medicine, Kyung Hee University, Seoul, South Korea

Maria Charikiopoulou and Aggeliki Rapti
Pulmonary Rehabilitation Department, General Hospital for Chest Diseases of Athens "SOTIRIA", Athens, Greece
2nd Pulmonary Department, General Hospital for Chest Diseases of Athens "SOTIRIA", Athens, Greece

Pantelis Theodoros Nikolaidis
Exercise Physiology Laboratory, Nikaia, Greece

Beat Knechtle and Thomas Rosemann
Institute of Primary Care, University of Zurich, Zurich, Switzerland

Georgia Trakada
Division of Pulmonology, Department of Clinical Therapeutics, School of Medicine, Alexandra Hospital, National and Kapodistrian University of Athens, Athens, Greece

Index

www.ingramcontent.com/pod-product-compliance
Lightning Source LLC
LaVergne TN
LVHW082129200926
848484LV00008B/2027